The 5-Minute Veterinary Consult Clinical Companion:
Small Animal Dermatology

The 5-Minute Veterinary Consult Clinical Companion: Small Animal Dermatology

Karen Helton Rhodes, DVM

Diplomate, American College of Veterinary Dermatology
Dermatology Consultations, Goshen, New York

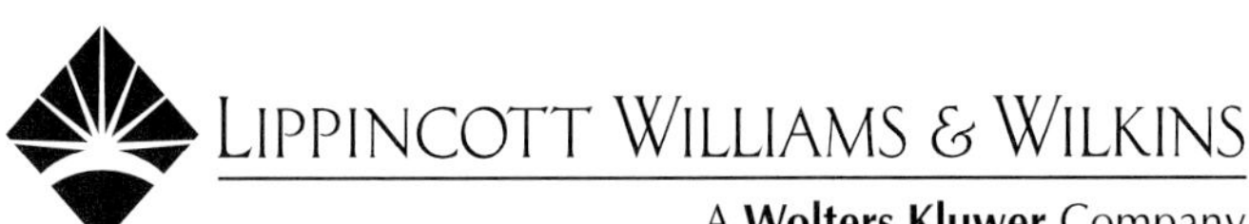

Lippincott Williams & Wilkins
A Wolters Kluwer Company

Philadelphia • Baltimore • New York • London
Buenos Aires • Hong Kong • Sydney • Tokyo

Editor: David Troy
Managing Editor: Dana Battaglia
Marketing Manager: Paul Jarecha
Production Editor: Jennifer Ajello
Designer: Armen Kojoyian
Compositor: Maryland Composition
Printer: Quebecor

351 West Camden Street
Baltimore, MD 21201

530 Walnut Street
Philadelphia, PA 19106

The publisher is not responsible (as a matter of product liability, negligence, or otherwise) for any injury resulting from any material contained herein. This publication contains information relating to general principles of medical care that should not be construed as specific instructions for individual patients. Manufacturers' product information and package inserts should be reviewed for current information, including contraindications, dosages, and precautions.

Printed in the United States of America

Library of Congress Cataloging-in-Publication Data

Rhodes, Karen Helton.
The 5-minute veterinary consult clinical companion: small animal dermatology / Karen Helton Rhodes.
p. cm.
ISBN 0-683-30574-3
1. Dogs–Diseases–Handbooks, manuals, etc. 2. Cats–Diseases–Handbooks, manuals, etc. 3. Exotic animals–Diseases–Handbooks, manuals, etc. 4. Veterinary dermatology–Handbooks, manuals, etc. I. Title: Five minute veterinary consult clinical companion. II. Title.

SF992.S55 R46 2002
636.7'08965–dc21 2001038313

The publishers have made every effort to trace the copyright holders for borrowed material. If they have inadvertently overlooked any, they will be pleased to make the necessary arrangements at the first opportunity.

To purchase additional copies of this book, call our customer service department at **(800) 638-3030** or fax orders to **(301) 824-7390.** International customers should call **(301) 714-2324.**

Visit Lippincott Williams & Wilkins on the Internet: http://www.LWW.com. Lippincott Williams & Wilkins customer service representatives are available from 8:30 am to 6:00 pm, EST.

04 05
2 3 4 5 6 7 8 9 10

To Arthur I. Hurvitz who, even in his absence, continues to be my mentor, friend, and muse.

Preface

The 5-Minute Veterinary Consult Clinical Companion: Small Animal Dermatology is designed as a quick reference text for the clinician and student of veterinary medicine. There are several excellent texts available in veterinary dermatology and dermatopathology. These books offer detailed information regarding structure and function of the skin, pathophysiology of disease, clinical descriptions of cutaneous diseases, diagnostic techniques, microscopic anatomy and pathology of the skin, and current therapy. Although these are excellent reference texts and are certainly required by all clinical and personal veterinary libraries, there was a need for a handbook to make this information readily accessible in the workplace.

This text is designed to aid the veterinary student and clinician in recognizing various skin disorders by acting as a guide through an extensive yet reasonable differential diagnostic list, providing direction in choosing the most appropriate and applicable diagnostic tests, and offering current therapeutic options. As clinicians, we often have a limited amount of time during appointments and are forced to make rapid, yet accurate decisions. This handbook is a condensed guide that can aid in those decisions. Several of the chapters have been adapted from the second edition of the *5-Minute Veterinary Consult, Canine and Feline,* for which I served as the dermatology section editor. All of the dermatology section chapters from the *5-Minute Consult* are included, plus pertinent chapters from other sections in the text. There are several features that are unique to the Handbook including chapters on cutaneous cytology, obtaining a diagnostic dermatopathology specimen, topical therapy, differential diagnostic lists for common clinical presentations, and sample client education handouts from a specialty dermatology practice (KHR). Also, a dermatologic drug formulary is added, and color photographs are coordinated with each chapter. Cutaneous disorders as a primary or concurrent owner complaint comprise a large percentage, 20–75%, of clinical cases in veterinary practices and the number of recognized diseases is rapidly expanding. Not only is the list of differentials extensive but the variety of species presented is also increasing. For this reason, a section describing common dermatologic disorders of *exotic pets* has been included.

The client education handouts are a great time-saving device. Client education handouts can offer extensive information on a specific disorder and thus act as an adjunct to the clinician's explanation and instructions. I have included some of my personal specialty practice handouts for use as a template, or they may be given to the client as is. I find that owners appreciate receiving written information that they can study at home in a stress-free environment.

The Clinical Companion is organized into (11) sections. Section 1, Diagnostics, includes chapters on techniques for practical cytology with multiple color plates and an informational guide for steps in obtaining a diagnostic biopsy sample. Section 2, Differential Diagnoses Based on Clinical Patterns, provides lists with brief descriptions of differentials to be considered in cases of alopecia, erosive and ulcerative disorders, scaling and crusting dermatoses, exfoliative disorders, papular and nodular dermatoses, and vesicular and pustular dermatoses—all complete with photographic examples. Section 3, Differential Diagnoses Based on Regional Lesions, organizes differentials based on body location such as pododermatoses and nailbed disorders, nasal dermatoses, depigmenting disorders, otitis, anal sac disorders and perianal fistulas, acne, and acral lick dermatitis. Section 4, Parasitic Dermatoses, addresses common cutaneous parasites such as ticks and associated diseases, fleas and various control products with individual advantages and disadvantages, cheyletiellosis, demodicosis, otodectes, and toxicities associated with common parasiticides. Section 5, Allergic and Hypersensitivity Dermatitis, includes chapters highlighting pathophysiology with emphasis on therapeutic control, anaphylaxis, inhalant/percutaneous allergic dermatitis, food hypersensitivity/intolerance, contact dermatitis, eosinophilic granuloma complex lesions, hypereosinophilic syndrome, and cutaneous drug eruptions. Section 6, Infectious Dermatoses, covers a broad range of agents encountered in veterinary dermatology. Section 7, Endocrine Dermatoses, includes hypothyroidism, hyperadrenocorticism, growth hormone–responsive dermatoses, sex hormone dermatoses, steroid hepatopathy, and feline skin fragility syndrome. Section 8, Immunologic/Autoimmune Disorders, addresses the common cutaneous diseases encountered in clinical practice (pemphigus complex, bullous pemphigoid, SLE, DLE, panniculitis, vasculitis, uveodermatologic syndrome—VKH-like disease). Section 9, Cutaneous Neoplasias, offers clinical photos, histopathologic descriptions, and therapeutic options for common cutaneous neoplasias. Section 10, Exotic Pet Dermatology, covers common dermatologic disorders of guinea pigs, ferrets, rabbits, and mice. Section 11, Selected Topics, is a compilation of unique dermatoses: and includes an explanation of the appropriate and efficacious use of topical therapy. Section 12, Laboratory Tests/Interpretation includes ACTH testing. The appendices include client education handouts and a dermatologic drug formulary for quick reference. In my practice, the handouts are selected for the individual client, completed *(fill in the blanks)*, and placed in a folder for the client to take home. This folder contains all information regarding phone/fax communication and medical information for the pet. Prescriptions are affixed to the folder so that all instructions are kept together in a package.

To my many friends and colleagues who agreed to participate in the project, were patient with the prolonged process, and readily shared their expertise and knowledge, I extend my sincere gratitude. A special thank you to Dr. Keith Baer, dermatopathologist, for his continued interest and support in the field of Veterinary Dermatology. Frank Smith and Larry Tilley have been a continued source of support and guidance for both *The 5-Minute Veterinary Consult* and its spin-off project, *The 5-Minute Veterinary Clinical Companion: Small Animal Dermatology*. I am most grateful for the insight offered by the staff at Lippincott Williams & Wilkins and their unfaltering support for the use of color kodachromes for the text. My last thank you is extended to Steven and Cameron for listening to ideas and helping with the routine activities at North Star Farm.

Karen Helton Rhodes

Table of Contents

SECTION 1 DIAGNOSTICS / 1

Chapter 1: Practical Cytology, James O. Noxon and Elizabeth E. Goldman / 3

Chapter 2: Dermatohistopathology: Obtaining a Diagnostic Biopsy, Karen Helton Rhodes / 19

SECTION 2 DIFFERENTIAL DIAGNOSES BASED ON CLINICAL PATTERNS / 25

Chapter 3: Alopecia, Canine, Karen Helton Rhodes, Karin M. Beale / 27

Chapter 4: Alopecia, Feline, Karen Helton Rhodes / 43

Chapter 5: Erosive and Ulcerative Dermatoses, Daniel O. Morris / 61

Chapter 6: Exfoliative Dermatoses, Alexander H. Werner and Linda Messinger / 74

Chapter 7: Papular and Nodular Dermatoses, Karen A. Kuhl and Jean Swingle Greek / 84

Chapter 8: Vesicular and Pustular Dermatoses, Ellen C. Codner and Karen Helton Rhodes / 88

SECTION 3 DIFFERENTIAL DIAGNOSES BASED ON REGIONAL LESION(S) / 99

Chapter 9: Pododermatitis, K. Marcia Murphy and Karen Helton Rhodes / 101

Chapter 10: Nail and Nailbed Disorders, Ellen C. Codner and Karen Helton Rhodes / 115
Chapter 11: Interdigital Dermatitis, David Duclos and Karen Helton Rhodes / 122
Chapter 12: Nasal Dermatosis, Ellen C. Codner and Karen Helton Rhodes / 128
Chapter 13: Depigmenting Disorders, John Gordon / 138
Chapter 14: Otitis Externa and Media, Alexander H. Werner / 144
Chapter 15: Otitis Media and Interna, Richard J. Joseph / 152
Chapter 16: Anal Sac Disorders, Jon D. Plant / 157
Chapter 17: Perianal Fistula, Michael A. Mitchell and James L. Cook / 160
Chapter 18: Canine and Feline Acne, David Duclos and Karen Helton Rhodes / 164
Chapter 19: Acral Lick Dermatitis, Karen A. Kuhl, Jean S. Greek, and Karen Helton Rhodes / 167

SECTION 4: PARASITIC DERMATOSES / 173
Chapter 20: Ticks and Tick Control, Steven A. Levy / 175
Chapter 21: Tick Bite Paralysis, Paul A. Cuddon / 180
Chapter 22: Fleas and Flea Control, Karen A. Kuhl and Jean S. Greek / 185
Chapter 23: Flea Control Products, John MacDonald / 190
Chapter 24: Cheyletiellosis, Alexander H. Werner / 194
Chapter 25: Sarcoptic Mange, Linda Medleau and Keith A. Hnilica / 198
Chapter 26: Demodicosis, Karen Helton Rhodes / 203
Chapter 27: Ear Mites, Karen A. Kuhl and Jean S. Greek/ 210
Chapter 28: Amitraz Toxicity, Steven R. Hansen / 213
Chapter 29: Ivermectin Toxicity, Allan J. Paul / 217
Chapter 30: Organophosphate and Carbamate Toxicity, Steven R. Hansen and Elizabeth A. Curry-Galvin / 220
Chapter 31: Pyrethrin and Pyrethroid Toxicity, Steven R. Hansen and Elizabeth A. Curry-Galvin / 225

SECTION 5 ALLERGIC AND HYPERSENSITIVITY DERMATITIS / 229
Chapter 32: Pruritus, W. Dunbar Gram / 231
Chapter 33: Clinical Management of Pruritic Inflammatory Skin Disease, Karen Helton Rhodes / 236
Chapter 34: Hypersensitivity Reaction: Anaphylaxis, Paul W. Snyder / 244
Chapter 35: Atopy, Jon D. Plant and Lloyd M. Reedy / 248
Chapter 36: Food Reactions, David Duclos / 253
Chapter 37: Contact Dermatitis, Alexander H. Werner and Margaret Swartout / 257
Chapter 38: Eosinophilic Granuloma Complex, Alexander H. Werner / 261

Chapter 39: Hypereosinophilic Syndrome, Karen M. Young / 268
Chapter 40: Cutaneous Drug Eruption, Daniel O. Morris / 271

SECTION 6 INFECTIOUS DERMATOSES / 275
Chapter 41: Sepsis and Bacteremia, Sharon K. Fooshee / 277
Chapter 42: Abscessation, Johnny D. Hoskins / 282
Chapter 43: Bacterial Pyoderma: Folliculitis and Furunculosis, Ellen C. Codner and Karen Helton Rhodes / 287
Chapter 44: Anaerobic Bacterial Infections, Sharon K. Fooshee / 294
Chapter 45: Mycobacterial Infections, Carol S. Foil / 297
Chapter 46: Dermatophilosis, Carol S. Foil / 305
Chapter 47: Nocardiosis, Gary D. Norsworthy / 309
Chapter 48: Malassezia Dermatitis, K. V. Mason / 314
Chapter 49: Dermatophytosis: Keratinophilic Mycosis, W. Dunbar Gram / 319
Chapter 50: Sporotrichosis: Subcutaneous Mycosis, W. Dunbar Gram / 325
Chapter 51: Cryptococcosis, Alfred M. Legendre / 329
Chapter 52: Coccidioidomycosis: Systemic Mycosis, Nita Kay Gulbas / 334
Chapter 53: Blastomycosis: Systemic Mycosis, Alfred M. Legendre / 340
Chapter 54: Leishmaniasis: Protozoan Dermatosis, Stephen C. Barr / 346
Chapter 55: Feline Calicivirus, Fred W. Scott / 350
Chapter 56: Feline Pox Virus Infection, J. Paul Woods / 354
Chapter 57: Canine Papillomatosis, Suzette M. Le Clerc and Edward G. Clark / 357

SECTION 7 ENDOCRINE DERMATOSES / 363
Chapter 58: Hypothyroidism, John W. Tyler / 365
Chapter 59: Hyperadrenocorticism, Peter P. Kintzer / 375
Chapter 60: Growth Hormone–Responsive Dermatoses, Margaret S. Swartout / 383
Chapter 61: Sex Hormone–Responsive Dermatoses, Margaret S. Swartout / 387
Chapter 62: Steroid Hepatopathy, Keith P. Richter / 394
Chapter 63: Feline Skin Fragility Syndrome, Karen Helton Rhodes / 400

SECTION 8 IMMUNOLOGIC/AUTOIMMUNE DISORDERS / 405
Chapter 64: Pemphigus, Margaret S. Swartout / 407
Chapter 65: Bullous Pemphigoid, Margaret S. Swartout / 415
Chapter 66: Discoid Lupus Erythematosus, Wayne S. Rosenkrantz / 420
Chapter 67: Systemic Lupus Erythematosus, Harm HogenEsch / 424

Chapter 68: Panniculitis, Kevin Shanley / 430
Chapter 69: Vasculitis, Karen A. Kuhl and Jean S. Greek / 436
Chapter 70: Uveodermatologic Syndrome, W. Dunbar Gram / 441

SECTION 9 CUTANEOUS NEOPLASIAS / 447
Chapter 71: Epidermotrophic Lymphoma, K. Marcia Murphy / 449
Chapter 72: Hair Follicle Tumors, Joanne C. Graham / 455
Chapter 73: Cutaneous Hemangiosarcoma, Robyn Elmslie / 457
Chapter 74: Histiocytoma, Joanne C. Graham / 461
Chapter 75: Mast Cell Tumors, Robyn Elmslie / 464
Chapter 76: Melanocytic Tumors of the Skin and Digit, Joanne C. Graham / 471
Chapter 77: Basal Cell Tumor, Robyn Elmslie / 476
Chapter 78: Squamous Cell Carcinoma, Skin, Joanne C. Graham / 478
Chapter 79: Ceruminous Gland Adenocarcinoma, Ear, Joanne C. Graham / 483
Chapter 80: Adenocarcinoma, Skin (Sweat gland, sebaceous), Robyn Elmslie / 486
Chapter 81: Feline Paraneoplastic Syndrome, Karen L. Campbell / 489

SECTION 10 EXOTIC PET DERMATOLOGY – KAREN ROSENTHAL / 495
Chapter 82: Guinea Pigs: Ectoparasite / 497
Chapter 83: Hedgehog: Chorioptes Mites / 499
Chapter 84: Rabbits: Urine Scald / 501
Chapter 85: Mice: Ectoparasites / 503
Chapter 86: Rabbits: Fur Mites / 505
Chapter 87: Guinea Pigs: Ovarian Cysts / 507
Chapter 88: Hamster Cushing Disease / 509
Chapter 89: Ferrets: Adrenal Gland Disease / 511
Chapter 90: Rabbits: Dermatophytosis / 513
Chapter 91: Ferrets: Mast Cell Tumors / 515
Chapter 92: Ferrets: Sarcoptic Mange / 517
Chapter 93: Rabbit Barbering / 519
Chapter 94: Ferret Canine Distemper Virus / 521

SECTION 11: SELECTED TOPICS / 523
Chapter 95: Canine Familial Dermatomyositis, Linda Medleau and Keith A. Hnilica / 525
Chapter 96: Canine Keratinization Disorders, Linda Messinger / 532
Chapter 97: Sterile Nodular/Granulomatous Dermatoses, Dawn E. Logas / 542
Chapter 98: Granulomatous Sebaceous Adenitis, Ellen C. Codner and Karen Helton Rhodes / 551
Chapter 99: Cutaneous Asthenia, Jon D. Plant and Karen Helton Rhodes / 554

Chapter 100: Feline Symmetrical Alopecia, David Duclos / 558
Chapter 101: Hepatocutaneous Syndrome, Sheila M. Torres / 562
Chapter 102: Lymphedema, Francis W.K. Smith, Jr. / 570
Chapter 103: Canine Juvenile Cellulitis (Puppy Strangles), Karen Helton Rhodes / 573
Chapter 104: Histiocytosis, Kenneth M. Rassnick /576
Chapter 105: Immunodeficiency Disorders, Primary, Paul W. Snyder / 582
Chapter 106: Shampoo Therapy, Anthony A. Yu / 586

SECTION 12 LABORATORY TESTS/INTERPRETATION / 593

Chapter 107: ACTH Response Test, Ellen N. Behrend and Robert Kemppainen / 595
Chapter 108: Low-Dose Dexamethasone Suppression Test, Ellen N. Behrend and Robert Kemppainen / 602
Chapter 109: High-Dose Dexamethasone Suppression Test and Plasma ACTH Levels, Peter P. Kintzer / 607
Chapter 110: Urine Cortisol: Creatinine Ratio, Ellen N. Behrend and Robert Kemppainen / 609
Chapter 111: Thyroid Hormones, Deborah S. Greco / 613
Chapter 112: Antinuclear Antibody (ANA) Titer/Lupus Erythematosus (LE) Cell Test, Albert H. Ahn and Francis W. K. Smith, Jr. / 617
Chapter 113: Coombs' Test, Albert H. Ahn / 622

APPENDIX I CLIENT EDUCATION HANDOUTS / 627

APPENDIX II DERMATOLOGIC FORMULARY / 653

APPENDIX III ENDOCRINE TESTING / 674

APPENDIX IV TESTS OF THE ENDOCRINE SYSTEM / 677

APPENDIX V CONVERSION TABLE FOR HORMONE ASSAY UNITS / 678

Contributors

ALBERT H. AHN, DVM
Clinician, Clinical Faculty, Tufts University
School of Veterinary Medicine
Manager, Veterinary Affairs
Hill's Pet Nutrition, Inc.
North Grafton, Massachusetts

STEPHEN C. BARR, BVSc, MVS, PhD, MACVSc
Diplomate, ACVIM (Internal Medicine)
Associate Professor of Medicine
Department of Clinical Sciences
Cornell University
College of Veterinary Medicine
Ithaca, New York

KARIN M. BEALE, DVM
Diplomate, ACVD
Staff Dermatologist
Gulf Coast Veterinary Specialists
Houston, Texas

ELLEN N. BEHREND, VMD
Diplomate, ACVIM (Internal Medicine)
Assistant Professor
Department of Clinical Sciences
College of Veterinary Medicine
Auburn University
Auburn, Alabama

KAREN L. CAMPBELL, DVM, MS
Diplomate, ACVIM (Internal Medicine)
Diplomate, ACVD
Department of Veterinary Clinical Medicine
University of Illinois
School of Veterinary Medicine
Urbana, Illinois

EDWARD G. CLARK, DVM
University of Saskatoon
Western College of Veterinary Medicine
Prairie Diagnostic Services
Saskatoon, SK
Canada

ELLEN C. CODNER, DVM
Diplomate, ACVIM, ACVD
Animal Dermatology Specialists
Martinez, California

JAMES L. COOK, DVM, PhD
Diplomate, ACVS
Assistant Professor, Small Animal Orthopedics
Assistant Professor, Orthopedic Surgery
Director, Comparative Orthopedic Laboratory
University of Missouri
Columbia, Missouri

PAUL A. CUDDON, BVSc
Diplomate, ACVIM (Neurology)
Veterinary Specialists of Northern Colorado
Loveland, Colorado

ELIZABETH A. CURRY-GALVIN, DVM
Assistant Director, Scientific Activities
American Veterinary Medical Association
Schaumburg, Illinois

DAVID DUCLOS, DVM
Diplomate, ACVD
Animal Skin and Allergy Clinic
West Lynnwood, Washington

ROBYN E. ELMSLIE, DVM
Diplomate, ACVIM (Oncology)
Veterinary Cancer Specialists
Englewood, Colorado

CAROL S. FOIL, DVM, MS,
Diplomate, ACVD
Professor of Dermatology
Department of Veterinary Clinical Sciences
Louisiana State University
School of Veterinary Medicine
Baton Rouge, Louisiana

SHARON F. GRACE, DVM
Diplomate, ACVIM (Internal Medicine), ABVP
Associate Clinical Professor
Department of Clinical Sciences
Mississippi State University
College of Veterinary Medicine
Mississippi State, Mississippi

ELIZABETH GOLDMAN, DVM
Arlington Heights, Illinois

JOHN G. GORDON, DVM
Diplomate, ACVD
MedVet Associates, Inc.
Columbus, Ohio

JOANNE C. GRAHAM, DVM
Diplomate, ACVIM (Internal Medicine)
Animal Medical Referral Center
Franklin Park Animal Hospital
Franklin Park, Illinois

W. DUNBAR GRAM, DVM
Diplomate, ACVD
Animal Allergy and Dermatology, P.C.
Virginia Beach, Virginia

DEBORAH GRECO, DVM, PhD
Diplomate, ACVIM (Internal Medicine)
Colorado State University
College of Veterinary Medicine
Veterinary Teaching Hospital
Fort Collins, Colorado

JEAN SWINGLE GREEK, DVM
Diplomate, ACVD
Veterinary Specialists of Kansas City
Overland Park, Kansas
Dermatology and Allergy Clinic for Animals
Santa Barbara, California

NITA KAY GULBAS, DVM
Phoenix, Arizona

STEVEN R. HANSEN, DVM
Diplomate, ABVT
Vice-President
ASPCA National Poison Control Center
Urbana, Illinois

KEITH A. HNILICA, DVM
Diplomate, ACVD
Assistant Professor, Veterinary Dermatology
Department of Small Animal Clinical Sciences
The University of Tennessee
College of Veterinary Medicine
Knoxville, Tennessee

HARM HOGENESCH, DVM, PHD
Diplomate, ACVP
Head of Veterinary Pathobiology
Purdue University
School of Veterinary Medicine
West Lafayette, Indiana

JOHNNY D. HOSKINS, DVM, PhD
Diplomate, ACVIM (Internal Medicine)
Professor Emeritus
Department of Clinical Sciences
School of Veterinary Medicine
Louisiana State University
Baton Rouge, Louisiana

RICHARD J. JOSEPH, DVM
Diplomate, ACVIM (Internal Medicine)
Staff Neurologist/Acupuncturist
Department of Medicine
The Animal Medical Center
New York, New York

ROBERT J. KEMPPAINEN, DVM, PhD
Professor, Department of Anatomy, Physiology and Pharmacology
College of Veterinary Medicine
Auburn University
Auburn, Alabama

PETER P. KINTZER, DVM
Diplomate, ACVIM (Internal Medicine)
Staff Internist
Boston Road Animal Hospital
Springfield, Massachusetts

KAREN ANN KUHL, DVM
Diplomate, ACVD
Veterinary Specialty Clinic
Midwest Veterinary Dermatology Center
Riverwoods, Illinois

SUZETTE M. LECLERC, DVM, MVETSc
Diplomate, ACVP
Clinical Associate
Prairie Diagnostic Services
Saskatoon, Saskatchewan, Canada

ALFRED M. LEGENDRE, DVM
Diplomate, ACVIM (Internal Medicine)
Professor of Medicine
Veterinary Teaching Hospital
University of Tennessee
College of Veterinary Medicine
Knoxville, Tennessee

STEVEN A. LEVY, VMD
Durham Veterinary Hospital PC
Durham, Connecticut

DAWN ELAINE LOGAS, DVM
Diplomate, ACVD
Staff Dermatologist
Veterinary Dermatology Clinic
Maitland, Florida

JOHN MACDONALD, DVM
Diplomate, ACVD
Associate Professor
Department of Small Animal Medicine and Surgery
Auburn University
College of Veterinary Medicine
Auburn, Alabama

KENNETH V. MASON, FACVSc
Animal Allergy and Dermatology Service
Albert Animal Hospital
Springwood, Australia

LINDA MEDLEAU, DVM
Diplomate, ACVD
Professor of Dermatology
Department of Small Animal Medicine
University of Georgia
College of Veterinary Medicine
Athens, Georgia

LINDA MESSINGER, DVM
Diplomate, ACVD
Veterinary Skin and Allergy Specialist PC
Veterinary Referral Center of Colorado
Englewood, Colorado

DANIEL O. MORRIS, DVM
Diplomate, ACVD
Assistant Professor of Dermatology
Veterinary Hospital
University of Pennsylvania
Philadelphia, Pennsylvania

K. MARCIA MURPHY, DVM
Raleigh, North Carolina

GARY D. NORSWORTHY, DVM
Diplomate, ABVP (Feline)
Practitioner, Alamo Feline Health Center
San Antonio, Texas

JAMES O. NOXON, DVM
Diplomate, ACVIM
Professor and Small Animal Section Leader
Veterinary Teaching Hospital
Department of Veterinary Medicine
Iowa State University
Ames, Iowa

ALLAN J. PAUL, DVM
Professor
Department of Veterinary Pathobiology
University of Illinois
College of Veterinary Medicine
Urbana, Illinois

JON D. PLANT, DVM
Diplomate, ACVD
Animal Dermatology Specialty Clinic
Marina del Ray, California

KENNETH M. RASSNICK, DVM
Diplomate, ACVIM (Oncology)
Assistant Professor
Comparative Cancer Program
Cornell University
College of Veterinary Medicine
Ithaca, New York

LLOYD M. REEDY, DVM†
Diplomate, ACVD

†Deceased.

KEITH P. RICHTER, DVM
Diplomate, ACVIM (Internal Medicine)
Internal Medicine Staff
Veterinary Specialty Hospital of San Diego
Rancho Santa Fe, California

WAYNE STEWART ROSENKRANTZ, DVM, Diplomate, ACVD
Animal Dermatology Clinics
Garden Grove, California

KAREN L. ROSENTHAL, DVM, MS, ABVP-Avian
Director of Special Species Medicine
Adjunct Assistant Professor of Special Species Medicine
University of Pennsylvania
School of Veterinary Medicine
Philadelphia, Pennsylvania

FRED W. SCOTT, DVM, PhD
Diplomate, ACVM, AFM
Department of Microbiology and Immunology
Cornell University
College of Veterinary Medicine
Ithaca, New York

KEVIN SHANLEY, DVM
Diplomate, ACVD
Staff Dermatologist
Metropolitan Veterinary Associates &
Delaware Veterinary Specialists Group
Dermatology Clinic for Animals
Valley Forge, Pennsylvania

FRANCIS W. K. SMITH, Jr., DVM
Diplomate, ACVIM (Internal Medicine & Cardiology)
Vice-President, Editor-in-Chief
VetMedCenter.com
San Francisco, California

Clinical Assistant Professor
Department of Medicine
Tufts University
School of Veterinary Medicine
North Grafton, Massachusetts

PAUL W. SNYDER, DVM, PhD
Diplomate, ACVP
Assistant Professor of Pathology
Department of Veterinary Pathobiology
School of Veterinary Medicine
Purdue University
West Lafayette, Indiana

MARGARET S. SWARTOUT, DVM
Diplomate, ACVIM (Internal Medicine)
Owner, Veterinary Specialty Consultation Service
Knoxville, Tennessee

SHEILA M. TORRES, DVM, PhD
Diplomate, ACVD
Assistant Professor, Small Animal Clinical Sciences
University of Minnesota
College of Veterinary Medicine
Minneapolis, Minnesota

JOHN WILLIAM TYLER, DVM
Diplomate, ACVIM (Internal Medicine)
Assistant Professor
Small Animal Internal Medicine
Animal Health Center
Mississippi State University
College of Veterinary Medicine
Mississippi State, Mississippi

ALEXANDER H. WERNER, VMD
Diplomate, ACVD
Staff Dermatologist
Valley Veterinary Specialty Services
Studio City, California

J. PAUL WOODS, DVM
Diplomate, ACVIM (Internal Medicine)
Certificate of Specialization in Small Animal Internal Medicine
Canadian Veterinary Medical Association
Associate Professor of Medicine
Department of Clinical Studies
Ontario Veterinary College
University of Guelph
Guelph, Ontario, Canada

KAREN M. YOUNG, VMD, PHD
Associate Professor
Department of Pathobiological Sciences
University of Wisconsin – Madison
School of Veterinary Medicine
West Madison, Wisconsin

ANTHONY YU, DVM, MS
Diplomate, ACVD
Animal Allergy & Skin Clinic
Beaverton, Oregon

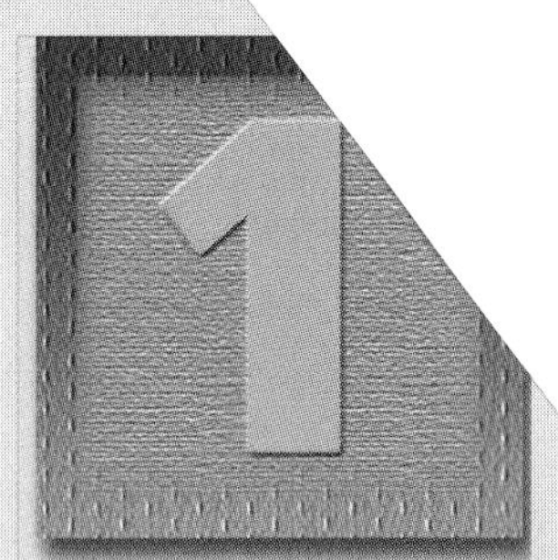

Diagnostics

Practical Cytology

James O. Noxon, Elizabeth E. Goldman

Cytology is an extremely useful diagnostic tool that is available to dermatologists and practitioners and is indicated in virtually every dermatology case. Cytologic examination of various tissue specimens is easy to perform, inexpensive, requires relatively few supplies and instruments, and provides excellent and often key diagnostic information to the clinician. The technical aspects of sample collection and slide preparation are critical aspects of this process. Poor technique will reduce the value of the procedure and lead to frustration on the part of the clinician. Poor slide preparation may destroy the diagnostic material that was collected and render the procedure worthless. As they say, "garbage in, garbage out."

Cytology of Cutaneous and Subcutaneous Lesions

Indications: Cytology is often helpful in determining the etiology of pustules, papules, nodules, tumors, draining tracts, chronic ulcerations, or plaques.

Materials: Cotton-tipped applicators, syringes, 22-, 23-, or 25-gauge needles, glass microscope slides, cover slips, a microscope, a camel-hair paintbrush, and various stains are needed.

Procedures—Sample Collection: Several techniques may be used to obtain samples. The best procedure may depend on the type and location of the lesion. Samples may be collected by 1) fine-needle aspiration of cells or material from lesions; 2) fine-needle biopsy of various lesions; 3) impression smears made from the surface of intact lesions; 4) impression smears made from cut surfaces of surgically excised lesions (e.g., nodules or tumors); and 5) impression smears made after lancing papules, pustules, or other lesions.

Fine-needle aspiration:

Many combinations of needles and syringes may be used to perform this procedure. Smaller needle and syringe combinations are used for softer tissues to be aspirated. The authors prefer a 23-gauge needle attached to a 3-cc syringe or a 22-gauge needle attached to a 6-cc syringe. Regardless of the combination used, the needle is carefully inserted into the center of the lesion. The plunger is pulled back 1–2 mls (or a comparable amount with larger syringes) to provide negative pressure within the syringe. The negative pressure is released and the needle may be redirected within the lesion and the process repeated. The negative pressure is completely released before withdrawing the needle from the lesion so that the collected sample will remain within the needle or needle hub. The needle is then detached from the syringe and air is drawn into the syringe. The needle is then replaced onto the syringe and the contents are expelled onto a clean microscope slide. The procedure may be repeated to collect material from various areas of the lesion, if it is large enough. An adequate sample may be collected from some tissues without the use of any negative pressure or vacuum, simply by inserting the needle into the lesion and then withdrawing it. This procedure works best for nodules, tumors, and for obtaining samples for lymph node cytology.

Fine-needle biopsy:

A 22- or 23-gauge needle is attached to a flexible intravenous infusion line or syringe pre-filled with 3–5 ml of air. Needles with stylets are not necessary, although the author uses a stylet when penetrating the thoracic wall during aspiration/biopsy of pulmonary masses. In dermatology cases, the tissue to be sampled is immobilized with one hand and the needle is rapidly inserted into the lesion and then moved rapidly back and forth with long strokes about 5–8 times. The needle tip should remain within the lesion. The contents of the needle are expelled immediately onto a glass slide and then spread over the slide as described below. It is important to have all the necessary materials at hand when performing this technique. The slide should NOT be allowed to dry. This technique works very well for solid masses and lymph nodes.

Surface impression smears (touch imprints):

In some cases, direct smears may be made from the surface of the skin. This procedure is also know as a Tzanck preparation. A clean glass slide is firmly pressed onto the skin lesion. When making touch imprints from the cut surface of a biopsy specimen, it is useful to gently blot excess blood from the surface of the lesion using a dry paper towel before making the imprint. Examination gloves should be worn to prevent the clinician from contaminating the slide with fingerprints, which can occasionally confuse the reader of the slide. If a copious amount of material is deposited onto the slide, it may need to be distributed using one of the techniques as described under Techniques of Slide Separation on the next page. Otherwise, the sample is allowed to dry for staining. This procedure works best for ulcers or plaques (e.g., eosinophilic plaque). It is important to consider that imprints made from the surface of the skin may only reflect changes or pathology on the surface and may miss underlying, deeper abnormalities (e.g., ulcerated neoplastic lesions).

Collecting the sample from a pustule or papule:

The surface of the lesion should be gently cleaned with a surgical scrub solution or alcohol, being careful not to rupture the lesion. If the lesion appears to be exceptionally friable, the lesion may be gently wiped once with alcohol and then allowed to dry before proceeding. Using a sterile injection needle, the lesion is carefully lanced to expose the contents. In some cases (e.g., large pustules), a sufficient amount of exudate may be collected (i.e., scooped) onto the needle for placement on the slide. In most cases, a clean microscope slide is pressed against the open lesion to collect the exudate. Care should be taken to avoid contaminating the slide with material from the adjacent areas of the skin. As with other techniques, the exudate (e.g., blood, cellular material, pus) should be quickly spread over the slide (see techniques described below) before the exudate dries.

TECHNIQUES OF SLIDE PREPARATION:

In some cases, the material is collected using one of the techniques described earlier, and then allowed to dry on the slide for examination. However, this often results in deposition of material on the slide in amounts too thick to properly evaluate. The preparation of the material and distribution onto the slide makes a huge difference in the quality of the slide, and thus, the value of the cytologic interpretation.

Samples may be distributed on a slide by non-traumatic imprints, squash preparations, or brush cytology. The *squash technique* involves placing the cytologic specimen on one end of a glass slide and then gently placing a second slide on the specimen at a right angle to the first slide. The weight of the second slide generally applies enough compression of the sample, and the top slide gently slides off the end of the first slide (Fig. 1-1). Once the technique is mastered, the specimen should be distributed in a thin layer over the slide. Unfortunately, cells collected from dermatologic lesions are often fragile and this technique can result in distortion of the cells in the sample.

The *brush technique* allows for more delicate distribution of the cells and fluid in the cytologic specimen. The sample is placed on a clean glass slide and then spread out (i.e., "painted") on the slide using a camel hair artist's brush (Fig. 1-2). The brush is then rinsed well with tap water and dried after each use. This technique gives single cell layer distribution on the slide, with a minimum of trauma to the sample (Fig. 1-3A,B). Alternatively, the tip of a sterile injection needle can be used to accomplish the same task, though there is more trauma to the cells.

Slides should then be fixed and stained. Heat fixing the slide with a match or lighter is beneficial when the slide contains waxy or greasy exudate, such as seen with most ear swabs or with impressions from seborrheic patients. Otherwise, the alcohol-based fixative used in most staining procedures is adequate. One slide should be left unstained in case a special stain is needed.

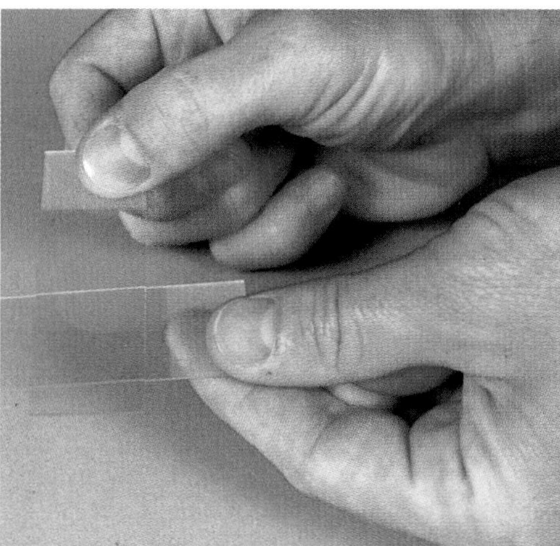

Figure 1-1 The *squash technique* involves placement of the cytologic specimen on a slide, covering the sample with another slide, and then gently pulling the two slides apart.

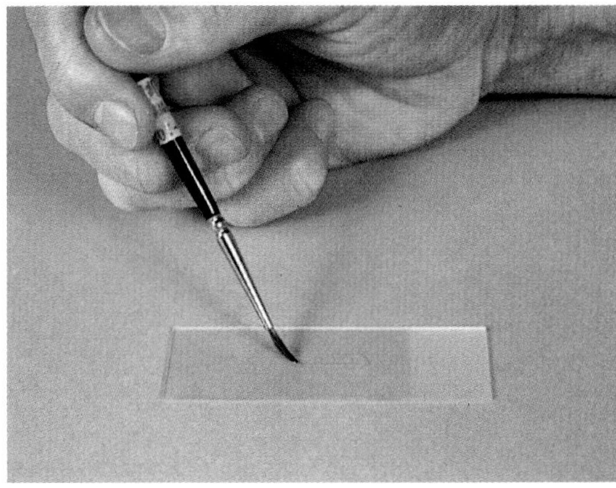

Figure 1-2 The brush technique uses a soft paintbrush to distribute cellular material on the slide.

Staining the Slide:

Several stains are available to stain material collected for examination. Romanowsky stains such as Wright's stain, and modified-Wright's stains (e.g., Diff-Quick Stain®-Baxter Scientific Products, Inc.[a]) are easily and quickly performed. They are excellent when permanent slides are desired. Supravital stains such as new methylene blue are also easy and rapid but are not as easily stored for future reference. Each clinician should choose a stain with which he/she is comfortable and become accustomed to its staining qualities. It is useful to save slides for future reference. To help preserve slides for storage, permanent cover slip-mounting medium is commercially available and easy to use.[b] These slides can make up an excellent reference set for the practitioner, especially if one sample is sent to a clinical pathologist and a second slide kept with a copy of the written report for future reference.

Stains used for fecal and urinalysis preparations should be kept separate from stains used for routine cytology to avoid bacterial contamination. All stains should be kept covered and changed on a routine basis (i.e., weekly, if possible) or whenever the stain appears contaminated or dirty.

Examination of the Slide:

It is absolutely essential to use a quality microscope that is properly tuned to view cytology specimens. Dirty or scratched objective or eyepieces will markedly decrease the quality of the procedure. It is outside the purvey of this chapter to review the process of microscope care and use, but it is critical to the success of any procedure requiring microscopy. A double-headed microscope is well worth the financial investment, as it will allow two clinicians or technicians to discuss or consult on various findings and allow the client to visualize key findings. The value of this client education should not be underestimated and is discussed in the summary.

When viewing a prepared slide, the entire slide should first be scanned using a low-power objective (2X or 4X, total magnification of 20–40X). Then the slide is examined more closely using a higher-power objective, such as 10X (total magnification 100X), and finally using high dry and/or oil immersion objectives. Most high dry objectives (40 power objective, total magnification of 400X) will not allow the user to focus on a slide unless the slide has a cover slip applied. The oil immersion objective (100X on most microscopes, total magnification of 1000X) is used primarily to identify micro-organisms and cellular inclusions (Table 1-1).

[a] Baxter Scientific Products, Inc., McGaw Park, IL 60085-6787
[b] Acrytol®: Surgipath Medical Industries, Inc. Richmond, IL 60071

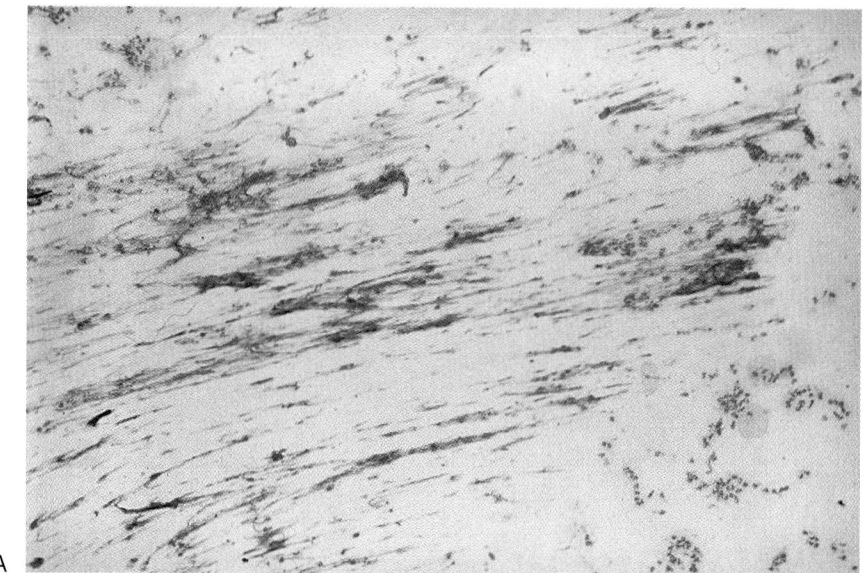

A

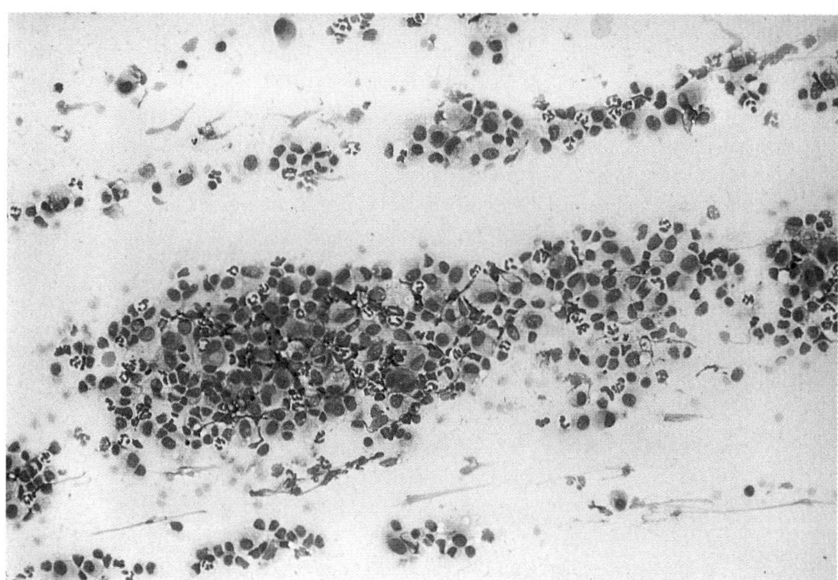

B

Figure 1-3 **A.** Example of a slide made with the squash technique. Notice the streaking of nuclear material, which can make interpretation of the slide difficult. **B.** Example of a slide made with the brush technique showing less cellular distortion and excellent distribution on the slide.

Keys to success:

1. Lesion selection is important. Pustules generally provide valuable information, whereas impressions made from the surface of a lesion may be difficult to interpret because of secondary inflammation and contamination.
2. Slide preparation and examination are critical to provide the clinician with good data. Slides should be air dried or dried with a hair dryer under low heat. Slides should *never* be dried using absorbent paper (i.e., bibulous paper) pressed onto the slide.

Table 1-1

Magnification Recommended for Cytologic Procedures†

Magnification	Use
20×	Skin scrapings, initial survey of cytology slides, survey of ear swabs for ectoparasites
40×	Same as for 20×, examination of hairs on trichogram
100×	Examination of hairs on trichogram, KOH preparation, closer view of cytology for pustules/impressions/etc., survey for *Malassezia* spp. yeasts
400×	KOH preparations, higher view of cytology specimens for cell detail, survey for bacterial/fungi/foreign objects, identification of *Malassezia* spp. yeast on impressions or scrapings
1000×	Confirmation of micro-organisms (e.g., bacterial), identification of yeast on impressions or scrapings

† (Total magnification = objective magnification times 10).

3. Stain maintenance is important to prevent poor-quality slides, artifacts, and contamination.
4. Care and tuning of a microscope is essential. It is simply impossible to make accurate assessments of samples when the instrument with which you view those samples is inferior or poorly maintained. Microscopes should be cleaned daily and adjusted for each slide that is viewed.

Table 1-2

Example of an Arbitrary Scale Useful for Evaluating Numbers of Infectious Agents in the External Ear Canal

Scale	High Power (400×)†
Bacteria	
0	None
1+	Less than 1–2 organisms
2+	2–5 organisms per field
3+	5–20 organisms per field
4+	Greater than 20 organisms per field
Yeast	
0	None
1+	Less than 1 organism per field
2+	Less than 5 per field
3+	5–10 organisms per field
4+	Greater than 10 organisms per field

† Represents averages. Some fields may have greater or less than the indicated numbers.

A
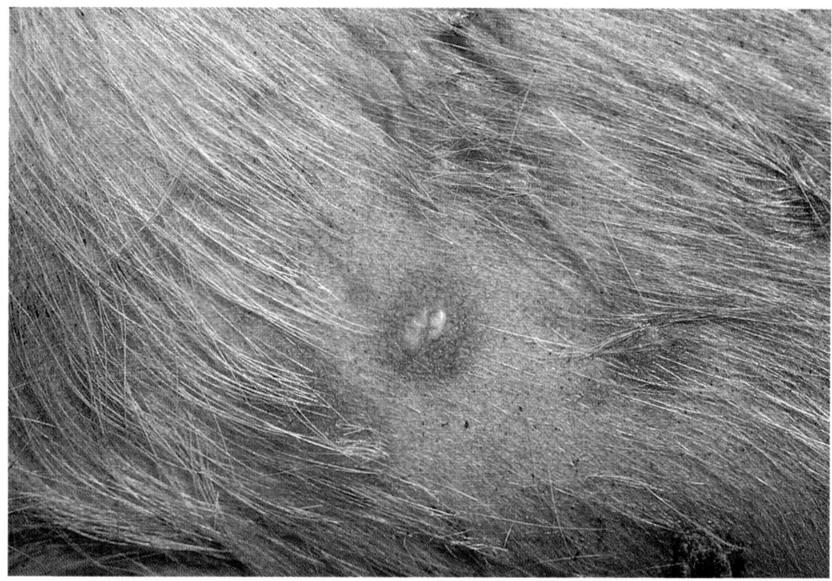

B
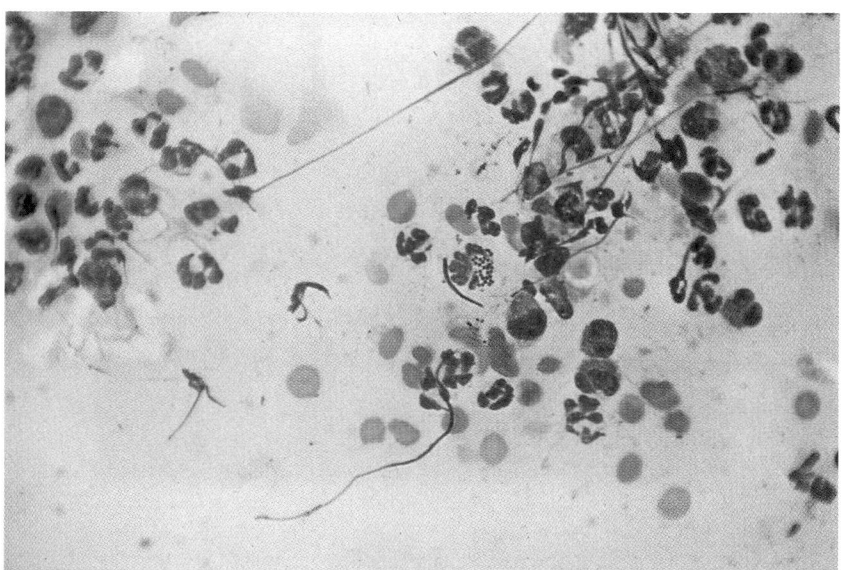

Figure 1-4 **A.** Pustule from a canine patient. **B.** Cytology from the same patient showing neutrophils and cocci within one of the neutrophils, signifying pyoderma.

5. Interpretation of cytology specimens requires good powers of observation and experience (Table1-2, Figs. 1-4 thru 1-6). Each slide should be thoroughly examined and the types of cells, types and relative numbers of micro-organisms, and other features noted and recorded in the medical record.

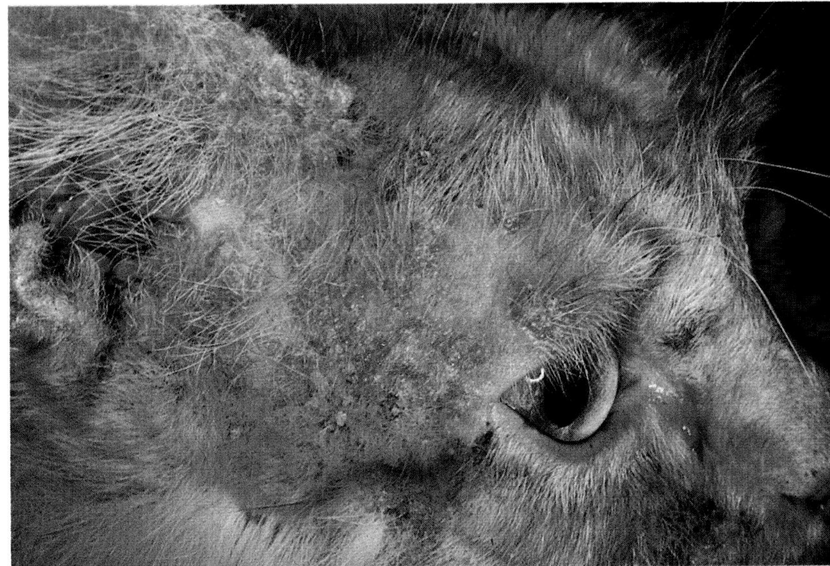
A

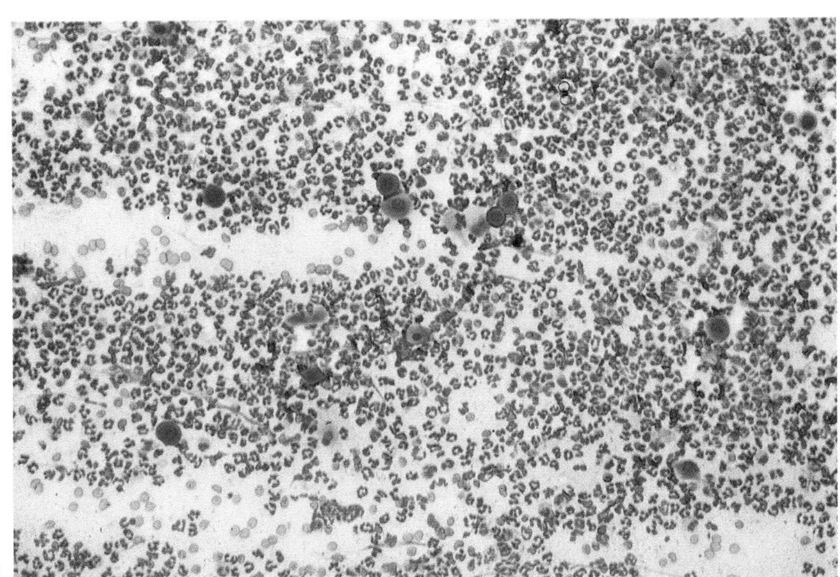
B

Figure 1-5 **A.** Feline patient with numerous crusts and pustules on the head. **B.** Cytology from this cat. Notice the numerous neutrophils without infectious agents and the numerous acantholytic cells, which are keratinocytes without their cellular attachments to other epithelial cells. This slide is strongly suggestive of pemphigus foliaceus.

A

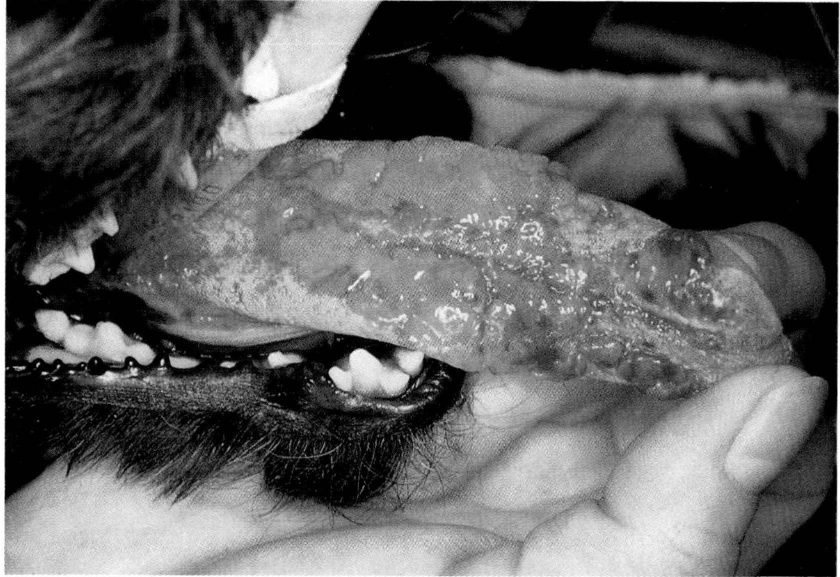

B

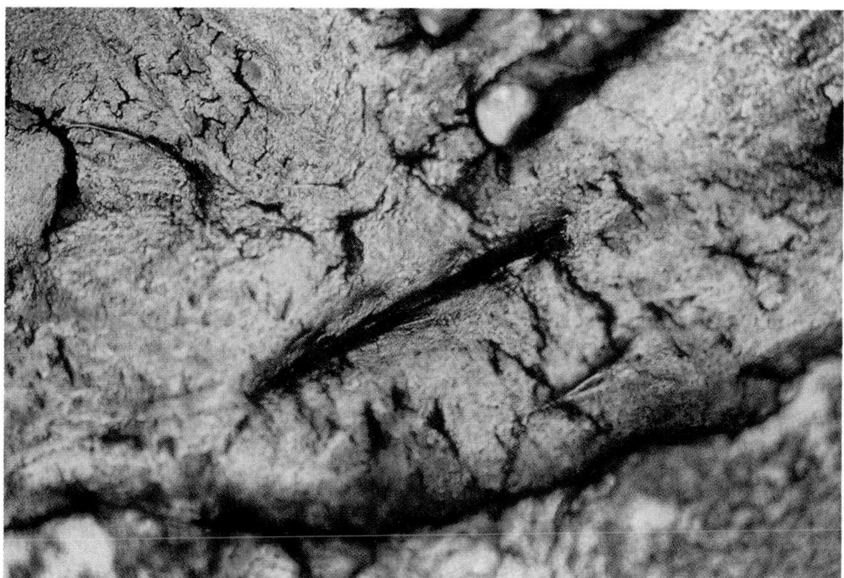

Figure 1-6 **A.** Tongue of a dog with chronic stomatitis. **B.** Cytologic specimen made by scraping the lesion with a scalpel blade and then brushing the material onto a microscope slide. Notice the barbed plant material. This is diagnostic of foreign body (plant) glossitis.

Ear Cytology

INDICATIONS: Cytology is a useful and valuable technique to assess current status and monitor response to therapy in patients with otitis externa. Ear cytology should be performed every time a patient is re-examined for an ear problem.

MATERIALS: Cotton swabs, glass microscope slides and cover slips, matches or lighter, Diff-Quik® stain, microscope, and immersion oil are needed.

PROCEDURE: A dry cotton swab is inserted into the horizontal ear canal or as far as possible without causing extreme discomfort to the patient and then rotated and removed from the ear. The swab is then gently rolled onto a glass slide, heat fixed by holding a match or lighter under the slide for 2–3 seconds, and then stained (Fig. 1-7). The slide should be handled gently during the staining process to avoid dislodging the cytology sample from the slide. After staining, the slide is examined as previously described under low power and under oil immersion.

Ear cytology always provides useful information. Special attention is paid to the following:

1. The presence and types of bacteria (rods and cocci) and yeast (*Malassezia* spp.)
2. The presence of a mixed bacterial and/or yeast infection versus the presence of a single type of bacteria or yeast. (Infections by single infectious agents may indicate a more serious infection and require culture and susceptibility testing.)
3. The presence of inflammatory cells. (If present, these suggest more severe damage to the external ear canal and indicate the need for systemic therapy.)

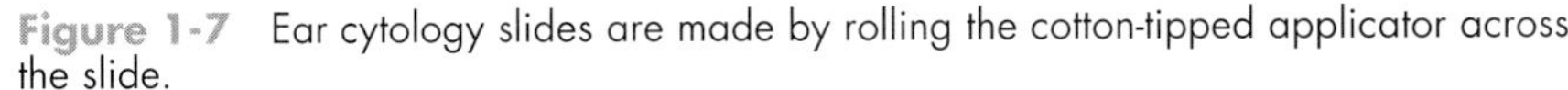
Figure 1-7 Ear cytology slides are made by rolling the cotton-tipped applicator across the slide.

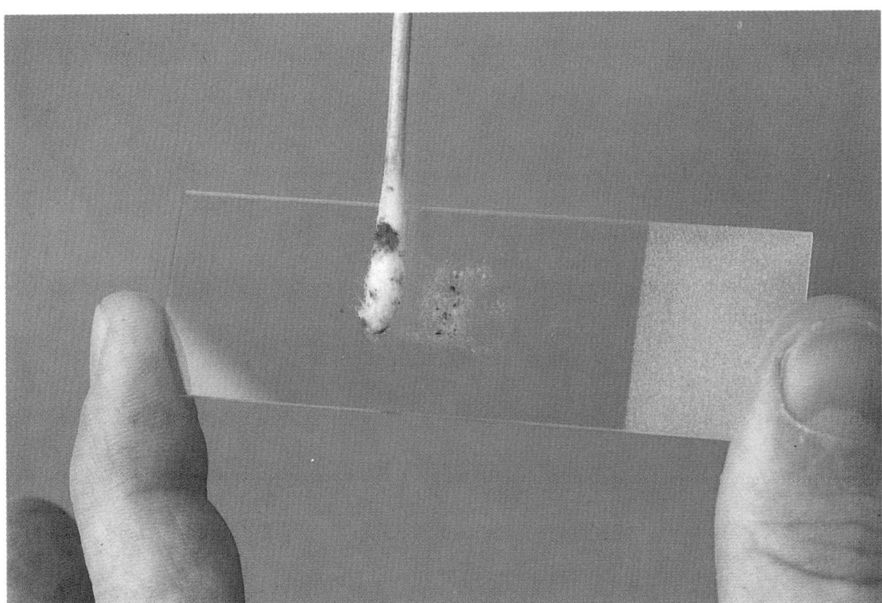

Keys to success: A major key is to obtain the specimen from the horizontal canal. This is most readily done if the pinna is pulled outward (i.e., away from the head) and downward to *straighten* out the external ear canal before the cotton-tipped applicator is inserted into the ear canal.

COMMENTS Squamous epithelial cells are usually seen in small numbers. Bacteria are seen in normal ears in low numbers and there are usually different types (rods, cocci) of bacteria present in normal ear canals. *Malassezia* spp. yeasts are considered normal inhabitants of the ear canal (up to 10 per high power field is normal). The relative number of bacteria, yeast, and epithelial cells may be recorded using an arbitrary scale that may vary from cytologist to cytologist (Table 1-2). However, a scale of this type will help to determine the efficacy of therapy when the patient is re-examined. The presence and relative number of neutrophils should also be noted. Neutrophils without bacteria may suggest a hypersensitivity reaction to medication being placed in the ear (e.g., neomycin or propylene glycol).

Skin Scrapings/Impression Smears for Yeast (*Malassezia* spp.)

INDICATIONS: Skin scrapings/smears for *Malassezia* are performed whenever yeast are suspected as a primary or secondary cause of pruritus, scaling, erythema, or seborrhea. They are part of a minimum database of information in patients with pruritus.

MATERIALS: A #10 scalpel blade, glass microscope slides or adhesive microscope slides, clippers to remove hair from areas to be sampled, cotton swab, and a microscope are needed. Adhesive microscope slides (Duro-Tak) are available from Delasco, Dermatologic Lab & Supply, 608 13th Avenue, Council Bluffs, IA 51501, 1-800-831-6273 or 1-888-335-2726 (Fig. 1-8).

PROCEDURES: Several procedures are useful to collect epithelial material to evaluate for yeast dermatitis. 1) Skin scrapings may be performed using the scalpel blade.

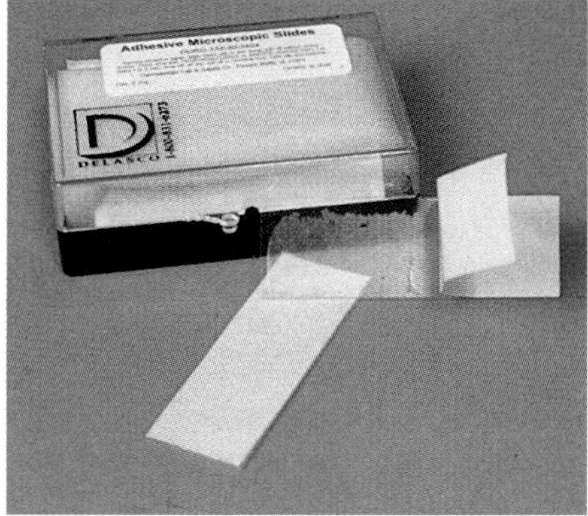

Figure 1-8 Adhesive microscope slides come with a paper covering that is removed before use.

Suspicious areas such as the interdigital spaces, flanks, fronts of the elbows, and perianal and perineal areas, should be carefully scraped with a dry scalpel blade (no mineral oil) to collect surface keratinocytes. It is not necessary nor desirable to induce capillary hemorrhage, as the yeast are found in the most superficial layers of the epidermis. This cellular material is pressed firmly onto the slide, heat fixed for 2–3 seconds, and stained (e.g., with Diff–Quik® stain). 2) A second technique involves the use of a cotton-tipped applicator swab to briskly swab the lesion. The swab is then rolled onto a slide, pressing firmly to adhere the epithelial material to the slide. The slide is heat fixed and stained. 3) In the direct impression technique, the glass slide may be firmly pressed against the skin to get impression smears of *Malassezia* from suspicious areas (Fig. 1-9). The slide should be imprinted several times in the same area to ensure adequate recovery of epithelial cells and debris. Examination gloves should be worn to prevent fingerprints (oils and epithelial cells) from causing confusion when you examine the slide. 4) If the adhesive slides are used, the slide should be pressed onto the affected area several times in each location. Heat fixing is not required. The slide should be gently stained and microscopically examined. Although yeast may be seen with 100X total magnification, it is best to evaluate the slide using the high dry or oil immersion objective as previously described.

Keys to success:

1. If regular glass slides are used, the sample must be forcefully pressed onto the slide for good adherence. The greater the amount of the sample that adheres to the slide, the better your chances are of having a significant and accurate test.

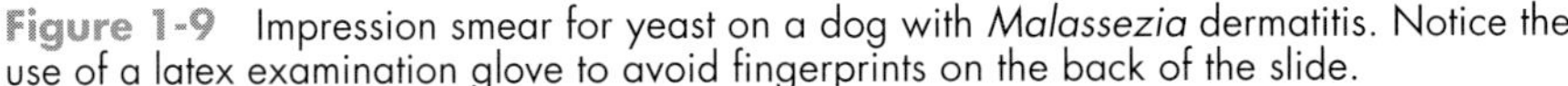

Figure 1-9 Impression smear for yeast on a dog with *Malassezia* dermatitis. Notice the use of a latex examination glove to avoid fingerprints on the back of the slide.

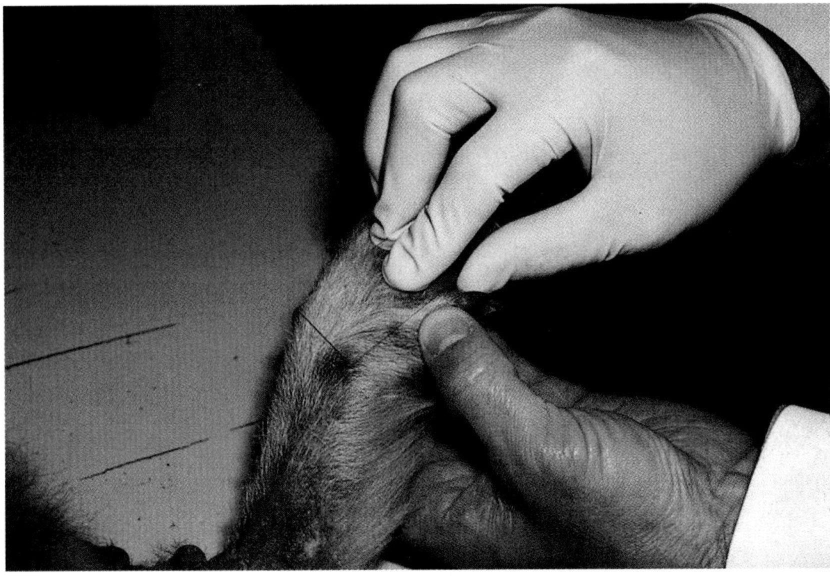

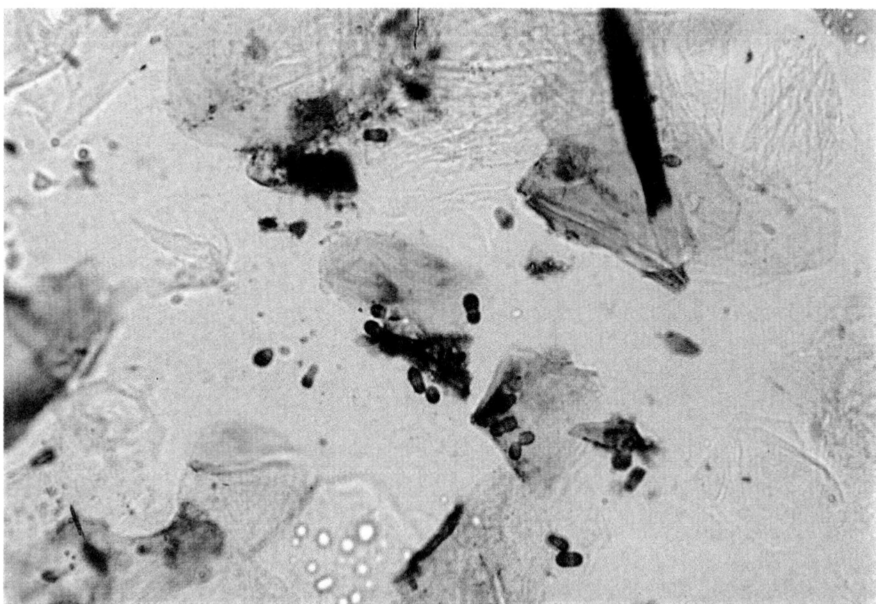

Figure 1-10 Cytologic specimen (oil immersion, 1000X) from a patient with *Malassezia* pododermatitis.

2. The cotton swab technique works well to collect samples from sensitive areas, such as perivulvar and perianal areas.
3. Heat fixation is not synonymous with *cooking*. Don't overheat the slide. If the slide is too warm to hold with your fingers, it is too warm for the sample.
4. The staining process should be done gently to avoid losing the sample when the slide is agitated during each step of the staining process. Instead of dipping the slide repeatedly, immersion of the slide in each fixative or stain and holding it in place for the same time it takes to dip the slide will improve the yield of the specimen.
5. Organisms are clearer under examination using high dry objectives (400X total magnification) when a drop of immersion oil is placed on the slide and then a cover slip applied on top of the oil (Fig. 1-10). Oil immersion (e.g., 1000X) magnification also works well.

COMMENTS 1) *Malassezia pachydermatis* is part of the normal flora of canine skin and ears, and acts as a perpetuating factor of otitis externa and various skin diseases (e.g., atopy) of the dog and cat. Both the skin and ear provide many physical characteristics (e.g., heat, humidity) associated with the ideal environment for growth of these organisms. 2) Organisms other than yeast may be recovered during this process. Pollens and saprophytic fungal hyphae are commonly found, as well as dermatophytes, plant pollens, and mold spores. Identification of these substances may be necessary to rule out a pathologic process. 3) As when examining cytology of the ear canal, it is useful to use an arbitrary, relative scale to evaluate the numbers of yeast found on the skin impressions or scrapings (Table 1-3). The scale tends to be arbitrary from one clinician to another because the technique used for sample collection may vary.

Table 1-3

Example of an Arbitrary Scale Useful for Evaluating Numbers of *Malassezia pachydermatis* found on cytology of the skin

Scale	High Power (400×)†
0	None
1+	Less than 1 organism per field
2+	Less than 5 per field
3+	5–10 organisms per field
4+	Greater than 10 organisms per field

† Represents averages. Some fields may have greater or less than the indicated numbers.

Cytologic Examination of the Fungal Culture

INDICATIONS: Fungal cultures should be run on all dermatology cases, especially if there are circular, crusted or scaly lesions, or if broken hairs are present. *Every* colony that grows on the fungal culture medium should be microscopically examined to determine if the colony is a pathogenic or saprophytic organism.

MATERIALS: Forceps, fungal culture media, glass slides, stains, cover slips, lactophenol cotton blue stain, and a microscope are needed. The technique of fungal culture and more information on that procedure is discussed later in this book.

PROCEDURE: A small amount of hyphae should be gently removed from the culture medium, placed onto a glass microscope slide, and a drop of lactophenol cotton blue stain placed on the specimen (Fig. 1-11). The hyphae should be gently teased apart with forceps or probes and a cover slip added. The sample should be examined microscopically and the fungus identified.

The hyphae should be examined under scanning (2–4X objectives) and high dry magnifications to look for the characteristics of the common pathogenic or saprophytic fungi. Several excellent reference texts have diagrams and photographs of the identifying traits of the various fungi. It is not clinically essential to determine which pathogen is present, but it is necessary to separate a pathogen from a saprophytic organism.

Another technique to distribute hyphae onto a slide for examination involves the use of a piece of clear acetate tape, which is touched to the surface of the fungal colony on the culture medium. A drop of stain (e.g., new methylene blue or lactophenol cotton blue) is placed on the slide, the tape pressed onto the slide, followed by a drop of immersion oil and a cover slip over the drop oil. The resulting "sandwich" of stain-tape with fungal elements-oil-cover slip allows the slide to be examined clearly with high dry objectives. Alternatively, adhesive slides may be used in lieu of tape.

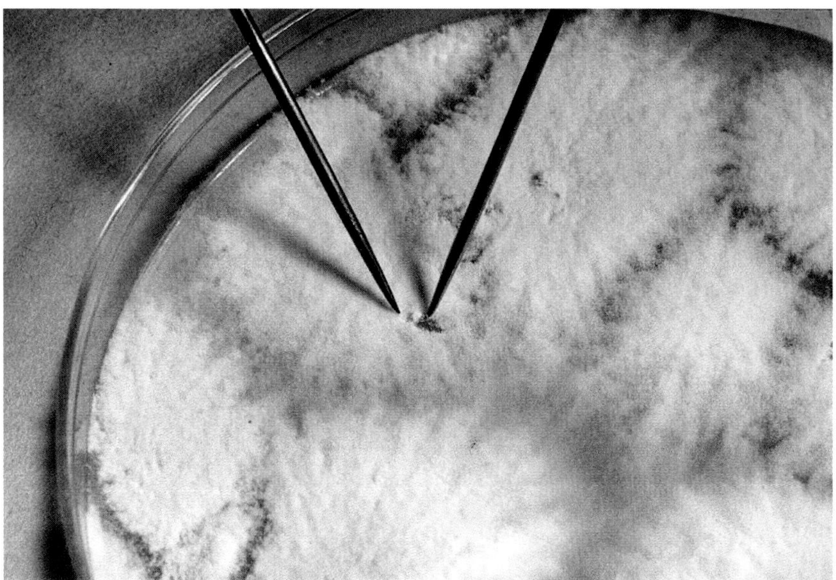

Figure 1-11 Teasing of fungal hyphae from the gross colony in preparation of microscopic examination to confirm the type of fungus growing from a patient with dermatitis.

Keys to success:

1. Colonies must have time to sporulate macroconidia, as that is the key characteristic used to identify organisms (Fig. 1-12). This may require extended times (3—4 weeks) depending on the media used for colony growth.

Figure 1-12 Hyphae and macroconidia or *Microsporum canis* showing characteristic canoe-shaped macroconidia.

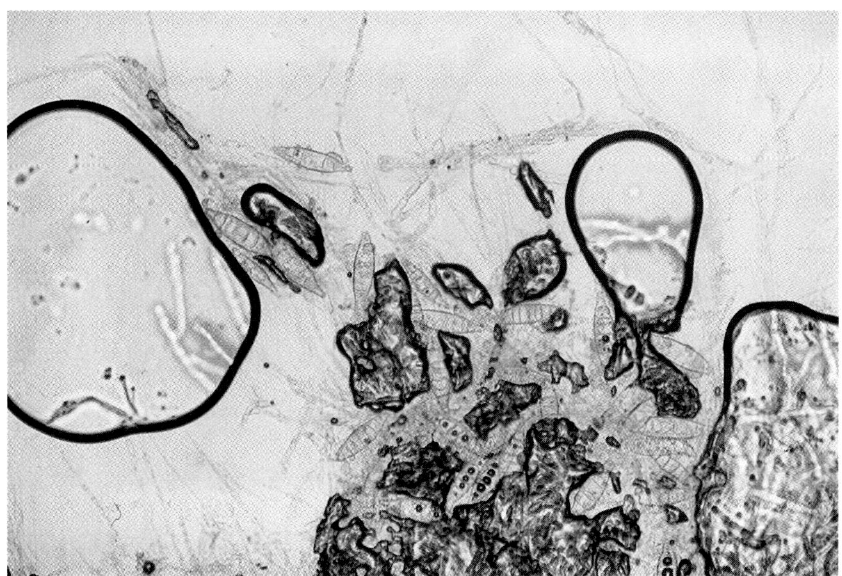

2. It is not necessary to stain the colony before microscopic examination, but it does help to define characteristics.
3. A reference text is helpful to confirm the identity of the organism. Several texts and manuals are available and some sites on the World Wide Web will also provide images and information to help in this process. Some veterinary dermatology textbooks provide adequate descriptions and photographs to assist in this process.

Summary

Cytologic examination of specimens collected from the skin and ears is not only rewarding to the clinician, but also has other practical applications. Allowing clients to visualize some of the specimens will enhance owner compliance, improve the veterinarian-client relationship, and increase the client's willingness to perform other diagnostic tests and procedures indicated in the case.

Recommended Reading

Myer DJ. The management of cytologic specimens. Comp Cont Ed 1987;9:10–16.

Barton CL. Cytologic diagnosis of cutaneous neoplasia: An algorithmic approach. Comp Cont Ed 1987;9:20–33.

Hall RL, MacWilliams PS. The cytologic examination of cutaneous and subcutaneous masses. Sem in Vet Med Surg 1988;3:94–108.

Valli VEO. Techniques in veterinary cytopathology. Sem Vet Med Surg 1988;3:85–93.

Scott D, Miller W, Griffin CE. Small animal dermatology, 5th ed. Philadelphia: Saunders, 1995:100–111.

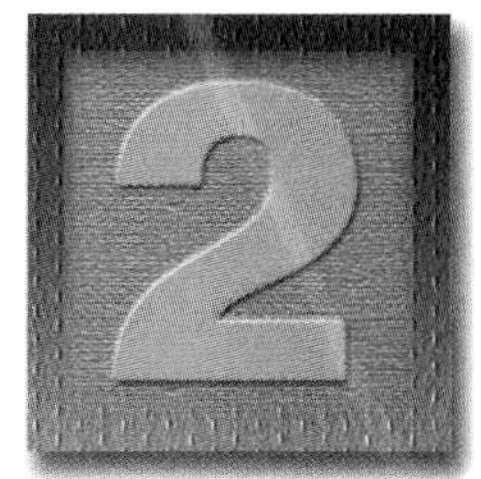

Dermatohistopathology: Obtaining a Diagnostic Biopsy

Karen Helton Rhodes

The skin biopsy is one of the most important diagnostic tools available. Three factors are key to obtaining a diagnostic biopsy: site selection, tissue handling, and a good dermatopathologist. There are a number of recognized dermatopathologists available through a variety of commercial and private laboratories. Your board-certified dermatologist(s) may be helpful in providing names and locations of laboratories. The art of site selection and tissue handling are the responsibility of the submitting veterinarian.

The Decision to Biopsy

There are a number of cutaneous disorders for which the biopsy is the only helpful diagnostic tool. The biopsy is equally important for what appears to be a "classic case" that continues to fail conventional therapy. The following "rules" apply to the question of

When to biopsy:

1. Persistent lesions
2. Any neoplastic or suspected neoplastic disorder
3. Any scaling dermatoses
4. Vesicular dermatosis
5. Undiagnosed alopecias
6. Any unusual dermatoses

Site Selection

It is often difficult to decide which area to biopsy. We have been taught to sample the periphery of the lesion so that both normal and abnormal areas will be available for inspection. This is a problem in many cases, and may facilitate a poor section when only a small portion of the pathology is present in the tissue. It is more productive to choose representative lesions and submit multiple pieces of skin for evaluation. Most laboratories will allow the clinician to submit up to four or five sections of skin for the same fee, as multiple sections will aid the pathologist in making a diagnosis. Remember, if the lesion is present on the planum nasale then submit a section of the planum nasale, not the surrounding skin. Although the area bleeds quite profusely when cut, it heals nicely with minimal scarring and increases the likelihood of an accurate diagnosis. The following "rules" apply to the question of

Where to biopsy:

1. Choose several representative lesions as they may represent various stages of the same disorder or multiple problems.
2. Include lesions characterized by scale, crust, erythema, erosion, ulceration, etc. (Fig. 2-1A–C)
3. It is not always necessary to biopsy the edge of a lesion, although a sample taken within the center of an ulcer is rarely diagnostic.
4. Pustules and vesicles should not be biopsied with a punch technique because the twisting motion of the punch will rupture or remove the roof of the lesion and disrupt the architecture of the sample; these lesions should be excised *in toto*.
5. Ulcers or deep draining lesions are best taken by excision, rather than by punch technique, because the twisting motion may separate the pathologic tissue from the more normal tissue, leaving important clues behind (i.e., vasculitis, panniculitis, etc.).
6. Do not be afraid to biopsy a footpad or the planum nasale—wedge samples are easier to close than circular punched samples.
7. Crusted lesions are good sites for biopsy. Remember, if the crust separates from the lesion during sampling be sure to include it in the formalin jar and make a notation for the technician to "please cut in the crust."
8. Heavily scaled areas are often good diagnostic sites.

Biopsy Technique

One of the most important points to remember is that cutaneous biopsy sites should not be scrubbed and cleaned, as this will remove clues regarding the diagnosis. It is often difficult for veterinarians to feel comfortable cutting through crust and scale without scrubbing the area. Most cutaneous biopsies can be done with local anesthesia via lidocaine injection into the subcutaneous region. (Fig. 2-2A,B) Some fractious animals may need a sedative (such as ketamine/valium). Avoid the 2- and 4-mm punches because the sections are too small for good sample size. The following "rules" apply to the question of

How to biopsy:

1. Never scrub or cleanse the area before excision—the surface crust may contain the pathologic changes necessary to make a diagnosis.
2. Use a surgical blade to obtain a wedge-shaped or elliptic biopsy specimen when sectioning the nose, footpad, vesicles, bullae, or deep lesions (vasculitis, panniculitis, etc.).

A

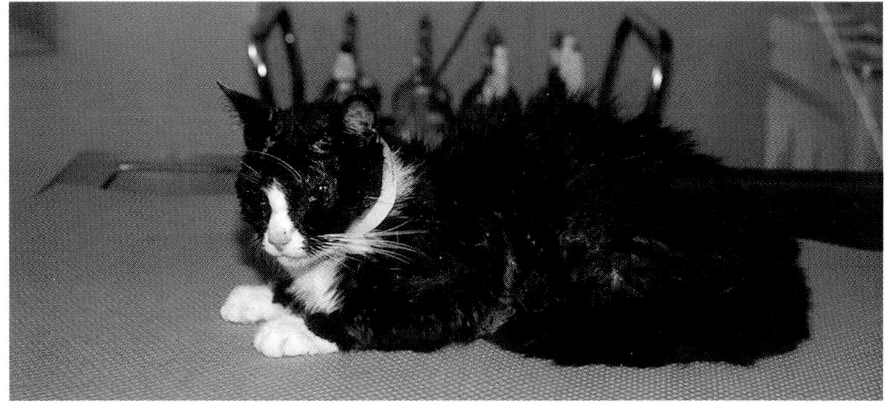

Figure 2-1A Ten-year-old DSH with a history of progressive, non-responsive, erosive, and ulcerative dermatosis with mild to moderate-reported pruritus.

B

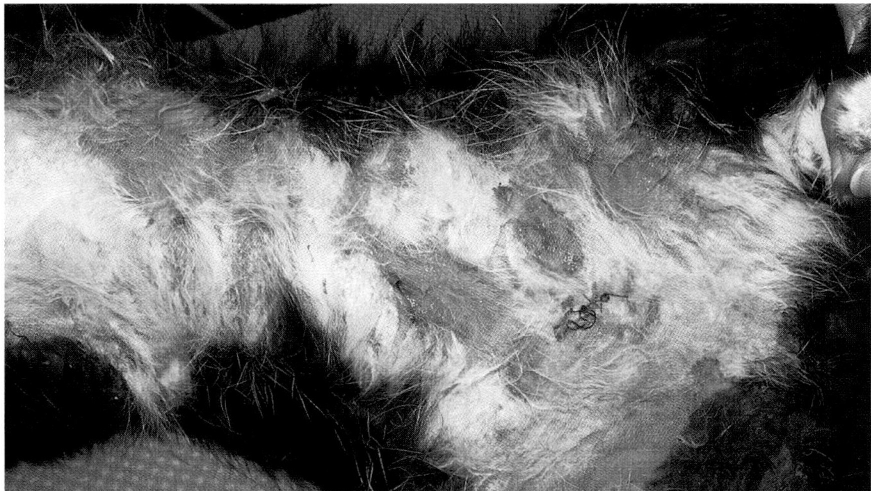

Figure 2-1B View of the ventrum of same cat revealing multifocal areas of erosions, ulcerations, and rare plaque-like lesions associated with generalized erythema.

C

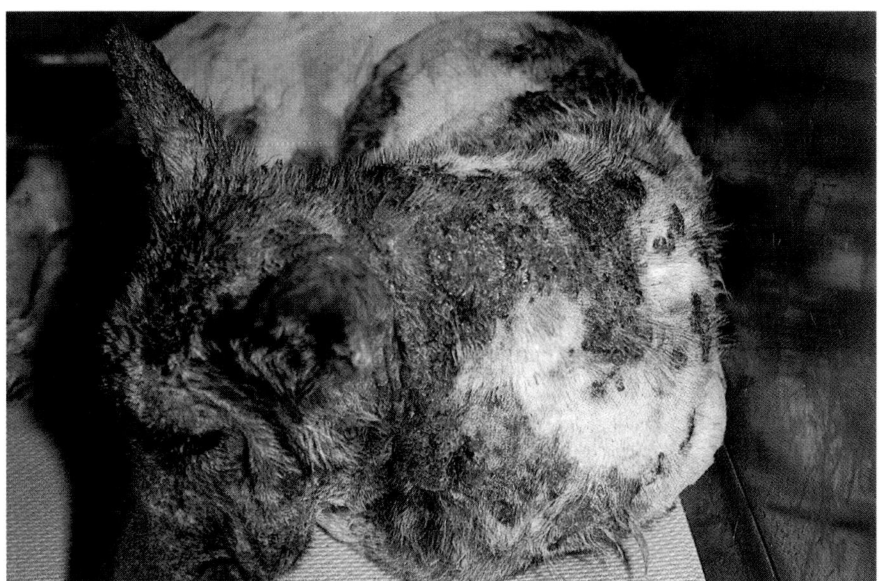

Figure 2-1C Eight-year-old German Shepherd with non-pruritic ulcerative and crusting dermatosis.

A

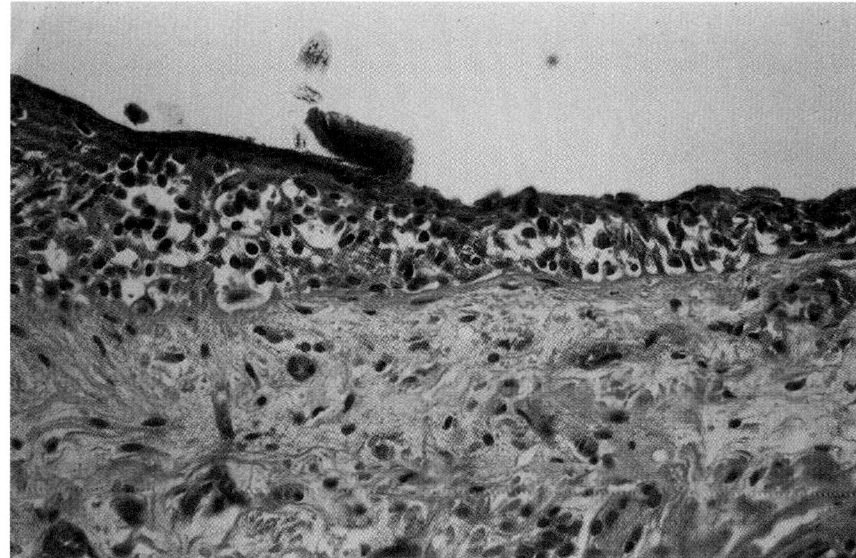

Figure 2-2A Cutaneous biopsy revealing epidermal lymphocytic exocytosis supporting a diagnosis of epidermotrophic lymphoma.

B

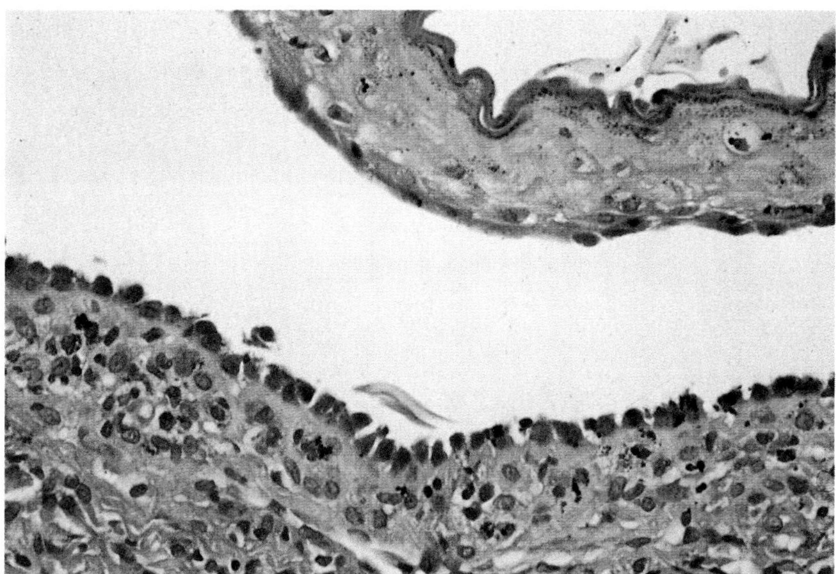

Figure 2-3B Eight cutaneous biopsy indicating the etiology as pemphigus vulgaris. Note the cleft of the epidermis leaving the cells of the stratum basale along the base of the vesicle ("Tombstone" appearance).

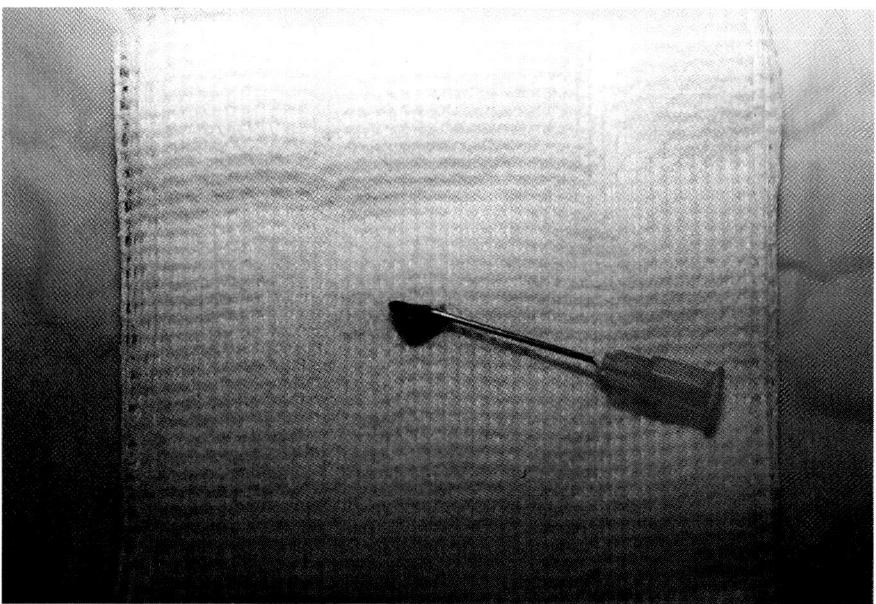

Figure 2-3 Avoid the use of forceps to handle the tissue as they are often associated with crushing the artifact.

3. When using a punch biopsy, choose the 6-mm size.
4. When using a punch biopsy, rotate in one direction only and do not re-use the tool as the blade is easily dulled and may cause the tissue to tear during the procedure.
5. When using lidocaine, place the anesthesia in the subcutaneous compartment, not intradermally.
6. Try not to handle the tissue with forceps (crushing artifact) but rather use a small-gauge needle to manipulate the tissue (Fig. 2-3).
7. Place the sample immediately in the formalin.
8. Small or thin specimens may be placed on a small piece of a tongue depressor with the haired portion to the outside to prevent curling and then floating upside down in the formalin.
9. Avoid freezing.

Remember to provide your pathologist with a thorough history and clinical description of the lesions. I routinely include a copy of the referral letter with the biopsy request. This letter outlines the history, clinical signs, differential diagnoses considered, and a plan. You and your pathologist should become a diagnostic team. It is unrealistic to expect the pathologist to consistently provide answers if we do not supply the appropriate tissue or information.

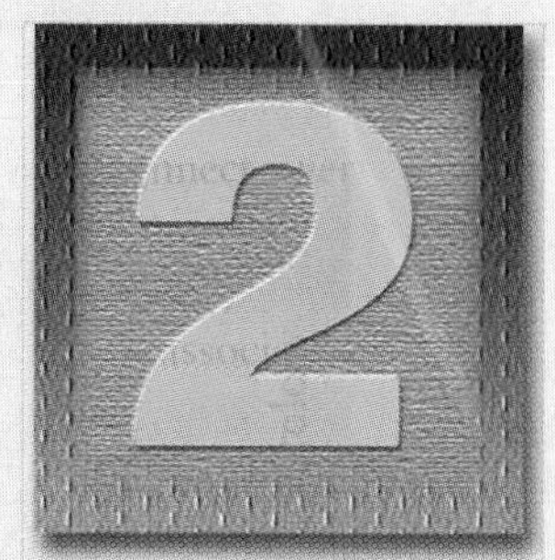

Differential Diagnoses Based on Clinical Patterns

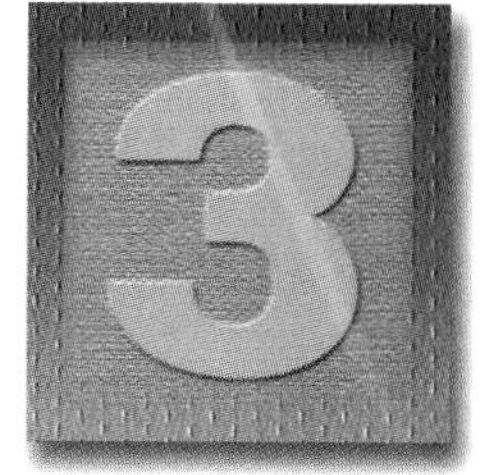

Alopecia, Canine

Karen Helton Rhodes and Karin M. Beale

Definition/Overview

- Common disorder
- Characterized by a complete or partial lack of hair in areas where it is normally present
- May be associated with a multifactorial cause
- May be the primary problem or only a secondary phenomenon

Pathophysiology/Etiology

- Multifactorial causes
- All of the disorders represent a disruption in the growth of the hair follicle from infection, trauma, immunologic attack, mechanical "plugging," endocrine abnormalities, or blockage of the receptor sites for stimulation of the cycle.

Signalment/History

No specific age, breed, or sex predilection

- The history (pruritis, acute/chronic onset, etc.) will vary with each specific disorder (see individual chapters).

Clinical Features

- May be acute in onset or slowly progressive
- Multifocal patches of circular alopecia—most frequently associated with folliculitis from bacterial infection or demodicosis
- Large, more diffuse areas of alopecia—may indicate a follicular dysplasia or metabolic component
- The pattern and degree of hair loss are important for establishing a differential diagnosis.

Differential Diagnosis

Multifocal

- Demodicosis—partial to complete alopecia with erythema and mild scaling; (Fig. 3-1) lesions may become inflamed and crusted (Fig. 3-2)
- Dermatophytosis—partial to complete alopecia with scaling; with or without erythema; not always ring-like
- Staphylococcal folliculitis—circular patterns of alopecia with papules epidermal collarettes, erythema, crusting, and hyperpigmented macules (Figs. 3-3 and 3-4)
- Injection reactions—inflammation with alopecia and/or cutaneous atrophy from scarring
- Rabies vaccine vasculitis—patch of alopecia observed 2–3 months postvaccination (Fig. 3-5)

Figure 3-1 Demodicosis characterized by multifocal patches of partial to complete alopecia.

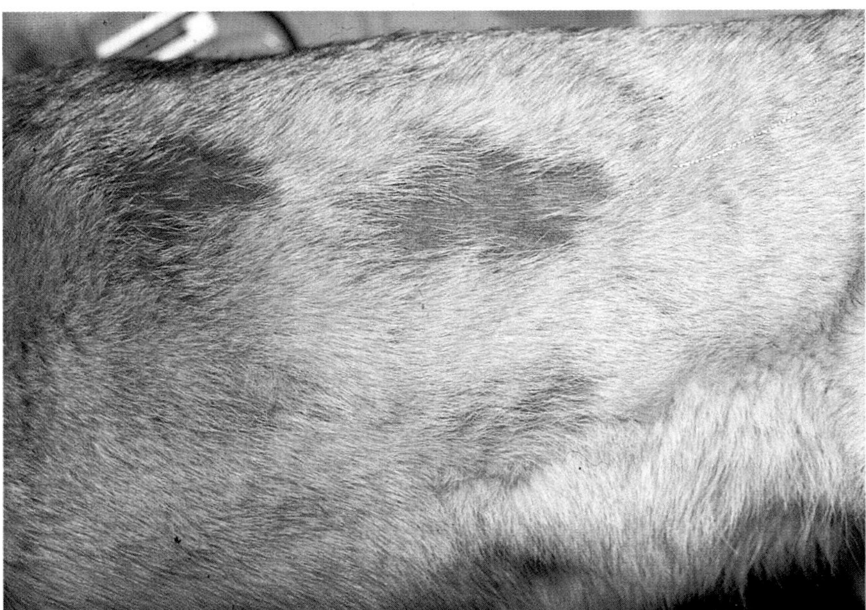

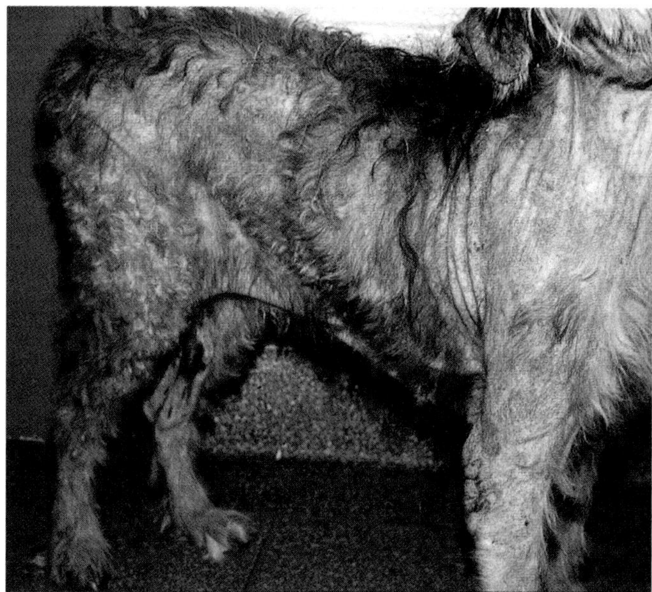

Figure 3-2 Generalized demodicosis causing severe erythroderma, partial to complete alopecia, and crusting.

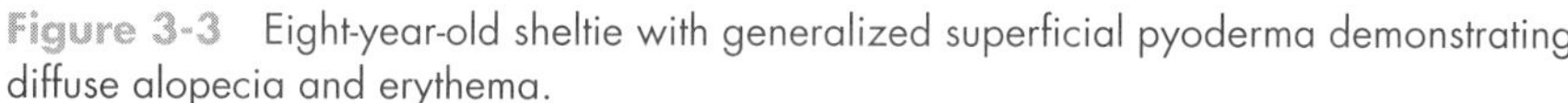

Figure 3-3 Eight-year-old sheltie with generalized superficial pyoderma demonstrating diffuse alopecia and erythema.

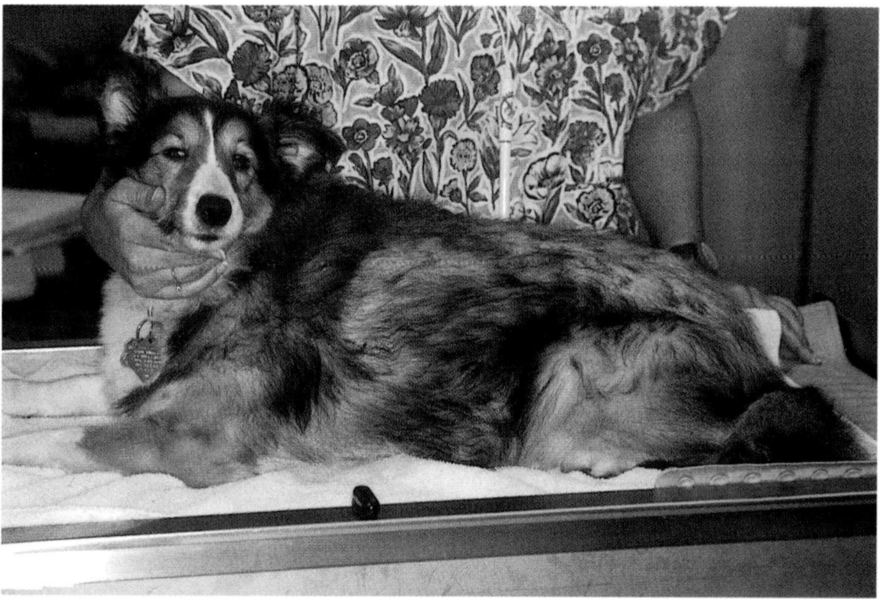

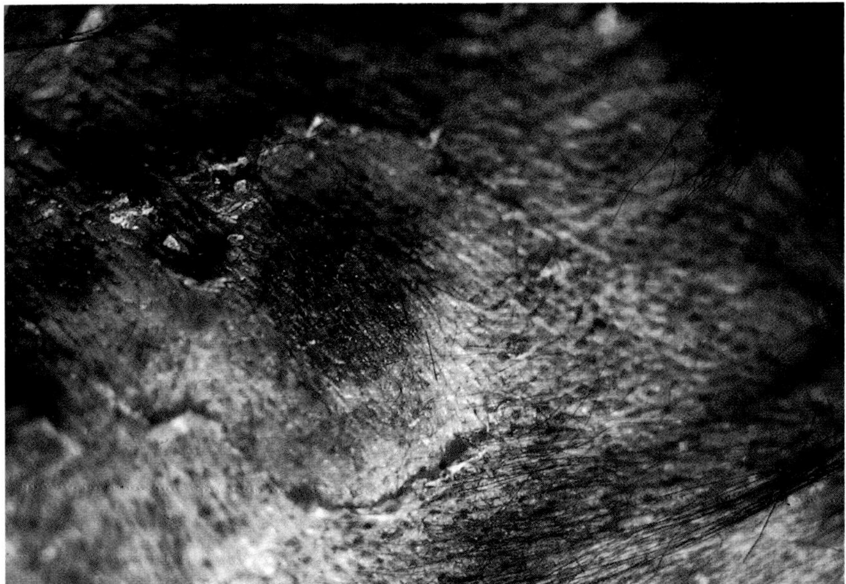

Figure 3-4 More typical pattern of superficial pyoderma demonstrating multifocal patches of alopecia (papules, pustules, epidermal collarettes, and hyperpigmented macules).

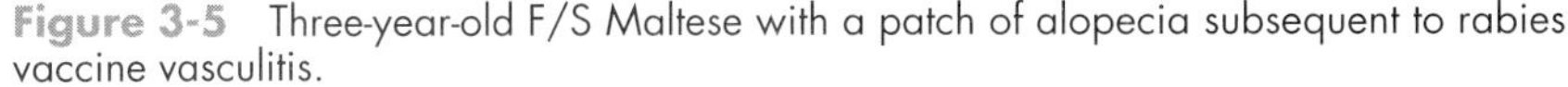

Figure 3-5 Three-year-old F/S Maltese with a patch of alopecia subsequent to rabies vaccine vasculitis.

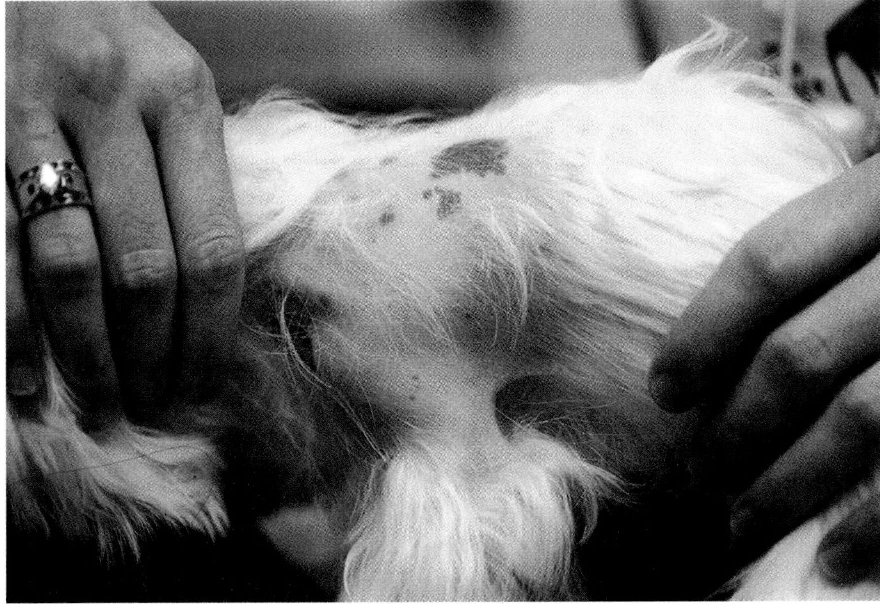

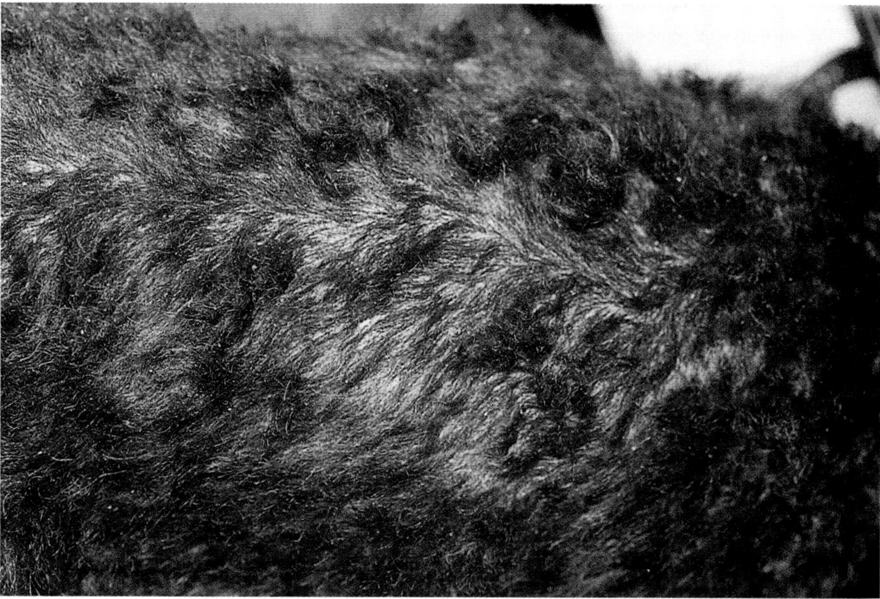

Figure 3-6 Dorsal trunk of a standard poodle demonstrating diffuse partial alopecia with matting of the hair by heavy adherent scale.

- Localized scleroderma—well-demarcated, shiny, smooth, alopecic, thickened plaque
- Alopecia areata—noninflammatory areas of complete alopecia
- Sebaceous adenitis (short-coated breeds)—annular to polycyclic areas of alopecia and scaling or generalized distribution along the dorsum and extremities (Fig. 3-6)

Symmetric

- Hyperadrenocorticism—trunkal alopecia associated with atrophic skin, comedones, and pyoderma (Figs. 3-7, 3-8)
- Hypothyroidism—alopecia is an uncommon presentation
- Growth hormone–responsive dermatosis—symmetric trunkal alopecia associated with hyperpigmentation; alopecia often starts along the collar area of the neck (Fig. 3-9)
- Hyperestrogenism (females)—symmetric alopecia of the flanks, perineal, and inguinal regions with enlarged vulva and mammary glands
- Hypogonadism in intact females—perineal, flank, and trunkal alopecia
- Testosterone-responsive dermatosis in castrated males—slowly progressive trunkal alopecia (Fig. 3-10)
- Male feminization from Sertoli cell tumor—alopecia of the perineum and genital region with gynecomastia (Fig. 3-11)
- Castration-responsive dermatosis—hair loss in the collar area, rump, perineum, and flanks
- Estrogen-responsive dermatosis in spayed female dogs—alopecia of the perineum and genital regions
- Seasonal flank alopecia—serpiginous flank alopecia with hyperpigmentation

Table 3-1

Differential Diagnosis of Canine Alopecia

Differential Diagnosis	Comments	Diagnostic Tests
Single Localized Area of Alopecia:		
Localized demodex	Often accompanied by hyperpigmentation, comedones, folliculitis, seborrhea	Deep skin scrapings
Dermatophytosis	Often accompanied by scaling, folliculitis	Dermatophyte culture, direct hair examination, woods lamp examination
Staphylococcal folliculitis	Often accompanied by collarette formation. Pustules, papules, crusts may be present.	Cytology, culture, response to treatment
Injection reaction	Most common with subcutaneous repositol corticosteroid injections. Cutaneous atrophy often present	History, histopathology
Rabies vaccine induced–vasculitis	Lesion may or may not be accompanied by visible inflammation. The lesion may not be observed until 2–3 months post vaccination	History, histopathology
Localized scleroderma	Well-demarcated, shiny, alopecic, smooth sclerotic plaque	Histopathology
Alopecia areata	Noninflammatory area of complete alopecia	Histopathology
Multifocal Areas of Alopecia:		
Staphylococcal folliculitis	Often accompanied by collarette formation. Papules, pustules, and crusts may also be present.	Cytology, culture, response to treatment
Dermatophytosis	Often accompanied by scaling, folliculitis	Direct hair examination, culture, woods lamp examination
Demodicosis	Hyperpigmentation, comedones, folliculitis, and seborrhea may be present	Deep skin scrapings
Sebaceous adenitis in short-coated breeds	Annular to polycyclic areas of alopecia and scaling	Histopathology
Alopecia areata	Noninflammatory areas of complete alopecia	Histopathology

Symmetric Alopecia:

Differential Diagnosis	Comments	Diagnostic Tests
Cushing's disease	Alopecia often accompanied by thin skin, comedone formation. Pyoderma may also be present.	(CBC, chemistry, urinalysis) Low-dose dexamethasone suppression test, ACTH stimulation test
Adrenal hyperplasia-like syndrome	Symmetric trunkal alopecia with hyperpigmentation	Rule out other endocrinopathies, histopathology, and ACTH stimulation with sex hormone profile.
Hypothyroidism	In the author's experience, this is a very uncommon presentation of hypothyroidism, but has been reported.	Free T4 by equilibrium dialysis and TSH levels
Growth hormone–responsive dermatosis	Symmetric trunkal alopecia accompanied by hyperpigmentation. Breed predispositions occur.	Rule out other endocrinopathies. Xylazine response test, response to therapy
Hyperestrogenism of female dogs.	Symmetric alopecia beginning in perineal, inguinal, and flank regions. May progress to trunkal hair loss. Nipples and vulva are enlarged.	Histopathology, ultrasonography (cystic ovaries), estrogen levels.
Hypogonadism in intact female dogs	Perineal and flank alopecia. May progress to trunkal alopecia.	Hair loss may be cyclic with a temporal relationship to estrus.
Testosterone-responsive dermatosis of male dogs	Slowly progressive trunkal alopecia in castrated male dogs.	Rule out other endocrinopathies and response to therapy.
Male feminization with Sertoli cell tumor	Alopecia of rump, perineum, and genital region. Alopecia is slowly progressive. Gynecomastia often present	History, physical examination, and response to castration, with histopathology of testicles
Castration-responsive dermatosis	Hair loss in collar area, rump, perineum, and caudomedial thighs. Flanks alone may be affected. May progress slowly to trunkal alopecia	Response to castration

(*continued*)

Table 3-1 (Continued)

Differential Diagnosis	Comments	Diagnostic Tests
Estrogen-responsive dermatosis of spayed female dogs	Alopecia beginning in perineal and genital regions. May progress to trunkal alopecia	Histopathology; rule out other endocrine dermatoses, and response to therapy
Patchy to Diffuse Hypotrichosis (Hair Thinning):		
Demodicosis	Often accompanied by hyperpigmentation, comedone formation, folliculitis, seborrhea	Deep skin scrapings
Staphylococcal folliculitis	May be accompanied by collarette formation, crusting, pustules, and papules	Cytology, culture, response to treatment
Dermatophytosis	Often accompanied by scaling, folliculitis	Dermatophyte culture, direct hair examination, woods lamp examination
Sebaceous adenitis	Accompanied by seborrhea, follicular casts. Breed predispositions occur.	Histopathology
Color mutant alopecia	Thinning of the hair coat. Often accompanied by recurrent folliculitis and comedone formation. Breed predispositions occur.	Histopathology, direct hair examination (trichogram)
Follicular dysplasia	Hair loss in puppies or adults that is slowly progressive. Breed predispositions occur.	Histopathology
Anagen defluxion Telogen defluxion	Hair loss occurs suddenly. In the case of telogen defluxion hair loss is usually associated with stressful event. With anagen defluxion, circumstances interfere with anagen (antimitotic drugs, etc.). No inflammation is present.	Direct hair examination (trichogram) Histopathology may be helpful with anagen defluxion.
Hypothyroidism	Diffuse hair thinning is most common. May also have pigmentation changes and comedone formation	Free T4 by equilibrium dialysis and TSH level
Cushing's disease	Trunkal hair loss often accompanied by thin skin and recurrent infections	(CBC, chemistry, UA), low-dose dexamethasone suppression test, ACTH stimulation test

Differential Diagnosis	Comments	Diagnostic Tests
Mycosis fungoides	Hair loss accompanied by scaling, erythema, pruritus, plaque or nodule formation	Histopathology
Pemphigus foliaceus	Hair loss often accompanied by crusts, scaling, collarette formation, and pustules	Histopathology
Primary keratinization defects	Examples include primary seborrhea of the cocker spaniel, springer spaniel, etc. Alopecia is accompanied by scaling and excessive greasiness.	Histopathology
Alopecic Conditions with Specific Locations:		
Pinnal alopecia	Alopecia of pinnae with miniaturization of hairs, and progressive hair loss. Breed predispositions occur.	Histopathology, signalment (rule out inflammatory and endocrine causes of pinnal alopecia)
Traction alopecia	Hair loss on the top or lateral aspects of cranium. Hair loss is related to prolonged use of barrettes or rubber bands in the hair applied too tightly.	History, physical examination, and histopathology
Post-clipping alopecia	Failure to regrow hair after clipping. Hair will usually regrow within 12 months.	History, physical examination
Melanoderma/alopecia of Yorkshire terriers	Symmetric hair loss and hyperpigmentation over pinnae, bridge of the nose, and sometimes tail or feet. Occurs in puppies and young adults	History, signalment, histopathology
Seasonal flank alopecia	Localized cyclic follicular dysplasia present on one or both flanks. Hair loss with hyperpigmentation	Histopathology, history
Black hair follicular dysplasia	Follicular dysplasia seen in only the black-haired areas of the coat	Histopathology
Dermatomyositis	Symmetric hair loss on face, tip of tail, digits, carpi, tarsi, and pinnae. Erythema, scaling, and mild crusting are common. Seen primarily in shelties and collies	Histopathology

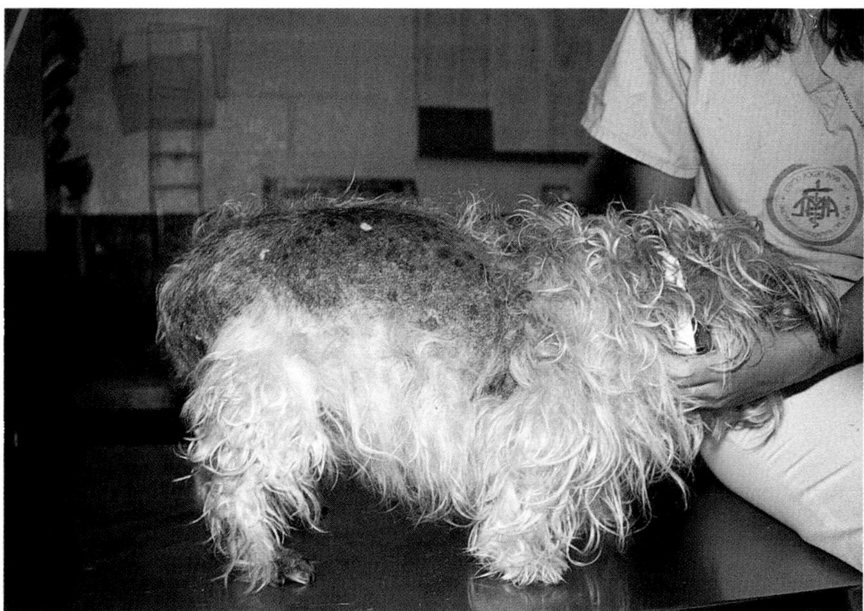

Figure 3-7 Hyperadrenocorticism: trunkal alopecia and hyperpigmentation.

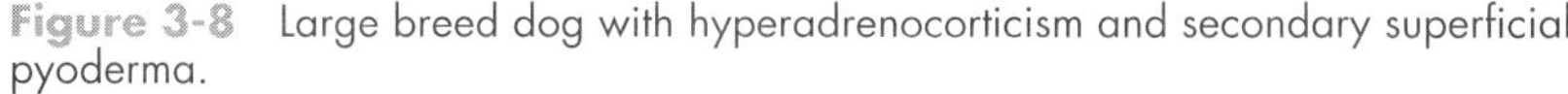

Figure 3-8 Large breed dog with hyperadrenocorticism and secondary superficial pyoderma.

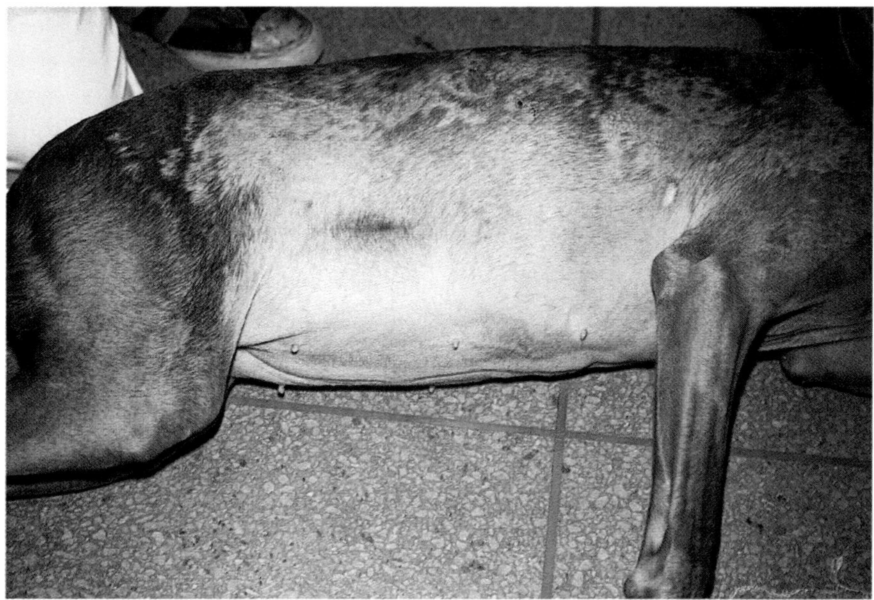

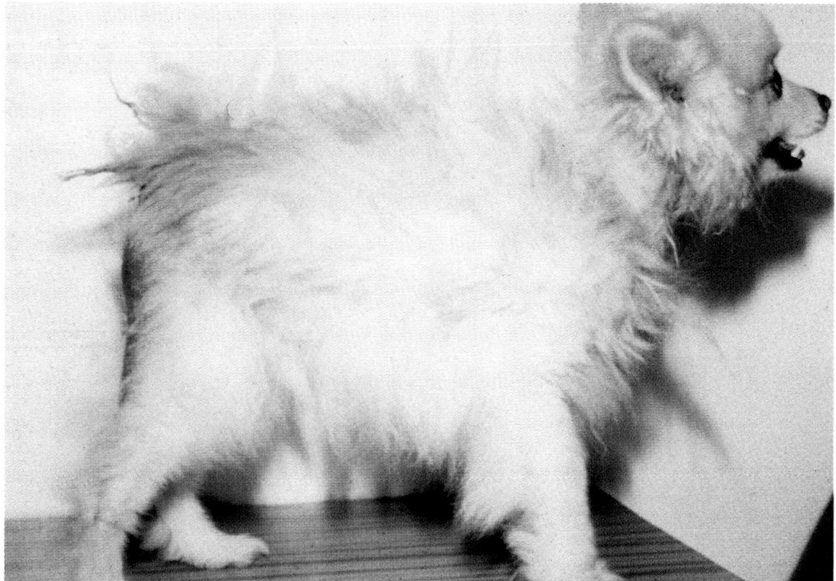

Figure 3-9 "Growth hormone–responsive" dermatosis. Note the predominance of alopecia around the neck region as well as the tail and perineum.

Figure 3-10 Five-year-old M/C pomeranian with adrenal sex hormone imbalance.

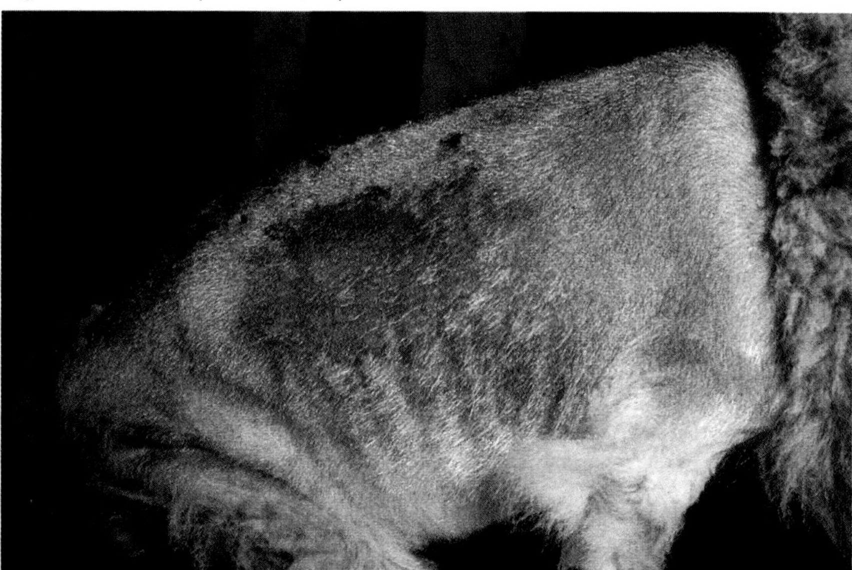

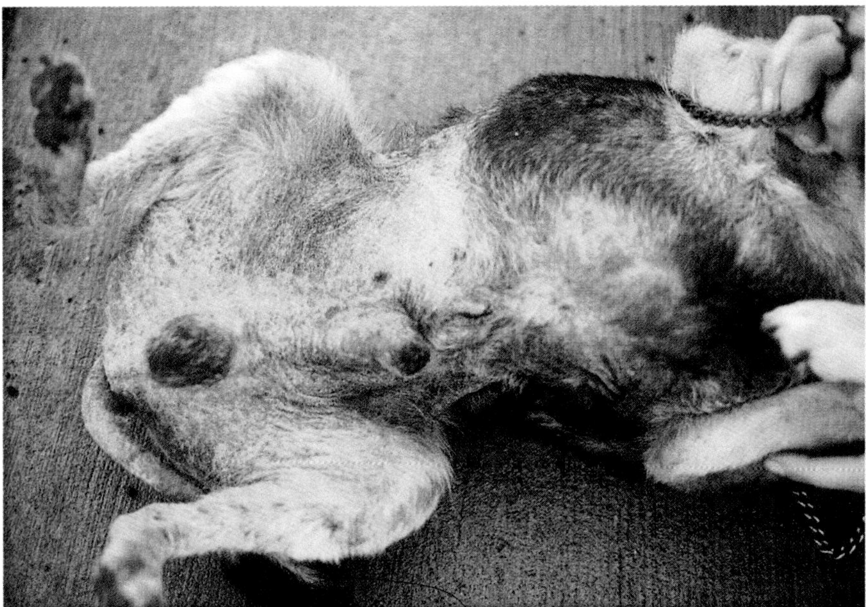

Figure 3-11 Sertoli cell tumor. Note the alopecia and associated hyperpigmentation.

Patchy to Diffuse

- Demodicosis—often associated with erythema, folliculitis, and hyperpigmentation
- Bacterial folliculitis—multifocal area of circular alopecia to coalescing large areas of hair loss; epidermal collarettes
- Dermatophytosis—often accompanied by scale
- Sebaceous adenitis—alopecia with a thick adherent scale; predominantly on the dorsum of the body, including the head and extremities
- Color mutant alopecia—thinning of the hair coat with secondary folliculitis
- Follicular dysplasia—slowly progressive alopecia
- Anagen defluxion and telogen defluxion—acute onset of alopecia
- Hypothyroidism—diffuse thinning of the hair coat (Fig. 3-12)
- Hyperadrenocorticism—trunkal alopecia with thin skin and formation of comedones
- Epidermotropic lymphoma—diffuse, generalized truncal alopecia with scaling and erythema, later nodule and plaque formation (Figs. 3-13,3-14)
- Pemphigus foliaceus—hair loss associated with scale and crust formation
- Keratinization disorders—alopecia associated with excessive scale and greasy surface texture (Fig. 3-15)

Specific Locations

- Pinnal alopecia—miniaturization of hairs and progressive alopecia
- Traction alopecia—hair loss on the top and lateral aspect of the cranium secondary to having barrettes or rubber bands applied to the hair
- Postclipping alopecia—failure to regrow after clipping

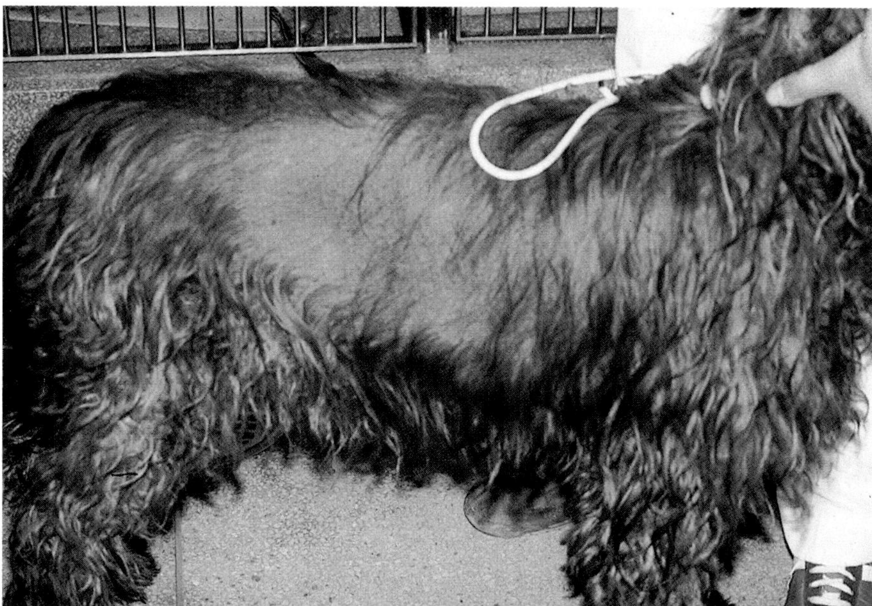

Figure 3-12 Partial to focally complete alopecia of the trunk associated with severe hypothyroidism (Note: hypothyroidism is often "overdiagnosed" as a cause for canine alopecia).

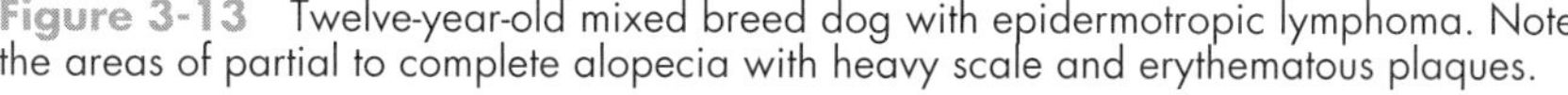

Figure 3-13 Twelve-year-old mixed breed dog with epidermotropic lymphoma. Note the areas of partial to complete alopecia with heavy scale and erythematous plaques.

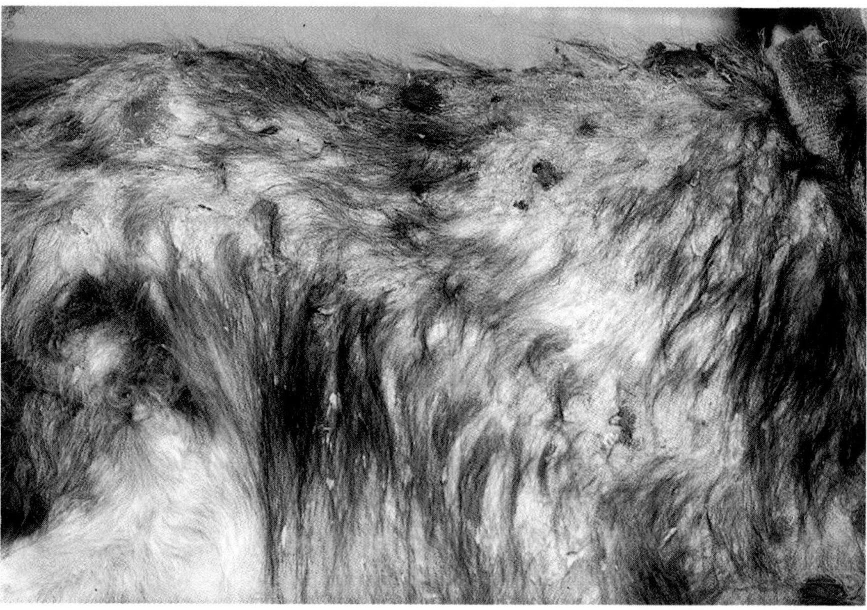

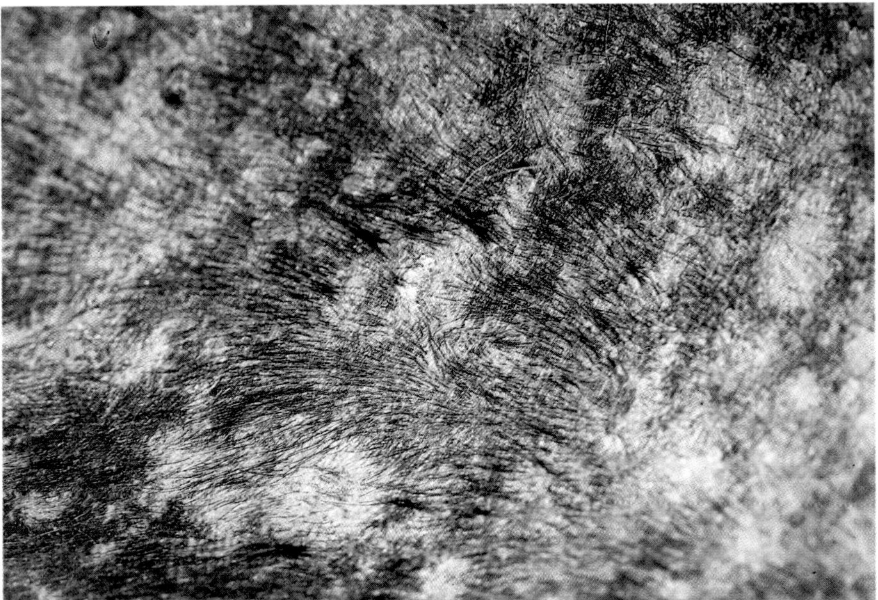

Figure 3-14 Fourteen-year-old cocker spaniel with epidermotropic lymphoma. Note the lack of plaques and nodules. Lesions consist of multifocal patches of alopecia (coat has been shaved) with adherent scale and mild erythema.

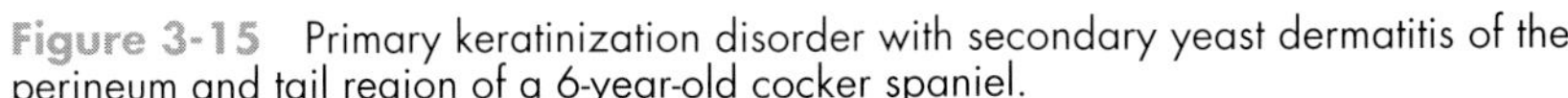

Figure 3-15 Primary keratinization disorder with secondary yeast dermatitis of the perineum and tail region of a 6-year-old cocker spaniel.

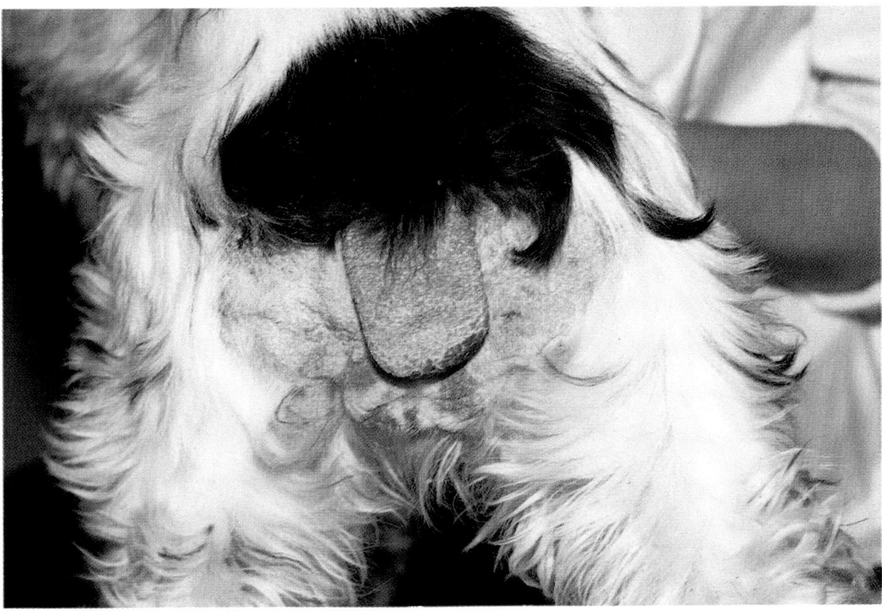

- Melanoderma (alopecia of Yorkshire terriers)—symmetric alopecia of the pinnae, bridge of the nose, tail, and feet
- Seasonal flank alopecia—serpiginous flank alopecia that may connect over the dorsum
- Black hair follicular dysplasia—alopecia of the black-haired areas only
- Dermatomyositis—alopecia of the face, tip of ears, tail, and digits; associated with scale and crusting

Diagnostics

CBC/Biochemistry/Urinalysis

Rule out metabolic causes such as hyperadrenocorticism.

Other Laboratory Tests

- Thyroid testing—diagnose hypothyroidism
- ACTH-response test, LDDST, and HDDST—evaluate for hyperadrenocorticism
- Sex hormone profiles (questionable validity)

Imaging

Ultrasonography—evaluate adrenal glands for evidence of hyperadrenocorticism

Diagnostic Procedures

- Response to therapy as a trial
- Fungal culture
- Skin scraping
- Cytology
- Skin biopsy

Therapeutics

- Demodicosis—Mitaban, ivermectin, interceptor
- Dermatophytosis—griseofulvin, ketoconazole, itraconazole, lime sulfur dips, lufenuron
- Staphylococcal folliculitis—shampoo and antibiotic therapy
- Sebaceous adenitis—keratolytic shampoo, essential fatty acid supplementation, retinoids
- Keratinization disorders—shampoos, retinoids, vitamin D, vitamin A
- Endocrine—ovariohysterectomy, castration, Lysodren, adrenalectomy

Precautions

Toxicity with griseofulvin, retinoids, and ivermectin

Comments

Zoonotic Potential

Dermatophytosis can cause skin lesions in people.

Pregnancy

Avoid retinoids and griseofulvin in pregnant animals.

Abbreviations

- HDDST = high-dose dexamethasone-suppression test
- LDDST = low-dose dexamethasone-suppression test

Suggested Reading

Helton-Rhodes KA. Cutaneous manifestations of canine and feline endocrinopathies. In: Nichols R, ed. Probl Vet Med 1990;12:617–627.

Schmeitzel LP. Growth hormone responsive alopecia and sex hormone associated dermatoses. In: Birchard SJ, Sherding RG, eds. Saunders manual of small animal practice. Philadelphia: Saunders, 1994:326–330.

Scott DW, Griffin CE, Miller BH. Acquired alopecia. In: Muller & Kirk's small animal dermatology. 5th ed. Philadelphia: Saunders, 1995:720–735.

Scott DW, Griffin CE, Miller BH. Endocrine and metabolic diseases. In: Muller & Kirk's small animal dermatology. 5th ed. Philadelphia: Saunders, 1995:627–719.

Scott DW, Griffin CE, Miller BH. Keratinization defects. In: Muller & Kirk's small animal dermatology. 5th ed. Philadelphia: Saunders, 1995:736–805.

Consulting Editor Karen Helton Rhodes

Alopecia, Feline

Karen Helton Rhodes

Definition/Overview

- Common problem
- Pattern of hair loss varied or symmetric
- Causes—multifactorial
- Often diagnostic dilemma

Pathophysiology/Etiology

Specific and unique for each cause, i.e.,

- Neurologic/behavioral—obsessive compulsive disorder
- Endocrine—sex hormone alopecia, hyperthyroidism, hyperadrenocorticism, diabetes mellitus
- Immunologic—allergic dermatitis, alopecia areata
- Parasitic—demodicosis, dermatophytosis
- Physiologic—sebaceous adenitis
- Neoplastic—paraneoplastic dermatitis, squamous cell carcinoma in situ, epidermotropic lymphoma
- Idiopathic/inherited—alopecia universalis, hypotrichosis, spontaneous pinnal alopecia, anagen, and telogen defluxion

Signalment/History

- No specific age, breed, or sex predilection
- Neoplastic and paraneoplastic associated alopecias—generally recognized in old cats
- History varies with specific cause

Clinical Features

- Neurologic and behavioral disorders tend to have minimal inflammation associated with the areas of alopecia.
- Allergic/hypersensitivity reactions are often characterized by erythema, alopecia, and excoriations.
- Endocrine diseases are rarely pruritic and tend to have a slow and progressive course.
- Feline dermatophytosis is frequently a scaling disorder associated with patchy or diffuse alopecia that may or may not be pruritic.
- The clinical presentation of neoplasia is quite varied: from diffuse scaling and alopecia in epidermotropic lymphoma to a focal plaque-like or papillated area with scale in squamous cell carcinoma "in situ."

Differential Diagnosis

Endocrine Alopecia/Sex Hormone

- Rare hormonal cases—primarily castrated males; alopecia along the caudal aspect of the hindlimbs, which may extend along the perineum

Figure 4-1 Feline "obsessive-compulsive disorder." Ventral abdominal alopecia with minimal erythema or trauma to the skin.

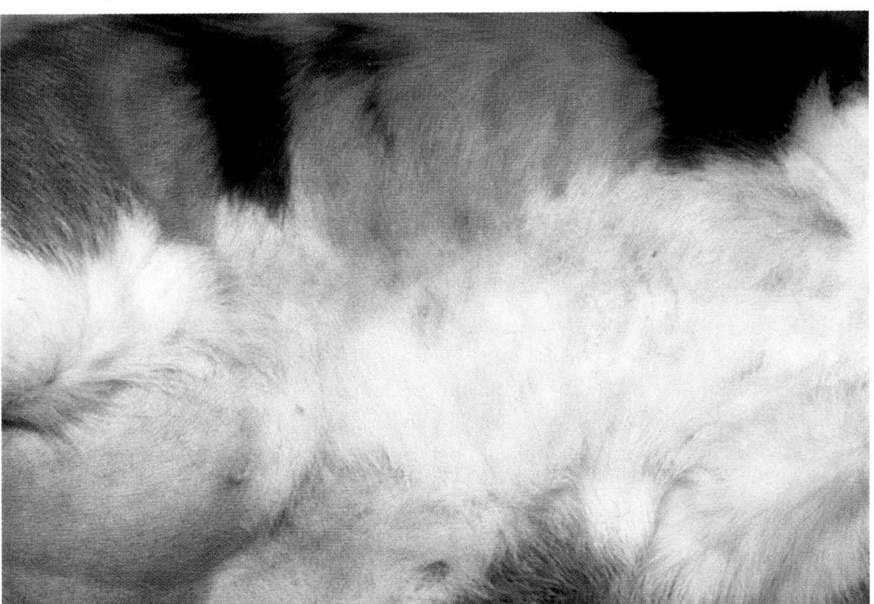

Obsessive-Compulsive Disorder

- Often misdiagnosed as endocrine
- The pattern of alopecia is frequently symmetric with minimal associated inflammation (Fig. 4-1).

Allergic Dermatitis

- Varies from mild partial alopecia with little inflammation to severe excoriation and ulceration
- Distribution—varied; often the head and neck region are most severely affected
- Food allergy and inhalant/percutaneous allergic dermatitis (Fig. 4-2).

Hyperthyroidism

- Partial to complete alopecia from self-barbering
- Varied pattern
- Middle-aged to old cats
- Often mistaken for allergic dermatoses, obsessive compulsive disorder, or hormonal (Figs. 4-3A, 4-3B).

Diabetes Mellitus

- Partial alopecia with an unkempt hair coat
- Poor wound healing
- Increased susceptibility to infections
- Cutaneous xanthomatosis secondary to hyperlipidemia nodular to linear, yellow-pink alopecic plaques that tend to ulcerate, (Figs. 4-4A, 4-4B).

Figure 4-2 Feline allergic dermatitis is often most severe along the head and neck region. Note the excoriations along the caudal aspect of the pinnae and neck region.

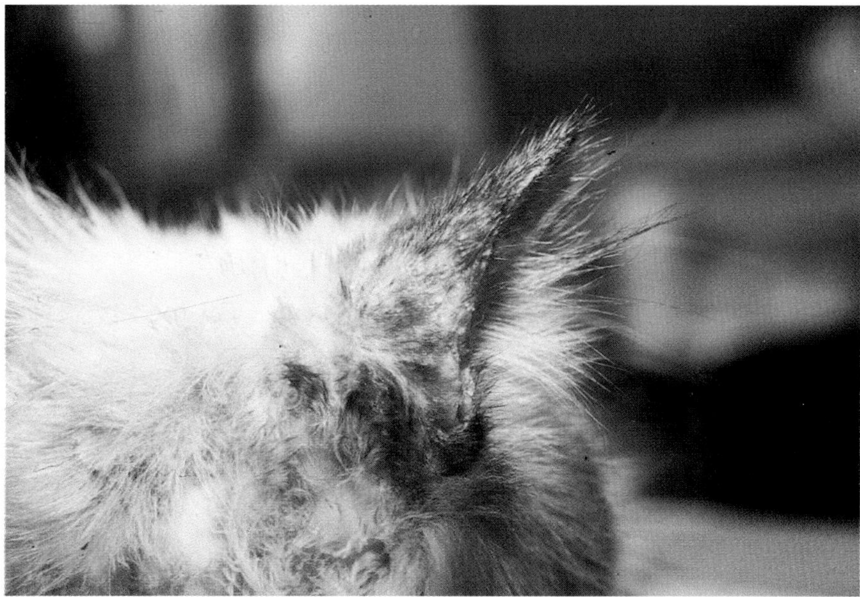

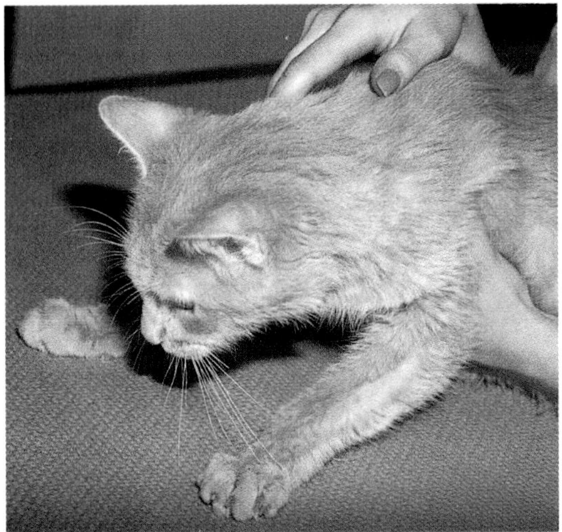

A

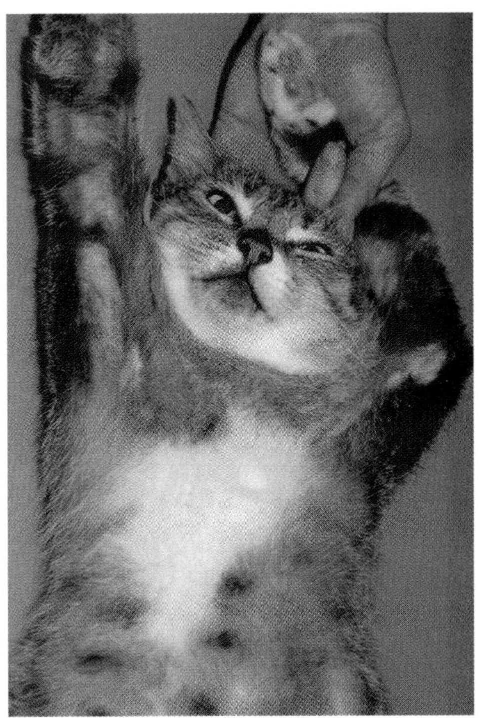

B

Figure 4-3A Feline hyperthyroidism is often associated with excess grooming, which may lead to focal areas of alopecia—as noted along the lateral aspect of the forelimbs.
Figure 4-3B Feline hyperthyroidism. This 9-year-old cat had no other clinical signs commonly recognized with hyperthyroidism other than excess grooming. Note the alopecia along the forelimbs.

Hyperadrenocorticism

- Rare; characterized by alopecia and extreme fragility of the skin
- Trunkal alopecia, with or without a rat tail and a curling of the pinnal tips (Figs. 4-5A, B, C).
- Extreme skin fragility noted in approximately 70% (Figs. 4-5D, 4-5E)
- Occurs secondary to pituitary or adrenal tumors
- Iatrogenic form less common in cats than in dogs

Paraneoplastic Alopecia

- Most cases associated with pancreatic exocrine adenocarcinomas
- Middle-aged to old cats (9–16 years)
- Acute onset
- Progresses rapidly
- Bilaterally symmetric, ventrally distributed (also located along the bridge of the nose and periocular (Fig. 4-6).
- Hair epilates in clumps.
- Rare pruritus
- Erythema with dry fissuring footpads
- Glistening appearance to the alopecic skin
- Skin is thin and hypotonic.
- Rapid weight loss

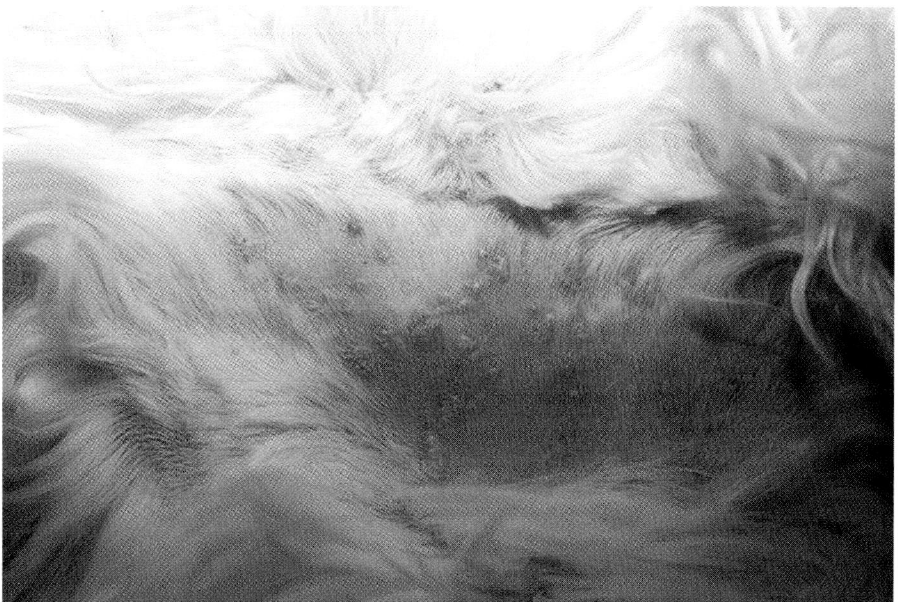

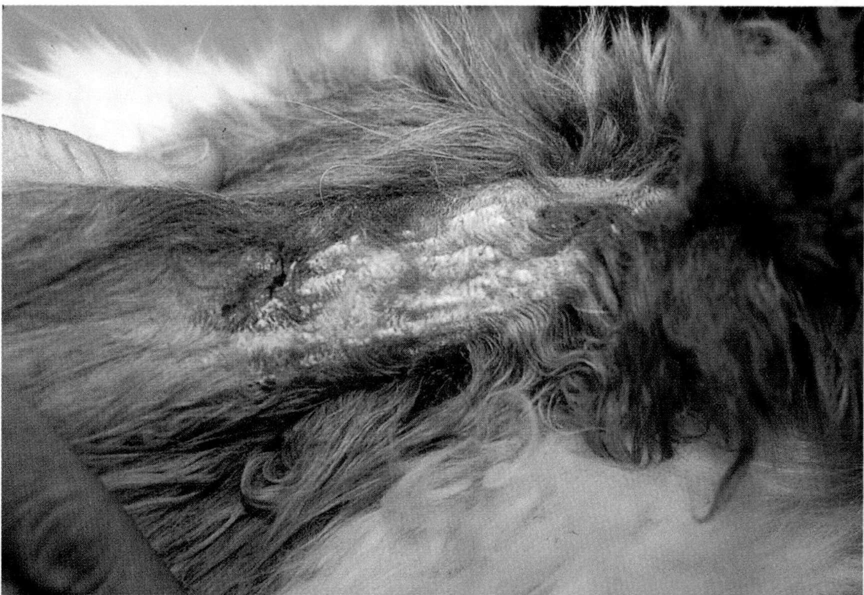

Figure 4-4A Cutaneous xanthomatosis may be associated with an endocrine imbalance (cortisol, thyroid, DM, etc.) or idiopathic hyperlipidemia. This 10-year-old DSH M/C cat demonstrates small coalescing yellow-pink nodules and plaques along the caudal ventral trunk.

Figure 4-4B Cutaneous xanthomatosis associated with diabetes mellitus. Note the linear to papular yellow-pink lesions along the ventral neck region of this 7-year-old DSH F/S cat.

Sebaceous Adenitis

- Slowly progressive partial alopecia associated with scaling along the dorsum of the body and the extremities (Fig. 4-7A).
- Sebaceous glands are selectively destroyed by toxic intermediate metabolites or immunologic mechanisms.

A
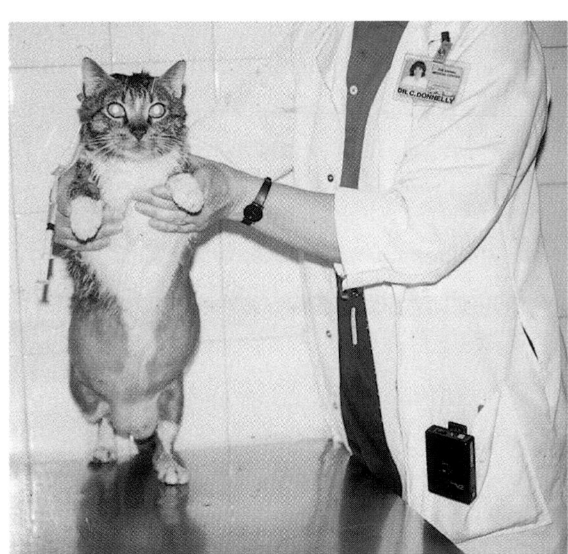

B
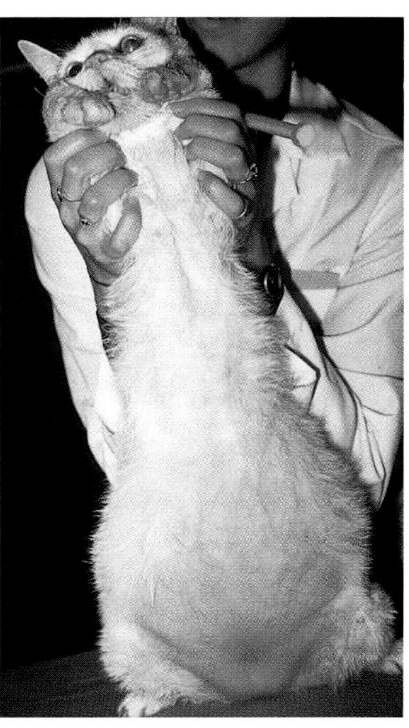

C
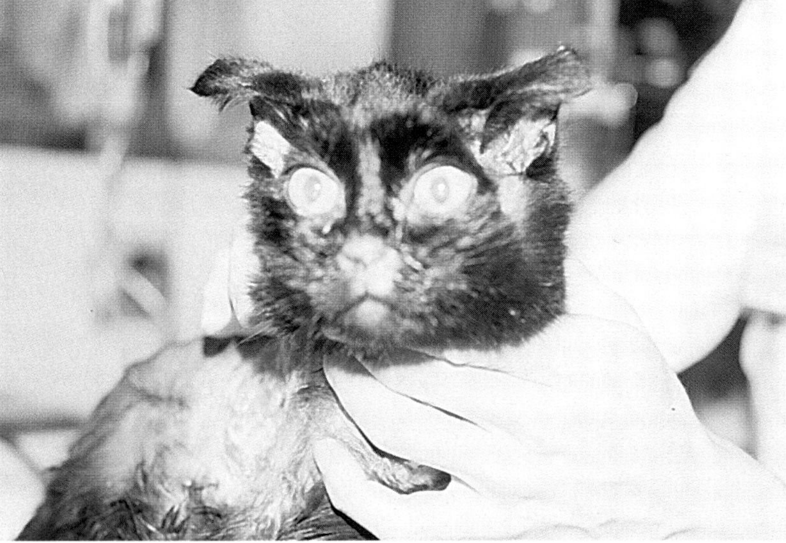

Figure 4-5A & 4-5B Feline hyperadrenocorticism. Note the "pot-bellied" appearance and the partial trunkal alopecia.
Figure 4-5C Feline hyperadrenocorticism. Note the curling of the tips of the pinnae.

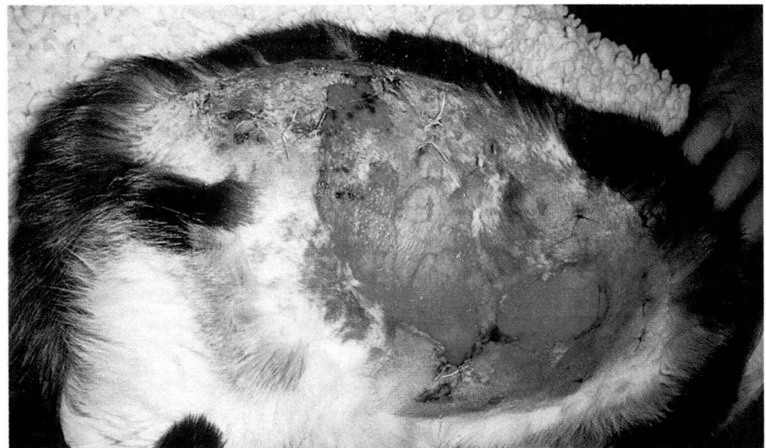
D

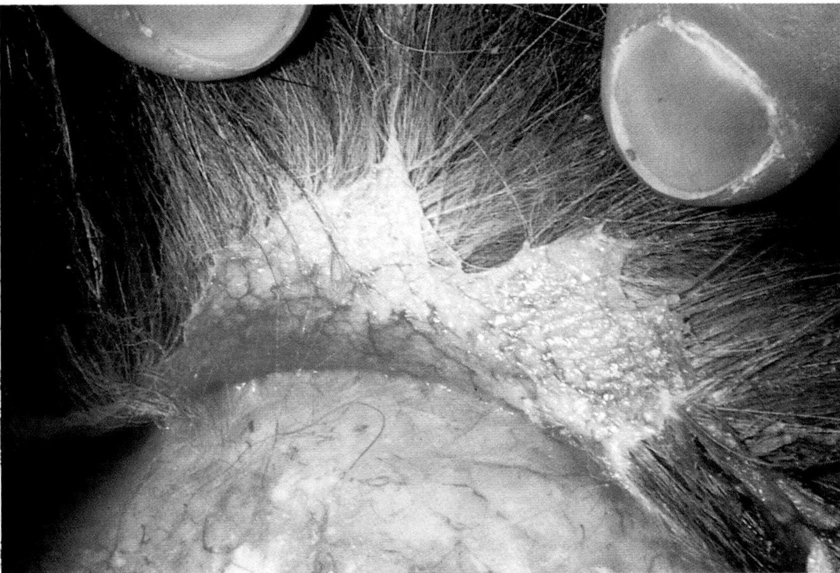
E

Figure 4-5D & 4-5E Feline skin fragility syndrome associated with hyperadrenocorticism. Note the large denuded area of the trunk and the ease with which the skin "peels." There is often minimal pain associated with these lesions, which may occur with routine gentle handling. (Courtesy of Dr. Rod Rosychuck)

- Possible dramatic pigment accumulation along the eyelid margins (Fig. 4-7B)
- Questionable association with systemic disease (e.g., inflammatory bowel disease, lupus-like syndromes, upper respiratory tract infections)

Squamous Cell Carcinoma In Situ

- Multicentric premalignant dermatosis in old cats
- Slightly elevated, plaque-like or papillated lesions with scaling and partially alopecic surfaces (Figs. 4-8A, 4-8B)
- Often misdiagnosed as seborrhea
- About 25% may convert to squamous cell carcinoma with in situ lesions along the borders (histologically).

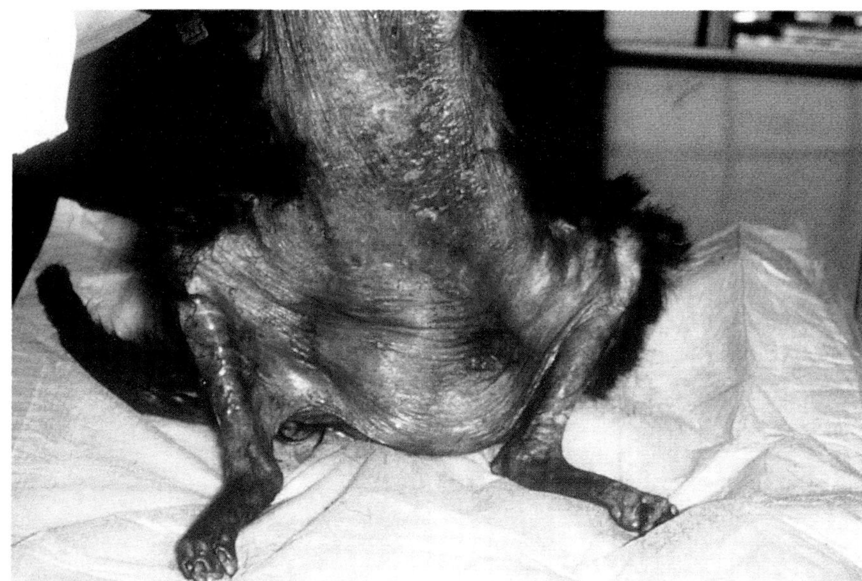

Figure 4-6 Paraneoplastic syndrome associated with pancreatic exocrine adenocarcinoma. Note the hyperpigmentation and the glistening appearance of the alopecic skin. Predominant ventral distribution common. (Courtesy of Dr. Karen Campbell)

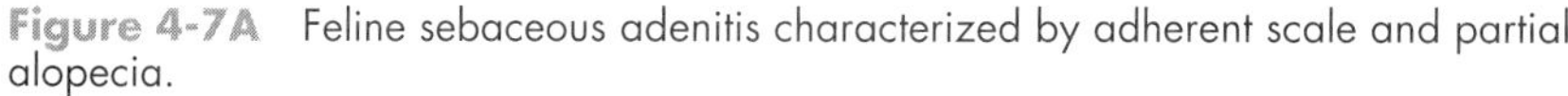

Figure 4-7A Feline sebaceous adenitis characterized by adherent scale and partial alopecia.

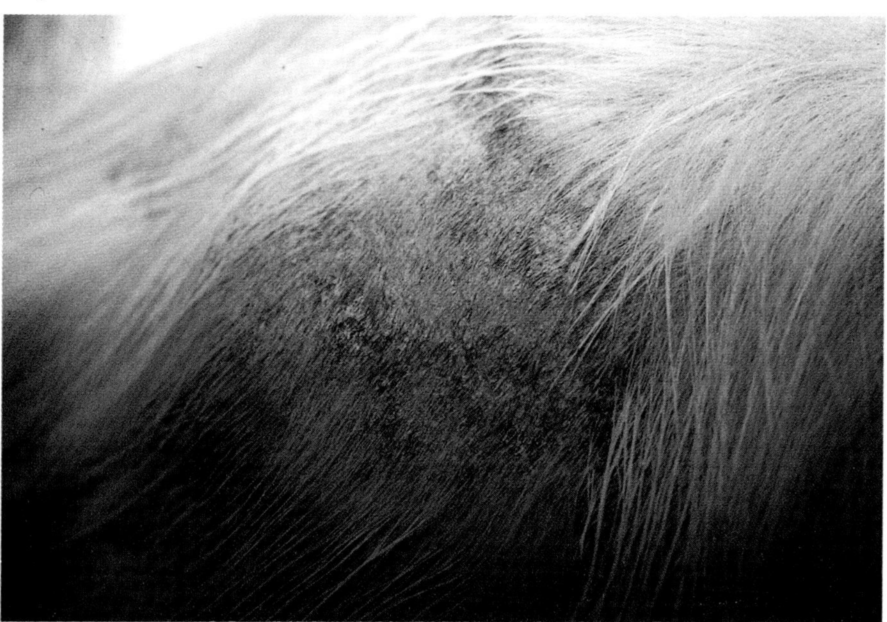

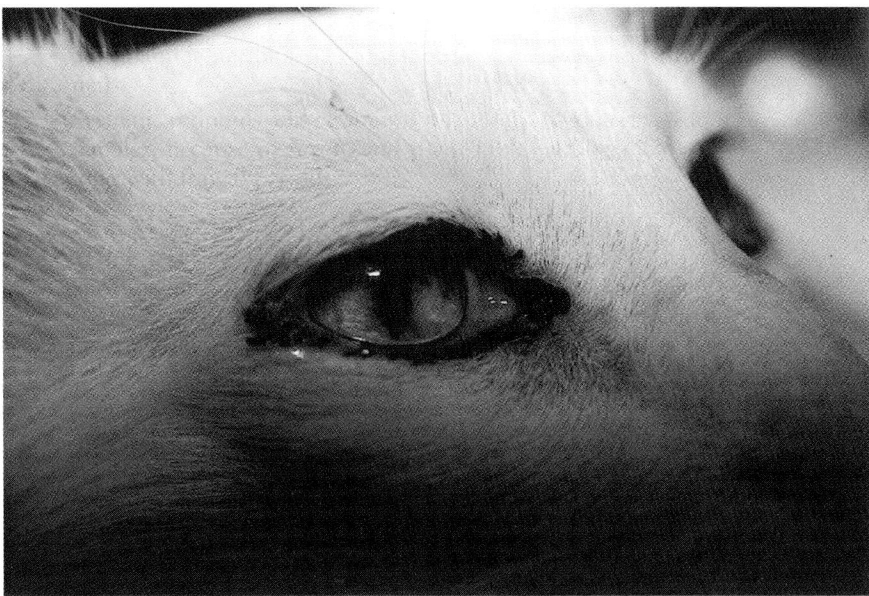

Figure 4-7B Pigment accumulation along the eyelid margins associated with sebaceous adenitis.

Figure 4-8A Feline squamous cell carcinoma "in situ" (Bowenoid carcinoma). Slightly elevated, pigmented, slightly scaled lesions are often overlooked by the owner until an advanced stage. Note the areas of partial alopecia with hyperpigmentation of the preauricular region.

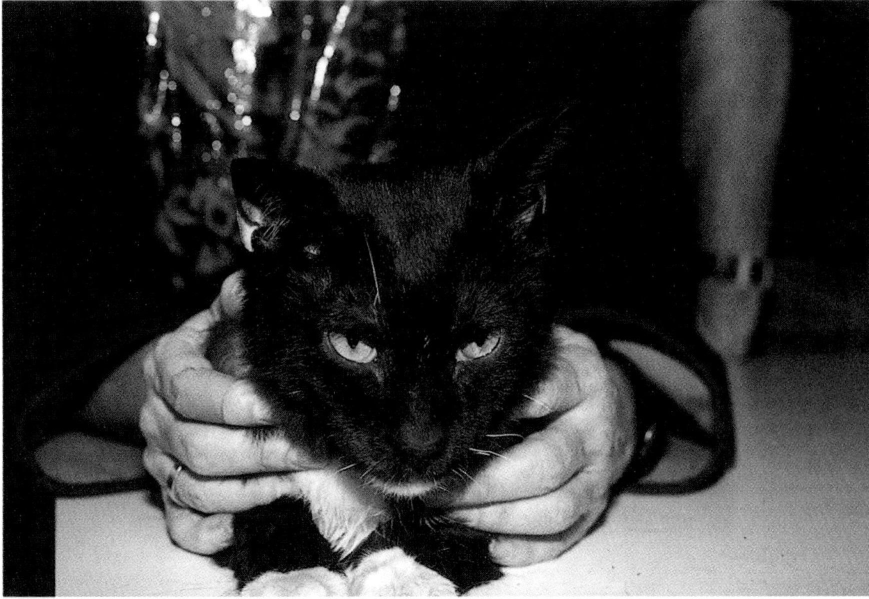

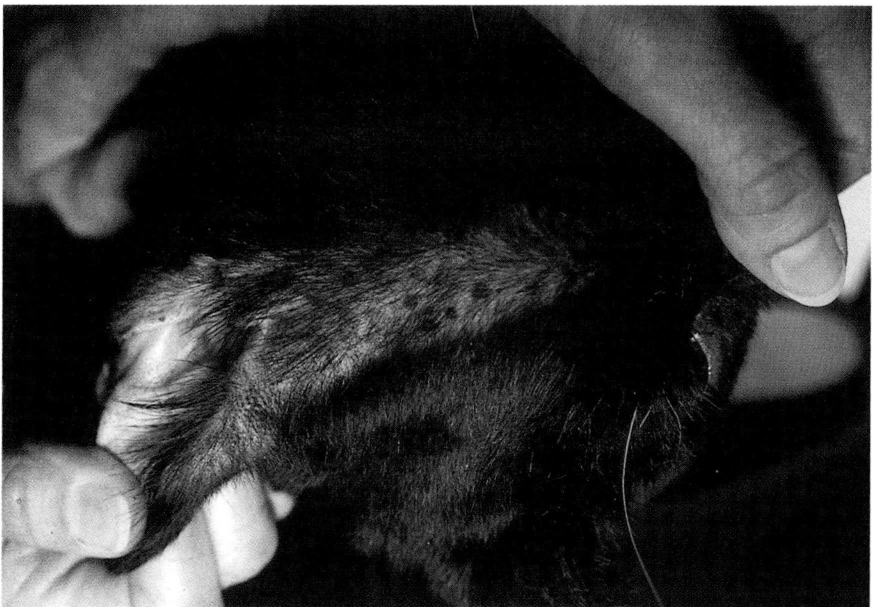

Figure 4-8B Feline squamous cell carinoma "in situ." Close-up view of the preauricular region in Figure 4-8A.

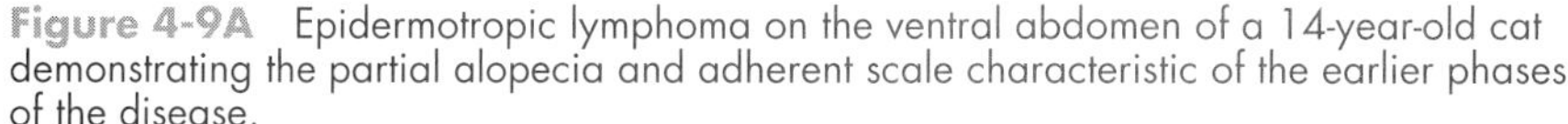

Figure 4-9A Epidermotropic lymphoma on the ventral abdomen of a 14-year-old cat demonstrating the partial alopecia and adherent scale characteristic of the earlier phases of the disease.

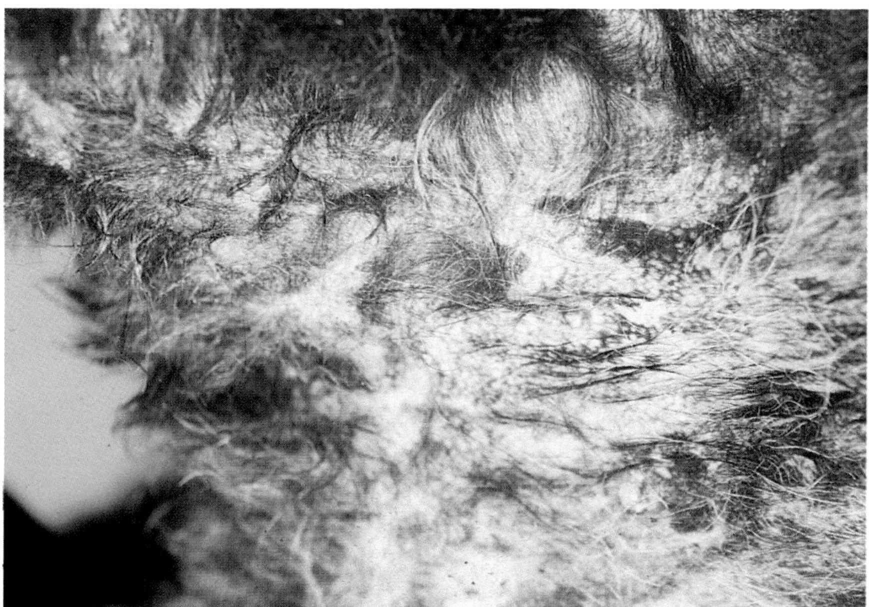

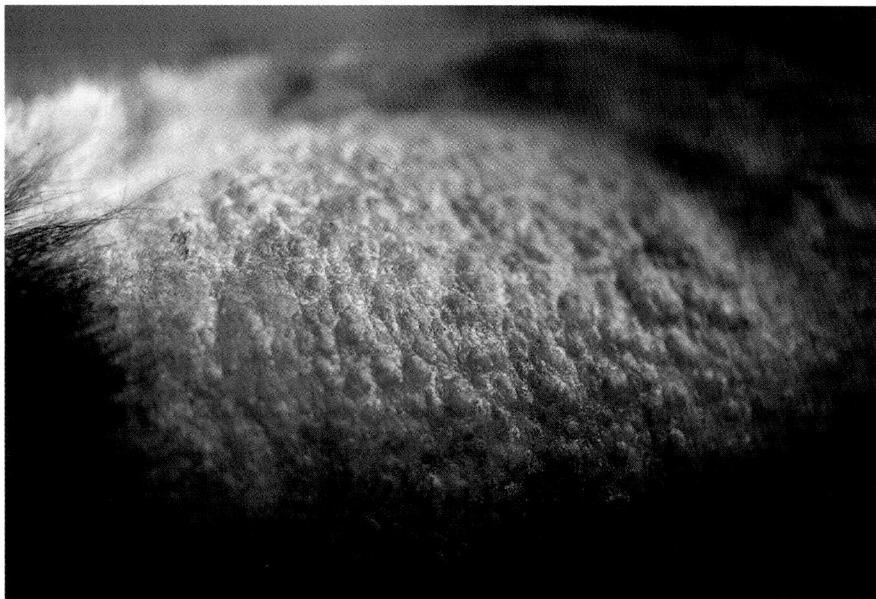

Figure 4-9B Epidermotropic lymphoma. Advanced stage of the disease demonstrating the plaque and nodular phase.

Epidermotropic Lymphoma

- Early stages—varying degrees of alopecia associated with scaling and erythema
- Later stages—plaques and nodules
- Old cats (Figs. 4-9A, 4-9B)

Alopecia Areata

Rare, complete alopecia in a patchy distribution with no inflammation (Figs. 4-10A, 4-10B)

Alopecia Universalis (Sphinx Cat)

- Hereditary
- Complete absence of primary hairs; decreased secondary hairs
- Thickened epidermis; normal dermis
- Sebaceous and apocrine ducts open directly onto the skin surface; oily feel to skin
- Wrinkled foreheads; gold eyes; no whiskers; downy fur on paws, tip of tail, and scrotum

Feline Hypotrichosis

- Siamese and Devon Rex cats (autosomal recessive alopecia)
- Poorly developed primary telogen hair follicles
- Born with a normal coat; thin and sparse by young adult

Spontaneous Pinnal Alopecia

- Siamese cats predisposed
- May represent form of alopecia areata or pattern baldness

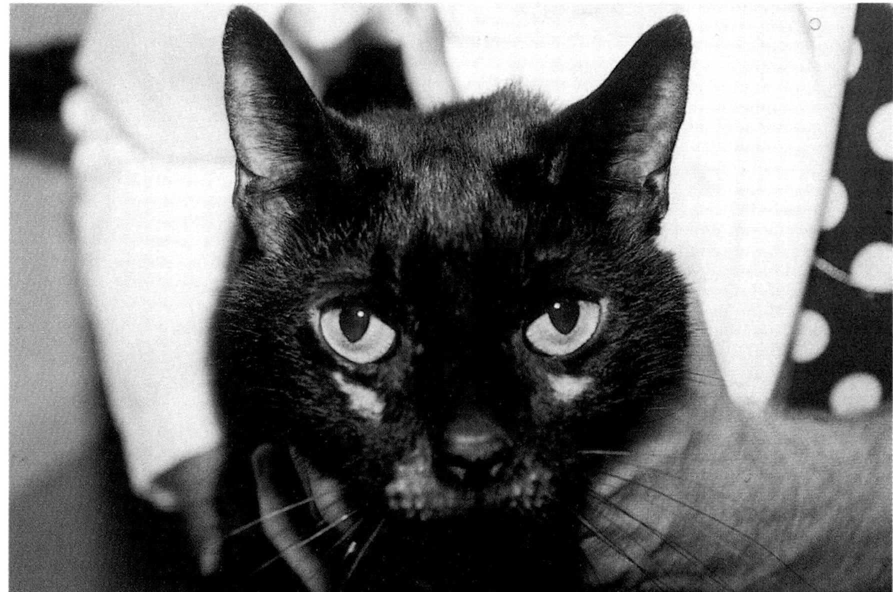

A

B

Figure 4-10A Feline alopecia areata. Noninflammatory complete alopecia in a patchy pattern. Note the areas of alopecia just below the eyes and along the muzzle.
Figure 4-10B Feline alopecia areata. Noninflammatory patch of alopecia of the trunk.

Anagen and Telogen Defluxion

- Acute loss of hair owing to interference with the growth cycle
- Causes—stress, infection, endocrine disorder, metabolic disorder, fever, surgery, anesthesia, pregnancy, drug therapy

Demodicosis

- Rare; unlike dogs
- Partial to complete multifocal alopecia of the eyelids, periocular region, head, and neck
- Variable pruritus with erythema, scale, and crust, and ceruminous otitis externa
- *Demodex cati* (elongated shape) often associated with metabolic disease (e.g., FIV, systemic lupus erythematosus, diabetes mellitus)
- Unnamed short/blunted *Demodex* mite is rarely a marker for metabolic disease; this form may be transferable from cat to cat and has been associated with pruritus

Dermatophytosis

Numerous clinical manifestations; always associated with alopecia of some degree

Diagnostics

CBC/Biochemistry/Urinalysis

Abnormalities may be noted with diabetes mellitus, hyperadrenocorticism, and hyperthyroidism.

Other Laboratory Tests

- FeLV and FIV—risk factors for demodicosis
- Thyroid hormones—document hyperthyroidism
- ANA titer—look for lupus-like syndromes
- ACTH-response test, LDDST, and HDDST—diagnose hyperadrenocorticism

Imaging

- Abdominal ultrasound—assess adrenals in hyperadrenocorticism and look for cancer in animals with paraneoplastic syndrome
- CT scan—look for pituitary tumors in animals with hyperadrenocorticism

Diagnostic Procedures

- Skin biopsy
- Skin scraping
- Fungal culture
- T-shirts to prove self-trauma
- Food elimination trials
- Intradermal skin testing

Table 4-1

Differential Diagnosis of Feline Alopecia

Differential Diagnosis	Comments	Diagnostic Tests
Single Localized Area		
Alopecia Areata	–Rare disorder in the cat –Focal area of alopecia with no inflammation –The affected skin appears normal –May be permanent or spontaneously resolve	Biopsy
Anagen and Telogen Defluxion	–Sudden loss of hair due to interference with hair follicle growth –Lack of inflammation	Biopsy
Dermatophytosis	–Focal area to diffuse –With or without inflammation –Usually characterized by excess scaling but may exhibit any clinical expression	Culture
Demodicosis	–Rare –Focal to diffuse lesions –May be pruritic –May be noninflamed or associated with erythema, scaling, and crusting	Skin scraping, biopsy
Injection Reaction	–Focal area of complete alopecia –Most common with subcutaneous repositol injection of corticosteroids	Biopsy, history
Multifocal to Diffuse Areas of Alopecia		
Pinnal Alopecia	–Spontaneous periodic or progressive permanent –Siamese cat	History, breed

Differential Diagnosis	Comments	Diagnostic Tests
Feline Hypotrichosis	–Autosomal recessive –Siamese and Devon Rex –Thin, sparse haircoat by the time the cat is a young adult	Biopsy
Feline Alopecia Universalis	–Hereditary defect characterized by complete absence of primary hairs, decreased numbers of secondary hairs, thickened epidermis, and normal dermis –Oily feel to the skin, lack of whiskers, downy fur at tip of tail, paws, and scrotum	Biopsy
Sebaceous Adenitis	–Partial alopecia associated with scaling and hyperpigmentation –Often the dorsum of the trunk and the head/neck region –May note excess secretions periocular	Biopsy
Diabetes Mellitus	–Partial diffuse alopecia –Often associated with secondary infection characterized as miliary dermatitis –Cutaneous xanthomatosis—yellow-pink plaques that may ulcerate	Hematology
Paraneoplastic Alopecia	–Acute onset of rapidly progressing, bilaterally symmetric, ventrally distributed alopecia –Hair epilates in large clumps –Skin is smooth and glistening –May have lesions along the nose, eyes, and footpads –Pancreatic exocrine adenocarcinoma and bile duct carcinomas	Hematology, biopsy
Feline Hyperadrenocorticism	–Bilateral symmetric trunkal alopecia –May be curling of the tips of the pinnae –Extreme skin fragility often noted	Hematology, biopsy
Feline Hyperthyroidism	–Unkempt haircoat with patchy partial alopecia –Often noted along the forelimbs from barbering –May mimic feline "endocrine" symmetric alopecia or OCD	Hematology

(continued)

Table 4-1 (Continued)

Differential Diagnosis	Comments	Diagnostic Tests
Feline Hypothyroidism	–Extremely rare –Most cases are poorly documented (response to Tx only) –Bilateral, symmetric, trunkal and cervical alopecia	Hematology
Feline "Endocrine" Alopecia	–Rare sex hormone imbalance, often misdiagnosed –More often allergic or psychogenic –Alopecia around the perineum and hindlimbs not associated with barbering	Biopsy, response to Tx
Feline Psychogenic Alopecia	–Often associated with partial to complete trunkal and ventral alopecia with no inflammation –Associated with self-plucking	Biopsy, T–shirts, response to Elavil
Feline Allergic Dermatitis	–Varying degrees of alopecia and erythema –May be associated with lesions of the eosinophilic granuloma complex or miliary dermatitis	Biopsy, response to Tx
Neoplasia	Epitheliotropic lymphoma: alopecia, erythema, scale, plaques, nodules	Biopsy
	Squamous cell carcinoma "in situ" (Bowen's): multifocal patches of alopecia with mounds of scale and hyperpigmentation	Biopsy

Therapeutics

- Therapy is limited for many of these disorders.
- Behavioral modification or application of a T-shirt may help prevent self-barbering.
- Removal of an offending dietary item may alleviate the symptoms of food allergy.
- If the pet is compliant, shampoo and topical therapy may help secondary problems, such as hyperkeratosis in sebaceous adenitis, crusting in demodicosis, secondary bacterial infections, and malodor for greasy conditions.

Drugs of Choice

- Obsessive compulsive disorder—amitriptyline (10 mg/cat/day for a 21-day trial)
- Endocrine alopecia (males)—testosterone supplementation
- Allergic dermatitis—antihistamines, diet, corticosteroids, hyposensitization vaccine
- Hyperthyroidism—oral medications such as methimazole (tapazole) or radioactive iodine therapy
- Diabetes mellitus—regulation of glucose levels (insulin)
- Hyperadrenocorticism—surgery; no known effective medical therapy
- Paraneoplastic alopecia—no therapy; often fatal
- Epidermotropic lymphoma—retinoids (isotretinoin), corticosteroids, interferon
- Sebaceous adenitis—retinoids, corticosteroids
- Squamous cell carcinoma in situ—surgical excision, retinoids (topical and oral)
- Alopecia areata—no therapy; possibly counterirritants
- Demodicosis—lime sulfur dips at weekly intervals for 4–6 dips; Mitaban and ivermectin have been tried with variable success (dose and frequency of application are questionable)
- Dermatophytosis—griseofulvin (CAUTION: idiosyncratic toxicity), ketoconazole, itraconazole (best choice), lym dip, lufenuron

Comments

Zoonotic Potential

Dermatophytosis—can cause skin lesions in humans

Pregnancy

Retinoids and griseofulvin should not be administered to pregnant animals.

See Also

- Demodicosis
- Dermatophytosis
- Diabetes Mellitus, Uncomplicated
- Epidermotropic Lymphoma
- Feline Paraneoplastic Syndrome

- Hyperthyroidism
- Sebaceous Adenitis

ABBREVIATIONS

- ANA = antinuclear antibody
- FeLV = feline leukemia virus
- FIV = feline immunodeficiency virus
- HDDST = high-dose dexamethasone suppression test
- LDDST = low-dose dexamethasone suppression test

Suggested Reading

Baer KE, Helton KA. Multicentric squamous cell carcinoma in situ resembling Bowen's disease in cats. Vet Pathol 1993;30:535–543.

Helton Rhodes KA, Wallace M, Baer KE. Cutaneous manifestations of feline hyperadrenocorticism. In: Ihrke PJ, Mason IS, White SD. Advances in veterinary dermatology. New York: Pergamon, 1993.

Scott DW, Griffin CE, Miller BH. Acquired alopecia. In: Muller & Kirk's small animal dermatology. 5th ed. Philadelphia: Saunders, 1995:720–735.

Scott DW, Griffin CE, Miller BH. Congenital and hereditary defects. In: Muller & Kirk's small animal dermatology. 5th ed. Philadelphia: Saunders, 1995:736–805.

Scott DW, Griffin CE, Miller BH. Endocrine and metabolic diseases. In: Muller & Kirk's small animal dermatology. 5th ed. Philadelphia: Saunders, 1995:627–719.

Author Karen Helton Rhodes

Consulting Editor Karen Helton Rhodes

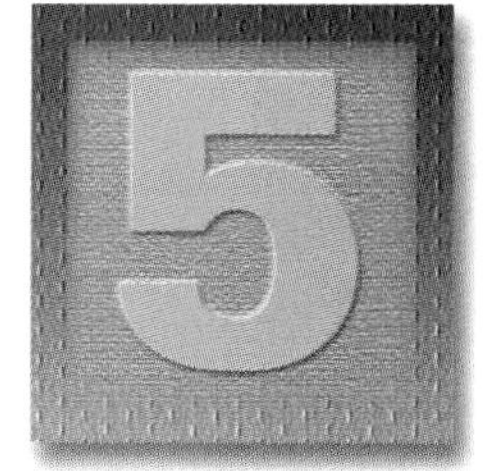

Erosive and Ulcerative Dermatoses

Daniel O. Morris

Definition

A heterogenous group of skin disorders characterized by disruption of the epidermis (erosions) or, if the basement membrane is compromised, the epidermis and dermis (ulcers)

Pathophysiology

Varies widely, depending on the cause; may include congenital or developmental disorders that compromise tissue cohesion; cell-mediated (inflammatory or neoplastic) injury; anoxic injury; destruction by trauma, toxins, irritants, contactants, microbial organisms, or parasitic migration; and antigen-specific autoimmune disorders

Signalment/History

Age, breed, and sex predispositions vary according to the disease in question.

- History and physical examination are especially important owing to the extensive differential list.
- Ascertain history of pruritus (self-induced ulcers or erosions), exposure to infectious organisms, travel history (for some fungal diseases), diet, and signs of systemic disease.

Clinical Features

- Many of the causes have subtle differences in appearance and distribution of lesions.
- Lesions may appear as "punched-out" holes or ulcers while others may be crusted; all are characterized by a disruption in the integrity of the epidermis.

Differential Diagnosis

Autoimmune

- Pemphigus foliaceus
- Pemphigus vulgaris (Figs. 5-1A, B)
- Bullous pemphigoid
- Systemic or discoid lupus erythematosus (Fig. 5-2)
- Cold agglutinin disease
- Lupus panniculitis

Immune-Mediated

- Erythema multiforme and toxic epidermal necrolysis (usually drug-induced or idiopathic) (Figs. 5-3, 5-4)
- Vasculitis separate bullet canine eosinophilic furunculosis of the face (may be insect-related)
- Canine juvenile cellulitis (puppy strangles)
- Cutaneous histiocytosis (Fig. 5-5)
- Feline indolent ulcer (rodent ulcer) (Fig. 5-6)
- Feline hypereosinophilic syndrome

Infectious

- Superficial or deep staphylococcal pyoderma (Fig. 5-7)
- Deep fungal (e.g., sporotrichosis, coccidioidomycosis) (Fig. 5-8)
- Superficial fungal (malasseziasis, dermatophytosis)
- Atypical mycobacteriosis
- Actinomycetic bacteria (e.g., *Nocardia* spp., *Actinomyces* spp., *Streptomyces* spp.)
- Pythiosis
- Protothecosis
- Leishmaniasis
- Feline cow pox
- FIV/FeLV-related

Parasitic

- Demodicosis
- Sarcoptic/notoedric and demodectic acariases
- Flea bite allergy
- Feline mosquito bite hypersensitivity (Fig. 5-9)
- Pelodera and hookworm migration

A

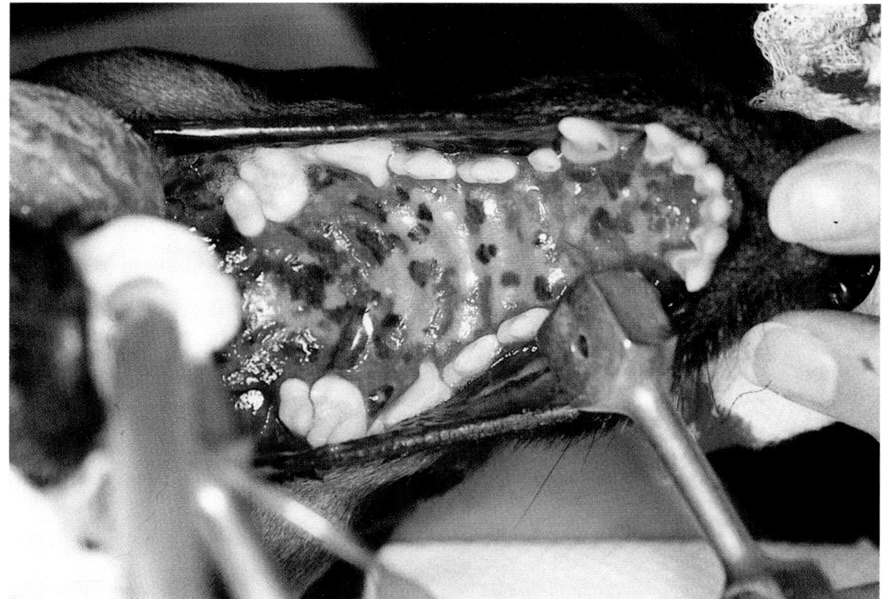

B

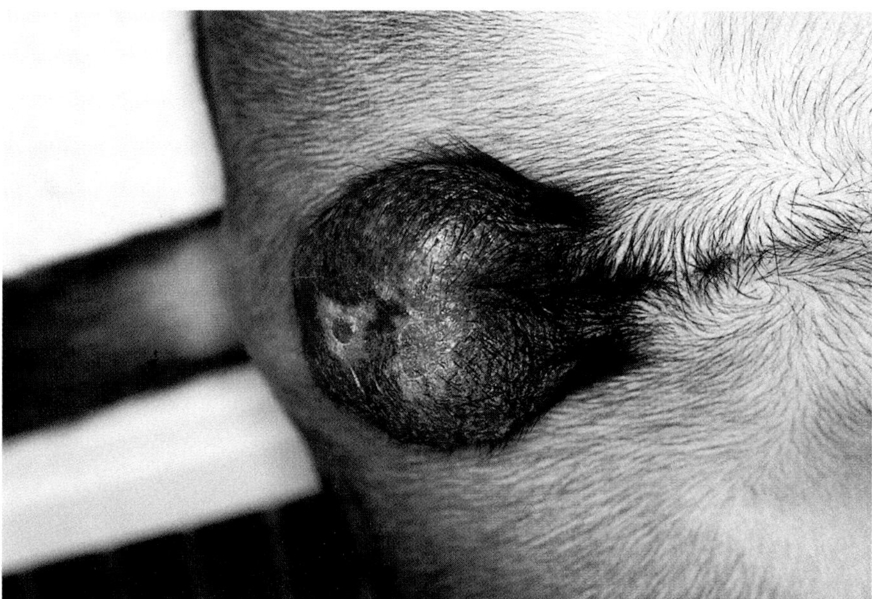

Figure 5-1 **A.** Eight-year-old male mixed breed dog with pemphigus vulgaris affecting the oral mucosa and **B.** scrotum.

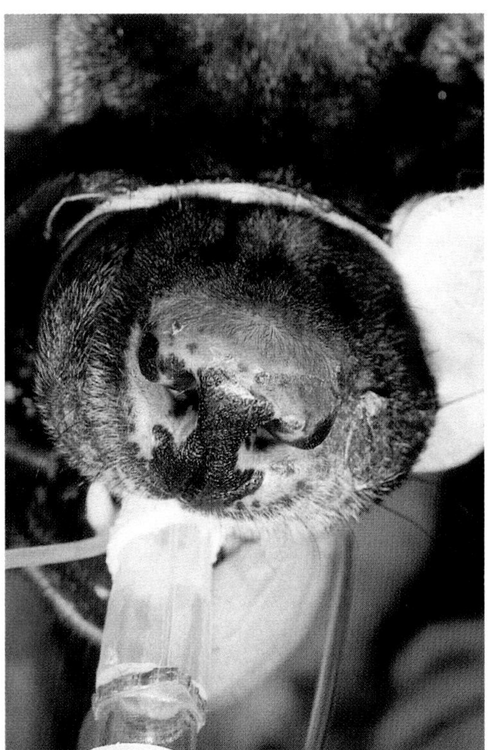

Figure 5-2 Five-year-old M(n) akita with discoid lupus erythematosus.

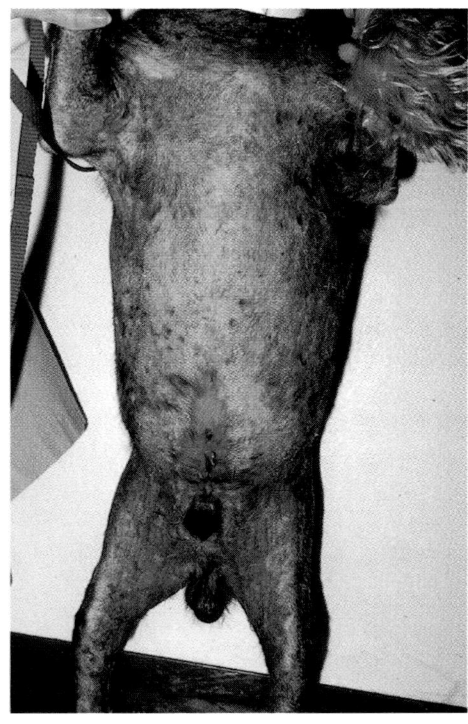

Figure 5-3 Five-year-old Male miniature schnauzer with tribrissen-induced toxic epidermal necrolysis of the ventrum.

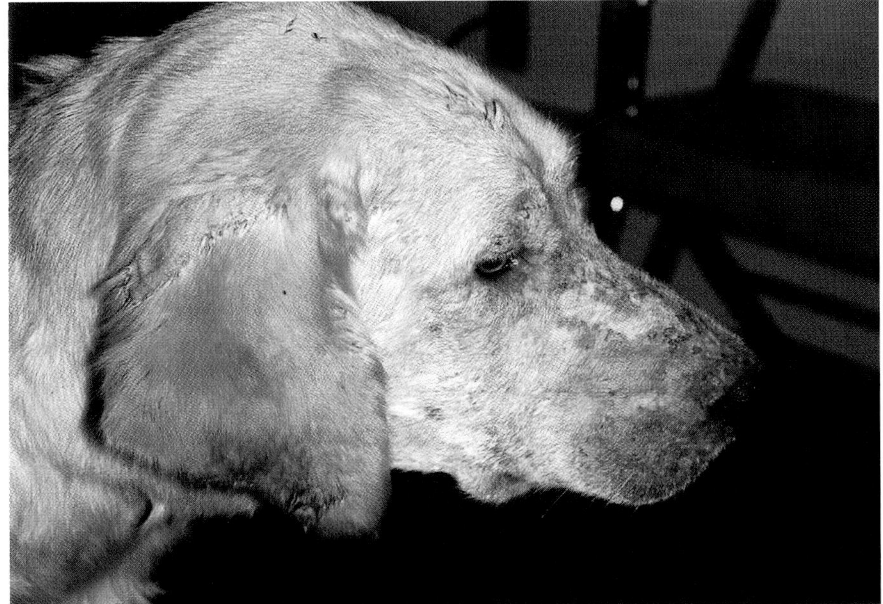
A

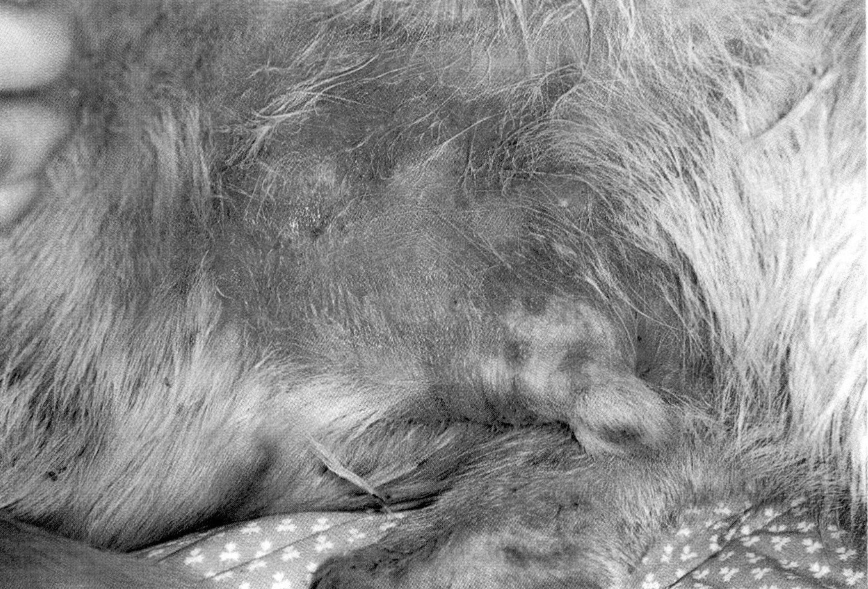
B

Figure 5-4 **A.** Two-year-old Male golden retriever with generalized erosive facial and **B.** groin dermatitis caused by drug-induced (cephalexin) pemphigus foliaceus–like dermatosis.

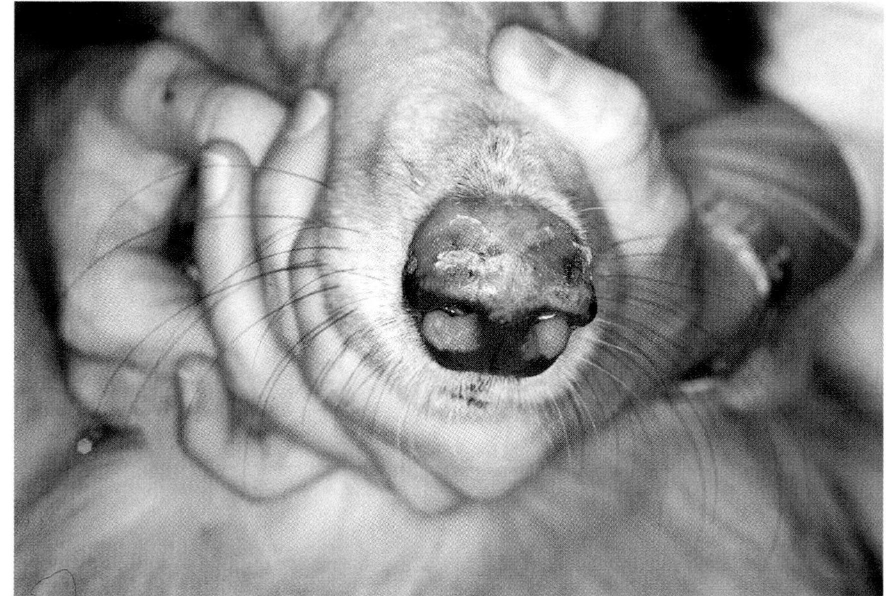

A

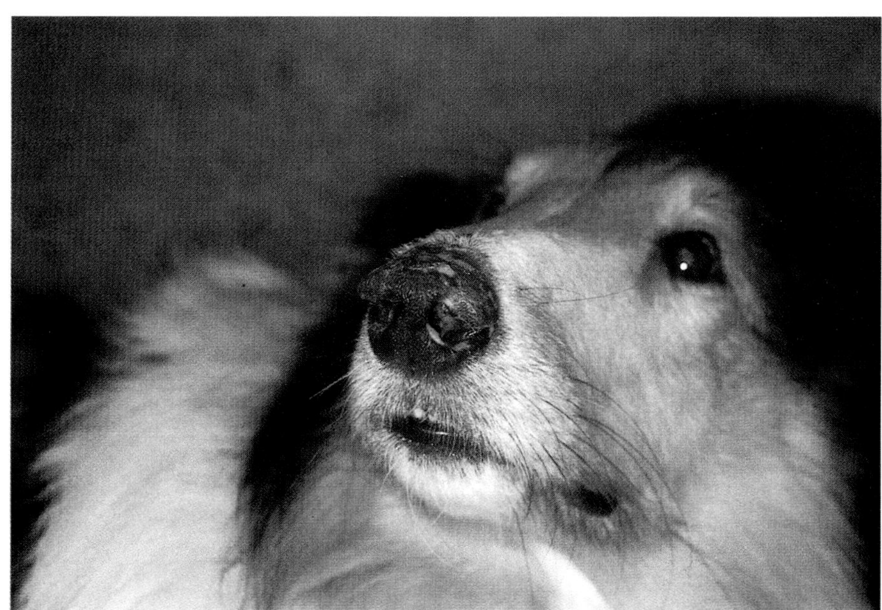

B

Figure 5-5 Seven-year-old M(n) collie with cutaneous histiocytosis. Before **A** and after **B** treatment with prednisone and chlorambucil.

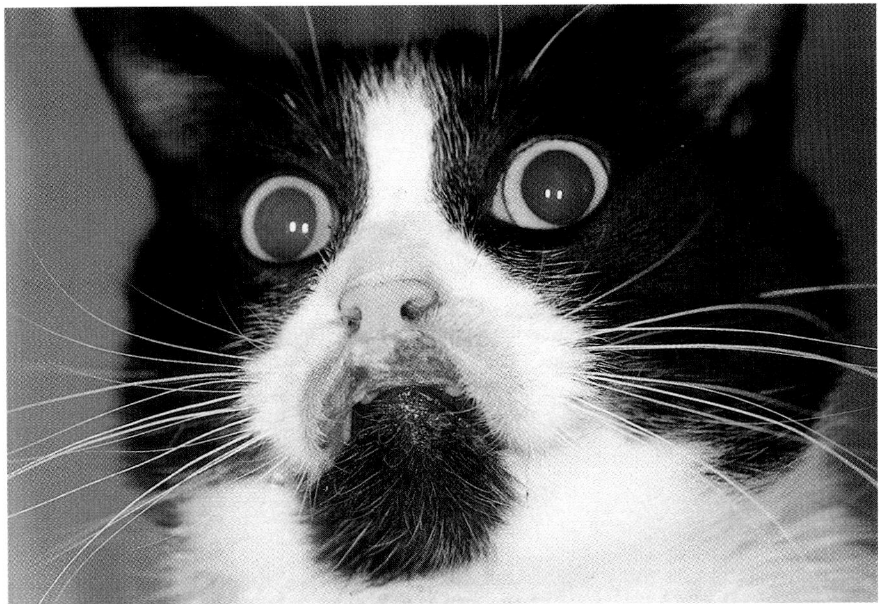

Figure 5-6 Five-year-old M(n) DSH with "rodent ulcer" of the upper lip.

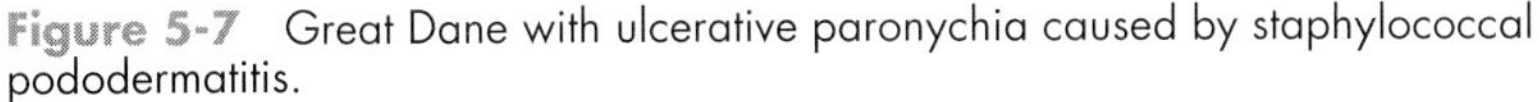

Figure 5-7 Great Dane with ulcerative paronychia caused by staphylococcal pododermatitis.

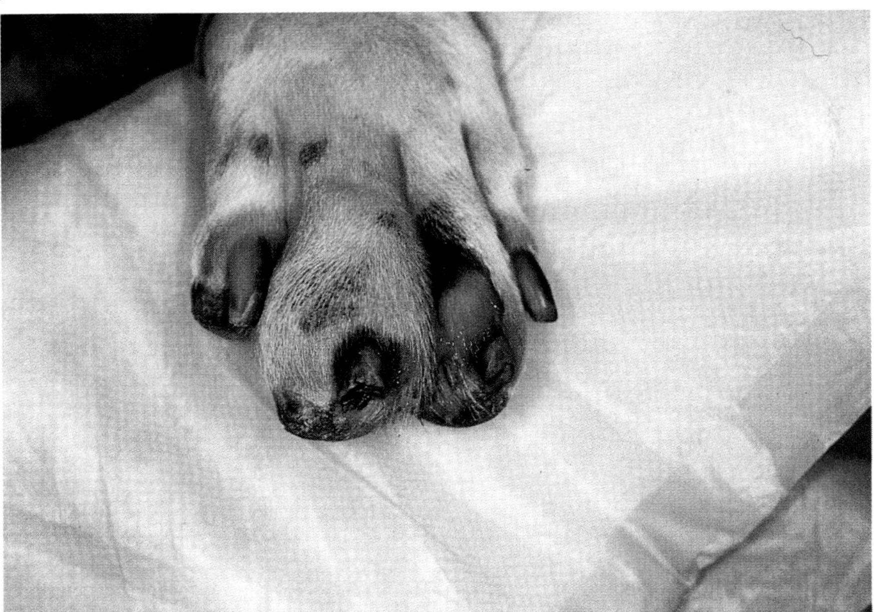

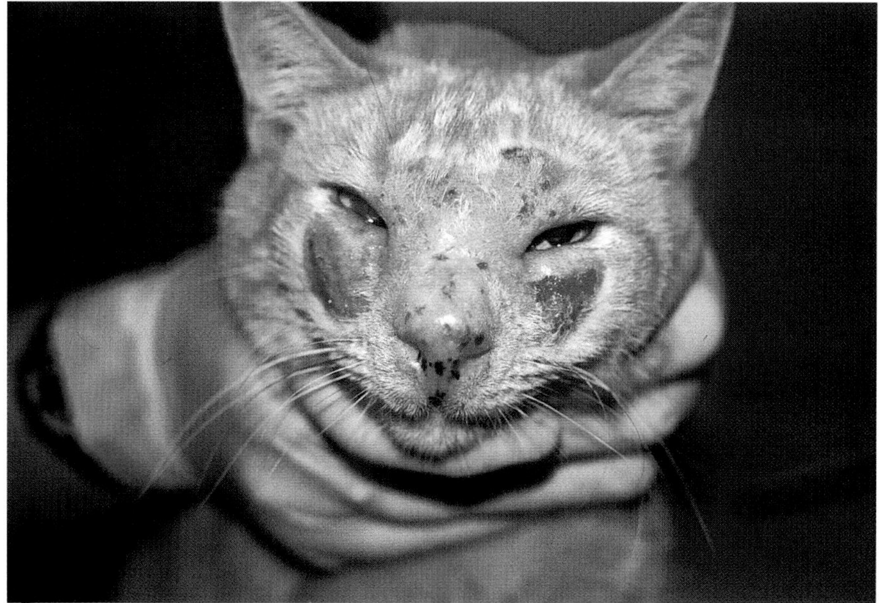

Figure 5-8 Seven-year-old M(n) DSH with ulcerative facial dermatitis caused by *Cryptococcus neoformans* infection.

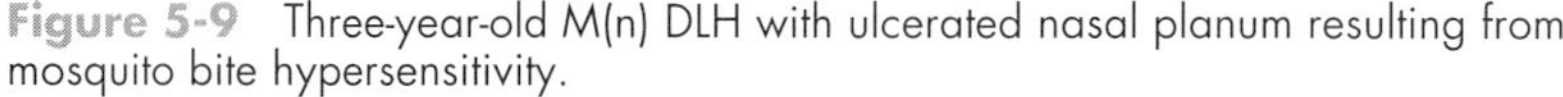

Figure 5-9 Three-year-old M(n) DLH with ulcerated nasal planum resulting from mosquito bite hypersensitivity.

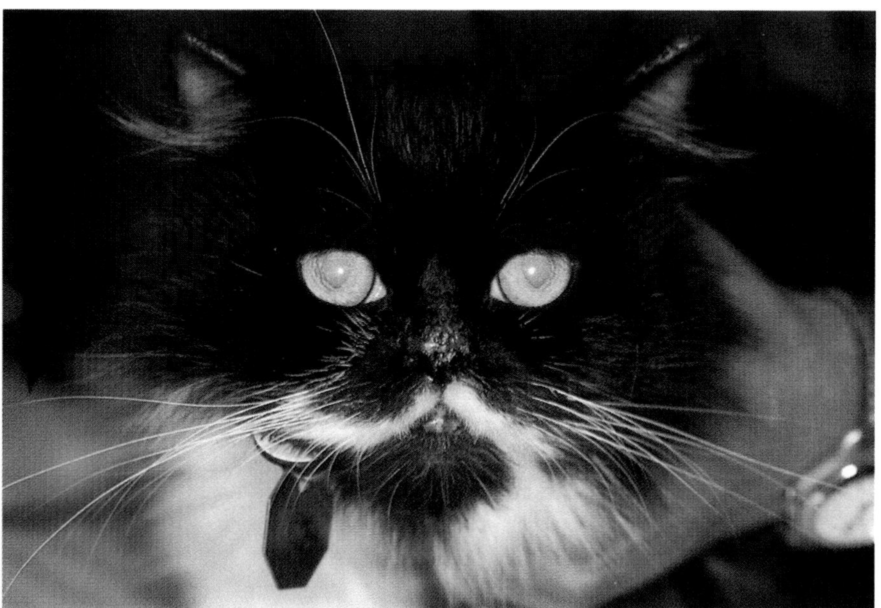

Congenital/Hereditary

- Canine juvenile dermatomyositis
- Junctional epidermolysis bullosa
- Cutaneous asthenia (Ehlers-Danlos syndrome)
- Aplasia cutis (epitheliogenesis imperfecta)

Metabolic

- Diabetes mellitus
- Necrolytic migratory erythema (hepatocutaneous syndrome)
- Hyperadrenocorticism (especially when complicated by secondary infections or calcinosis cutis)
- Uremia (mucous membranes)

Neoplastic

- Squamous cell carcinoma
- Squamous cell carcinoma in situ (Bowen's disease)
- Mast cell tumors
- Cutaneous T-cell lymphoma (mycosis fungoides) (Fig. 5-10)

Nutritional

- Zinc-responsive dermatosis
- Generic dog food dermatosis

Physical/Conformational Dermatoses

- Pressure point ulcers
- Intertrigo
- Self-trauma as a result of pruritic dermatoses (Fig. 5-11)

Figure 5-10 Nine-year-old F(s) Shetland sheepdog with mucocutaneous nodule-stage mycosis fungoides (epitheliotropic cutaneous T-cell lymphoma).

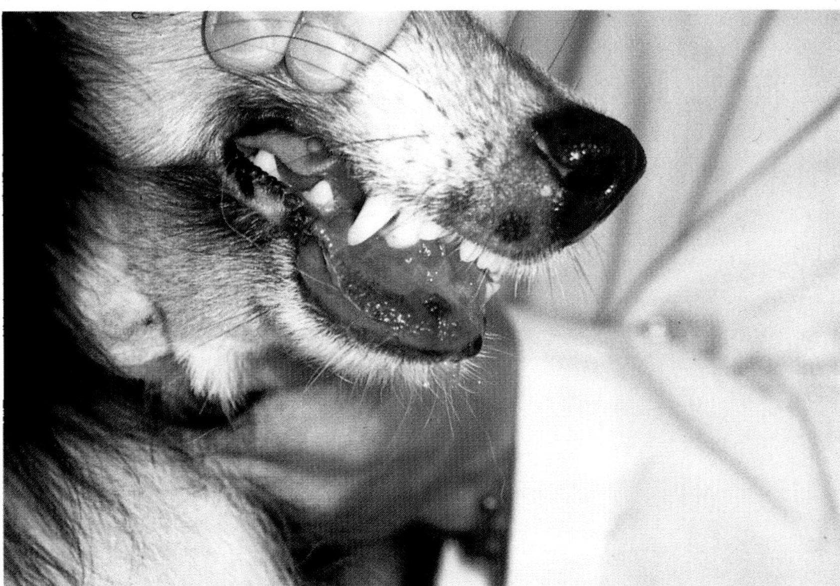

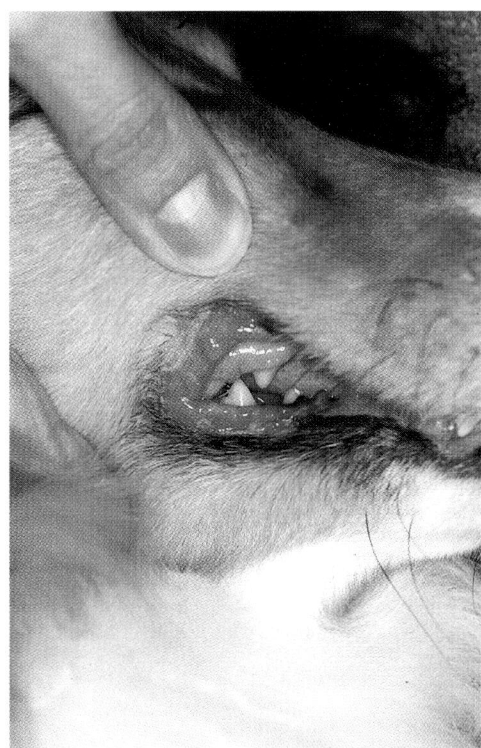

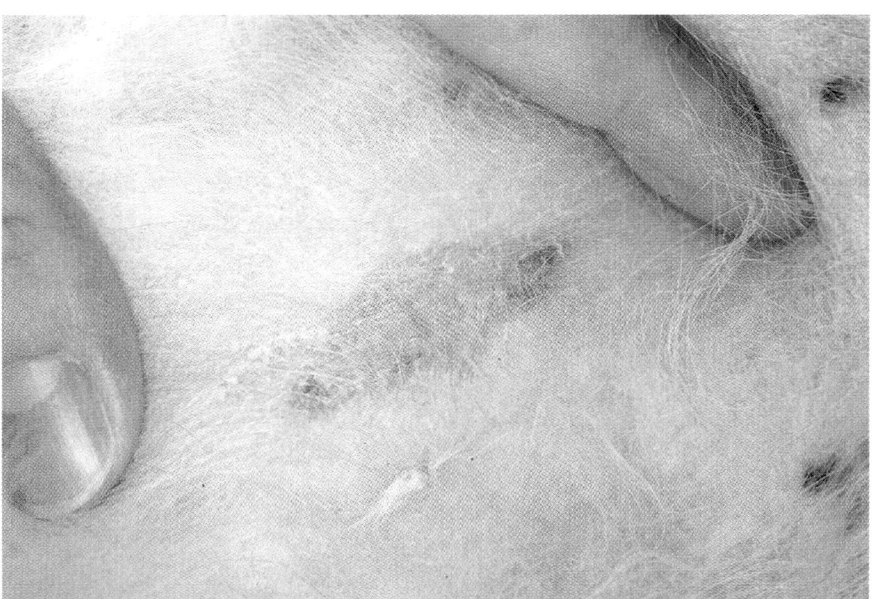

Figure 5-11 **A.** One-year-old F(s) Shetland sheepdog with "ulcerative dermatosis of the Shetland sheepdog" affecting the oral mucosa and groin **B**.

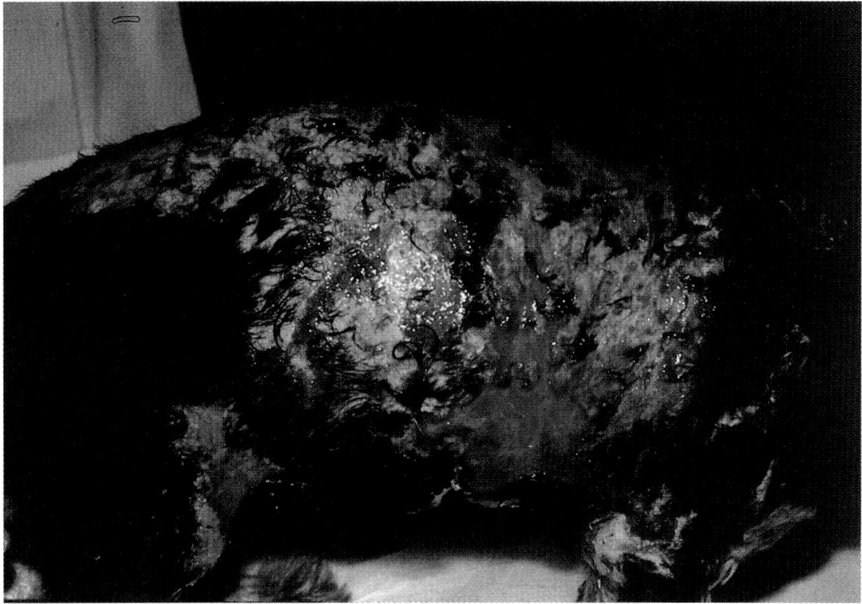

Figure 5-12 Mixed breed dog with a thermal burn of the dorsum resulting from heating pad injury.

Idiopathic

- Ulcerative dermatosis of collies and shelties
- Feline ulcerative dermatosis with linear subepidermal fibrosis
- Lupoid dermatosis of German short-haired pointers
- Canine and feline acne
- Feline plasma cell pododermatitis
- Idiopathic nodular panniculitis

Miscellaneous

- Thermal, electrical, solar, or chemical burns (Fig. 5-12)
- Frost bite
- Chemical irritants
- Venomous snake and insect bites
- Thallium toxicosis

Diagnostics

CBC/Biochemistry/Urinalysis

Most helpful when metabolic disease is suspected or in any patient with signs of systemic disease

Other Laboratory Tests

Fungal serology and tests for immune-mediated diseases (e.g., ANA titer) may be indicated on a case-by-case basis.

Imaging

- Rarely indicated
- Thoracic radiographs—for deep/systemic fungal disease
- Thoracic or abdominal radiographs—identify calcinosis associated with hyperadrenocorticism

Diagnostic Procedures

- Skin scrapings—suspected parasitism
- Direct impression cytology (Tzanck prep)—identify acantholytic cells if pemphigus is suspected
- Fine needle aspirate with cytology—indurated or nodular lesions
- Bacterial (aerobic and anaerobic), mycobacterial, and/or fungal cultures—suspected infectious disease (especially in cats with ulcers or draining tracts)
- Skin biopsy for histopathology—most informative test; for cavitary lesions, the leading edge should be harvested with a scalpel blade if the defect is too large to be excised in total; punch biopsy sufficient for diffuse erosive lesions

Therapeutics

- Outpatient for most diseases
- Varies widely according to the cause
- Supportive therapy with fluid and nutritional supplementation is indicated in cases with severe fluid and protein loss through transepidermal exudation.

Drugs of Choice

Vary widely according to cause

Contraindications

A definitive diagnosis can be imperative, because some immune-mediated cases that require immunosuppression may mimic infectious diseases that require specific antimicrobial chemotherapy (and for which immunosuppression could be fatal).

Precautions

Side effects—associated with many antimicrobial, immunosuppressive, and antineoplastic drugs; consult a veterinary drug text

Comments

Zoonotic Potential

- Sarcoptic acariasis
- Dermatophytosis
- Sporotrichosis
- Mycelial phase of some fungi (e.g., *Coccidioides immitis, Blastomyces dermatitidis*), when grown on culture media, can be infectious to humans through inhalation.
- In-clinic fungal culturing (other than for dermatophytes) is not advised.

- Some diseases are potentially life-threatening.
- Some diseases have zoonotic potential.
- Superinfections and drug side effects are possible in cases requiring immunosuppression.
- Some infectious diseases (nocardiosis, atypical mycobacteriosis) may be controlled but not cured.

ABBREVIATIONS

- ANA = antinuclear antibody
- FeLV = feline leukemia virus
- FIV = feline immunodeficiency virus

Suggested Reading

Angarano DW. Erosive and ulcerative skin disease. In: Kunkle GA, ed. Veterinary clinics of North America: small animal practice. Feline dermatology. Philadelphia: Saunders, 1995:871–885.

Beale KM. Nodules and draining tracts. In: Kunkle GA, ed. Veterinary clinics of North America: small animal practice. Feline dermatology. Philadelphia: Saunders, 1995:887–900.

Scott DW, Miller WH, Griffin CE, eds. Muller & Kirk's small animal dermatology. 5th ed. Philadelphia: Saunders, 1995.

Consulting Editor Karen Helton Rhodes

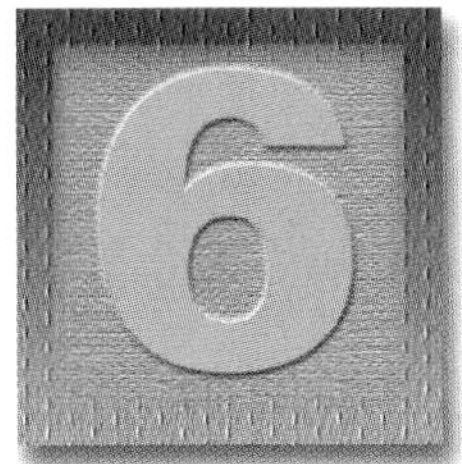

Exfoliative Dermatoses

Alexander H. Werner and Linda Messinger

Definition/Overview

Excessive production or abnormal shedding of epidermal cells resulting in the clinical presentation of cutaneous scaling (See flow chart on page 80)

Pathophysiology/Etiology

- An increase in the production, a decrease in the desquamation, or an increase in the cohesion of keratinocytes results in abnormal shedding of epidermal cells individually (fine scale) and in sheets (coarse scale).
- Primary exfoliative disorders—keratinization defects, in which the genetic control of epidermal cell proliferation and maturation is abnormal (via enzyme abnormalities, etc.)
- Secondary exfoliative disorders—from the effects of disease states on the normal maturation and proliferation of epidermal cells

Signalment/History

- Primary—apparent by 2 years of age; characteristic in affected breeds (see Causes)
- Secondary—any age; any breed of dog or cat
- Owners often complain of progressive deterioration of the coat, excessive scaling, malodorous skin, and variable degrees of pruritus.
- Rarely an acute onset
- Paramount in distinguishing the possible causes of defects in exfoliation

Clinical Features

- Dry or greasy accumulations of fine scale or coarse rafts of epidermal cells located diffusely throughout the hair coat or focally in keratinaceous plaques
- "Rancid fat" odor common
- Comedones
- Follicular casts (accumulation of adherent debris around the hair shaft)
- Alopecia
- Pruritus
- Secondary pyoderma
- *Malassezia* overgrowth infrequent finding
- Occurrence of pruritus—assists in determining the possibility of a cutaneous hypersensitivity; primary keratinization defects are often nonpruritic, unless secondary pyoderma develops.
- Concurrent signs (e.g., lethargy, weight gain, polyuria/polydipsia, reproductive failure, change in body conformation, and lack of hair regrowth), with or without inflammation, can assist in differentiation.

Differential Diagnosis

Primary

- Primary idiopathic seborrhea (primary keratinization disorder)—primary cellular defect; accelerated epidermopoiesis and hyperproliferation of the seborrheic epidermis, follicular infundibulum, and sebaceous glands identified in some breeds; breeds at highest risk: cocker and springer spaniels, West Highland white terriers, basset hounds, Doberman pinschers, Irish setters, and Labrador retrievers; dry (sicca) and greasy (oleosa) forms exist, but determination of type has little prognostic value. (Fig. 6-1)

Figure 6-1 Primary keratinization disorder of a 4-year-old f/s cocker spaniel. Note the patches of hyperkeratosis over the eyes and along the bridge of the nose (also, biopsy site).

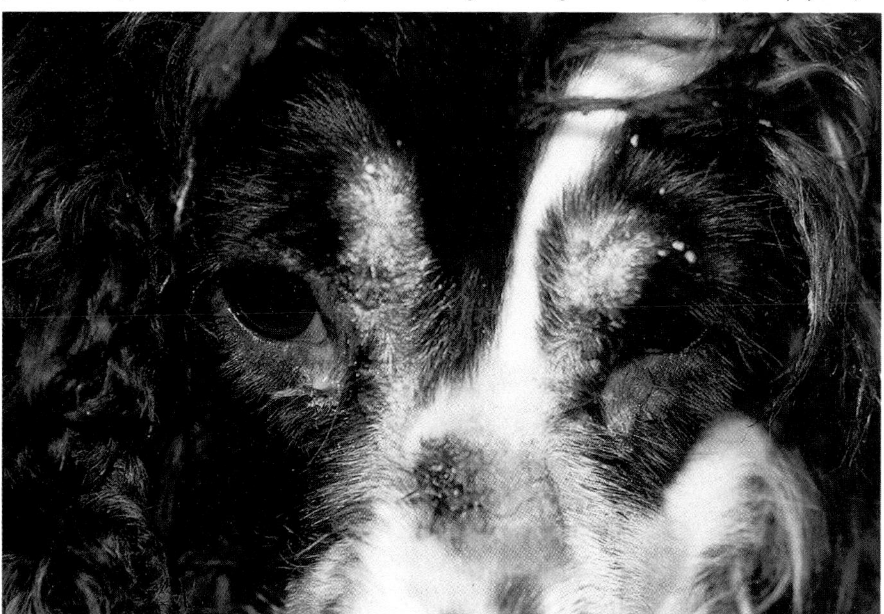

- Vitamin A–responsive dermatosis—nutritionally responsive; seen primarily in young cocker spaniels; clinical signs similar to severe idiopathic seborrhea; distinguished by the response to dietary vitamin A supplementation (Fig. 6-2)
- Zinc-responsive dermatosis—nutritionally responsive; results in alopecia, scaling, crusting, and erythema around the eyes, ears, feet, lips, and other external orifices; two syndromes: young adult dogs (especially Siberian huskies and Alaskan malamutes) and rapidly growing, large-breed puppies
- Ectodermal defects—follicular dysplasias; seen as color mutant or dilution alopecia; represent abnormalities in melanization of the hair shaft and structural hair growth; keratinization defects theorized as causative for several syndromes; breeds commonly affected: blue and fawn Doberman pinschers, Irish setters, dachshunds, chow chows, Yorkshire terriers, poodles, great Danes, whippets, salukis, and Italian greyhounds; signs include the failure to regrow blue or fawn hair with normal "point" hair growth, excessive scaliness, comedone formation, and secondary pyoderma
- Idiopathic nasodigital hyperkeratosis—excessive accumulation of scale and crusts on the nasal planum and footpad margins; common in middle-aged spaniels; lesions generally asymptomatic, unless severe enough to result in cracking and secondary bacterial infection
- Sebaceous adenitis—inflammatory disease; breeds: middle-aged standard poodles, akitas, and Samoyeds; characteristic diffuse hair loss and excessive scaling; tightly adherent follicular casts; most dogs are generally healthy and asymptomatic; akitas: frequently develop severe and deep bacterial pyoderma; Vizslas: disease appears distinctly different and granulomatous (Fig. 6-3)

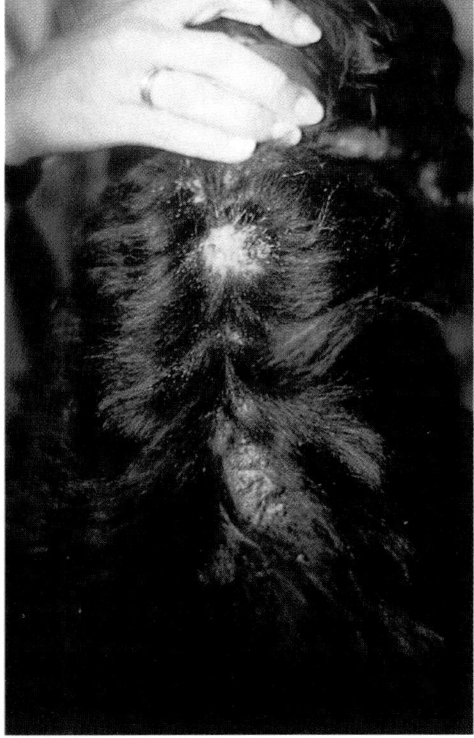

Figure 6-2 Vitamin A–responsive dermatosis characterized by multifocal patches of excess keratin.

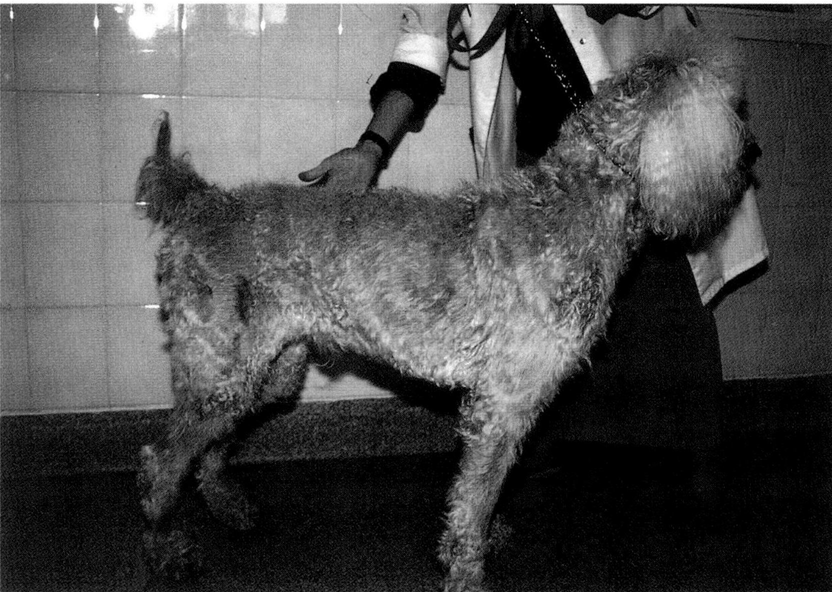

Figure 6-3 Standard poodle with generalized granulomatous sebaceous adenitis demonstrating follicular casting of keratin that effectively mats the hair down onto the skin and gives the clinical appearance of alopecia.

- Epidermal dysplasia and ichthyosis—rare and severe congenital disorder of keratinization; reported in West Highland White Terriers; generalized accumulations of scale and crusts at an early age; secondary infections (bacterial and yeast) common; prognosis in severe cases is poor

Secondary

- Cutaneous hypersensitivity—atopy, flea allergic dermatitis, food allergy, and contact dermatitis; pruritus and resultant skin trauma and irritation
- Ectoparasitism—scabies, demodicosis, and cheyletiellosis; inflammation and exfoliation (Fig. 6-4)
- Pyoderma—skin infection; bacterial enzymatic dyshesion and increased exfoliation of keratinocytes in the attempt to shed pathogenic organisms
- Dermatophytosis—commonly exfoliative; increased shedding of affected keratinocytes is a primary skin mechanism in resolving fungal infection. (Fig. 6-5)
- Endocrinopathy—hypothyroidism and hyperadrenocorticism commonly produce excessive scaling; hypothyroidism: abnormalities in keratinization, failure to regrow hair, and excessive sebum production; hyperadrenocorticism: abnormal keratinization and decreased follicular activity; secondary pyoderma common in both syndromes; other hormonal abnormalities (e.g., sex hormone abnormalities, hyperthyroidism, and diabetes mellitus) may also be associated with excessive scaling
- Age—geriatric animals may have a dull, brittle, and scaly hair coat; changes may be caused by natural alterations in epidermal metabolism associated with age; no specific defect identified
- Nutritional disorders—malnutrition and generic dog food dermatosis; result in scaling from abnormalities in keratinization
- Autoimmune skin diseases—pemphigus complex: may appear exfoliative owing to rupturing of fragile vesicles and secondary pyoderma; cutaneous and

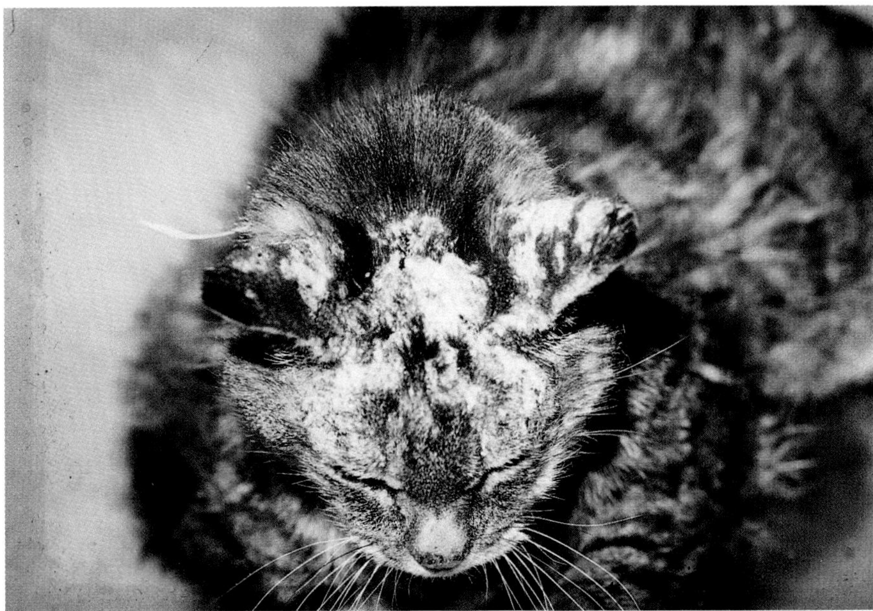

Figure 6-4 *Notoedres* infestation manifesting as a marked hyperkeratotic disorder in a cat.

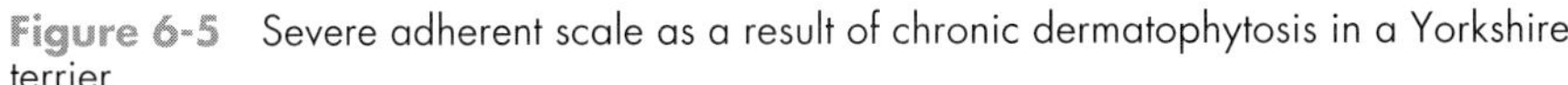

Figure 6-5 Severe adherent scale as a result of chronic dermatophytosis in a Yorkshire terrier.

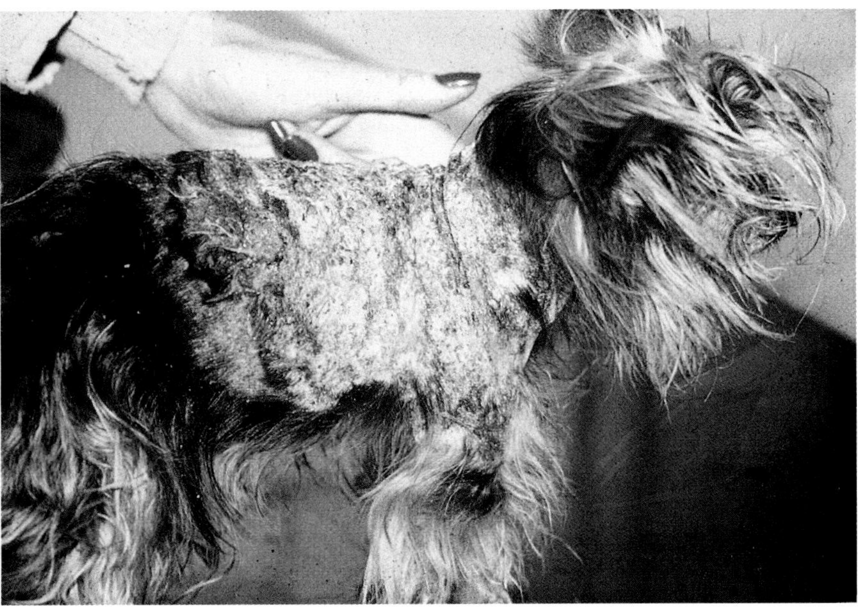

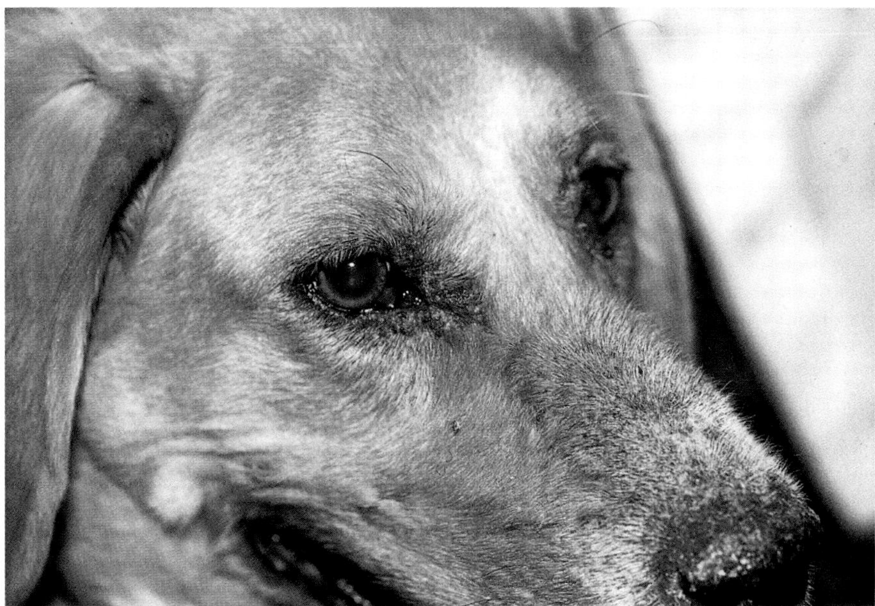

Figure 6-6 Pemphigus foliaceus in a 6-year-old mixed breed dog. Note the scaling along the bridge of the nose and the periocular region.

systemic lupus erythematosus: cutaneous signs frequently appear as regions of alopecia and scaling (Fig. 6-6)

- Neoplasia—primary epidermal neoplasia (epidermotropic lymphoma): may produce alopecia and scaling as epidermal structures are damaged; preneoplastic conditions (alopecia mucinosis, actinic keratosis): initially appear exfoliative (Fig. 6-7)

Figure 6-7 Epidermotropic lymphoma in a cocker spaniel. Note the areas of depigmentation and diffuse scaling on the shaved skin of this dog.

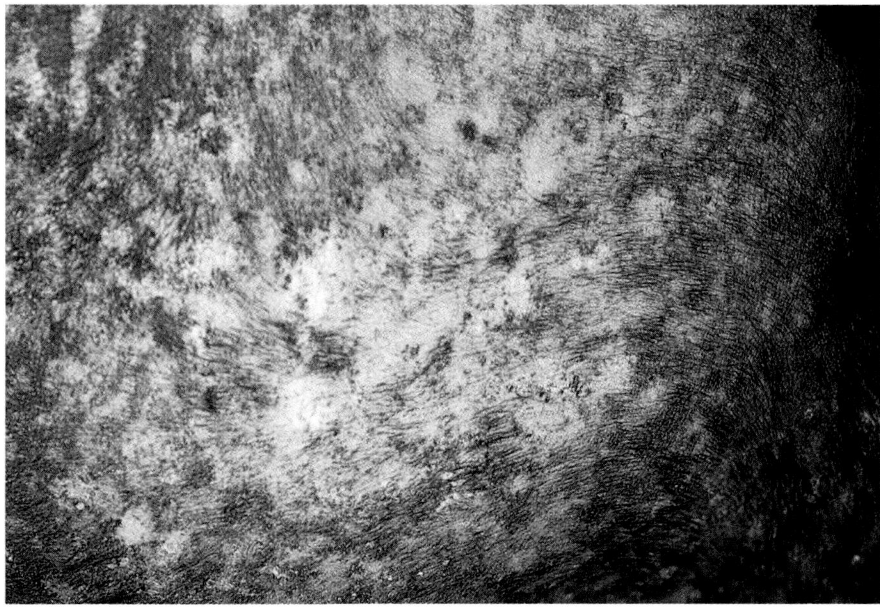

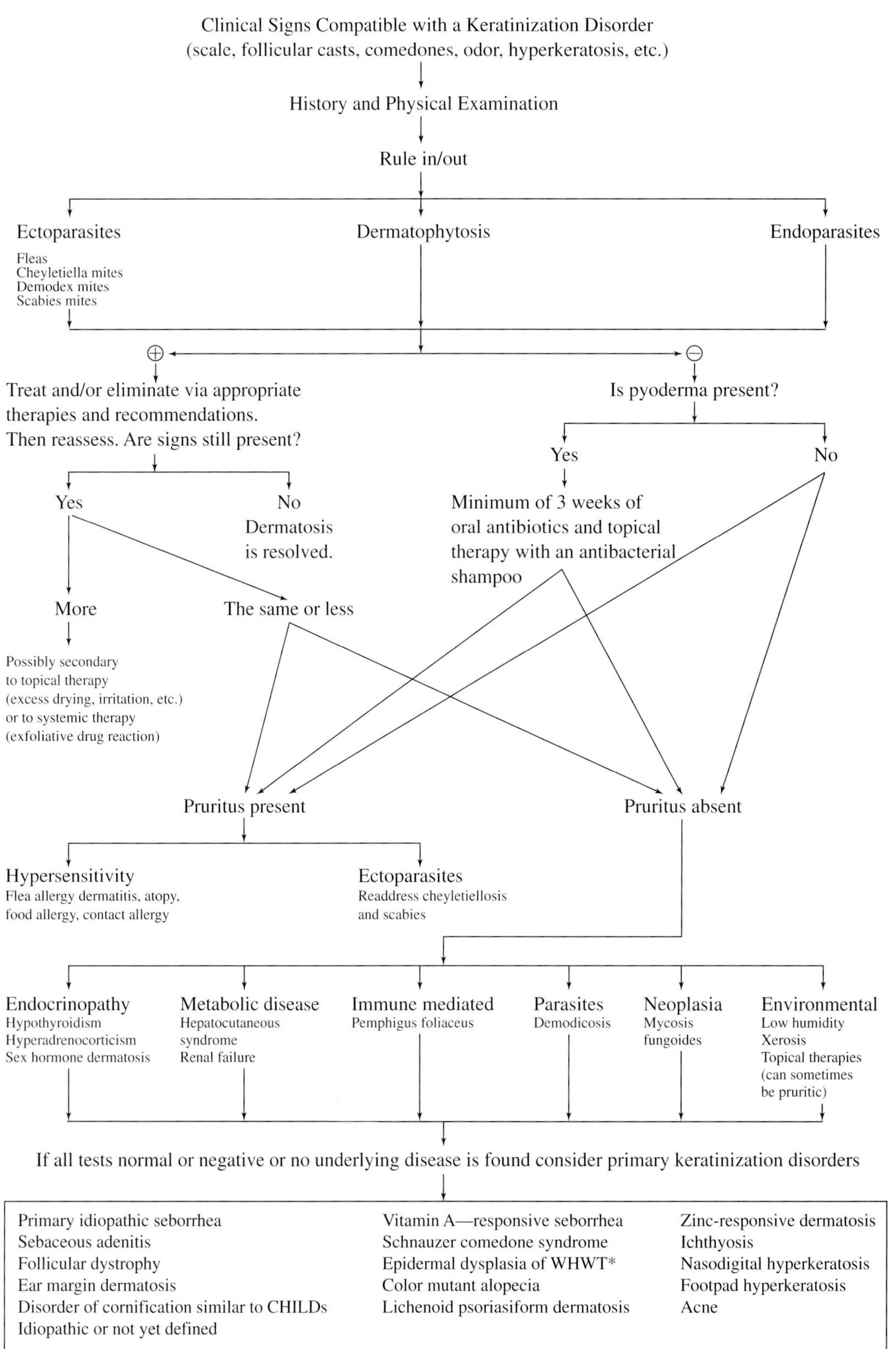

Primary idiopathic seborrhea	Vitamin A—responsive seborrhea	Zinc-responsive dermatosis
Sebaceous adenitis	Schnauzer comedone syndrome	Ichthyosis
Follicular dystrophy	Epidermal dysplasia of WHWT*	Nasodigital hyperkeratosis
Ear margin dermatosis	Color mutant alopecia	Footpad hyperkeratosis
Disorder of cornification similar to CHILDs	Lichenoid psoriasiform dermatosis	Acne
Idiopathic or not yet defined		

*West Highland White Terrier

Source: Flow Chart Courtesy of Dr. Linda Messinger

- Miscellaneous—any disease process may result in excessive scale formation owing to metabolic dyscrasia or cutaneous inflammation

Diagnostics

CBC/Biochemistry/Urinalysis

- Normal with primary keratinization disorders
- Mild, nonregenerative anemia and hypercholesterolemia are consistent with hypothyroidism.
- Neutrophilia, monocytosis, eosinopenia, lymphopenia, elevated serum alkaline phosphatase, hypercholesterolemia, and hyposthenuria suggest hyperadrenocorticism.

Other Laboratory Tests

Thyroid hormone levels and adrenal function tests if an endocrinopathy is suspected; see specific chapters for test recommendations

Diagnostic Procedures

- Skin scrapings—diagnose ectoparasitism
- Skin biopsy—rule out particular differential diagnoses; strongly recommended for most cases
- Intradermal skin testing—identify atopy
- Food-elimination trial—identify food allergy
- Epidermal exudate preparations—determine type of microflora on the skin

Therapeutics

- Frequent and appropriate topical therapy—cornerstone of proper treatment
- Underbathing, rather than overbathing, is a common error.
- Diagnose and control all treatable primary and secondary diseases.
- Recurrence of secondary pyoderma may require repeated therapy and further diagnostics.
- Maintaining control is often lifelong.

Drugs of Choice

Shampoos

- Contact time—5–15 min required; >15 min discouraged, because it results in epidermal maceration, loss of barrier function, and excessive epidermal drying
- Hypoallergenic (soap free)—useful only in mild cases of dry scale and to maintain secondary exfoliation after the primary disease has been controlled
- Sulfur/salicylic acid—keratolytic, keratoplastic, and bacteriostatic; an excellent first choice for the moderately scaly patient; not overly drying
- Benzoyl peroxide—strongly keratolytic, antimicrobial, and follicle flushing; may cause irritation and severe dryness; benzoyl peroxide best for recurrent bacterial infection and/or extreme greasiness
- Ethyl lactate—less effective than benzoyl peroxide for follicular flushing and antimicrobial activity, but not as irritating or drying; most useful for moderate pyoderma and dry scale

- Tar—keratolytic, keratoplastic, and antipruritic; degreasing, but less so than benzoyl peroxide; use for moderate scale associated with pruritus

Moisturizers

- Excellent for restoring skin hydration (frequent shampooing may result in excessive dryness and discomfort) and increasing effectiveness of subsequent shampoos
- Humectants—encourage hydration of the stratum corneum by attracting water from the dermis; at high concentrations may be keratolytic
- Microencapsulation—recent advances may improve the residual activity of moisturizers by permitting sustained release after bathing
- Emollients—coat the skin; smooth the roughened surfaces produced by excessive scaling; usually combined with occlusives to encourage hydration of the epidermis

Systemic Therapy

- Specific causes require specific treatments (i.e., thyroxine replacement for hypothyroidism; zinc supplements for zinc-responsive dermatosis).
- Systemic antibiotics—always indicated for secondary pyoderma
- Retinoid drugs—varied success for idiopathic or primary seborrhea; reports of individual response to retinoids (especially cocker spaniels with a primary keratinization defect); generally, topical therapy provides more benefits for dogs than does retinoid administration; vitamin A analogues (etretinate, soriatane, and isotretinoin) used in limited studies; vitamin D analogues are currently being evaluated for use in keratinization defects

Precautions

- Corticosteroids—may be used judiciously to control the inflammation resulting from many exfoliative disorders; will mask signs of pyoderma and prevent accurate diagnosis of primary disease
- Vitamin A and D analogues—side effects can be severe; thus, patients should be referred to a dermatologist before being treated with these experimental drugs

Comments

Patient Monitoring

- Antibiotics and topical therapy—recheck every 3 weeks to monitor response; patients may respond differently to the various topical therapies
- Seasonal changes, development of additional diseases (especially cutaneous hypersensitivity), and recurrence of pyoderma—may cause previously controlled patients to worsen; re-evaluation critical for determining if new factors are involved and if changes in therapy are necessary
- Endocrinopathies—after pill administration (routine 4–6-hr) thyroid monitoring or ACTH-stimulation tests should be used for proper management
- Autoimmune disorders—re-evaluate frequently during the initial phase of induction; less often after remission; clinical evaluation and laboratory data required

Zoonotic Potential

Dermatophytosis and several ectoparasites have either zoonotic potential or the ability to produce human lesions.

Pregnancy

- Sulfonamide antibiotics and chloramphenicol—do not use in pregnant animals
- Systemic retinoids and vitamin A in therapeutic dosages—do not use in intact females, because of severe and predictable teratogenicity and the extremely long withdrawal period

Synonyms

Keratinization disorders—seborrhea, idiopathic seborrhea, keratinization defect, dyskeratinization, and incorrect human terms (eczema and psoriasis); sebopsoriasis: correct term to describe the similarities between some human and canine keratinization defects

See Also

- Atopy
- Demodicosis
- Hyperadrenocorticism (Cushing Disease)
- Hypothyroidism
- *Malassezia* Dermatitis
- Pyoderma
- Sarcoptic Mange

Suggested Reading

Griffin CE, Kwochka KW, Macdonald JM. Current veterinary dermatology: the science and art of therapy. St. Louis: Mosby, 1993.

Consulting Editor Karen Helton Rhodes

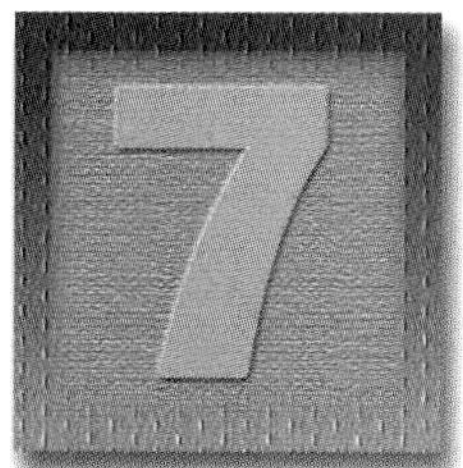

Papular and Nodular Dermatoses

Karen A. Kuhl and Jean Swingle Greek

Definition/Overview

Diseases whose primary lesions may manifest as papules and nodules, which are solid, elevated lesions of the skin

Etiology/Pathophysiology

- Papules—usually the result of tissue infiltration by inflammatory cells; accompanying intraepidermal edema or epidermal hyperplasia and dermal edema
- Nodules—larger than papules; usually the result of a massive infiltration of inflammatory cells into the dermis or subcutis

Signalment/History

Any age, breed, or sex

- May be an acute onset of lesions or a recurring insidious problem

Differential Diagnosis

- Superficial and deep bacterial folliculitis
- Dermatophytosis
- Sebaceous adenitis
- Sterile eosinophilic pustulosis

- Canine and feline acne
- Kerions
- Demodicosis
- Rhabditic dermatitis
- Actinic conditions
- Folliculitis, dermatophytosis, and demodicosis—any disease or medication that causes immune compromise predisposes animals
- Rhabditic dermatitis—may be associated with contact with decaying organic debris (straw or hay) containing *Pelodera strongyloides*
- Actinic conditions—seen more frequently in outdoor, short-haired dogs living in areas with ample sunlight

Diagnostics

CBC/Biochemistry/Urinalysis

- Should be within normal range in most patients
- A circulating eosinophilia may be present with sterile eosinophilic pustulosis.

Diagnostic Procedures

- Skin scrapings—identify possible *Demodex* mites or rhabditiform larvae
- Dermatophyte cultures—identify possible dermatophytosis
- Tzanck preparations—determine if bacteria and degenerative neutrophils are present; compatible with bacterial folliculitis; eosinophils indicate eosinophilic pustulosis or furunculosis is more likely.
- Skin biopsy—if none of these tests has revealed a definitive diagnosis or the lesions are nonresponsive to conventional therapy

Therapeutics

- For nearly all causes, animal can be treated as an outpatient.
- Generalized demodicosis and secondary sepsis require hospitalization.
- Alteration of activity or diet should not be necessary.

Drugs of Choice

Bacterial Folliculitis

- Superficial pyoderma—appropriate antibiotics based on bacterial culture and sensitivity should be given for 3–4 weeks
- Deep pyoderma—appropriate antibiotics based on bacterial culture and sensitivity should be given for 6–8 weeks or more

Sebaceous Adenitis

- A 50–75% mixture of propylene glycol and water once daily as a spray to affected areas or bathing and soaking in baby oil weekly
- Essential fatty acid dietary supplements (PO q12h) in addition to evening primrose oil (500 mg PO q12h)
- Refractory cases—isotretinoin (1 mg/kg PO q12–24h); if response is seen, taper dosage (1 mg/kg q48h or 0.5 mg/kg q24h)
- Cyclosporine has also been used (5 mg/kg PO q12h).
- Most cases are refractory to corticosteroids.

Canine Acne

- May resolve without therapy in mild cases
- More severe cases—benzoyl peroxide shampoos and gels every 24 hr until lesions resolve; then as needed
- Mupirocin—topical antibiotic; apply every 24 hr or alternate with the benzoyl peroxide therapies
- Recurrent or very deep infection (furunculosis)—systemic antibiotics and warm water soaks
- Very refractory cases—topical tretinoin (q12h) or isotretinoin (1–2 mg/kg PO q24h)

Feline Acne

- Underlying cause should be sought and treated accordingly
- No underlying cause found—Stri-Dex pads or benzoyl peroxide gels used daily or alternated daily
- Cats can be sensitive to the irritant effects of benzoyl peroxide.
- Refractory cases—try systemic antibiotics

Rhabditic Dermatitis

- Remove and destroy bedding.
- Wash kennels, beds, and cages and treat with a premise insecticide or flea spray.
- Bathe affected animal and remove crusts.
- Parasiticidal dip—at least 2 times at weekly intervals
- Severe infection—antibiotics may be necessary

Actinic Conditions

- Sunlight—avoid between 10 A.M. and 4 P.M.; apply sunscreen with an SPF ≥ 15 every 12 hr
- Severe inflammation—topical or systemic corticosteroids may provide comfort; topical, 1–2.5% hydrocortisone usually sufficient; systemic, prednisone (initially, 1 mg/kg PO for 3–5 days)
- Secondary infection—antibiotics may be necessary
- Squamous cell carcinoma—prognosis is guarded to poor, depending on the stage of the disease; therapy includes synthetic retinoids, hyperthermia, cryosurgery, photochemotherapy, radiation therapy, and surgical excision

Other

- Dermatophytosis—see specific chapter
- Sterile eosinophilic pustulosis—prednisolone/prednisone (2.2–4.4 mg/kg q24h; then taper to an alternate-day low dosage)
- Kerion—see Dermatophytosis
- Demodicosis—see specific chapter

CONTRAINDICATIONS

Corticosteroids and other immune suppressants should be avoided with folliculitis, dermatophytosis, kerions, and demodicosis.

PRECAUTIONS

- Fatty acids—use with caution in dogs with inflammatory bowel disease or recurrent bouts of pancreatitis

- Isotretinoin—may cause keratoconjunctivitis sicca, hyperactivity, ear pruritus, erythematous mucocutaneous junction, lethargy with vomiting, abdominal distension and erythema, anorexia with lethargy, collapse, and swollen tongue; CBC and chemistry screen abnormalities include high platelet count, hypertriglyceridemia, hypercholesterolemia, and high alanine transaminase
- Cyclosporine—may cause vomiting and diarrhea, gingival hyperplasia, B-lymphocyte hyperplasia, hirsutism, papillomatous skin lesions, and high incidence of infection; potential toxic reactions include nephrotoxicity and hepatotoxicity

Comments

Patient Monitoring

- CBC, chemistry screen, and urinalysis—monitor monthly for 4–6 months in patients receiving cyclosporine or synthetic retinoid therapy
- Tear production—monitor monthly for 4–6 months, then every 6 months in patients receiving synthetic retinoid therapy
- Skin scrapings—monitor therapy in patients with demodicosis (see Demodicosis)
- Repeat fungal cultures—monitor therapy in patients with dermatophytosis (see Dermatophytosis)
- Resolution of lesions—monitor progress of sebaceous adenitis, actinic conditions, and all other diseases

Possible Complications

Actinic conditions may progress to squamous cell carcinoma.

Zoonotic Potential

Dermatophytosis—contagious to humans in 30–50% of cases of *Microsporum canis*

Pregnancy

- Synthetic retinoids—very teratogenic; do not use in pregnant animals, animals intended for reproduction, or intact animals; should not be used by women of childbearing age
- Corticosteroids—do not use in pregnant animals

See Also

- Demodicosis
- Dermatophytosis
- Pyoderma

Suggested Reading

Griffin CE, Kwochka KW, MacDonald JM, eds. Current veterinary dermatology. St. Louis: Mosby, 1993.

Gross TL, Ihrke PJ, Walder EJ. Veterinary dermatopathology. St. Louis: Mosby, 1992.

Muller GH, Kirk RW, Scott DW, eds. Small animal dermatology. 4th ed. Philadelphia: Saunders, 1989.

Consulting Editor Karen Helton Rhodes

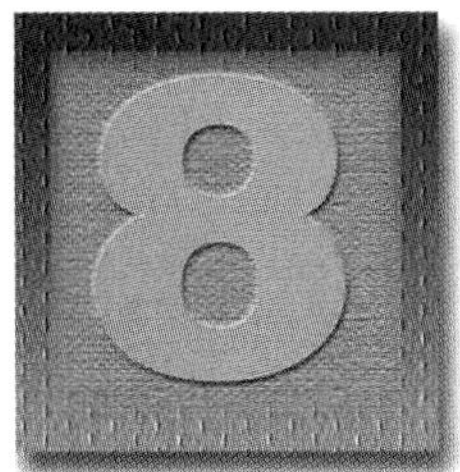

Vesicular and Pustular Dermatoses

Ellen C. Codner and Karen Helton Rhodes

Definition/Overview

- Pustule—small, circumscribed elevation of the epidermis filled with pus
- Vesicle—small, circumscribed elevation of the epidermis filled with clear fluid

Etiology/Pathophysiology

Pustules and vesicles—produced by edema, acantholysis (pemphigus), ballooning degeneration (viral infections), proteolytic enzymes from neutrophils (pyoderma), degeneration of basal cells (lupus), or dermoepidermal separation (bullous pemphigoid)

Signalment/History

- Many of these disorders have a breed predilection as listed below
- The history is rarely helpful, with most information gained via clinical features and histopathologic findings
- Lupus—collies, shelties, and German shepherds may be predisposed
- Pemphigus erythematosus—collies and German shepherds may be predisposed
- Pemphigus foliaceus—akitas, chow chows, dachshunds, bearded collies, Newfoundlands, Doberman pinschers, and schipperkes may be predisposed
- Bullous pemphigoid—collies and Doberman pinschers may be predisposed

- Dermatomyositis—young collies and shelties
- Subcorneal pustular dermatosis—schnauzers affected most frequently
- Linear IgA dermatosis—dachshunds exclusively
- Dermatophytosis—young animals

Risk Factors

- Drug exposure—SLE and bullous pemphigoid (Fig. 8-1)
- Pyodermas are usually secondary to a predisposing factor (e.g., demodicosis, hypothyroidism, allergy, or steroid administration).
- Sunlight—pemphigus erythematosus, bullous pemphigoid, SLE, DLE, and dermatomyositis

Clinical Features

- Some vesicles and pustules are friable, which may confuse the differential list by appearing as more of an adherent scale or crust rather than an intact vesicle or pustule.

Differential Diagnosis

Pustular

Superficial Pyodermas

- Most common cause
- Readily respond to appropriate antibiotic therapy if the underlying cause is effectively managed
- Intact pustule—direct smear reveals neutrophils engulfing bacteria; culture usually yields *Staphylococcus intermedius;* biopsy shows intraepidermal neutrophilic pustules or folliculitis (Figs. 8-2, 8-3)

Figure 8-1 Vesicular eruption secondary to griseofulvin exposure.

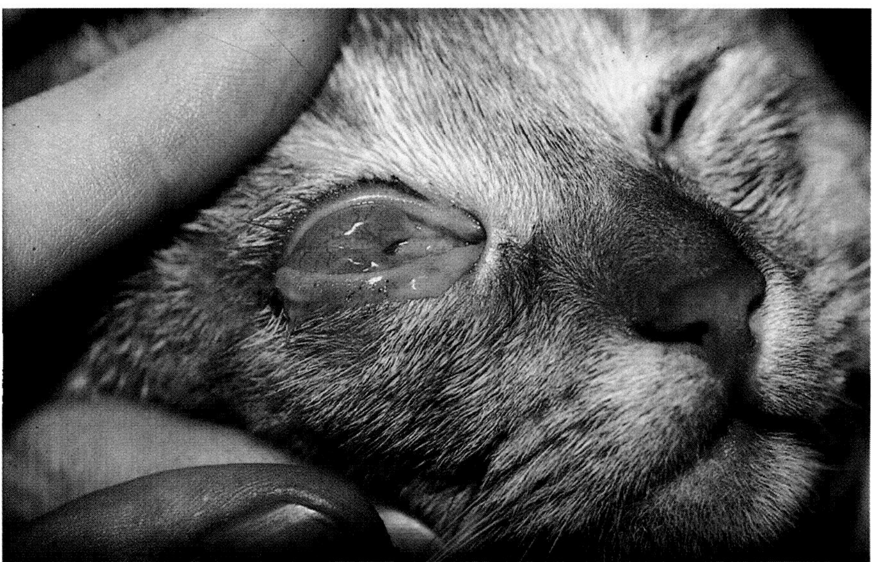

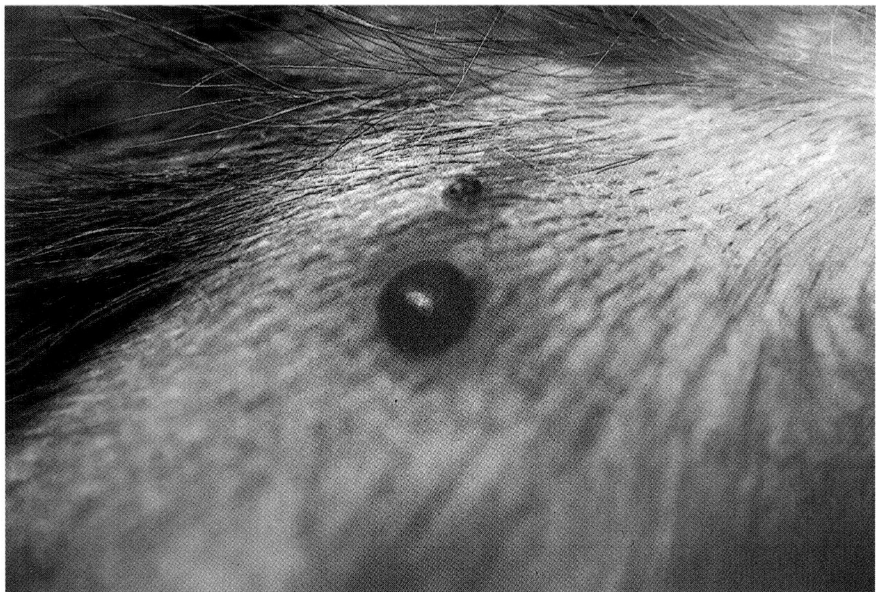

Figure 8-2 Intact pustule associated with canine superficial pyoderma.

Pemphigus Complex

- A group of immune-mediated diseases characterized histologically by acantholytic cells (Figs. 8-4, 8-5)
- Direct smears—many acantholytic cells, nondegenerate neutrophils, and no bacteria
- Culture of an intact pustule negative

Figure 8-3 Papules, pustules, epidermal collarettes, and hyperpigmented macule characteristic of superficial pyoderma.

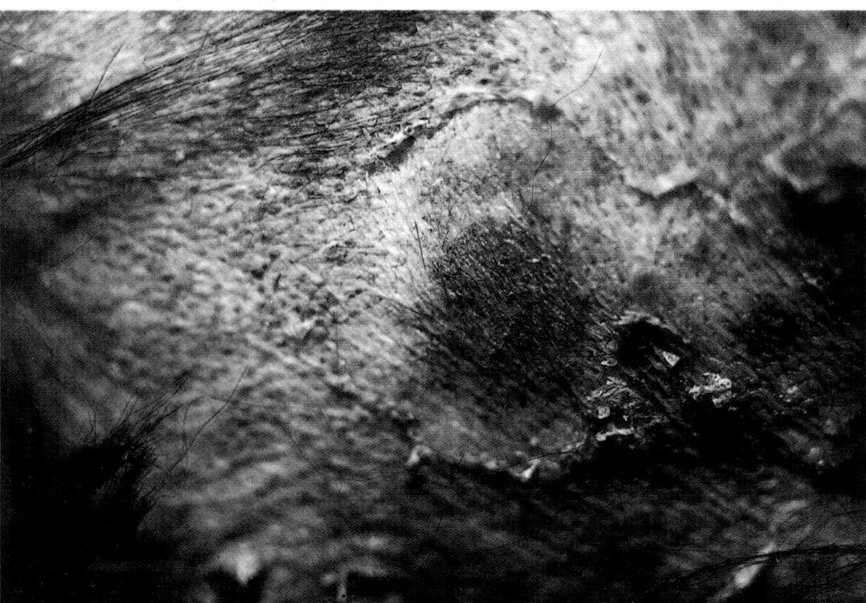

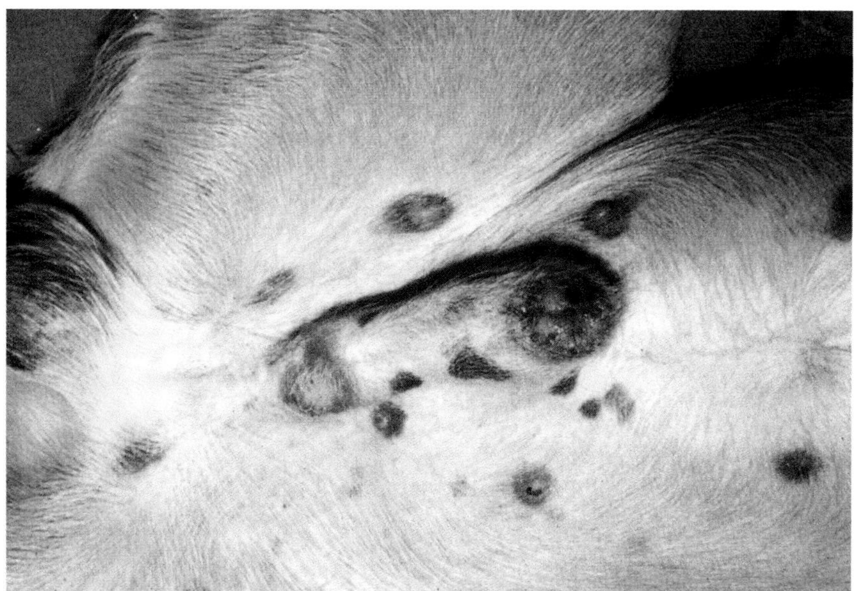

Figure 8-4 Intact pustules on the ventrum of a dog with pemphigus foliaceus.

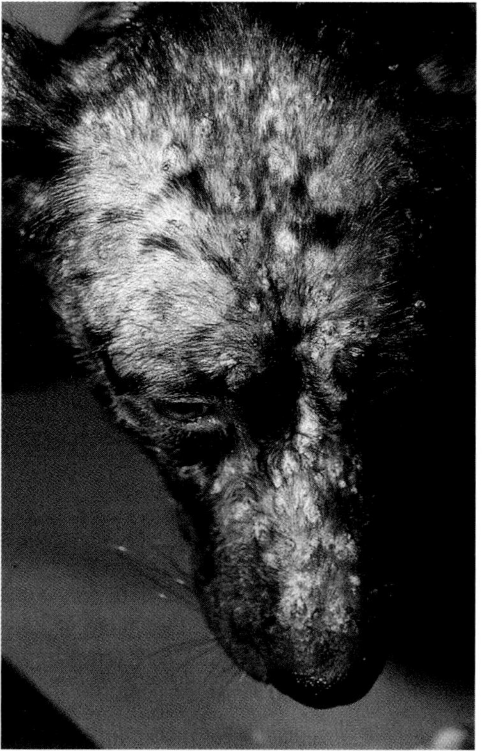

Figure 8-5 Pustules and crusts representative of pemphigus foliaceus.

- Direct immunofluorescence—deposits in the intercellular spaces of the epidermis in approximately 50% of the cases
- Tends to wax and wane irrespective of antibiotic therapy; responds to immunosuppressive therapy

Subcorneal Pustular Dermatosis

- A rare idiopathic pustular dermatosis of dogs (Fig. 8-6)
- Tends to wax and wane
- Intact pustules—direct smears reveal numerous neutrophils, no bacteria, and occasional acantholytic cells; cultures negative
- Direct immunofluorescence negative
- Poor response to glucocorticoids and antibiotics

Dermatophytosis

- Common disease of both dogs and cats
- Dermatophyte culture positive
- Secondary bacterial infection common
- Biopsy—folliculitis with fungal elements

Sterile Eosinophilic Pustulosis

- A rare idiopathic dermatosis of dogs
- Direct smears—numerous eosinophils, nondegenerate neutrophils, occasional acantholytic cells, and no bacteria
- Biopsy—eosinophilic intraepidermal pustules, folliculitis, and furunculosis
- Direct immunofluorescence negative
- Rapid response to glucocorticoids

Figure 8-6 Subcorneal pustular dermatosis with both intact and ruptured lesions along the tail of a dog.

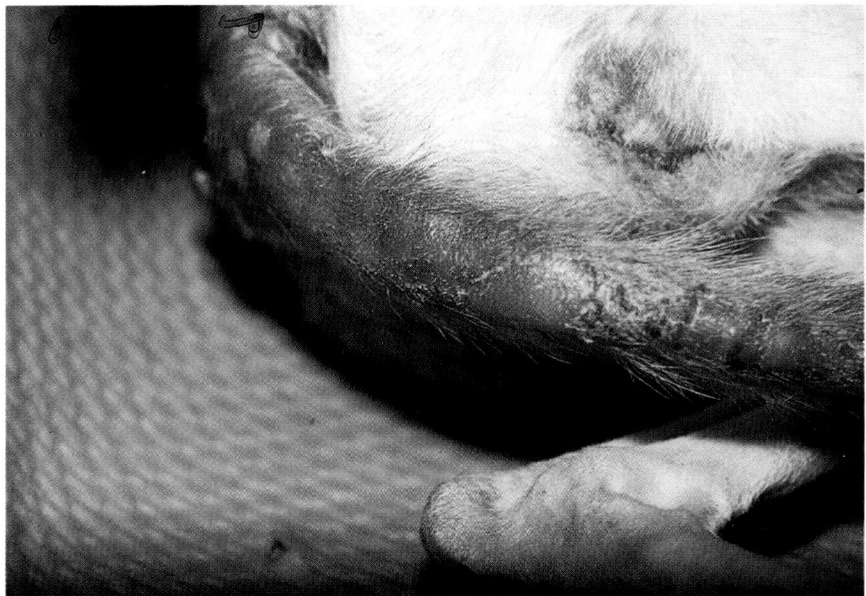

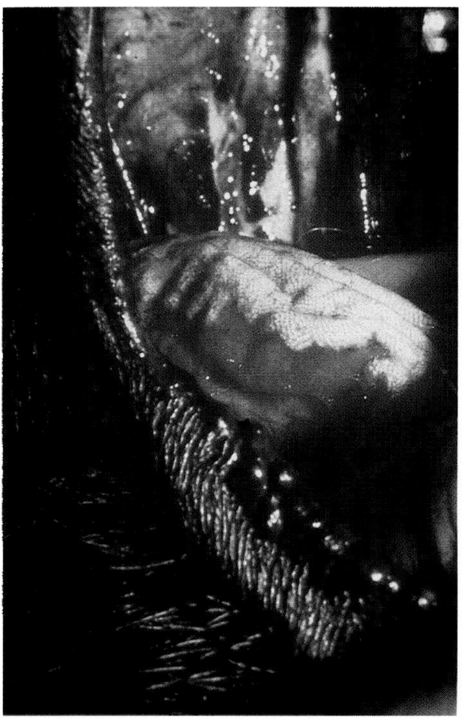

Figure 8-7 Ulcerations of the lateral aspect of the tongue representative of SLE.

Linear IgA Dermatosis

- A rare idiopathic dermatosis of dachshunds
- Tends to wax and wane
- Pustules—sterile and subcorneal
- Direct immunofluorescence positive for IgA at the basement membrane zone

VESICLES/ULCERATION

SLE

- A multisystemic disease with variable clinical signs and cutaneous manifestations, including mucocutaneous ulceration (Fig. 8-7)
- Direct immunofluorescence positive at the basement membrane zone
- ANA positive

DLE

- Affects only the skin; lesions usually confined to the face
- Depigmentation, erythema, and ulceration of the nasal planum common
- Biopsy—interface dermatitis
- Direct immunofluorescence positive at the basement membrane zone
- ANA negative, rarely positive

Bullous Pemphigoid

- Ulcerative disorder of the skin and/or mucous membranes
- Biopsy—subepidermal cleft formation

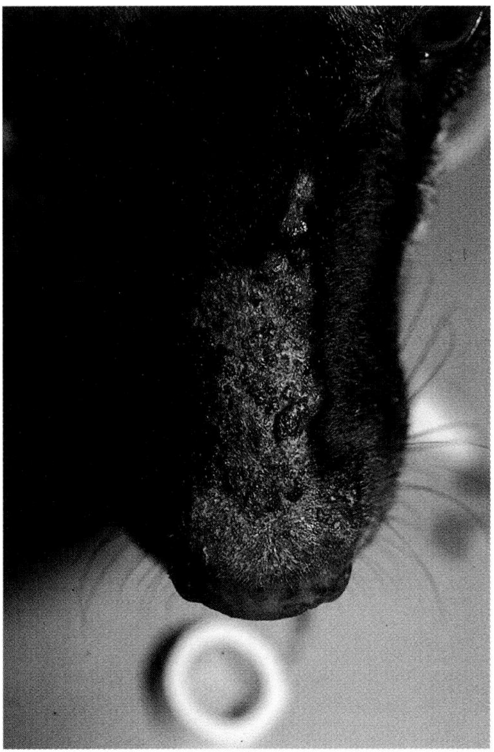

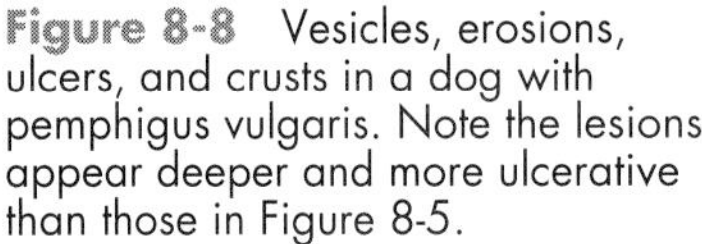

Figure 8-8 Vesicles, erosions, ulcers, and crusts in a dog with pemphigus vulgaris. Note the lesions appear deeper and more ulcerative than those in Figure 8-5.

Figure 8-9 Dermatomyositis in a collie dog. Note the areas of scarring and hyperpigmentation.

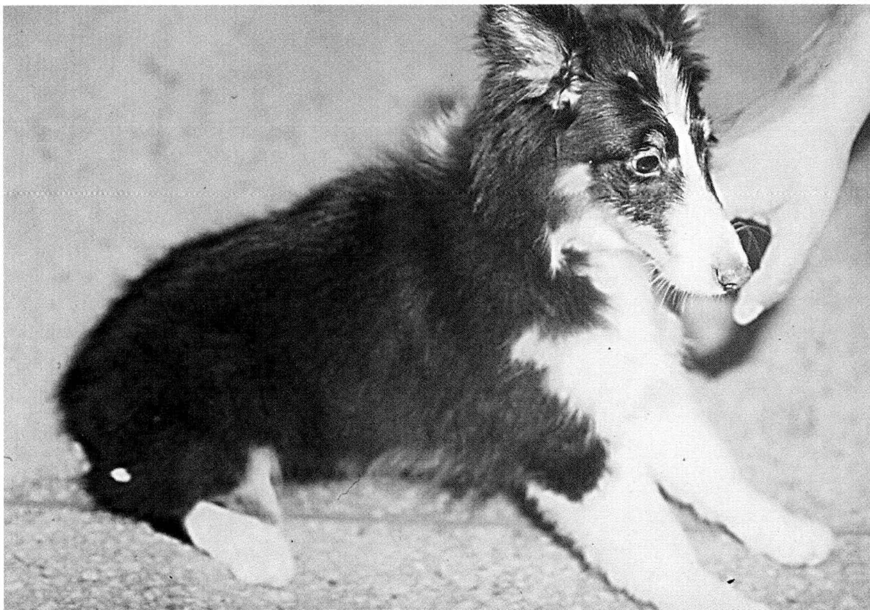

- Direct immunofluorescence positive at the basement membrane zone
- Acantholysis is not seen.

Pemphigus Vulgaris

- Most severe form of pemphigus (Fig. 8-8)
- Characterized by ulceration of the oral cavity, mucocutaneous junction, and skin
- Biopsy—suprabasal acantholysis and cleft formation
- Direct immunofluorescence positive at the intercellular spaces of the epidermis

Dermatomyositis

- An idiopathic inflammatory disease of the skin and muscle of young collies and shelties
- Lesions affect the face, ear tips, tail tip, and pressure points of the extremities (Fig. 8-9).
- Characterized by alopecia, crusting, pigmentation disturbances, erosions/ulceration, and scarring
- Biopsy—follicular atrophy, perifolliculitis, and hydropic degeneration of the basal cells
- Direct immunofluorescence negative
- Muscle biopsy and EMG—evidence of inflammation

Diagnostics

CBC/Biochemistry/Urinalysis

- Results usually unremarkable
- SLE—anemia, thrombocytopenia, or glomerulonephritis may develop
- Eosinophilic pustular dermatosis—most affected dogs have peripheral eosinophilia

Diagnostic Procedures

- Direct smear from intact pustule
- Culture of intact pustule
- Biopsy for histopathology
- Direct immunofluorescence, including IgA
- ANA titer
- EMG
- Muscle biopsy

Therapeutics

- Periodic bathing with an antimicrobial shampoo—helps remove surface debris and control secondary bacterial infections
- Usually treated as an outpatient
- SLE, pemphigus vulgaris, and bullous pemphigoid may be life-threatening and require inpatient intensive care.

Drugs of Choice

Subcorneal Pustular Dermatosis

- Dapsone—1 mg/kg PO q8h until remission (usually 1–4 weeks); then tapered to 1 mg/kg q24h or twice weekly
- Sulfasalazine (Azulfidine)—10–20 mg/kg PO q8h until remission; then as needed

Linear IgA Dermatosis

- Prednisolone—2.2–4.4 mg/kg PO q24h until remission; then taper to alternate-day therapy
- Dapsone—1 mg/kg PO q8h until remission; then taper and give as needed; individual patients may respond to one drug and not the other

Sterile Eosinophilic Pustulosis

- Prednisolone: 2.2–4.4 mg/kg PO q24h until remission (usually 5–10 days); then as needed to prevent relapses (usually long-term, alternate-day therapy required)

Precautions

Prednisolone

- Secondary infections
- Iatrogenic Cushing's disease
- Muscle wasting
- Steroid hepatopathy
- Behavioral changes
- Polydipsia, polyuria
- Polyphagia

Dapsone

- Dogs—mild anemia, mild leukopenia, and mild elevation of ALT, which are not associated with clinical signs, are frequently noted; usually return to normal when dosage is reduced for maintenance
- Occasionally, fatal thrombocytopenia or severe leukopenia
- Occasional vomiting, diarrhea, or pruritic skin eruption
- Cats—more susceptible to dapsone toxicity; hemolytic anemia and neurotoxicity reported

Sulfasalazine

Keratoconjunctivitis sicca

Patient Monitoring

- Dapsone—monitor hemogram, platelet count, and ALT every 2 weeks initially and if any clinical side effects develop
- Long-term sulfasalazine therapy—monitor tear production
- Immunosuppressive therapy—monitor every 1–2 weeks initially; then every 3–4 months during maintenance therapy

Comments

- Many of these disorders are not curable but can be effectively controlled with appropriate maintenance medications.
- Client education is an important aspect in maintaining good control.

See Also

- Acne—Cats; Acne—Dogs
- Dermatomyositis
- Dermatophytosis
- Lupus Erythematosus, Cutaneous (Discoid)
- Lupus Erythematosus, Systemic (SLE)
- Pemphigoid, Bullous
- Pemphigus
- Pyoderma

Abbreviations

- ALT = alanine aminotransferase
- ANA = antinuclear antibody
- DLE = discoid lupus erythematosus
- EMG = electromyography
- SLE = systemic lupus erythematosus

Suggested Reading

Muller GH, Kirk RW, Scott DW. Small animal dermatology. 4th ed. Philadelphia: Saunders, 1989.

Consulting Editor Karen Helton Rhodes

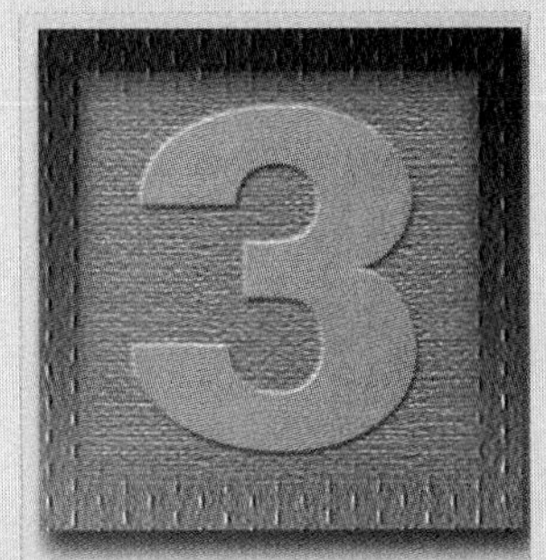

Differential Diagnoses Based on Regional Lesion(s)

Pododermatitis

K. Marcia Murphy and Karen Helton Rhodes

Definition/Overview

An inflammatory, multifaceted complex of diseases that involves the feet of dogs and, less commonly, cats

Etiology/Pathophysiology

- Depends on the underlying cause
- Causes include infectious, allergic, autoimmune, endocrine/metabolic, neoplastic, and environmental diseases
- Psychogenic dermatoses rarely involved

Signalment/History

Breed Predilections

- Short-coated breeds (dogs)—most commonly affected; English bulldogs, great Danes, basset hounds, mastiffs, bull terriers, boxers, dachshunds, Dalmatians, German short-haired pointers, and weimaraners
- Long-coated breeds (dogs)—German shepherds, Labrador retrievers, golden retrievers, Irish setters, and Pekingese
- Cats—none

Historical Findings

- History—extremely important; determine environment and general husbandry (e.g., indoor vs. outdoor, working dog vs. pet, unsanitary conditions, other pets affected, trauma, contact irritants, hookworms)
- Seasonality—suggests atopic dermatitis, allergic contact dermatitis, or irritant contact dermatitis
- Lesions elsewhere on the body—may aid in diagnosis of cause
- Response to previous therapy—antibiotics, antifungals, and corticosteroids
- Diet, travel history, and other medical problems—important in investigation

Clinical Features

Infectious (Dogs)

- Tissues—may be erythematous and edematous, nodules, inflammatory plaques (fungal "kerions"), ulcers, fistulae, hemorrhagic bullae, or serosanguineous or seropurulent discharge
- Feet—may be grossly swollen, may have pitting edema of the metacarpal and metatarsal areas
- Skin—may be alopecic and moist owing to constant licking; patient may have some degree of pain, pruritus, and paronychia
- Regional lymph nodes may be enlarged (Fig. 9-1).

Infectious (Cats)

- Painful paronychia, involving one or more claws
- Higher incidence of nodular, often ulcerated lesions, compared with dog

Figure 9-1 Pododermatitis caused by bacterial folliculitis and furunculosis with demodicosis. Note the involvement of the entire digit, nailbed region, and interdigital spaces with edema of the tissues, alopecia, hyperkeratosis, and focal erosions and ulcerations.

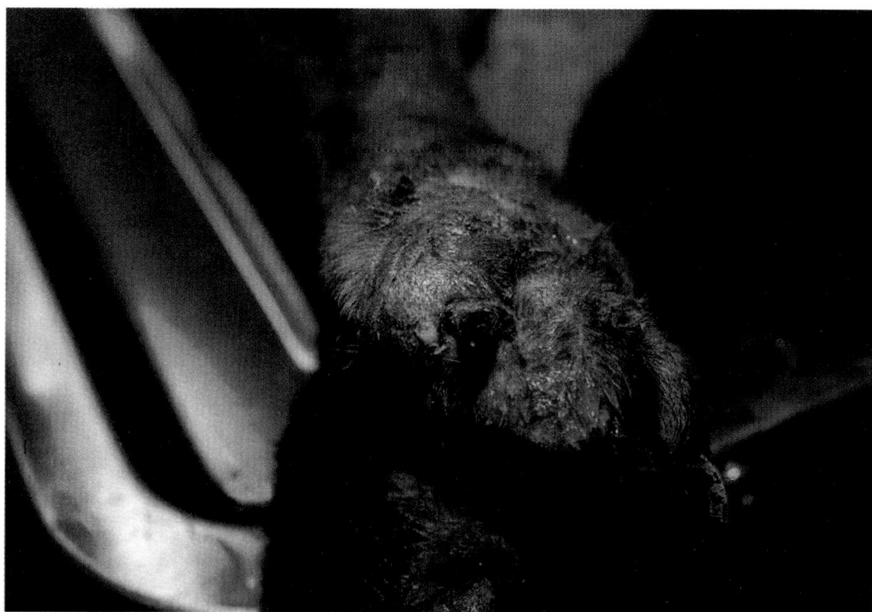

- Footpads and periungual areas—commonly involved
- Interdigital spaces—seldom affected
- Scaly and crusted lesions—occasionally seen

Allergic (Dogs)

- Feet—erythematous and alopecic, secondary to pruritus; dorsal surface usually more severely affected
- Salivary staining may be evident.
- Allergic contact dermatitis—uncommon cause; dermatitis of the ventral interdigital surfaces is usually worse, although the whole paw may be involved

Allergic (Cats)

Single or multiple, exudative or ulcerated, eosinophilic, pruritic plaques of the digits, and periungual and interdigital spaces (Fig. 9-2)

Immune-Mediated (Dogs)

- Crusts and ulcerations—most common lesions; occasionally vesicles or bullae are seen
- All four feet may be affected, especially the nailbeds and footpads.
- Hyperkeratotic and erosive dermatitis of the footpads—common finding in pemphigus foliaceus (Figs. 9-3, 9-4)

Immune-Mediated (Cats)

- Lesions—generally involve the footpad, including hyperkeratosis and ulceration
- Lameness and paronychia—may occur
- Pyonychia common in feline pemphigus foliaceus

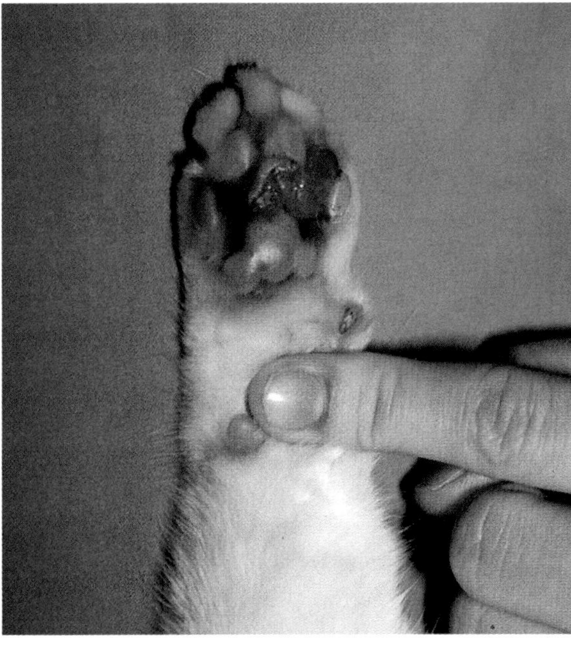

Figure 9-2 Eosinophilic plaque (feline eosinophilic granuloma complex) involving the digital and metacarpal pads.

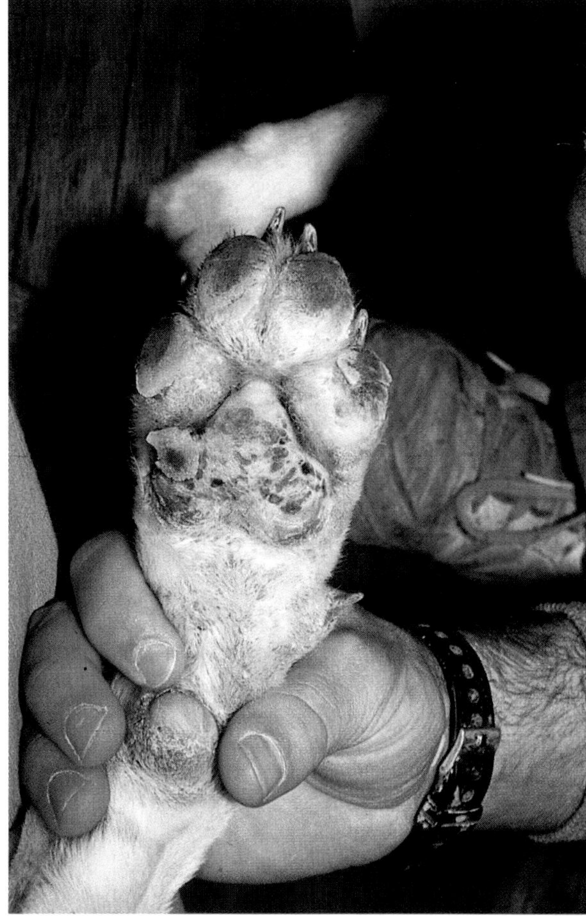

Figure 9-3 Pemphigus foliaceus in a 3-year-old Dalmatian. These lesions are within 3 weeks of the onset of clinical signs. Note the erosions, superficial separation of the pads, and mild-to-moderate erythema.

ENDOCRINE/METABOLIC (DOGS)

- Lesions—usually consistent with secondary infectious pododermatitis
- Hepatocutaneous syndrome—rare condition; signs of skin disease precede the onset of signs of internal disease; lesions include hyperkeratosis and ulceration of the footpads (Fig. 9-5) Exact etiology unknown

ENDOCRINE/METABOLIC (CATS)

Whitish nodules resembling candle wax; may be caused by cutaneous xanthomatosis; seen with diabetes mellitus and hyperlipidemia (Fig. 9-6)

NEOPLASTIC

- Dogs—lesions usually nodules, possible ulceration or pruritus; usually only one foot is involved; multiple foot involvement with nailbed squamous cell carcinoma reported

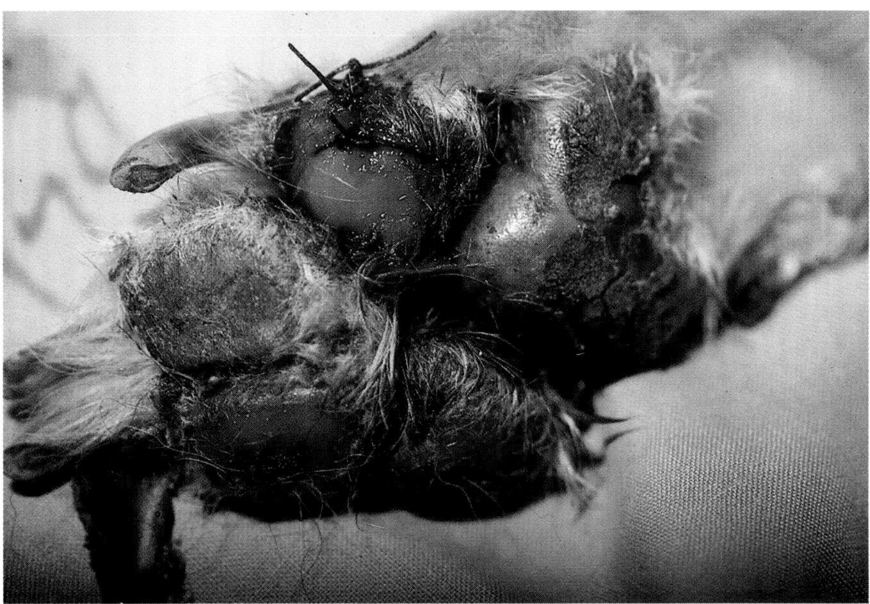

Figure 9-4 Pemphigus vulgaris in a 9-year-old mixed breed dog. Note the marked degree of ulceration of the pads with peripheral hyperkeratosis and crusting.

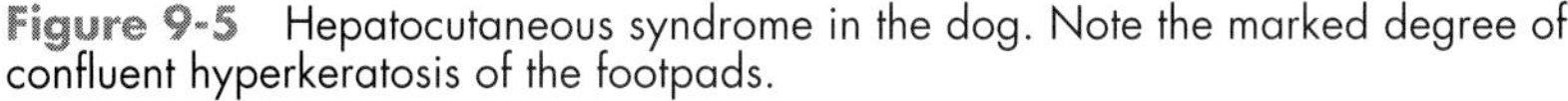

Figure 9-5 Hepatocutaneous syndrome in the dog. Note the marked degree of confluent hyperkeratosis of the footpads.

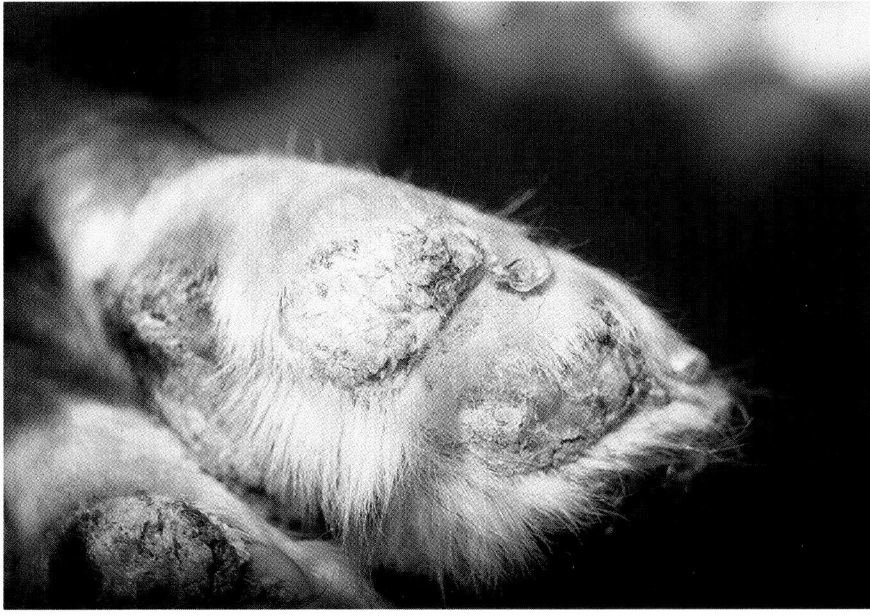

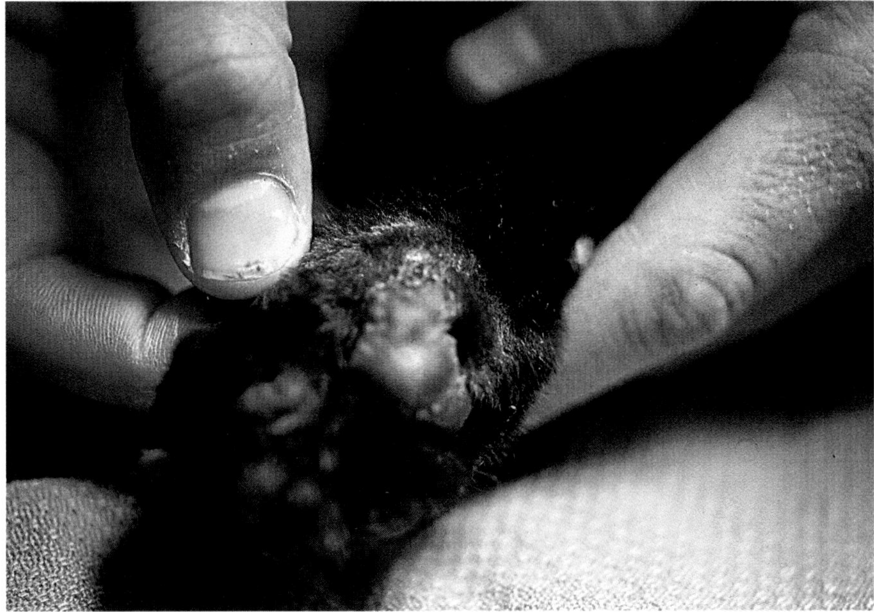

Figure 9-6 Cutaneous xanthomatosis of the footpads in a cat associated with idiopathic hyperlipidemia. Note the yellow-pink plaques along the margins of the footpads.

- Cats—tumors appear as nodules; variably ulcerated and painful; localized destruction variable, depends on the tumor type (Fig. 9-7)

Environmental (Dogs and Cats)

- Depends on underlying cause
- Lesions—involve one digit or foot (foreign body, trauma) or multiple digits (irritant contact dermatitis, thallium toxicity, housed on rough surface or in moist environment)
- Chronic interdigital inflammation, ulceration, pyogranulomatous abscesses, draining tracts, or swelling, with or without pruritus

Figure 9-7 Cutaneous lymphoma affecting the digits of a cat. No lesions were noted in any other areas of the body.

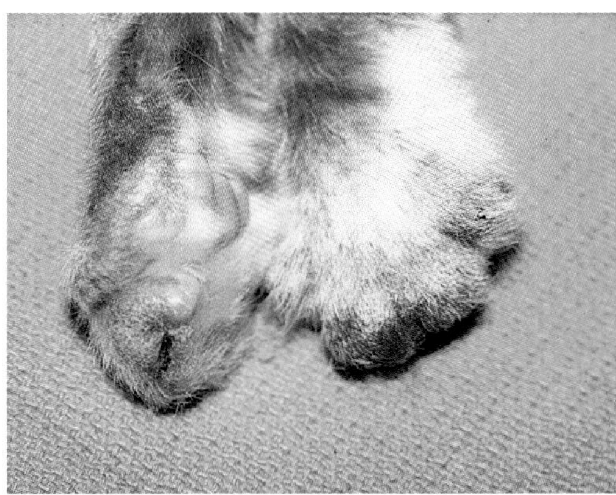

MISCELLANEOUS

- Hyperkeratosis of the footpads (dogs)—associated with several diseases (e.g., zinc-responsive dermatosis, generic dog food dermatosis, and idiopathic digital hyperkeratosis)
- Nodules without draining tracts (dogs)—associated with sterile pyogranulomas in several breeds and nodular dermatofibrosis of the German shepherds and golden retrievers
- Hypomelanosis of the footpads (cats)—associated with vitiligo
- Hypermelanosis of the footpads (cats)—associated with lentigo simplex
- Polydactylism and syndactylism (cats)—common in certain families

Differential Diagnosis (Table 9-1)

INFECTIOUS (DOGS)

- Bacterial—*Staphylococcus intermedius, Pseudomonas* spp., *Proteus* spp., *Mycobacterium* spp., *Nocardia* spp., or *Actinomyces* spp.
- Fungal—dermatophytes, intermediate mycoses (sporotrichosis, mycetoma), or deep mycoses (blastomycosis, cryptococcosis)
- Parasitic—*Demodex canis, Pelodera strongyloides,* and hookworms
- Protozoal—leishmaniasis

INFECTIOUS (CATS)

- Bacterial—same as dog, plus *Pasteurella* spp.
- Fungal—same as dog, excluding blastomycosis
- Parasitic—*Neotrombicula autumnalis, Notoedres cati,* or *Demodex* spp.
- Protozoal—*Anatrichosoma cutaneum*

ALLERGIC

- Dogs—atopy; food hypersensitivity; allergic contact dermatitis
- Cats—atopy; rare for flea allergy dermatitis, adverse food reaction (food hypersensitivity), or contact dermatitis to involve paws

IMMUNE-MEDIATED

- Dogs—pemphigus foliaceus; systemic lupus erythematosus; erythema multiforme; toxic epidermal necrolysis; vasculitis; cold agglutinin disease; pemphigus vulgaris; bullous pemphigoid; epidermolysis bullosa acquisita
- Cats—pemphigus foliaceus; systemic lupus erythematosus; erythema multiforme; toxic epidermal necrolysis; vasculitis; cold agglutinin disease; plasma cell pododermatitis (Figs. 9-8, 9-9)

ENDOCRINE/METABOLIC

- Dogs—hypothyroidism; hyperadrenocorticism; hepatocutaneous syndrome (necrolytic migratory erythema)
- Cats—hypothyroidism; hyperadrenocorticism; cutaneous xanthomatosis (secondary to diabetes mellitus or idiopathic); endocrine pododermatitis rare

Table 9-1

Differential Diagnosis of Footpad and Claw Disorders

There are a number of disorders that affect the footpads, interdigital spaces, nail, and nailbeds of both dogs and cats. The following information is presented as a simplistic chart that may be helpful in narrowing the differentials included for the individual case. More detailed information can be found in subsequent portions of the text.

Footpads

Differential Diagnosis	Comments	Diagnostic Tests	Treatment
Traumatic/Irritant	–Rough ground surfaces predispose to erosions –Caustic cleaning agents –Cat litter with deodorizers, etc.	–History	–Avoidance –Rest from exercise –Booties
Idiopathic Hyperkeratosis	–May be coupled with nasal hyperkeratosis –"Feathers" or fronds of keratin at margins –May fissure or cause pain	–History/clinical ± biopsy	–Kerasolv*DVM –RetinA –Vitamin E topical
Neoplastic	–Bronchogenic adenocarcinoma (mass) –Epitheliotropic lymphoma—depigmentation, ulceration, etc. –Squamous cell carcinoma –Melanomas –Mast cell tumors –Keratoacanthomas –Inverted papillomas –Eccrine adenocarcinomas –Spinocellular epithelioma –Malignant fibrous histiocytoma –Fibrosarcoma	–Biopsy/radiographs	–Variable

Differential Diagnosis	Comments	Diagnostic Tests	Treatment
Zinc Responsive	–Recognized in the dog –Marked hyperkeratosis	–Biopsy	–Zinc methionine @ 2 mg/kg/day –Zinc sulfate @ 10 mg/kg/day ± EFA
Pemphigus Complex	–Mild to severe hyperkeratosis with focal crusts secondary to ruptured pustules –Thick exudative paronychia/pyonychia (cat)	–Cytology for acantholysis –Biopsy to confirm Dx	–Prednisone @ 1 mg/# divided bid –Imuran (dog) @ 1 mg/kg/day –Leukeran (cat) 0.2 mg/kg/day or every other day
Bullous Pemphigoid	–Hyperkeratosis, ulceration, depigmentation	–Biopsy	–Same as above
Superficial Necrolytic Dermatitis (hepatocutaneous syndrome)	–Severe hyperkeratosis, ulceration, erosion –Rarely, associated with diabetes, gastric carcinoma, pancreatic adenocarcinoma; commonly, associated with hepatic disease –Interdigital regions also affected –Claws may slough in severe cases	–Biopsy –Ultrasound –Serum chemistry	–No cure to date –Supportive Tx –Corticosteroids
Vasculitis	–Ulceration/erosions –"Punched-out" lesions on pads –Central portions of pads often affected rather than periphery	–Serum chemistry –ANA (SLE) –Tick serology –Cutaneous "deep" biopsy	–Corticosteroids –Dapsone –Trental –Imuran/Leukeran –Tetracycline/niacinamide
Drug Eruption	–Crusting, erosion, ulceration, erythema, sloughing (toxic epidermal necrolysis)	–Biopsy	–Withdrawal of drug –Corticosteroids are debatable
Acrodermatitis	–Autosomal recessive trait in bull terriers –Hyperkeratosis and fissuring of the pads –Interdigital and nailfold inflammation	–Signalment –Biopsy	–Zinc supplementation –Supportive care

(*continued*)

Table 9-1 (Continued)

Differential Diagnosis	Comments	Diagnostic Tests	Treatment
Calcinosis Circumscripta	–Rare, idiopathic –Most cases associated with renal failure or parathyroid hyperplasia –Swollen pads with chalky white infiltrate	–Serum chemistry –Biopsy	–DMSO topical
Cutaneous Horns	–More common in the cat –May be associated with FeLV & FIV –Rarely, may have neoplastic base	–FeLV & FIV –Clinical/biopsy	–Excision, if needed
Feline Eosinophilic Granuloma Complex	–Plaques and granulomas on the footpads	–Biopsy	–Allergy work-up –Corticosteroids
Cutaneous Xanthomatosis	–Primarily cats –Idiopathic or associated with diabetes –Abnormal lipid metabolism –Yellow-pink plaques that may ulcerate	–Biopsy –Hematology	–Correct metabolic disease –Diet manipulation
Feline Plasma Cell Pododermatitis	–Swollen metacarpal & metatarsal pads –May ulcerate –May be associated with FIV	–Biopsy –Hematology	–Corticosteroids –Leukeran –Gold salts
Feline Paraneoplastic Syndrome	–Pancreatic adenocarcinoma –Bile duct carcinoma –Scale/crust/fissures	–Biopsy	–No Tx
Noninflammatory Hypomelanosis	–Loss of pigment without inflammation –Often associated with "vitiligo" or idiopathic leukoderma/leukotrichia	–Clinical or biopsy	–No Tx

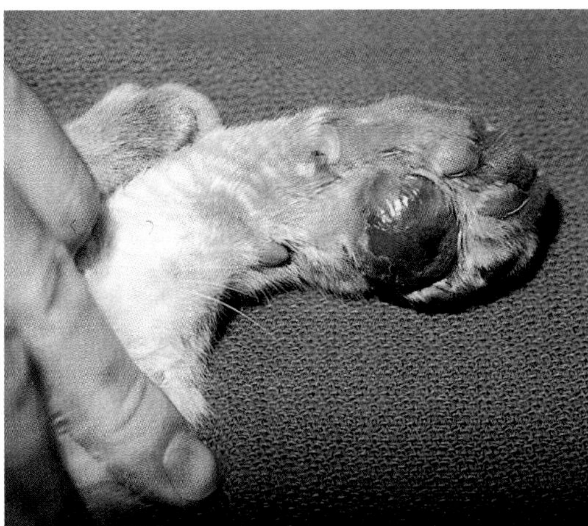

Figure 9-8 Plasma cell pododermatitis. Primarily affects the metacarpal and metatarsal pads, leaving the digital pads within normal limits. Affected pads are swollen and spongy and may or may not have focal erosions and ulcerations.

NEOPLASTIC

- Higher incidence in cats than in dogs
- Dogs—squamous cell carcinomas; melanomas; mast cell tumors; keratoacanthomas; inverted papillomas, eccrine adenocarcinomas
- Cats—papillomas; spinocellular epithelioma; trichoepithelioma; fibrosarcoma; malignant fibrous histiocytoma; metastatic primary adenocarcinoma of the lung; other metastatic carcinomas

ENVIRONMENTAL

- Dogs—irritant contact dermatitis; trauma; concrete and gravel dog runs; excessive exercise; clipper burn; foreign bodies (grass awns, bristle-like hairs of short-coated dogs); thallium toxicity; rock-salt exposure (Fig. 9-10)
- Cats—irritant contact dermatitis; foreign bodies; thallium toxicity

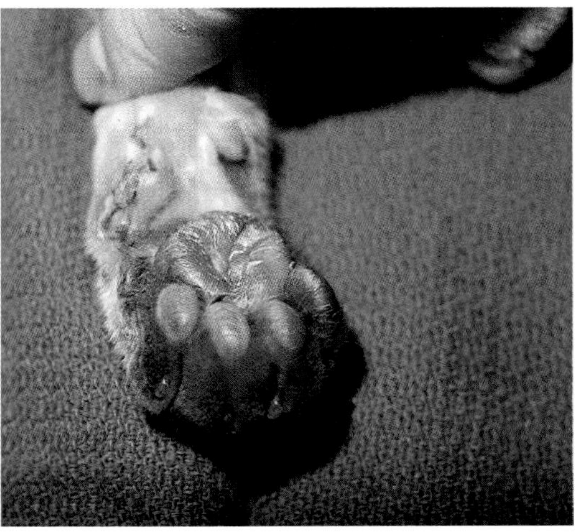

Figure 9-9 Plasma cell pododermatitis. Note how easy the affected pads compress.

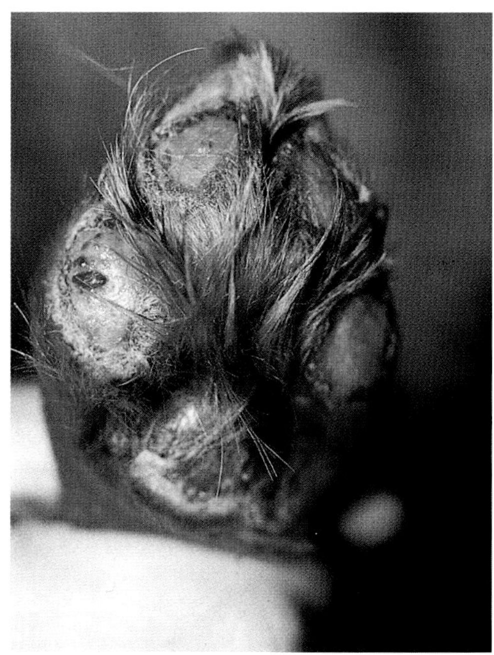

Figure 9-10 Footpad erosion and ulceration secondary to rock salt exposure along the streets of New York City after a snowstorm.

Diagnostics

CBC/Biochemistry/Urinalysis

Depend on the underlying cause

Other Laboratory Tests

Endocrine tests, serology, or immune studies

Imaging

- Radiographs and ultrasound
- Neoplastic—depending on the underlying cause, may be necessary to confirm systemic disease or stage tumors

Diagnostic Procedures

- Skin scrapings, fungal culture, and a stained smear of any exudate or pustule contents
- Biopsy—histopathology very helpful; immunohistochemical staining may be necessary; immunoperoxidase or immunofluorescence
- Food elimination diet
- Intradermal skin testing
- Endocrine tests
- Dogs—biopsies indicated if skin scrapings are negative and lesions (nodules, draining tracts) are seen

- Cats—biopsies may be indicated in all cases, because pedal dermatosis is relatively rare

Therapeutics

Nursing Care

Foot soaks, hot packing, and/or bandaging may be necessary, depending on cause.

Diet

Hypoallergenic diet—determine food hypersensitivity

Client Education

- Depends on underlying cause and severity of condition
- Discuss husbandry, lifestyle, and preventative medical practices.
- For allergic, immune-mediated, or endocrine causes, client must understand that condition will be managed, not cured.

Surgical Considerations

- Melanomas and squamous cell carcinomas—very poor prognosis; early diagnosis necessitates removal of the digit, digits, or paw
- Infectious—may benefit from surgical débridement of devitalized tissue before medical therapy

Drugs of Choice

- Long-term antibiotics, antifungals, anti-inflammatory or immunosuppressive levels of corticosteroids, chemotherapeutic agents, hormone-replacement therapy, or zinc supplementation
- Depend on the underlying cause and secondary infections

Comments

Patient Monitoring

Depends on the underlying cause and treatment protocol selected

Prevention/Avoidance

- Environmental cause—good husbandry and preventative medical practices should avoid recurrence
- Allergic cause—important to avoid the allergen (inhalant or food), if possible

Expected Course and Prognosis

- Success of therapy depends on finding the underlying cause; often the cause is unknown; even when the cause is known, management can be frustrating owing to relapses or lack of affordable therapeutics.
- Often the disease can only be managed and not cured.
- Surgical intervention is sometimes the only option.

PREGNANCY

Avoid systemically administered corticosteroids, antifungals, chemotherapeutic agents, azathioprine, and certain antimicrobials (e.g., enrofloxacin) in pregnant animals.

Suggested Reading

Foil CS. Disorders of the feet and claws. Paper presented at the 11th Kal Kan Symposium.

Guaguere E, Hubert B, Delabre C. Feline pyodermatoses. Vet Dermatol 1992;3:1–12.

White SD. Pododermatitis. Vet Dermatol 1989;1:1–18.

Consulting Editor Karen Helton Rhodes

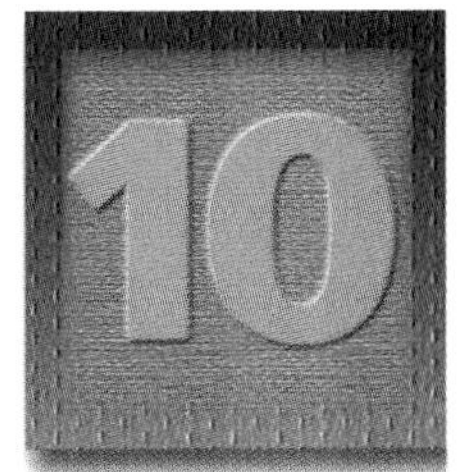

Nail and Nailbed Disorders

Ellen C. Codner and Karen Helton Rhodes

Definition/Overview

- Paronychia/pyonychia inflammation of soft tissue around the nail
- Onychomycosis—fungal infection of the nail
- Onychorrhexis—brittle nails that tend to split or break
- Onychomadesis—sloughing of the nail
- Nail dystrophy—deformity caused by abnormal growth

Etiology/Pathophysiology

- Nails and nailfolds—subject to trauma, infection, vascular insufficiency, immune-mediated disease, neoplasia, defects in keratinization, and congenital abnormalities
- A particular nail deformity may be caused by a variety of diseases.
- A single disease can present with various nail lesions.
- Sometimes, the cause is unknown.

Signalment/History

- Dachshund—predisposed to onychorrhexis
- Large breed dogs seem to be predisposed to lupoid onychodystrophy.

- History is variable and dependent on the specific etiology
- May be slowly progressive or acute in onset

Clinical Features

- Licking of the area
- Lameness
- Pain
- Swelling, erythema, and exudate of nailfold
- Deformity or sloughing of nail

Differential Diagnosis

Paronychia/Pyonychia (Table 10-1)

- Infection—bacteria, dermatophyte, yeast (*Candida*), demodicosis, leishmaniasis
- Immune-mediated—pemphigus, bullous pemphigoid, SLE, drug eruption, lupoid onychodystrophy
- Neoplasia—squamous cell carcinoma, melanoma, eccrine carcinoma, osteosarcoma, subungual keratoacanthoma, inverted squamous papilloma
- Arteriovenous fistula
- Immune-mediated disease (cat)

Onychomycosis

- Dogs—*Trichophyton mentagrophytes*—usually generalized (Fig. 10-1)
- Cats—*Microsporum canis*

Onychorrhexis

- Idiopathic—especially in dachshunds; multiple nails
- Trauma
- Infection—dermatophytosis, leishmaniasis

Onychomadesis

- Trauma
- Infection
- Immune-mediated—pemphigus, bullous pemphigoid, SLE, drug eruption, lupoid onychodystrophy
- Vascular insufficiency—vasculitis, cold agglutinin disease
- Neoplasia—see above
- Idiopathic

Nail Dystrophy

- Acromegaly
- Feline hyperthyroidism
- Zinc-responsive dermatosis
- Congenital malformations

Table 10-1

Nail and Nailbed Disorders

Differential Diagnosis	Comments	Diagnostic Tests	Treatment
Fungal Infections	–Rare –One or two affected nails –Trichophyton most often –Friable, misshapen nail	–Difficult to culture, shave off portions of proximal nail	–Oral and topical antifungals –Aggressive Tx –Severe; P3 digit amputation
Bacterial Infections	–Secondary, opportunistic –Rare, primary –Paronychia, swelling, pain –Severe case, slough nail –Extension osteomyelitis –Usually one or two nails	–Biopsy –Culture & sensitivity	–Avulsion of affected nails –Systemic and topical antibiotics
"Lupoid" Onychodystrophy	–Common to see all nails affected –Nails seem to separate, lift, and fall off ± pain –Paronychia absent	–Clinical –Biopsy (P3 digit amp.) –ANA negative	–Antibiotics, secondary –EFA –Tetracycline/niacinamide –Corticosteroids –Trental
Immune-Mediated Skin Disease	–Pemphigus, BP, SLE, vasculitis –Pyonychia; PF cats –Sloughing of nails with paronychia	–CBC, SMA, ANA –Biopsy	–Corticosteroids –Chemotherapeutic agents

(*continued*)

Table 10-1 (Continued)

Differential Diagnosis	Comments	Diagnostic Tests	Treatment
Neoplasia	–Squamous cell carcinoma, melanoma, MCT, keratoacanthoma, neurofibrosarcoma, hemangiopericytoma, osteosarcoma, myxosarcoma, lymphosarcoma –Originate from distal digit/claw or claw fold –Digit swelling, paronychia, dystrophic claw or sloughed claw	–Biopsy	–Digit amputation, etc.
Idiopathic Onychodystrophy	–Deformed brittle nails (onychorrhexis) –Deformed soft nails (onychomalacia) –Reported in: dachshund, husky, Rhodesian ridgeback, German shepherd		

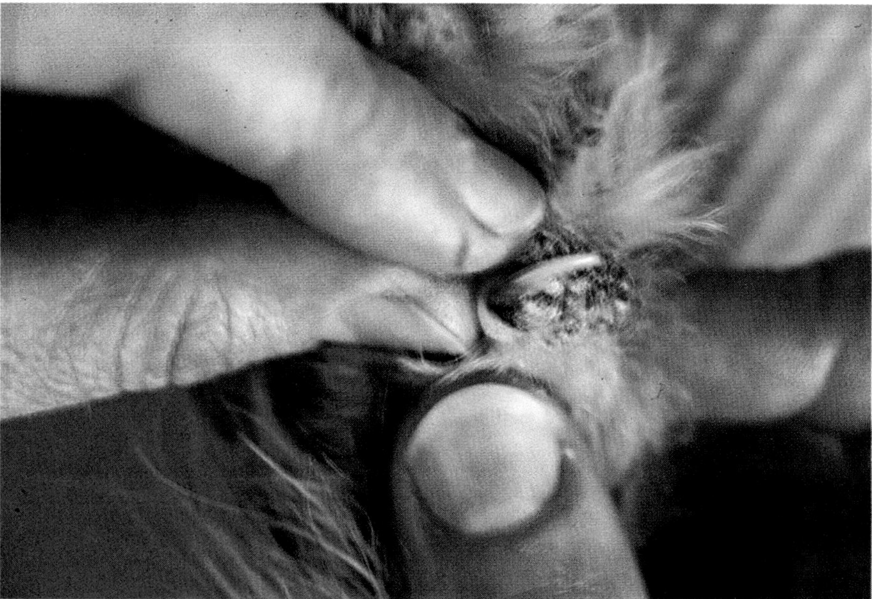

Figure 10-1 Paronychia/pyonychia of a cat with pemphigus foliaceus (PF). PF in cats is often characterized by a cheesy exudate that is expressed when the nail is extruded.

Diagnostics

CBC/Biochemistry/Urinalysis

May show evidence of SLE, diabetes mellitus, hyperthyroidism, or other systemic illness

Other Laboratory Tests

- FeLV
- T_4
- ANA titer

Imaging

Radiographs—osteomyelitis of third phalanx

Other Diagnostic Procedures

- Biopsy—histopathology and direct immunofluorescence; often involves a third phalanx amputation
- Cytology of exudate
- Skin scraping
- Bacterial and fungal culture

Therapeutics

Paronychia

- Surgical removal of nail plate (shell)—provide adequate drainage; grasp nail firmly with hemostat and strip it from its attachments with one swift downward motion; bandage foot following procedure

- Antimicrobial soaks
- Identify underlying condition and treat specifically.

Onychomycosis

- Antifungal soaks—chlorhexidine, povidone iodine, lime sulfur
- Surgical removal of nail plate—may improve response to systemic medication
- Amputation of third phalanx

Onychorrhexis

- Repair with fingernail glue (type used to attach false nails in humans).
- Remove splintered pieces.
- Amputation of third phalanx
- Treat underlying cause.

Onychomadesis

- Antimicrobial soaks
- Treat underlying cause.

Neoplasia

- Depends on biologic behavior of specific tumor
- Surgical excision
- Amputation of digit
- Amputation of leg
- Chemotherapy
- Radiation therapy

Nail Dystrophy

Treat underlying cause.

Drugs of Choice

- Bacterial paronychia—systemic antibiotics based on culture and sensitivity; cephalosporins pending culture result
- *Candida paronychia*—ketoconazole (10 mg/kg PO q12h); topical nystatin or miconazole
- Onychomycosis—griseofulvin (50–150 mg/kg PO per day) or ketoconazole (10 mg/kg PO q12h) for 6–12 months until negative cultures; itraconazole (10 mg/kg PO daily) for 3 weeks and then pulse therapy twice a week until resolved
- Onychomadesis—depends on cause; immunosuppressive therapy for immune-mediated diseases

Medication Precautions

- Griseofulvin—may cause bone marrow suppression, anorexia, vomiting, and diarrhea (cats); absorption enhanced if given with a high-fat meal; do not use in pregnant animals
- Ketoconazole—may cause anorexia, gastric irritation, hepatic toxicity, and lightening of the hair coat

Comments

- Trauma or neoplasia often affects a single nail.
- Involvement of multiple nails suggests a systemic disease.
- Immune-mediated diseases (except lupoid onychodystrophy) usually have other skin lesions in addition to nail/nailfold lesions.
- Paronychia (infectious)—immunosuppression (endogenous or exogenous), FeLV infection, trauma, and diabetes mellitus
- Bacterial onychomadesis—excessively short nail trimming (into the quick)

Expected Course and Prognosis

- Bacterial or fungal paronychia and onychomycosis—treatment may be prolonged and response may be influenced by underlying immunosuppressive factors
- Onychomycosis and onychorrhexis—may require amputation of the third phalanx for resolution
- Nail dystrophy—prognosis is good when underlying cause can be effectively treated (e.g., hyperthyroidism, zinc-responsive dermatosis)
- Onychomadesis—prognosis depends on underlying cause; immune-mediated diseases and vascular problems carry a more guarded prognosis than do trauma or infectious causes
- Neoplasia—some can be totally excised or removed by amputation of the digit; others are highly malignant and may have already spread by the time of diagnosis

Abbreviations

- ANA = antinuclear antibody
- FeLV = feline leukemia virus
- SLE = systemic lupus erythematosus

Suggested Reading

Muller GH, Kirk RW, Scott DW. Small animal dermatology. 4th ed. Philadelphia: Saunders, 1989.

Authors Ellen C. Codner and Karen Helton Rhodes
Consulting Editor Karen Helton Rhodes

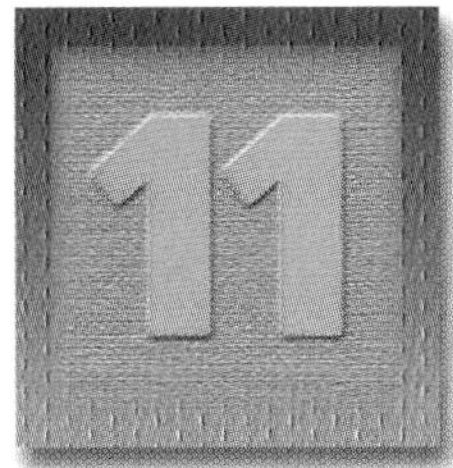

Interdigital Dermatitis

David Duclos and Karen Helton Rhodes

Definition/Overview

- Disease of the feet of dogs
- Also known as pododermatitis, interdigital pyoderma, pedal folliculitis, and furunculosis

Etiology/Pathophysiology

- Infectious—bacterial and fungal; bacterial most common and may be primary or secondary; often recurrent; immunosuppression/immunodeficiency always a question
- Allergic, metabolic, trauma, irritant, parasitic, immune-mediated, nutritional, idiopathic (See Table 11-1)

Signalment/History

- Dogs of any age, sex, or breed
- Short-coated male dogs (e.g., English bulldogs, Great Danes, basset hounds, mastiffs, bull terriers, boxers, dachshunds, Dalmatians, German short-haired pointers, and Weimaraners) may be predisposed.
- Some long-coated breeds (e.g., German shepherds, Labrador retrievers, golden retrievers, Irish setters, and Pekingese) are possibly predisposed.

Clinical Features

- May affect one foot and one interdigital space or multiple interdigital spaces and feet
- Diseased tissue—usually erythematous and swollen; has either intact bullae, ruptured draining tracts, or both (often appears cystic)
- Sometimes mild to severe swelling of the affected feet
- Mild to severe lameness may be seen.

Differential Diagnosis

One Affected Foot

- Foreign bodies (e.g., grass awns, wood slivers, suture material)
- Osteomyelitis
- Neoplasia
- Infection—bacterial or fungal

More Than One Affected Foot

- Hypersensitivity reaction—food, atopy, contact dermatitis (Fig. 11-1)
- Infection—bacterial, fungal, yeast (Fig. 11-2)
- Trauma—clipper burns, cuts
- Chemical—contact irritant dermatitis
- Metabolic—hypothyroidism, hyperadrenocorticism
- Parasitic—demodicosis often complicated by the presence of furunculosis and draining tracts; heartworm, hookworm, and pelodera result in erythema, pruritus, and patchy alopecia of the feet; pelodera affects the limbs and the ventral abdomen (Fig. 11-3)

Figure 11-1 Interdigital dermatitis characterized by erythema and secondary bacterial infection as a result of allergic dermatitis.

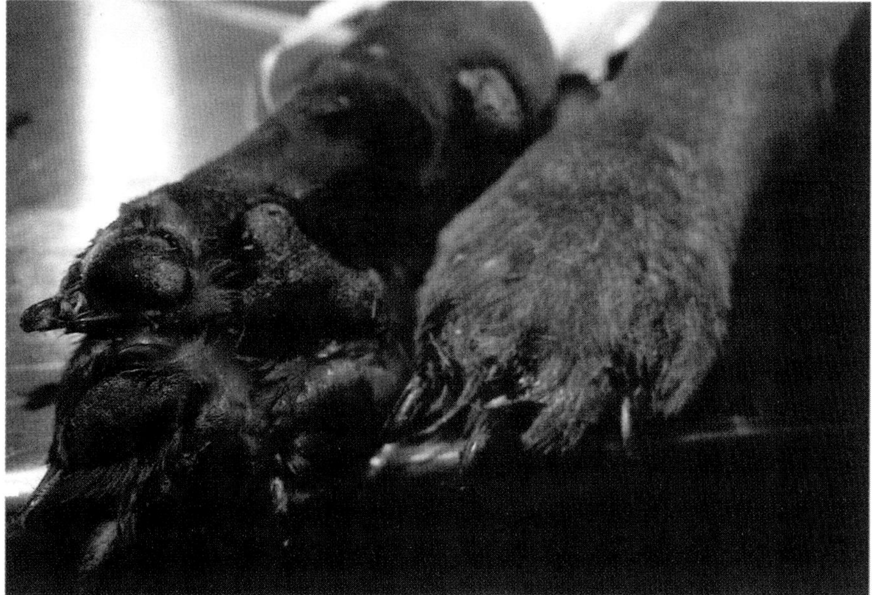

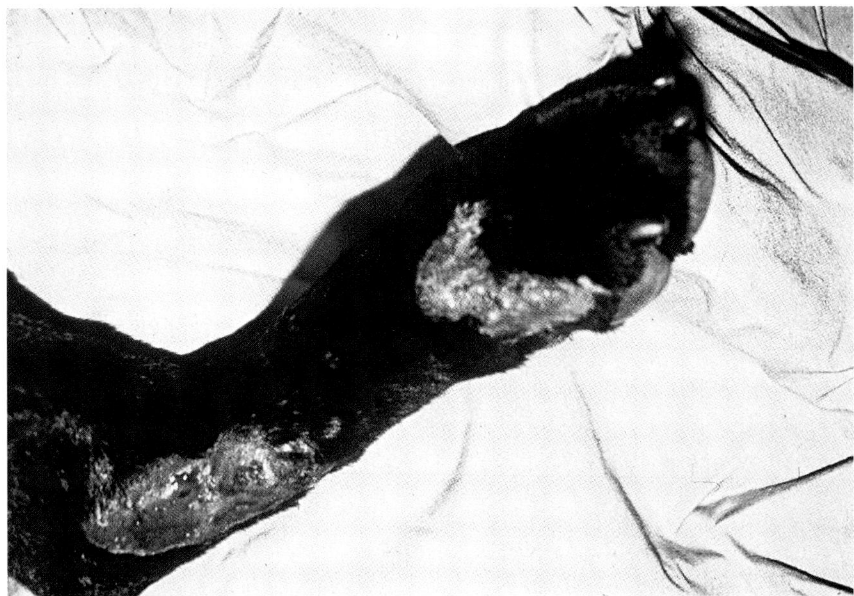

Figure 11-2 Folliculitis and furunculosis with associated alopecia of the extremity of this young dog with deep staphylococcal infection.

Figure 11-3 Pododemodicosis and bacterial furunculosis.

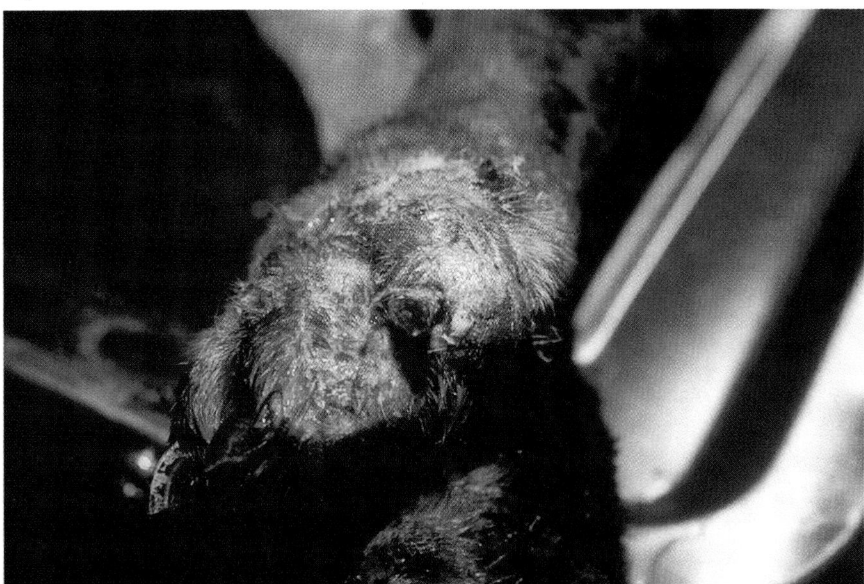

- Idiopathic
- Immune mediated—pemphigus, pemphigoid, systemic lupus erythematosus
- Zinc deficiency or zinc responsive
- Superficial necrolytic dermatitis (hepatocutaneous syndrome)
- Foreign body reaction—(e.g., grass awns); often one foot yet may be multiple

Diagnostics

CBC/Biochemistry/Urinalysis

- Usually normal
- Superficial necrolytic dermatitis—may have high liver and pancreatic enzyme activities

Other Laboratory Tests

- Blood tests—heartworm microfilaria
- Thyroid hormone tests—hypothyroidism
- Adrenal response tests (low-dose dexamethasone-suppression test, urine cortisol: creatinine ratio, ACTH stimulation)—hyperadrenocorticism

Imaging

Radiographs—underlying osteomyelitis

Diagnostic Procedures

- Biopsies—foreign bodies, demodicosis, neoplasia, infectious agents (fungi, bacteria) or other parasites (heartworm and, rarely, hookworm); other than causal findings listed above (e.g., parasites and bacteria), the reaction pattern is a folliculitis, perifolliculitis, and pyogranulomatous dermatitis if the follicles have ruptured
- Skin scrapings—identify parasites (demodicosis), pelodera, or fungi (dermatophytosis)
- Fecal flotation—identify hookworm ova
- Cytologic examination of the exudate with Wright-Giemsa stain—identify yeast, bacteria, and (rarely) parasites; evaluate the type of inflammatory response (e.g., eosinophils may suggest parasites or hypersensitivity)
- Culture—bacterial and fungal

Therapeutics

- Treatments are directed at an underlying cause, if determined.
- If a bacterial cause is suspected, then start immediate treatment with a broad-spectrum antibiotic while pending culture and sensitivity results (i.e., amoxicillin with clavulanate or cephalosporins).
- Antibiotic therapy must be used for an extended period of time (minimum of 6–8 weeks).
- Most infections are gram-positive *Staphylococcus intermedius* yet gram-negative infections may also occur (e.g., *Pseudomonas*) and may be difficult to control.

Table 11-1

Interdigital Dermatitis

Infectious Bacterial/Fungal	–Erythema, swelling, exudation, draining tracts –Fungal "kerions" –Primary or secondary –Often "mistakenly" called cysts owing to granuloma formation	–Biopsy –Culture & Sensitivity	–Long-term antibiotics or antifungals –Aggressive topical Tx
Foreign Bodies	–Plant awns, glass, etc.	–Surgical exploration –Biopsy	
Allergic Dermatitis	–Alopecia, erythema, salivary staining of the dorsum of the digits –Pruritus always a feature	–Skin scraping –Allergy work-up	–Antihistamines –Corticosteroids –Hyposensitization –EFA –Topicals
Demodicosis	–Erythema, swelling, alopecia –Common secondary bacterial component	–Skin scraping –Biopsy, if furunculosis	–Ivermectin –Mitaban dips –Milbemycin (LymDip—cat)
Parasitic	–Erythema, alopecia	–Biopsy	–Parasiticides
Neoplasia	Squamous cell carcinoma, melanoma, MCT, keratoacanthoma, neurofibrosarcoma, hemangiopericytoma, osteosarcoma, myxosarcoma, lymphosarcoma –Originate from distal digit/claw or claw fold –Digit swelling, paronychia, dystrophic claw or sloughed claw	–Biopsy	–Digit amputation, etc.
Idiopathic Onychodystrophy	–Deformed brittle nails (onychorrhexis) –Deformed soft nails (onychomalacia) –Reported in: dachshund, husky, Rhodesian ridgeback, German Shepherd		

- Choice of antibiotic depends on sensitivity: frequent options with good clinical results include cephalosporins, fluoroquinolones, dicloxacillin, carbenicillin, ciprofloxacin, etc.
- Draining lesions—twice-daily foot soaks with a mild astringent such as Burrows solution (10–15 minutes)
- Shampooing the feet daily with a benzoyl peroxide product is often very helpful.
- Topical therapy with mupirocin ointment or benzoyl peroxide gel tid
- May be beneficial to restrict activity or protect the feet
- Severe refractory cases may require surgical debridement and removal of the interdigital web (fusion podoplasty).

Comments

- Rifampin—use with caution for short periods (30–60 days) at 5–10 mg/kg q24h; penetrates deep lesions well owing to its lipid solubility; must be accompanied by a good antibiotic, because bacteria rapidly develop resistance
- Monitor liver enzymes and CBC every 2 weeks.
- Do not use with liver disease.
- Stimulates liver enzymes involved in drug metabolism and thus can influence the metabolism of concurrently administered drugs; concentrations of anticoagulants, digioxin, corticosteroids, and other drugs become subtherapeutic.
- When rifampin and ketoconazole are administered concurrently, both drugs are subtherapeutic.
- Use caution when concurrently administering other drugs.
- Monitor closely to detect the underlying cause; though often tedious, it is essential for complete resolution and healing.
- Medication should be continued for extended periods of time; 6–8 weeks is often the minimum.
- Because of extensive furunculosis the lesions are often markedly granulomatous. This granulation tissue tends to "wall off" the bacteria and "protect" the organisms from antibiotics. Rifampin has the ability to penetrate granulation tissue and may be an adjunct to therapy.

Suggested Reading

Scott DW. Canine pododermatitis. In: Kirk RW, ed. Current veterinary therapy, small animal practice VII. Philadelphia: Saunders, 1980:467–469

Consulting Editor Karen Helton Rhodes

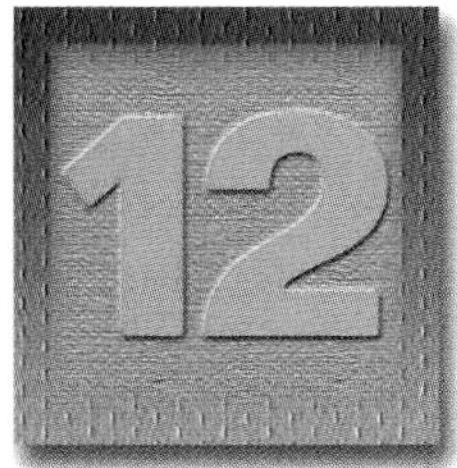

Nasal Dermatosis

Ellen C. Codner and Karen Helton Rhodes

Definition/Overview

Pathologic condition of the nasal skin involving either the haired portion (bridge of the nose) or nonhaired portion (nasal planum)

Etiology/Pathophysiology

- Bacterial
- Fungal: dermatophytosis, sporotrichosis, cryptococcosis, aspergillosis
- Immunologic: DLE/SLE, pemphigus complex, uveodermatologic syndrome
- Environmental: sun exposure
- Drug eruption/reaction
- Neoplasia
- Nutritional: zinc-responsive dermatosis, generic dog-food–induced hyperkeratosis
- Miscellaneous: trauma, idiopathic sterile granuloma, vitiligo (idiopathic leukoderma/leukotrichia), nasal hypopigmentation, dermatomyositis

Signalment/History

- Dermatophytosis, zinc-responsive dermatosis, dermatomyositis, and demodicosis—more likely in dogs < 1 year of age
- Zinc-responsive dermatosis—Siberian huskies, Alaskan malamutes

- Dermatomyositis—collies, Shetland sheepdogs
- Uveodermatologic syndrome—akitas, Samoyeds, Siberian huskies
- SLE and DLE—collies, Shetland sheepdogs, German shepherds; DLE may occur more often in females
- Epidermotropic lymphoma—old dogs

Risk Factors

- Adult cats—may be inapparent carriers of dermatophytes
- Rooting behavior—pyoderma, dermatophytosis
- Sun exposure—nasal solar dermatitis, DLE, SLE, pemphigus erythematosus
- Poorly pigmented nose—nasal solar dermatitis, squamous cell carcinoma
- Large, rapidly growing breeds oversupplemented with calcium or fed high-cereal diet—zinc-responsive dermatosis
- Immunosuppression—demodicosis, pyoderma, dermatophytosis

Clinical Features

- Depigmentation
- Hyperpigmentation
- Erythema
- Erosion/ulceration
- Vesicles/pustules
- Crusts
- Scarring
- Alopecia
- Nodules/plaques

Differential Diagnosis

Nasal Solar Dermatitis

- Lesions—confined to nose; precipitated by heavy sunlight exposure
- Begins in poorly pigmented skin at junction of nasal planum and bridge of nose
- Negative DIF

DLE

- Primarily affects nasal area (Figs. 12-1, 12-2, 12-3)
- Exacerbated by sunlight
- Positive DIF at basement membrane zone
- Biopsy—interface dermatitis

SLE

- Multisystemic disease
- Skin lesions—often involve nose, face, mucocutaneous junctions; multifocal or generalized (Figs. 12-4, 12-5)
- ANA positive
- Positive DIF at basement membrane zone
- Biopsy—Interface dermatitis and vasculitis (may be variable)

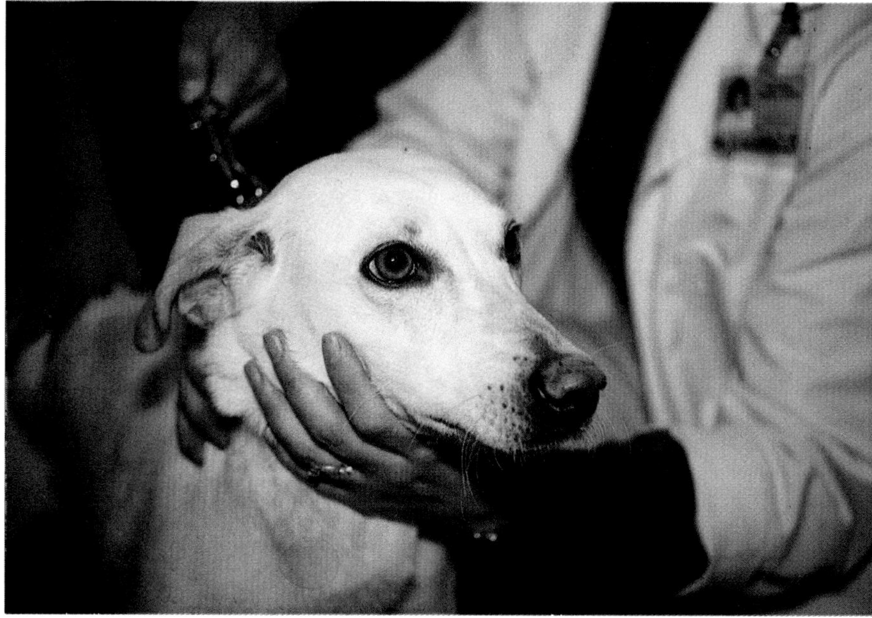

Figure 12-1 Three-year-old lab mix with progressive depigmentation with associated erythema and ulceration of the planum nasale characteristic of discoid lupus erythematosus.

Figure 12-2 Close-up view of Figure 12-1. Discoid lupus erythematosus.

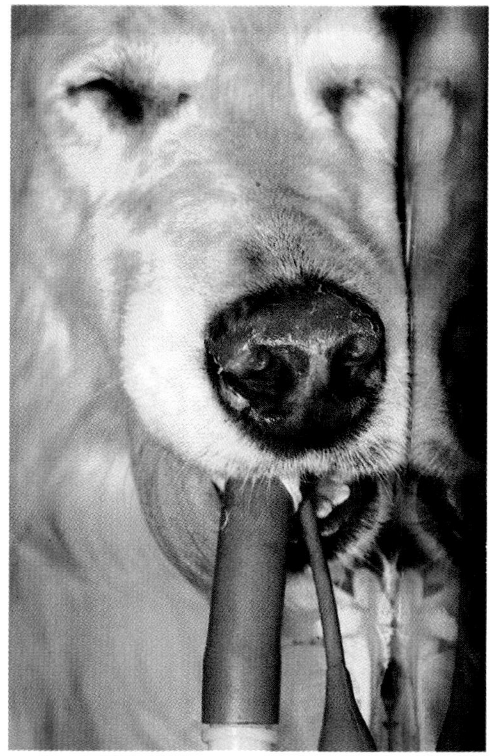

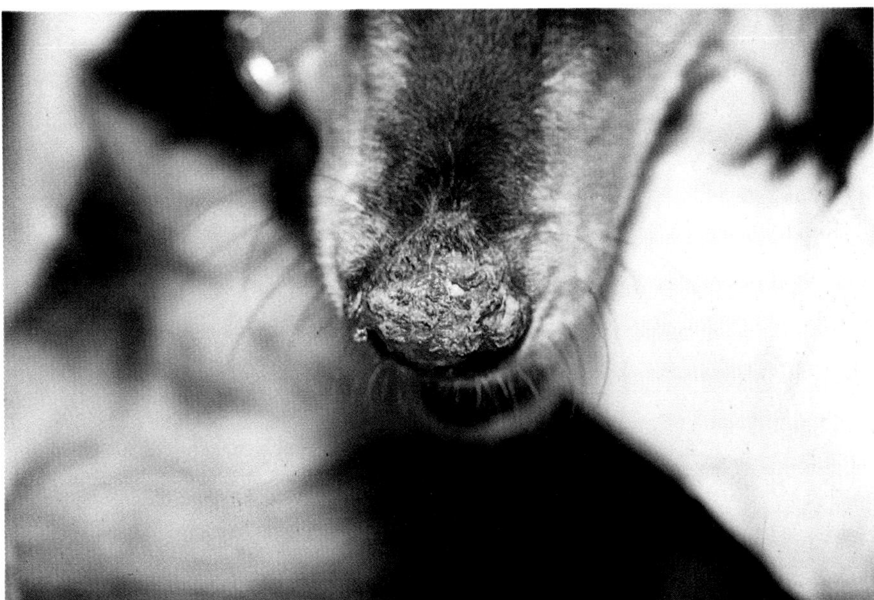

Figure 12-3 Advanced case of DLE demonstrating the remodeling of the planum nasale characteristic of chronic changes.

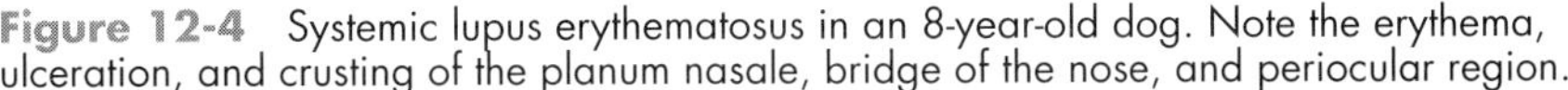

Figure 12-4 Systemic lupus erythematosus in an 8-year-old dog. Note the erythema, ulceration, and crusting of the planum nasale, bridge of the nose, and periocular region.

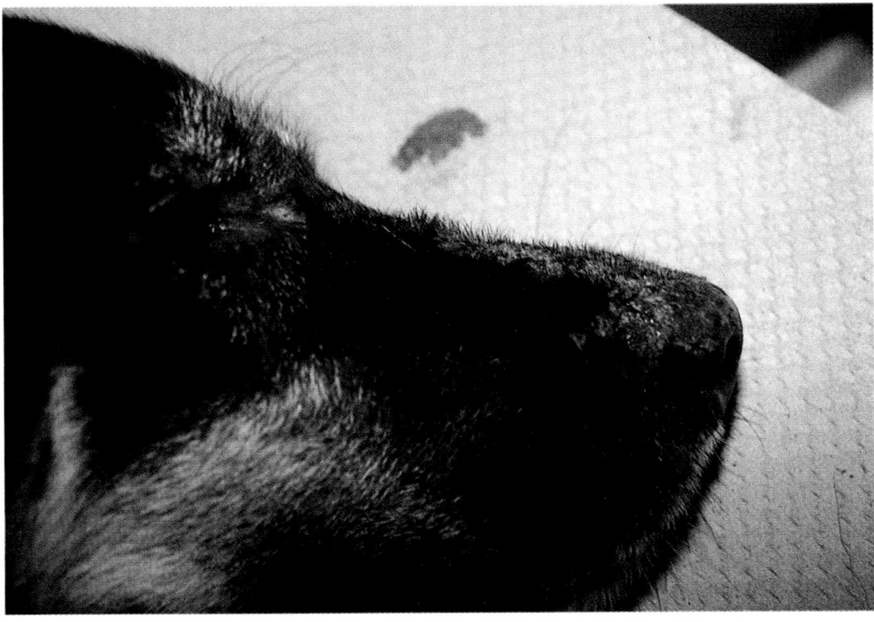

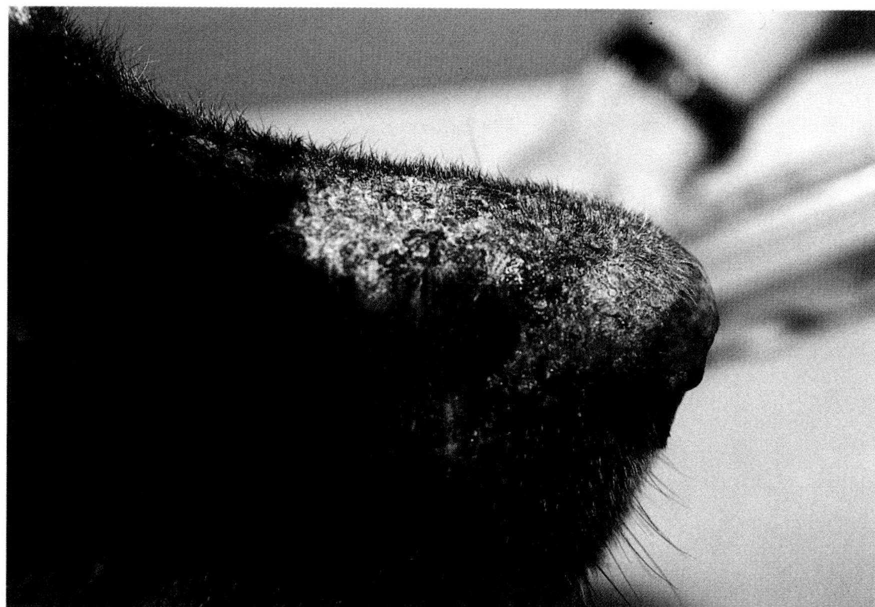

Figure 12-5 SLE. Close-up view of the bridge of the nose from Figure 12-3.

Pemphigus Foliaceus

- Lesions—usually start on face and ears; commonly involve footpads; eventually generalize (Fig. 12-6)
- Biopsy—subcorneal pustules with acantholysis
- Positive DIF in intercellular spaces of epidermis

Figure 12-6 Pemphigus foliaceus demonstrating the typical pattern of cutaneous involvement along the bridge of the nose and periocular region.

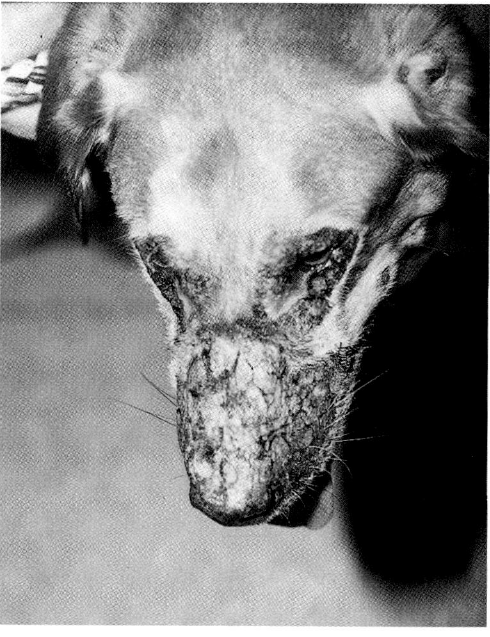

Pemphigus Erythematosus

- Lesions—primarily confined to face and ears
- Biopsy—intraepidermal pustules with acantholysis
- Positive DIF at basement membrane zone and intercellular spaces

Demodicosis

- Often starts on face or forelimbs
- May generalize
- Diagnose with skin scrapings

Plastic (or Rubber) Dish Dermatitis

- Depigmentation and erythema of anterior nasal planum and anterior lips
- No ulceration or crusting
- History of exposure, rare

Dermatomyositis

- Typical breed
- Nasal, facial, and extremity lesions—characterized by erosion, alopecia, scarring, and hyperpigmentation
- Polymyositis or megaesophagus may be seen.
- Biopsy—interface dermatitis with follicular atrophy
- Negative DIF

Uveodermatologic Syndrome

- Typical breed
- Uveitis and cutaneous macular depigmentation without inflammation—nose, lips, and eyelids (Fig. 12-7)
- Biopsy of early lesions—interface dermatitis, pigmentary incontinence

Zinc-responsive Dermatosis

- Typical signalment or diet (i.e., high-fiber or calcium supplementation)
- Crusted lesions—face, mucocutaneous junctions, pressure points, footpads
- Biopsy—parakeratotic hyperkeratosis

Other

- Nasal pyoderma—acute onset of folliculitis on haired portion of nose
- Dermatophytosis—haired portion of the nose; diagnose with culture or biopsy
- Vitiligo—cutaneous macular depigmentation without inflammation on nose, lips, eyelids, footpads, and nails; leukotrichia with leukoderma may be seen. (Figs. 12-8, 12-9)
- Nasal hypopigmentation—normal black coloration of nasal planum fades to light brown or whitish color; may be seasonal or wax and wane
- Topical drug hypersensitivity (neomycin)
- Tumors—SCC, basal cell carcinoma, mycosis fungoides, fibrosarcoma (Fig. 12-10)
- Trauma
- Idiopathic sterile granuloma
- Idiopathic nasal hyperkeratosis—dry, horny growths of keratin localized to nasal planum

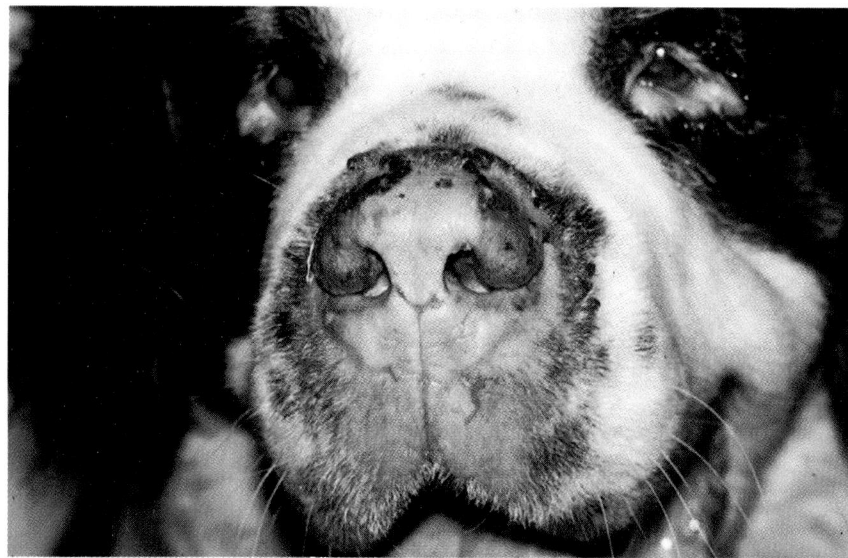

Figure 12-7 Uveodermatologic syndrome (Vogt Kayanagi Harada–like syndrome). Note the characteristic pattern of depigmentation and lack of associated inflammation, common in the early phases of the disease.

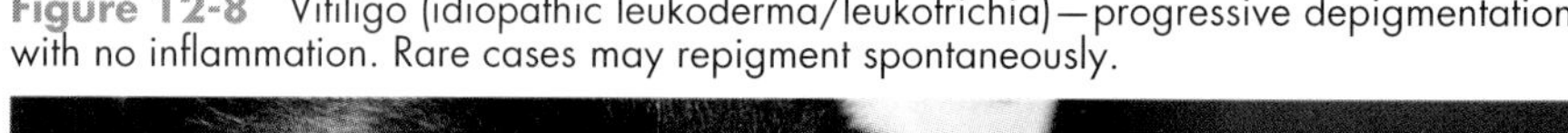

Figure 12-8 Vitiligo (idiopathic leukoderma/leukotrichia)—progressive depigmentation with no inflammation. Rare cases may repigment spontaneously.

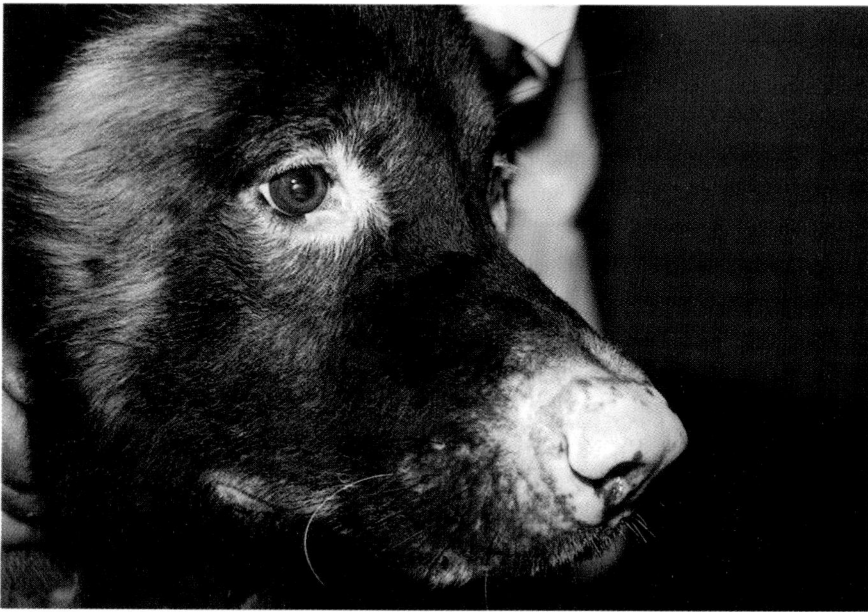

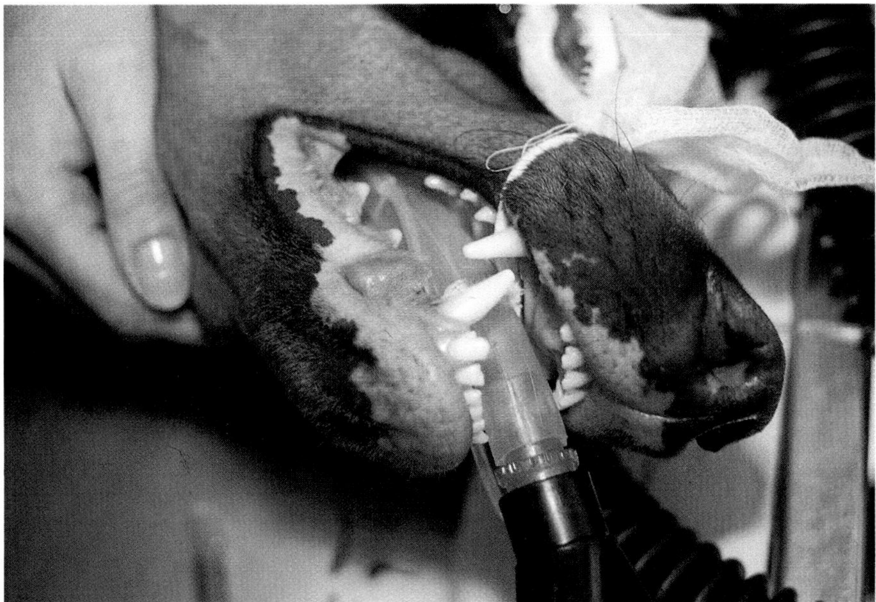

Figure 12-9 Vitiligo. Note the depigmentation of the mucocutaneous junction regions.

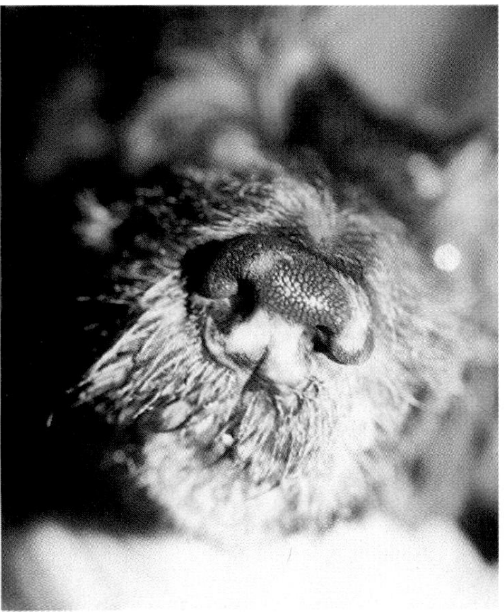

Figure 12-10 Cutaneous lymphoma in an 11-year-old dog with generalized scaling and depigmentation of the planum nasale.

Diagnostics

CBC/Biochemistry/Urinalysis

- Usually normal
- SLE—may see hemolytic anemia, thrombocytopenia, or evidence of glomerulonephritis (high BUN, proteinuria)

Diagnostic Procedures

- Skin scrapings—*Demodex*
- Cytology—fungal organisms, bacteria, or acantholytic cells (pemphigus)
- Dermatophyte test medium—dermatophytosis
- Culture on Sabouraud agar—other fungal infections
- Bacterial culture and sensitivity or cytologic evaluation—pyoderma
- Joint tap—evidence of polyarthritis in SLE
- ANA—positive in most cases of SLE
- Ocular examination—uveitis in uveodermatologic syndrome
- ECG—evidence of myocarditis in SLE
- EMG—evidence of polymyositis in SLE and dermatomyositis
- DIF—deposition of immunoglobulin at the basement membrane zone in DLE, SLE, and pemphigus erythematosus and intercellular spaces of epidermis in pemphigus foliaceus and pemphigus erythematosus
- Skin biopsy

Pathologic Findings

- Folliculitis/furunculosis (± mites, bacteria, or fungal elements)—demodicosis, dermatophytosis, nasal pyoderma
- Follicular atrophy and perifollicular fibrosis—dermatomyositis
- Interface dermatitis—DLE, SLE, dermatomyositis, uveodermatologic syndrome
- Intraepidermal pustules with acantholysis—pemphigus foliaceus and pemphigus erythematosus
- Parakeratotic hyperkeratosis—zinc-responsive dermatosis
- Hypomelanosis—vitiligo, uveodermatologic syndrome
- Granulomatous/pyogranulomatous dermatitis—pyoderma, fungal, foreign body, idiopathic sterile granuloma

Therapeutics

- Outpatient, except SLE with severe multiorgan dysfunction or tumors requiring surgical excision or radiation therapy
- Reduce exposure to sunlight—DLE, SLE, pemphigus erythematosus, nasal solar dermatitis, squamous cell carcinoma
- Discourage rooting behavior—pyoderma, dermatophytosis
- Warm soaks—aid removal of exudate and crusts
- Replace plastic or rubber dish and avoid contact with topical drug or other agent causing hypersensitivity reaction.

Drugs

- Fungal infections—systemic antifungals: griseofulvin, ketoconazole, itraconazole (drug of choice in the cat); topical enilconazole for aspergillosis; surgical excision of early discrete lesions
- Nasal solar dermatitis—topical corticosteroids; antibiotics for secondary infection; sunscreens; tattoo hypopigmented skin (not currently used)
- Idiopathic sterile granuloma—surgical excision when feasible; immunosuppressive therapy with glucocorticoids ± azathioprine or leukeran; trental; tetracycline: niacinamide
- SLE—immunosuppressive therapy with prednisolone ± azathioprine (dogs), chlorambucil, or gold salts (cats)
- Vitiligo/nasal depigmentation—no treatment
- Tumors—surgical excision; chemotherapy; radiation therapy
- Idiopathic nasal hyperkeratosis—antibiotic-corticosteroid cream for fissures
- Other diseases—see specific disease

Contraindications

- Avoid chrysotherapy in patients with renal disease.
- Azathioprine—use cautiously in cats; may cause fatal leukopenia or thrombocytopenia; leukeran is a better choice.

Precautions

- Griseofulvin—can cause anorexia, vomiting, diarrhea, and bone marrow suppression; feed with high-fat diet, teratogenic
- Ketoconazole—may cause anorexia, gastric irritation, hepatotoxicity, and lightening of hair coat

Comments

- Epidermotropic lymphoma is often associated with nasal depigmentation. An early clue may be generalized scaling (mild or severe) with depigmentation of the planum nasale or mucocutaneous junctions (eyes, mouth, etc.).
- Nasal pyoderma is often very acute in onset and may be quite painful.
- A cutaneous biopsy is often necessary in cases of nasal dermatosis. Remember, if the lesion occurs on the planum nasale then you must biopsy the actual tissue and not the skin around the nose to obtain an accurate diagnosis.

Abbreviations

- ANA = antinuclear antibody
- DIF = direct immunofluorescence
- DLE = discoid lupus erythematosus
- EMG = electromyography
- SLE = systemic lupus erythematosus

Suggested Reading

Muller GH, Kirk RW, Scott DW. Small animal dermatology. 4th ed. Philadelphia: Saunders, 1989.

Authors Ellen C. Codner and Karen Helton Rhodes
Consulting Editor Karen Helton Rhodes

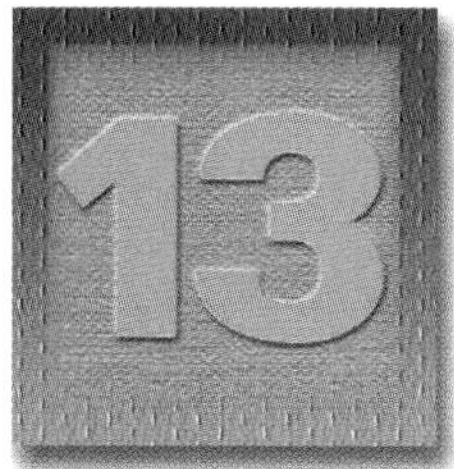

Depigmenting Disorders

John N. Gordon

Definition/Overview

Pathologic or cosmetic condition involving depigmentation of the skin and/or hair coat

Signalment/History

- SLE and DLE—collies, Shetland sheepdogs, German shepherds
- DLE—may occur more often in females
- Pemphigus foliaceus—chow chows, akitas
- Uveodermatologic syndrome—akitas, Samoyeds, Siberian huskies
- Vitiligo—Dobermans and Rottweilers, typically < 3 years old
- Seasonal nasal hypopigmentation—Siberian huskies, Alaskan malamutes, Labrador retrievers
- Cutaneous T-cell lymphoma (mycosis fungoides)—typically dogs > 10 years old

Clinical Features

- Leukotrichia
- Leukoderma
- Erythema
- Erosion and ulcerations

Differential Diagnosis

Nasal Solar Dermatitis

- Lesions confined to nose and precipitated by heavy sunlight exposure
- Begins in poorly pigmented skin at the junction of the nasal planum and dorsal muzzle
- Negative for direct immunofluorescence

DLE

- Primarily affects nasal area
- Exacerbated by sunlight
- Positive direct immunofluorescence at basement membrane zone
- Biopsy—interface dermatitis

SLE

- Multisystemic disease
- Skin lesions—often involve nose, face, and mucocutaneous junctions; multifocal or generalized
- ANA—positive
- Positive direct immunofluorescence at basement membrane zone

Pemphigus Foliaceus

- Lesions—usually start on face and ears; commonly involve footpads; eventually generalized
- Biopsy—subcorneal pustules with acantholysis
- Positive direct immunofluorescence in intercellular spaces of epidermis

Pemphigus Erythematosus

- Lesions—primarily confined to face and ears (Figs. 13-1, 13-2)

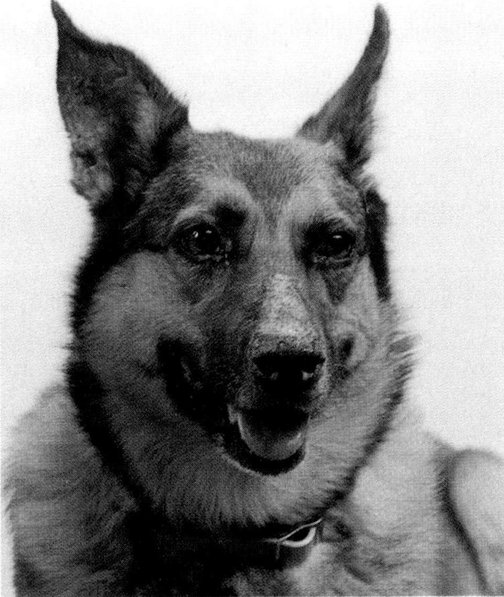

Figure 13-1 Pemphigus erythematosus with depigmentation of the bridge of the nose.

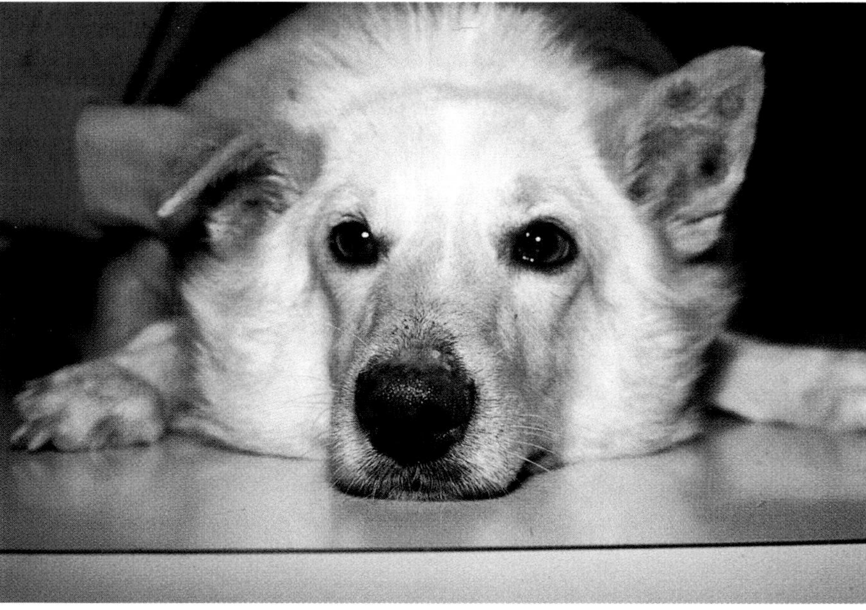

Figure 13-2 Pemphigus erythematosus showing mild depigmentation and erythema of the junction of the planum nasale and the bridge of the nose.

- Biopsy—intraepidermal pustules with acantholysis and interface dermatitis
- Positive direct immunofluorescence at basement membrane zone and intercellular spaces
- ANA—positive

Uveodermatologic Syndrome

- Typical breed
- Uveitis and cutaneous macular depigmentation with inflammation on nose, lips, and eyelids (Fig. 13-3)
- Biopsy of early lesions—interface dermatitis, pigmentary incontinence
- Neoplasia-epidermotropic lymphoma (CTLL) will often cause depigmentation of the MCJ as well as the affected skin and footpads.

Others

- Plastic or rubber dish dermatitis—depigmentation and erythema of the rostral nasal planum and lips; no ulceration and minimal crusting; history of exposure (Fig. 13-4)
- Vitiligo—cutaneous macular depigmentation without inflammation on nose, lips, eyelids, footpads, and nails; leukotrichia may be present with leukoderma (Fig. 13-5)
- Seasonal nasal hypopigmentation—normal black coloration of nasal planum fades to light tan or pink; usually seasonal or slowly progressive with age
- Albinism—hereditary lack of pigment of the skin, hair coat, and irises
- Schnauzer gilding syndrome—young miniature schnauzers may develop idiopathic golden hair coat coloration, primarily of the trunk.
- Drug reaction—may resemble various cutaneous disorders such as DLE, SLE, pemphigus foliaceus, and pemphigus erythematosus; pruritus is variable; onset of signs is usually within 2 weeks of administration.

HISTORICAL FINDINGS

- Pain
- Head shaking
- Scratching at the pinnae
- Malodorous ears

RISK FACTORS

- Abnormal or breed-related conformation of the external canal (e.g., stenosis, hirsutism, and pendulous pinnae) restricts proper air flow into the canal.
- Excessive moisture (e.g., from swimming or frequent cleanings) can lead to infection; overzealous client compliance with recommendations for ear cleanings common
- Topical drug reaction and irritation and trauma from abrasive cleaning techniques
- Underlying systemic diseases produce abnormalities in the environment and ear canal immune response.

Clinical Features

- Otitis externa—often a secondary symptom of an underlying disease
- Infection—purulent and malodorous exudate
- Inflammation—exudation, pain, pruritus, and erythema
- Chronic otitis externa (dogs)—results in tympanic membrane rupture (71%) and otitis media (82%)

PHYSICAL EXAMINATION FINDINGS

- Redness and swelling of the external canal, leading to stenosis
- Scaling and exudation—may result in malodor and canal obstruction
- Cats—hold the pinna down or tilt the head
- Vestibular signs (with head tilt, nystagmus, anorexia, ataxia, and infrequent vomiting) indicate development of otitis media/interna.

Differential Diagnosis

PRIMARY CAUSES

- Parasites (otitis externa)—*Otodectes cynotis, Demodex* spp., *Sarcoptes* and *Notoedres,* and *Otobius megnini*
- Hypersensitivities—atopy, food allergy, contact allergy, and systemic or local drug reaction (Fig. 14-1)
- Foreign bodies—plant awns
- Obstructions—neoplasia, polyps, cerumen gland hyperplasia, and accumulation of hair; may also be a secondary event
- Keratinization disorders and increased cerumen production—functional obstruction of the ear canal (Fig. 14-2)
- Autoimmune diseases—frequently affect the pinnae; sometimes affect the external ear canal

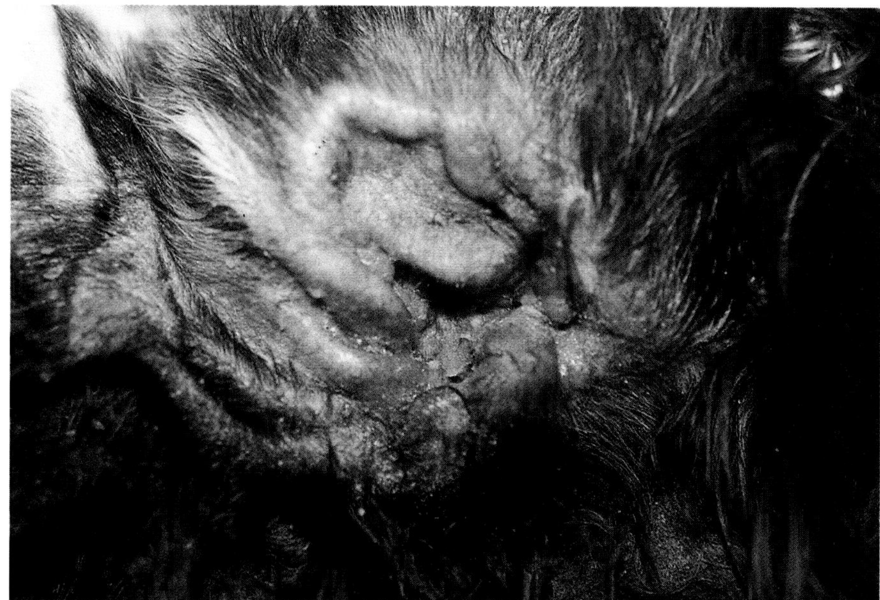

Figure 14-1 Erythema of the pinna and canal with excess wax production and ceruminous gland hyperplasia secondary to allergic dermatitis. (Courtesy of Kevin Shanley.)

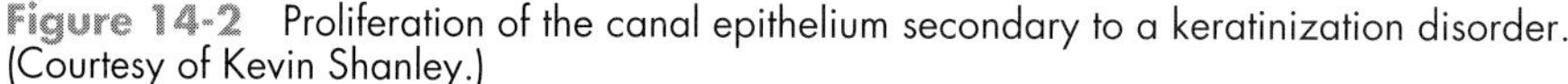

Figure 14-2 Proliferation of the canal epithelium secondary to a keratinization disorder. (Courtesy of Kevin Shanley.)

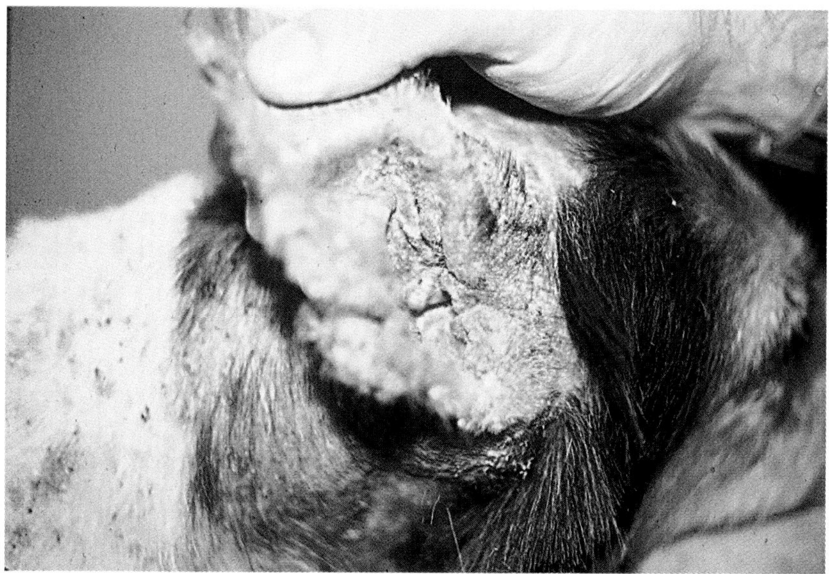

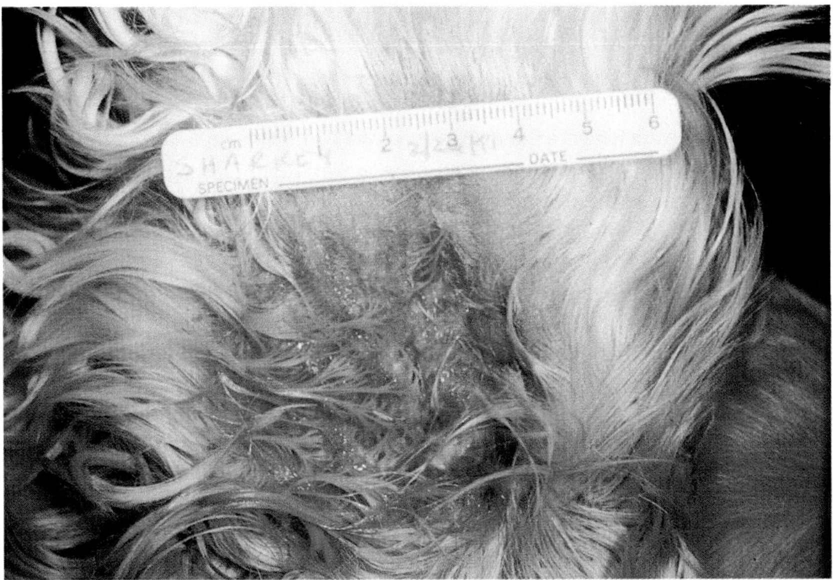

Figure 14-3 Allergic otitis externa with secondary yeast overgrowth. Note the copious amounts of a creamy yellow exudate. The canal was extremely malodorous. (Courtesy of Kevin Shanley.)

Perpetuating Factors

- Secondary bacterial infections—common; *Staphylococcus intermedius* most often cultured from the horizontal canal in otitis externa; *Pseudomonas* spp., *Proteus* spp., *Corynebacterium* spp., and *Escherichia coli* frequently reported; *Pseudomonas* spp. most often cultured in otitis media

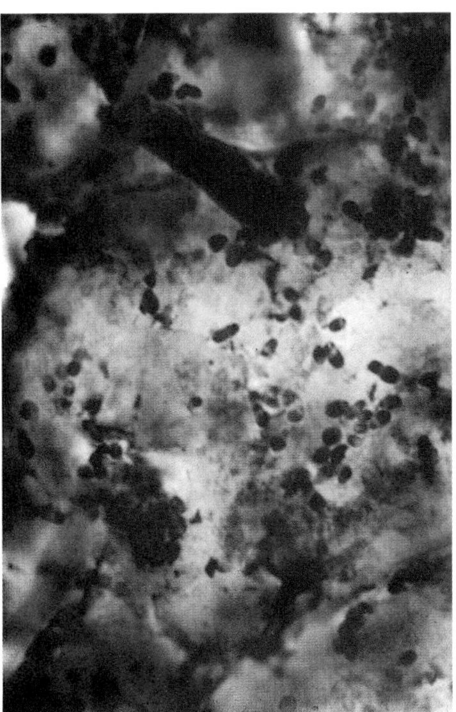

Figure 14-4 Direct smear of the exudate from the canal in Figure 14-3. Note the characteristic "peanut"-shaped *Malassezia* organisms. (Courtesy of Kevin Shanley.)

- Infections—often mixed with, or entirely the result of, *Malassezia pachydermatis;* other yeast (*Candida*) or fungal species rare (Figs. 14-3,14-4)
- Progressive changes—canal hypertrophy, cerumen gland hyperplasia and adenitis, fibrosis, and cartilage calcification; cause recalcitrant otitis externa; prevent return to a normal ear canal even with proper treatment
- Otitis media—can produce symptoms on its own; can act as a reservoir for organisms, causing recurrent condition

Diagnostics

CBC/Biochemistry/Urinalysis

May indicate a primary underlying disease

Imaging

Bullae radiographs—otitis media

Diagnostic Procedures

- Skin scrapings from the pinna—parasites
- Skin biopsy—autoimmune disease, neoplasia, or cerumen gland hyperplasia
- Culture of exudate—often reserve for resistant infection, cytology often more important
- Microscopic examination of aural exudate—single most important diagnostic tool after complete examination of the ear canal
- Appearance of the exudate—yeast infections commonly produce a yellow-tan thick exudate; bacterial infections commonly produce a brownish-black thin exudate; however, appearance does not allow an accurate diagnosis of the type of infection; microscopic examination necessary
- Infections within the canal can change with prolonged or recurrent therapy; repeat examination of aural exudate is required in chronic cases.

Figure 14-5 Direct smear demonstrating *Malassezia pachydermatis* organisms. (Courtesy of Kevin Shanley.)

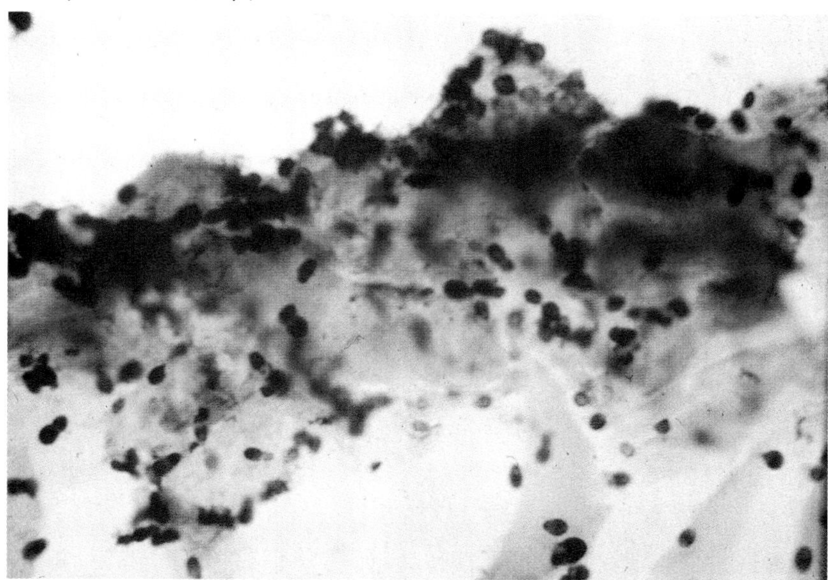

Microscopic Examination

- Preparations—make from both canals (the contents of the canals may not be the same); spread samples thinly on a glass microscope slide; examine both unstained and modified Wright-stained samples.
- May need to heat-fix sample if the exudate is very waxy
- Mites—presumptive diagnosis
- Type(s) of bacteria or yeast—assist in the choice of therapy (Fig. 14-5)
- Findings (types of organisms; WBCs)—note in the record; rank the number of organisms and cell types on a scale of 0–4 to allow treatment monitoring
- WBCs within the exudate—active infection; systemic antibiotic therapy may be warranted

Therapeutics

DIET

No restrictions unless a food allergy is suspected

CLIENT EDUCATION

Teach clients, by demonstration, the proper method for cleaning ears.

SURGICAL CONSIDERATIONS

- Indicated when the canal is severely stenotic or obstructed or when neoplasia or a polyp is diagnosed
- Severe, unresponsive otitis media may require a bullae osteotomy.

DRUGS OF CHOICE

Systemic

- Antibiotics—useful in severe cases of bacterial otitis externa; mandatory when the tympanum has ruptured; trimethoprim-potentiated sulfonamides (dosage varies by preparation), cephalexin (25 mg/kg q8-12h), enrofloxacin (2.5 mg/kg q12h), or clindamycin (10 mg/kg q12h)
- Antifungals—use with overwhelming yeast or fungal infection; ketoconazole (5–10 mg/kg q12h)
- Corticosteroids—reduce swelling and pain; anti-inflammatory dosages of prednisone (0.25–0.5 mg/kg q12h); use sparingly and for short durations only
- Ivermectin—various external ear parasites; 300 μg/kg SC weekly for 4 weeks eliminates *Otodectes* infestation, "Revolution"

Topical

- Topical therapy paramount for resolution and control of otitis externa
- First, completely clean the external ear canal of debris; complete flushing under general anesthesia reserved for uncooperative patients or severe cases, including otitis media.
- Second, thoroughly clean the ear daily during initial therapy, then every 3–7 days once signs resolve.
- Finally, apply appropriate topical medications frequently and in sufficient quantity to completely treat the entire canal.

- Not recommended—combination ointments (e.g., Otomax, Panalog, Liquachlor), which often accumulate and perpetuate the condition
- Recommended—antibacterial (e.g., gentocin) or antiyeast drops (miconazole), with or without corticosteroid; commercial ear cleansers with cerumenolytics, antiseptics, and astringents; Alocetic for routine cleaning or when the competence of the tympanic membrane is in question; chlorhexidine-containing solutions (e.g., Chlorhexiderm Flush, Hexadene Flush) for more severe cases when the tympanic membrane is intact (controversial)
- Cerumenolytics—dioctyl sodium sulfosuccinate or carbamide peroxide; emulsify wax, facilitating removal
- Antiseptics—acetic acid or chlorhexidine gluconate; reduce or eliminate infectious organisms
- Astringents—isopropyl alcohol, boric acid, or salicylic acid; reduce moisture
- Antibiotics, antifungals, and/or parasiticides—use only when presence of organism(s) has been confirmed.
- Ivermectin—effective for ear mites in cats, but recurrence rates higher than with other parasiticides; use only for large numbers of animals (kennels) or when a persistent carrier state is suspected
- Resistance to medications—perform a culture and sensitivity of the aural exudate; recently, suspensions of silver sulfadiazine and of enrofloxacin have been shown to be effective
- Generally, ingredients should be limited to those needed to treat a specific infection (i.e., antibiotics only for a bacterial infection).

Contraindications

- Ivermectin—not FDA approved for treating ear mites; client disclosure and consent are paramount before administration; herding breeds (dogs) have increased sensitivity and should not be treated with this drug
- Ruptured tympanum—use caution with topical cleansers and medications other than sterile saline or dilute acetic acid; potential for ototoxicity is a concern; controversial

Comments

- Use extreme caution when cleaning the external ear canals of all animals with severe and chronic otitis externa, because the tympanum can easily be ruptured.
- Postflushing vestibular complications are common in cats, although usually temporary; warn clients of possible complications and residual effects.
- Several topical medications infrequently induce contact irritation or allergic response; re-evaluate all worsening cases.
- Uncontrolled otitis externa can lead to otitis media, deafness, vestibular disease, cellulitis, facial nerve paralysis, progression to otitis interna, and rarely, meningoencephalitis.
- Otitis externa—with proper therapy, most cases resolve in 3–4 weeks; failure to correct underlying primary cause results in recurrence
- Perpetuating factors (e.g., stenosis of the ear canal and calcification of the auricular cartilage) will not resolve and may result in recurrence
- Otitis media—may take 6+ weeks of systemic antibiotics until all signs have resolved and the tympanic membrane has healed

Suggested Reading

Griffin CE. Otitis externa and otitis media. In: Griffin CE, Griffin CE, Kwochka KW, MacDonald JM, eds. Current veterinary dermatology: the science and art of therapy. St. Louis: Mosby 1993.

Consulting Editor Karen Helton Rhodes

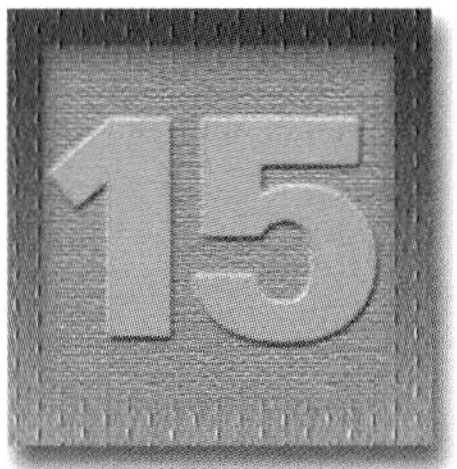

Otitis Media and Interna

Richard J. Joseph

Definition/Overview

Inflammation of the middle (otitis media) and inner (otitis interna) ear, most commonly caused by bacterial infection

Etiology/Pathophysiology

- Most often arises from extension of infection of the external ear through the tympanic membrane; may extend from the oral and nasopharyngeal cavities via the eustachian tube
- Interna—may also result from hematogenous spread of a systemic infection
- Nervous—vestibulocochlear receptors in the inner ear and the facial nerve and sympathetic chain in the middle ear (peripheral) with possible extension of infection intracranially (central)
- Ophthalmic—cornea and conjunctiva; from exposure and/or lack of tear production after nerve damage
- Gastrointestinal—taste; from damage to the parasympathetic branch of the facial nerve (chordae tympani) supplying the ipsilateral rostral two thirds of the tongue

Signalment/History

Breed Predilections

- Cocker spaniels and other long-eared breeds
- Poodles with chronic otitis or pharyngitis from dental disease

Historical Findings

- Pain when opening the mouth; reluctance to chew; shaking the head; pawing at the affected ear
- Head tilt
- Patient may lean, veer, or roll toward the side affected with peripheral vestibulitis.
- Vestibular deficits—may be transient and episodic
- Bilateral involvement—may note wide head excursions, truncal ataxia, and deafness
- Vomiting and nausea—may occur during the acute phase
- Facial nerve damage—saliva and food dropping from the corner of the mouth; an inability to blink; ocular discharge
- Anisocoria and/or protrusion of the third eyelid (Horners syndrome) may be noted.

Risk Factors

- Nasopharyngeal polyps and inner, middle, or outer ear neoplasia—may predispose patient to bacterial infection
- Vigorous ear flush
- Ear cleaning solutions (e.g., chlorhexidine)—may be irritating to the middle and inner ear; avoid if the tympanum is ruptured
- Inhalant anesthesia and traveling by airplane—change middle ear pressures

Clinical Features

- Related to the severity and extent of the infection; may range from none to those related to bulla discomfort and nervous system involvement
- Evidence of aural erythema, discharge, and thick and stenotic canals support otitis externa.
- Gray, dull, opaque, and bulging tympanic membrane on otoscopic examination indicates a middle ear exudate.
- Dental tartar, gingivitis, tonsillitis, or pharyngitis—may be associated
- Ipsilateral mandibular lymphadenopathy—may occur with severe infections
- Pain—upon opening the mouth or bulla, palpation may be detected
- Corneal ulcer—may be caused by inability to blink or a dry eye

Neurologic Examination Findings

- Damage to the associated neurologic structures depends on the severity and location.
- Vestibular portion of cranial nerve VIII—when vestibular portion is affected, there is always an ipsilateral head tilt.
- Bilateral damage of cranial nerve VIII—rare; patient is reluctant to move and may stay in a crouched posture with wide head excursions; physiologic nystagmus poor to absent
- Nystagmus—resting or positional and rotatory or horizontal; may be seen
- Vestibular strabismus—ipsilateral ventral deviation of eyeball with neck extension; may be noted
- Ipsilateral leaning, veering, falling, or rolling—may occur
- Facial nerve damage—ipsilateral paresis/paralysis of the ear, eyelids, lips, and nares; may be reduced tear production (indicated by the Schirmer tear test);

with chronic facial nerve paralysis, contracture of the affected side of the face caused by fibrosis of the denervated muscles; deficits can be bilateral.

- Affected sympathetic chain—Horners syndrome; always miosis of the affected pupil; may note protrusion of the third eyelid, ptosis, and enophthalmos

Differential Diagnosis

- Bacteria—primary agents
- Yeast (*Malassezia* spp., *Candida* spp.) and *Aspergillus*—agents to consider
- Mites—predispose patient to secondary bacterial infections
- Unilateral disease—foreign bodies, trauma, polyps, and tumors (e.g., fibromas, squamous cell carcinoma, ceruminous gland carcinoma, and primary bone tumors)
- Signs associated with congenital vestibular anomalies are present from birth.
- Hypothyroidism—may cause a polyneuropathy with a predilection for cranial nerves VII and VIII; abnormal thyroid profile (T_4, free T_4, TSH level or response) supports the diagnosis
- Central vestibular diseases—differentiated by occurrence of lethargy, somnolence, stupor, and other brainstem signs
- Neoplasia and nasopharyngeal polyps—common causes of refractory and relapsing otitis media and interna; diagnosed by imaging of the head
- Thiamine deficiency (cats)—bilateral central vestibular signs; history of an all-fish diet or persistent anorexia helps the diagnosis
- Metronidazole toxicity—bilateral central vestibular signs after high dosage or prolonged use
- Trauma—history and physical evidence of injury
- Idiopathic vestibular disease (old dogs and young to middle-aged cats), idiopathic facial paralysis, and idiopathic Horners syndrome—diagnoses made by exclusion

Diagnostics

CBC/Biochemistry/Urinalysis

- Leukocytosis with a left shift—may be noted
- Globulins—may be high if infection is chronic
- Urinalysis—usually normal; pyuria and bacteria in the urine may be seen if the bacterial infection is hematogenous

Other Laboratory Tests

- Blood and/or urine cultures—may be positive with a hematogenous source of infection
- Low T_4, free T_4 with a high TSH level, or inadequate elevation of T_4 levels after a TSH response test—hypothyroidism

Imaging

- Bullae radiographs—tympanic bullae may appear cloudy if exudate is present; may see thickening of the bullae and petrous temporal bone with chronic disease; may see lysis of the bone with severe cases of osteomyelitis; may be normal

- CT and MRI—detailed evidence of fluid and soft tissue density within the middle ear and the extent of involvement of the adjacent structures; CT better at revealing associated bony changes

Diagnostic Procedures

- Myringotomy—insert a spinal needle (20 gauge; 2.5–3.5 in.) through the otoscope and tympanic membrane to aspirate middle ear fluid for cytologic examination and culture and sensitivity
- BAER—test the functional integrity of the peripheral and central auditory pathways; detect any associated hearing loss
- CSF analysis—if neutrophilic pleocytosis and increased protein with intracranial extension of the infection are noted, perform culture and sensitivity

Pathologic Findings

Purulent exudate within the middle ear cavity surrounded by a thickened bullae and microscopic evidence of degenerative neutrophils with intracellular bacteria characteristic

Therapeutics

- Inpatient—severe debilitating infection; neurologic signs
- Discharge stable patients, pending further diagnostics and surgery, if indicated.
- Fluid therapy—if unable to eat or drink owing to vomiting and disorientation
- Concurrent otitis externa—culture and clean the ear; use warm normal saline if the tympanum is ruptured; if a cleaning solution is used, follow with a thorough flush with normal saline; dry the ear canal with a cotton swab and low vacuum suction; astringents (e.g., Otic Domeboro or boric acid) can be effective
- Restrict activity with substantial vestibular signs to avoid injury.
- Vomiting from vestibulitis—withhold food and water for 12–24 hr
- Severe disorientation—hand feed and water small amounts frequently; elevate head to avoid aspiration pneumonia
- Inform client that most bacterial infections resolve with an early aggressive course of broad-spectrum antibiotics and do not recur.
- Warn client that relapsing signs may occur and may require surgical drainage if bony structure changes and/or middle ear effusion are evident on imaging studies.
- Reserve surgery for relapsing or nonresponsive patients.
- Do not rely on severity of neurologic signs as an indication for surgical intervention; reserve surgery for patients with evidence of middle ear exudate, osteomyelitis refractory to medical management, and nasopharyngeal polyps or neoplasia.
- Bullae osteotomy—allows drainage of the middle ear cavity
- Ear ablation through the horizontal ear canal—indicated when otitis media is associated with recurrent otitis externa or neoplasia
- Cytologic examination and culture and sensitivity of middle ear effusion and histopathologic evaluation of samples of abnormal tissue—perform at the time of surgery

- Topical water-based or ophthalmic antibiotic solutions—chloramphenicol or a triple antibiotic preparation preferred
- Antibiotics—long-term (6–8 weeks); broad-spectrum systemic agents; select on basis of culture and sensitivity, if available
- Penicillinase-resistant penicillin and cephalosporins—good initial drugs
- Ruptured tympanum or associated neurologic deficits—avoid oil-based or irritating external ear preparations (e.g., chlorhexidine) and aminoglycosides, which are toxic to inner ear structures
- Otitis media or interna—topical and systemic corticosteroids contraindicated; may exacerbate the signs associated with infection

Comments

- Avoid rigorously flushing the external ear; may result in or exacerbate signs of otitis media or interna.
- Evaluate for resolution of signs after 10–14 days—or sooner if the patient is deteriorating.
- Routine ear cleaning and dental prophylaxis—may reduce chances of infection
- Signs associated with vestibular and facial nerve damage or Horners syndrome—may remain
- Severe infections—may spread to the brainstem
- Osteomyelitis of the petrous temporal bone and middle ear cavity effusion—common sequela to severe, chronic infections
- Bulla osteotomy— postoperative complications include Horners syndrome, facial paralysis, and onset or exacerbation of vestibular dysfunction
- Cats—consider avoiding bilateral bullae osteotomies in patients with bilateral effusions; may be an increased incidence of death after surgery
- Otitis media and interna—usually responsive to medical management
- When medical management is ineffective, a surgical evaluation for lateral ear resection should be explored.
- Vestibular signs—improvement in 2–6 weeks; more rapid in small dogs and in cats

Abbreviations

- BAER = brainstem auditory-evoked response
- CSF = cerebrospinal fluid
- TSH = thyroid-stimulating hormone

Suggested Reading

Bruyette DS, Lorenz MD. Otitis externa and media: diagnostic and medical aspects. Semin Vet Med Surg Small Anim 1993;8:3–9.

Schunk KL, Averill DR. Peripheral vestibular syndrome in the dog: a review of 83 cases. J Am Vet Med Assoc 1983;182:1354–1358.

Author Richard J. Joseph

Consulting Editor Karen Helton Rhodes

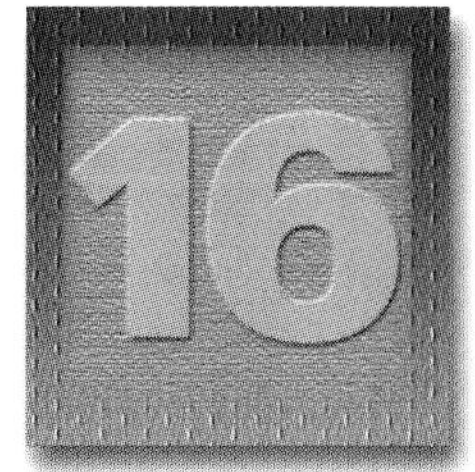

Anal Sac Disorders

Jon D. Plant

Definition/Overview

- Dogs—three types (impaction, sacculitis, and abscess), which are probably stages of the same disease process
- Cats—rare; impaction occasionally noted

Etiology/Pathophysiology

- Infection
- Trauma
- Idiopathic
- Immunologic
- Parasitic
- Seborrheic

Signalment/History

- Dogs
- Rarely cats
- Small breeds—miniature poodles, toy poodles, and Chihuahuas reportedly predisposed
- No age or sex predispositions

- Possible predisposing factors—chronically soft feces, recent diarrhea, excessive glandular secretions, and poor muscle tone
- Retained secretions may lead to infection and abscess formation.

Clinical Features

- Scooting
- Tenesmus
- Perianal pruritus
- Tail chasing
- Perianal discharge, if abscess ruptures
- Behavioral changes
- Pyotraumatic dermatitis

Differential Diagnosis

- Erythema and swelling of the perineum—anal sac neoplasia
- Perianal pruritus—food hypersensitivity, flea allergy dermatitis, atopy, tapeworms, tail-fold pyoderma, and seborrheic skin disorders affecting the perineum
- Anal sac abscesses must be differentiated from perianal fistulas.

Diagnostics

- History and digital palpation examination—establish diagnosis; if easily palpated through the skin, sacs are considered enlarged
- Normal anal sacs—clear or pale yellow-brown secretion
- Impaction—thick, pasty brown secretion
- Anal sacculitis—creamy yellow or thin green-yellow secretion
- Abscessed—red-brown exudate, fever, swelling, and erythema over the anal sacs
- Ruptured—discharging sinus
- Cytology of anal sac contents—number of leukocytes and bacteria indicate infection
- Bacterial culture and sensitivity—may help for animals with chronic or recurrent anal sac infections

Therapeutics

- Express contents for impaction or sacculitis.
- Instill an antibiotic/corticosteroid ointment for infected anal sacs.
- If necessary, establish drainage in abscesses; clean and flush anal sacs.
- Recurrent abscesses—consider anal sac excision.

Suggested Reading

Burrows CF, Ellison GW. Recto-anal diseases. In: Ettinger SJ, ed. Textbook of veterinary internal medicine. 3rd ed. Philadelphia: Saunders, 1989:1570–1572.

Consulting Editor Karen Helton Rhodes

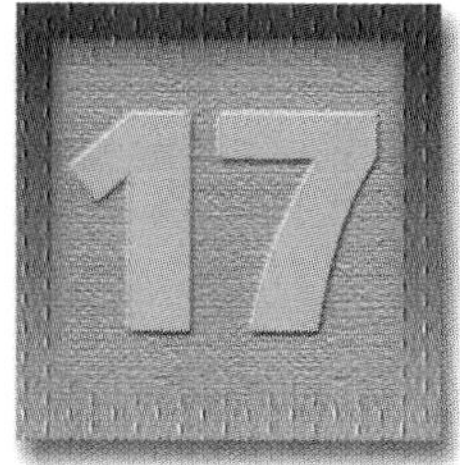

Perianal Fistula

Michael A. Mitchell and James L. Cook

Definition/Overview

Characterized by multiple chronic fistulous tracts or ulcerating sinuses involving the perianal region

Etiology/Pathophysiology

- Not known; apocrine gland inflammation (hidradenitis suppurativa), impaction and infection of the anal sinuses and crypts, infection of the circumanal glands and hair follicles, and anal sacculitis have all been implicated.
- An association with colitis in German shepherd dogs has been proposed.
- The gastrointestinal system becomes involved when excessive scar tissue formation around the anus results in tenesmus, dyschezia, or other problems associated with defecation.
- Self-mutilation can be a major problem.
- Low tail carriage and a broad tail base—proposed risk factors predisposing the dog to inflammation and infection because of poor ventilation, accumulation of feces, moisture, and secretions
- High density of apocrine sweat glands in the cutaneous zone of the anal canal of German shepherd dogs
- Hidradenitis suppurativa may be associated with immune or endocrine dysfunction, genetic factors, and poor hygiene.

Signalment/History

- Dogs
- German shepherd dog and Irish setter most commonly affected breeds
- Mean age, 7 years; range, 7 months to 12 years
- No gender predisposition reported; sexually intact dogs have a higher prevalence
- A genetic basis has been proposed but not proven.

Clinical Features

- Vary with the severity and extent of involvement
- Dyschezia
- Tenesmus
- Hematochezia
- Constipation
- Diarrhea
- Malodorous mucopurulent anal discharge
- Painful tail movements
- Licking and self-mutilation
- Reluctance to sit, posturing difficulties, and personality changes
- Fecal incontinence
- Anorexia
- Weight loss
- Perianal fistulous tracts

Differential Diagnosis

- Chronic anal sac abscess
- Perianal adenoma or adenocarcinoma with ulceration and drainage
- Rectal fistula

Diagnostics

CBC/Biochemistry/Urinalysis

- Usually normal
- Patients with inflammation may have an inflammatory leukogram.

Diagnostic Procedures

- Presumptive diagnosis—based on clinical signs and results of physical examination
- Definitive diagnosis—made by biopsy of the affected area
- Colonoscopy with biopsy may reveal associated colitis

Therapeutics

- Clipping hair from the affected area
- Daily antiseptic lavage
- Systemic and topical antibiotics
- Hydrotherapy
- Elevation of the tail
- Analgesics
- Dietary modification—stool softeners if pain/tenesmus; fiber-enhanced or hypoallergenic diet if associated colitis/proctitis
- Postoperative nursing care may also include warm-packing the affected area.
- Surgery is considered the most effective treatment if medical therapy is unsuccessful.
- Which surgical method to use is controversial; none of those currently used consistently resolves the problem.
- Surgical options include electrosurgery, cryosurgery, surgical debridement with fulguration by chemical cautery, exteriorization and fulguration by electrocautery, surgical resection, radical excision of the rectal ring, tail setting, tail amputation, and laser surgery.
- Perform anal sacculectomy with the above-selected procedure.
- Each technique has advantages and disadvantages that must be weighed when making a choice.
- Primary objective of surgery is complete removal or destruction of diseased tissue while preserving normal tissue and function.
- Multiple procedures may be necessary for complete resolution.

Drugs

- Cyclosporine (2–3 mg/kg PO q24h × 12 weeks)—most dogs improve; up to 50% may clear completely; 50% still require surgery because of inadequate clearing of fistulas or anal stricture
- Assess cyclosporine levels every 3 weeks; appropriate levels are 200–300 ng/mL.
- Unsuccessful medical treatment can be detrimental by delaying surgery.
- Antibiotics and analgesics may be indicated in some cases.
- Corticosteroids (2 mg/kg PO q12h) and a hypoallergenic diet for 6 weeks may yield partial or complete resolution (about 33% of cases); most dogs do not improve; corticosteroid side effects are common.

Comments

Possible Complications

- Recurrence
- Failure to heal
- Dehiscence of surgical site
- Tenesmus
- Fecal incontinence
- Anal stricture

- Flatulence
- The incidence of postoperative complications is directly related to severity of disease.

Expected Course/Prognosis

- Guarded for complete resolution except in mildly affected patients
- Clients often become frustrated with the difficulty of attaining definitive resolution.

Suggested Reading

Harkin KR, Walshaw R, Mullaney TP. Association of perianal fistula and colitis in the German shepherd dog: response to high-dose prednisone and dietary therapy. J Am Anim Hosp Assoc 1996;32:515–520.

Matthews KA, Sukhiani HR. OL27–400 (cyclosporin) treatment of canine perianal fistulas: a prospective, randomized, double-blind, controlled study. Proceedings, 6th Ann ACVS Symposium, San Francisco, CA, 1997:15–16.

Matthiesen DT, Marretta SM. Diseases of the anus and rectum. In: Slatter D, ed. Textbook of small animal surgery. 2nd ed. Philadelphia: Saunders, 1993:627–644.

van Ee RT. Perianal fistulas. In: Bojrab MJ, ed. Disease mechanisms in small animal surgery. 2nd ed. Philadelphia: Lea & Febiger, 1993:285–286.

Consulting Editor Karen Helton Rhodes

CANINE AND FELINE ACNE

David Duclos and Karen Helton Rhodes

Definition/Overview

- Chronic inflammatory disorder of the chin and lips of young animals that can become chronic and progressive
- Characterized by folliculitis and furunculosis
- Some animals have a single episode; many have a lifelong recurrent problem; for a few, the disease process is continual; frequency and severity of each occurrence varies with the individual

Etiology/Pathophysiology

- Unknown
- Poor grooming
- Abnormalities in keratinization, sebum production, or immune barrier function
- Once thought that hormones played a triggering role; now speculated that genetic predisposition plays a more important role

Signalment/History

- Some short-coated dog breeds appear to be genetically predisposed to follicular keratosis and secondary bacterial infection—boxers, Great Danes, doberman pinschers, English bulldogs, weimeraners, mastiffs, Rottweilers, and German short-haired pointers
- No breed predilection noted in cats

Clinical Features

- The area may be minimally to markedly swollen with numerous erythematous papules.
- Advanced stages—lesions may be exudative and indicate a secondary deep bacterial infection
- Lesions may be painful on palpation
- Chronic resolved lesions may be scarred and lichenified.
- Comedones, mild erythematous papules, and serous crusts develop on the chin and less commonly on the lips.
- Sometimes swelling of the chin
- More severe cases—nodules, hemorrhagic crusts, pustules, severe erythema, alopecia, and pain

Differential Diagnosis

- Dermatophytosis
- Demodicosis
- Foreign body
- Contact dermatitis
- *Malassezia* infection
- Feline leprosy
- Neoplasia of the sebaceous glands and other follicular and epidermal neoplasia
- Allergy (including eosinophilic granuloma complex)

Diagnostics

- Bacterial culture and sensitivity testing—in patients with suppurative folliculitis and furunculosis that are responsive to initial antibiotic selection
- Biopsy—histologic confirmation for cases in which diagnosis is in question
- Clinical signs and histopathologic findings are diagnostic.
- Initial lesions—hairless follicular papules; characterized histopathologically by marked follicular keratosis, plugging, dilatation, and perifolliculitis
- Bacteria—in the early stages: not seen and cannot be isolated from lesions; as disease progresses: papules enlarge and rupture, promoting a suppurative folliculitis and furunculosis

Therapeutics

- Depends on the severity and chronicity of the disease
- Reduce behavioral trauma to the chin (e.g., rubbing on the carpet, chewing bones that increase salivation).
- Frequent cleaning with benzoyl peroxide shampoo or gel or mupirocin ointment to reduce the bacterial numbers on the surface of the skin
- Instruct owners to avoid expressing the lesions, which may cause internal rupture of the papule and massive inflammation.

TOPICAL

- Benzoyl peroxide shampoo or gel (antibacterial)
- Mupirocin ointment (antibacterial-staph)
- Isotretinoin (Retin-A) or tretinoin (vitamin A acid, retinoic acid gel)—may reduce follicular keratosis
- Corticosteroids—may be necessary to reduce inflammation
- Other topical—clindamycin or erythromycin solution; benzamycin (benzoyl peroxide—antibiotic gel)

SYSTEMIC

- Antibiotics appropriate for deep bacterial infection—especially cephalosporins (Cephalexin, 22 mg/kg PO q8h for 6–8 weeks)
- May need to perform bacterial culture and sensitivity test
- Systemic isotretinoin—use with caution, if animal will not allow application of topical medications; CAUTION: inform owners that it can have potential deleterious side effects in humans (drug interactions and teratogenic) if taken by mistake; container should be labeled for animal use only and kept separate from human medications to avoid accidental use

Comments

- Benzoyl peroxide—may bleach carpets and fabrics; may be irritating
- Mupirocin ointments—greasy
- Topical retinoids—may be drying and irritating
- Topical steroids—may cause adrenal suppression with repeated use

Suggested Reading

Scott DW, Miller WH, Griffin CE. Bacterial skin diseases. In: Kirk's small animal dermatology. 5th ed. Philadelphia: Saunders, 1995:304–305.

Authors Karen Helton Rhodes/David Duclos

Consulting Editor Karen Helton Rhodes

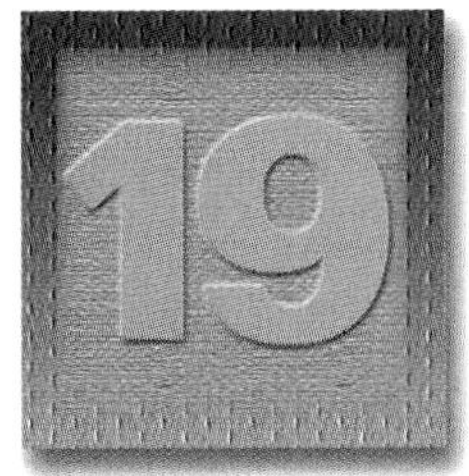

ACRAL LICK DERMATITIS

Karen A. Kuhl, Jean S. Greek and
Karen Helton Rhodes

Definition/Overview

A firm, raised, ulcerative, or thickened plaque that is usually located on the dorsal aspect of the carpus, metacarpus, tarsus, or metatarsus (Fig. 19-1)

Etiology/Pathophysiology

- Trauma (fractures, etc.)
- Arthritis
- Neoplasia
- Foreign body
- Behavioral
- Infection

Signalment/History

- Primarily dogs
- Most common in large-breeds—especially Doberman pinschers, Labrador retrievers, Great Danes, Irish and English setters, golden retrievers, akitas, Dalmatians, sharpeis, and Weimaraners (Fig. 19-2)
- Age at onset—varies with the cause
- Sex predilection—some sources suggest more common in males; others indicate no preference

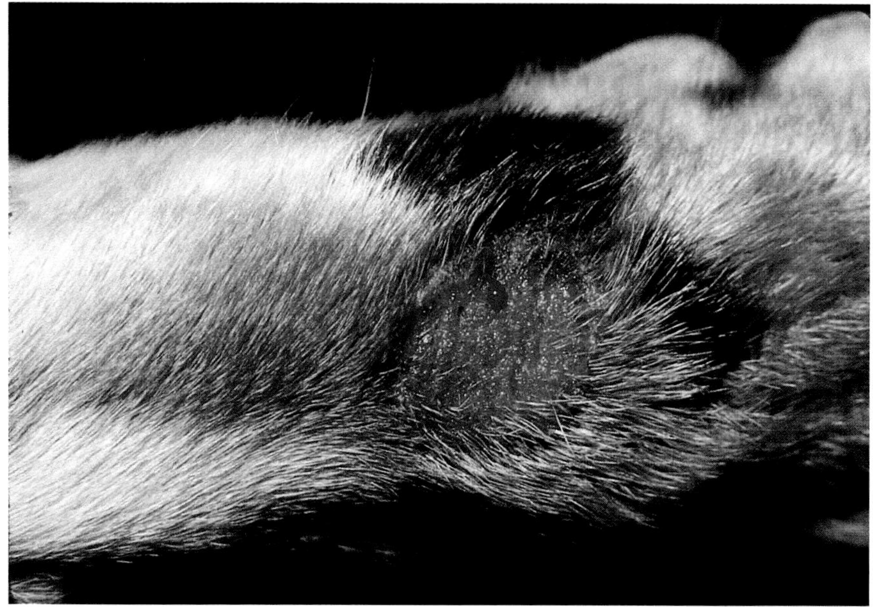

Figure 19-1 Acral lick granuloma on the metacarpus of a young dog.

Figure 19-2 Acral lick granuloma on the forelimb of a golden retriever.

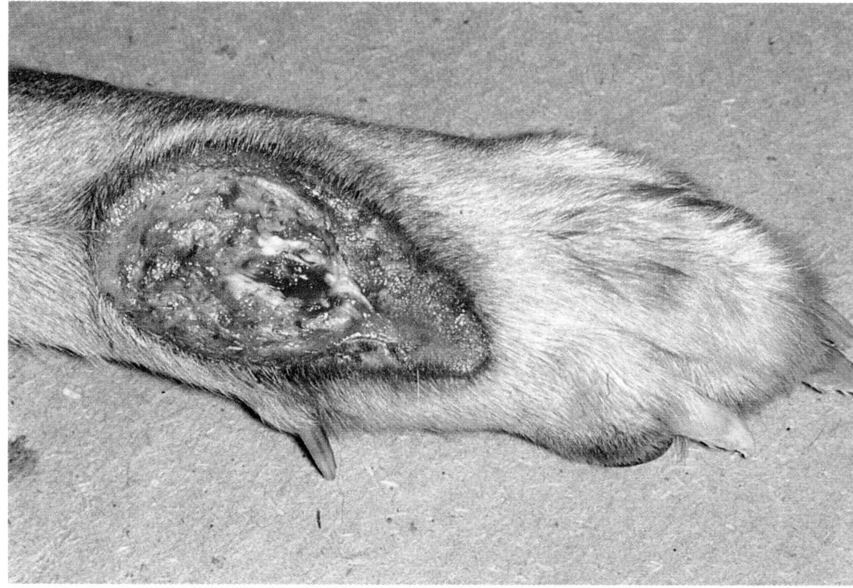

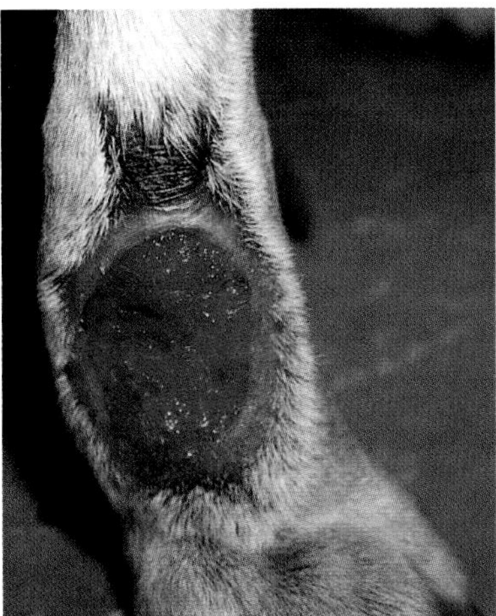

Figure 19-3 Radiographs revealed marked arthritis in the joint, which may have induced excessive licking in this case.

Clinical Features

- Excessive licking and chewing of the affected area
- Occasionally a history of trauma to the affected area
- Alopecic, ulcerative, thickened, and raised firm plaques, usually located on the dorsal aspect of the carpus, metacarpus, tarsus, or metatarsus
- Lesions often occur singly, although they may occur in more than one location.

Differential Diagnosis

- Allergic animals often have multiple lick granulomas and other areas of pruritus compatible with the specific allergy.
- Endocrinopathies, demodicosis, and dermatophytosis—determined on the basis of laboratory test results
- Staphylococcal furunculosis
- Dermatophytosis; Majocchi's granuloma
- Arthritis of the area inducing excessive licking (Fig. 19-3)
- Trauma (fractures, sensory nerve dysfunction, etc.) (Fig. 19-4)
- Foreign body reaction
- Neoplasia
- Psychogenic

Diagnostics

CBC/Biochemistry/Urinalysis

Normal except in cases of hyperadrenocorticism

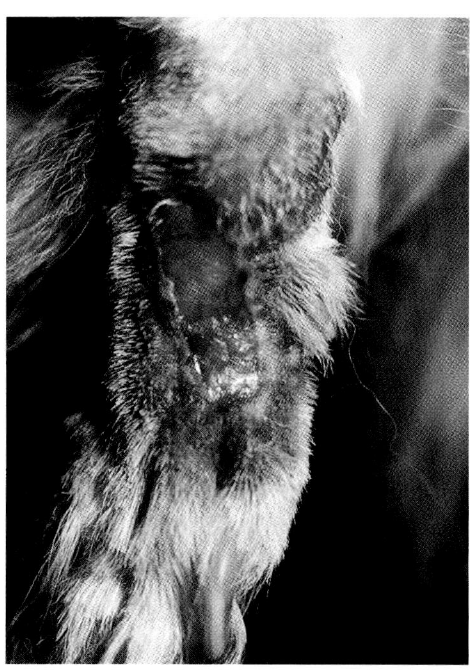

Figure 19-4 A hairline fracture induced to this acral lick granuloma.

Other Laboratory Tests

- Low thyroid levels—suggests hypothyroidism
- Abnormal ACTH-stimulation test or abnormal LDDST—suggests hyperadrenocorticism

Imaging

Radiology—neoplasia; some forms of trauma; radiopaque foreign bodies; bony proliferation may be seen secondary to the chronic irritation

Diagnostic Procedures

- Examine skin scrapings, dermatophyte culture, and Tzanck preparations—rule out demodicosis, dermatophytosis, or a bacterial infection
- Bacterial culture and sensitivity (if indicated)—determine appropriate antibiotics
- Food-elimination diet—determine food allergy
- Intradermal allergy testing—helpful for atopic animals
- Biopsy—to rule out neoplasia, if necessary

Pathologic Findings

Histopathology—ulcerative, hyperplastic epidermis with mild perivascular dermatitis; varying degrees of fibroplasia

Therapeutics

- Affected animal must get plenty of attention and exercise.
- Diet—no modification unless an allergy is suspected

- Difficult to treat, especially if no underlying cause is found; warn owner that patience and time are necessary.
- Surgery—do not consider until all other therapies have been exhausted; will often cause increased licking and attention to the affected area, resulting in poor wound closure; if underlying causes are not addressed, recurrence is likely.

DRUGS

Antibiotics

- Based on bacterial culture and sensitivity
- Give until infection is completely resolved, often at least 6 weeks.

Systemic

- Hydroxyzine HCl (1–2 mg/kg PO q8h)
- Chlorpheniramine (4–8 mg/dog q12h PO; maximum of 0.5 mg/kg q12h)
- Naltrexone (2.2 mg/kg PO q12–24h)
- Amitriptyline HCl (1.1–2.2 mg/kg PO q12h); used at the lower dosage for 10 days; if no improvement, use at the higher dosage for 10 days
- Doxepin may also be tried (3–5 mg/kg PO q12h; maximum, 150 mg q12h).
- **CAUTION:** none of these medications should be used concurrently.

Topical

- Flunixin meglumine and fluocinolone in dimethyl sulfoxide (combined), mupirocin, topical 5% benzoyl peroxide, and products capsaicin
- Intralesional corticosteroids may be used in early or very small lesions; rarely of any use in chronic lesions
- Topical medications should be applied with gloves.
- Animals should be kept from licking the area for 10–15 min.

Other

- After all other underlying diseases have been ruled out or treated, therapies for psychogenic dermatoses may be tried.
- Psychotropic drugs—fluoxetine hydrochloride (1 mg/kg PO q24h) or clomipramine hydrochloride (1–3 mg/kg PO q24h)
- Physical restraints—Elizabethan collars and bandaging; short-term use

Comments

- Doxepin—do not use with monoamine oxidase inhibitors, clonidine, anticonvulsants, oral anticoagulants, steroid hormones, antihistamines, or aspirin.
- Antihistamines—do not use more than one at a time.
- Monitor level of licking and chewing closely.
- Treat underlying disease to prevent recurrence.
- If no underlying disease is detected, suspect psychogenic causes (obsessive-compulsive or self-mutilation disorder); prognosis is guarded.
- Animals receiving tricyclic antidepressants—CBC, chemistry profile, ECG every 1–2 months, because of potential for cardiotoxicity and hepatotoxicity

Age-Related Factors

Dogs > 5 years old—strongly consider allergy

Zoonotic Potential

Transmitted to humans only if dermatophytosis is the underlying cause; exceedingly rare

Abbreviation

LDDST = low-dose dexamethasone-suppression test

Suggested Reading

Shanley K, Overall K. Psychogenic dermatoses. In: Kirk RW, Bonagura JD, eds. Current veterinary therapy XI. Philadelphia: Saunders, 1992:552–557.

Consulting Editor Karen Helton Rhodes

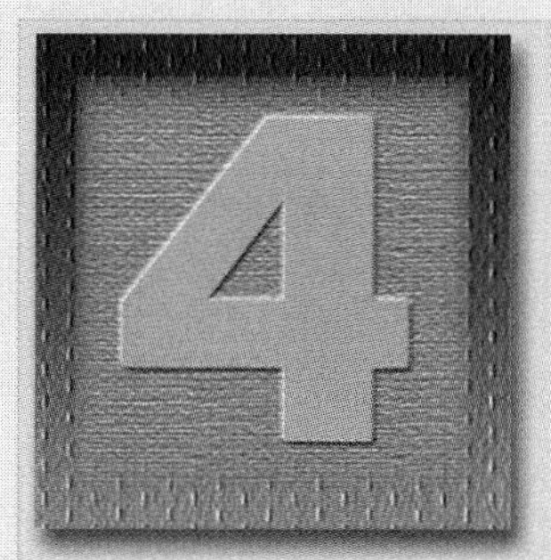

Parasitic Dermatoses

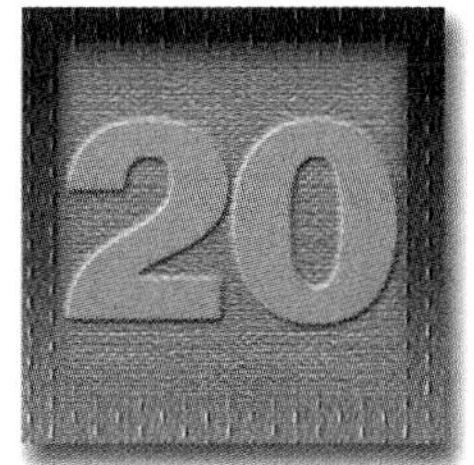

Ticks and Tick Control

Steven A. Levy

Definition/Overview

- Dogs and cats may be parasitized by hard ticks of the family Ixodidae.
- Ectoparasites that feed only on the blood of their hosts; arthropods; closely related to scorpions, spiders, and mites
- Transmitted microbial pathogens—protozoa, helminths, fungi, bacteria, rickettsiae, and viruses
- May cause toxicosis, hypersensitivity, paralysis, and blood-loss anemia

Etiology/Pathophysiology

- Hard ticks—four life stages: egg, larva, nymph, and adult; larvae and nymphs must feed to repletion before detaching and molting; as adult female ixodid ticks engorge, they may increase their weight by more than 100-fold; after detachment females may lay thousands of eggs.
- Blood-loss anemia—from heavy infestations
- Damage to the integument—tick mouth parts cut through the host's skin; bites are generally painless; local irritation and infection may occur
- Salivary secretion of neurotoxins—may lead to systemic signs (tick paralysis); local action may cause impaired hemostasis and immune suppression.
- Pathogens—acquired when ticks feed on infected reservoir hosts (often rodents and small feral mammals); sometimes transovarial transmission occurs and infected eggs hatch and produce infected larvae; greatest potential for systemic disease occurs when infections acquired in early life stages are trans-

mitted to new hosts when the next stage feeds; may affect virtually any organ system
- Transmission of pathogens and toxins—often requires periods of attachment from hours to days; the essentially painless bite allows adequate feeding times.

Signalment/History

Geographic Distribution

- Strong geographic specificities exist for some tick species; thus geographic prevalence of associated diseases
- *Ixodes scapularis*—Lyme disease; midwest, northeast, and parts of the southeast
- *Ixodes pacificus*—western coastal states
- *Rhipicephalus sanguineus*—found throughout the continental U.S.; but canine ehrlichiosis and babesiosis most common in the southeast

Species

- Dogs and cats
- Cats are thought to be quite efficient at removing ticks, but tick attachment and subsequent tick-vectored diseases are routinely diagnosed.

Risk Factors

- Large hunting breeds (dogs)—considered to be at high risk, because they are likely to come in contact with environments harboring questing ticks
- Domestic animals—can be in close contact with ticks owing to encroachment of ticks into suburban environments and expansion of suburban environment into surrounding forests, prairies, and coastline areas

Clinical Features

- Attached ticks or tick feeding cavities from which ticks have detached may be seen on the skin.
- Associated tick-borne diseases (borreliosis, ehrlichiosis, babesiosis, Rocky Mountain Spotted Fever, and others)—vary with the organ system(s) affected
- Irritation caused by ticks and subsequent self-trauma—may lead to pyotraumatic dermatitis ("hot spots") in dogs

Diagnostics

- Ticks—examine the skin for attached ticks or tick feeding cavities
- Tick-borne diseases—evaluate epidemiologic considerations for each disease, history of tick parasitism, and complete clinical examination

Therapeutics

- Outpatient after removal of ticks
- Removal—do as soon as possible to limit time available for neurotoxin or pathogen transmission; grasp ticks close to the skin with fine-pointed tweez-

ers and gently pull free; species with short, strong mouth parts (e.g., *Dermacentor*) usually pull free with host skin attached; species with long, fragile mouth parts (e.g., *Ixodes*) often leave fragments of mouth parts embedded in the feeding cavity.
- Wash feeding cavity with soap and water; generally sufficient to prevent local inflammation or secondary infection
- Inform client that application of hot matches, Vaseline, or other materials not only fails to cause tick detachment but allows for longer periods of attachment and feeding.

PREVENTION/AVOIDANCE

- Avoid environments that harbor ticks; may be difficult except for pets kept strictly indoors
- Tick control—essential to realize that this does not always equal control of tick-borne diseases; often the goal is the perceived absence of ticks on the host animal
- Pets—owners report complete tick control even though there may be some period of attachment and tick feeding or live ticks may spend some time crawling on the animal after they have been exposed to lethal levels of an acaricide; immature ticks of some species (*R. sanguineus* and *I. scapularis*) may be undetected because of their minute size
- Tick-borne pathogens—may be transmitted very rapidly (viruses) or may require several hours (*Rickettsia rickettsii*) or days (*Borrelia burgdorferi*)

Insecticides and Acaricides

- In the U.S., the EPA licenses agents as effective against various species of pests.
- Control—inferred as providing control of diseases carried by that species; although this may be correct in some or all cases, veterinarians should be sophisticated enough to require demonstration of efficacy in prevention of disease transmission before accepting a disease-control claim at face value; challenging because ticks are widely dispersed in the environment, spend a relatively short time on their hosts, poses great reproductive capacities, and have long lifetimes
- Acaricidal collars (Preventic) and spot treatment (Frontline)—have gained wide use; ease of application is as important as efficacy; direct marketing to pet owners of veterinarian-dispensed products has been a major factor in shifting tick control away from OTC formulations
- Bathing, spraying, or powdering with appropriate organophosphate or pyrethrin-containing products has become far less common with the advent of new convenient and effective products.

Comments

CONDITIONS

- Canine babesiosis—vectored by *R. sanguineus;* caused by protozoan parasite *Babesia canis;* infects canine RBCs, leading to sludging in capillaries and destruction in the spleen
- Rocky Mountain Spotted Fever—vectored by *Dermacentor variabilis;* caused by *R. rickettsii;* invades vascular endothelial tissues, leading to necrotizing vasculitis

- Canine ehrlichiosis—vectored by *R. sanguineus;* caused by *Ehrlichia canis;* infects mononuclear cells and platelets
- Granulocytic ehrlichiosis—emerging disease; caused by *E. equi* (also called *E. phagocytophila*); infects granulocytes, leading to nonspecific signs and fever
- Lyme disease—vectored by *I. scapularis* and *I. pacificus;* caused by *Borrelia burgdorferi;* dogs may develop fevers associated with arthritis or syndromes leading to complete heart block, protein-losing nephropathy, and neurologic abnormalities
- Canine hepatozoonosis—caused by protozoal organism *Hepatozoon canis* after the dog ingests an infected *R. sanguineus;* cysts and pyogranulomas in the muscles and other tissues associated with myositis and renal failure, often leading to death in chronic cases
- Tick paralysis—caused by a neurotoxin; affects acetylcholine synthesis and/or liberation at the neuromuscular junction of the host animal; signs (typified by ascending flaccid paralysis often initially affecting the pelvic limbs) develop 5–9 days after tick attachment

Vaccines

- Currently for "prevention" of only Lyme disease; two types for dogs: whole-cell, killed bacterin (since 1990) and Osp A (since 1996)
- Safety and efficacy—peer-reviewed published data for dogs naturally exposed to *B. burgdorferi* available only for bacterin; 1969 dogs received a total of 4033 doses of bacterin during a 20-month period; 4498 control dogs were not vaccinated; immunization was found to be safe regardless of previous history of Lyme disease or exposure to *B. burgdorferi;* 38 (1.9%) of vaccinated dogs had minor reactions that resolved without complications immediately or within 72 hr after vaccination; cumulative incidence of Lyme disease was 1.0% in vaccinated dogs and 4.7% in control dogs; 40% of vaccinated dogs had serologic evidence of infection with *B. burgdorferi* before vaccination but the incidence of Lyme disease was only 2%; incidence of Lyme disease in infected control dogs was 4.8%; thus, vaccination of infected dogs was associated with about a 50% decrease in the incidence of Lyme disease; some clinical experiences have not shown this high degree of efficacy and have reported potentially harmful side effects (e.g., immune-mediated phenomena)

Zoonotic Potential

- Ticks may parasitize many different species of mammals, birds, and reptiles at different stages in their developmental cycles; infections acquired in early life stages may be transmitted when ticks feed again in the next stage.
- Humans, if parasitized, may be exposed to babesiosis, Rocky Mountain Spotted Fever, ehrlichiosis, borreliosis, or tick paralysis.

See also

- Babesiosis
- Ehrlichiosis
- Hepatozoonosis
- Lyme Disease (Borreliosis)
- Rocky Mountain Spotted Fever
- Tick Bite Paralysis

Suggested Reading

Hoskins JD, ed. Tick-transmitted disease. Vet Clin North Am 1991:21.

Levy SA, Barthold SW, Dombach DM, et al. Canine borreliosis. Compend Contin Educ 1993;15:833–848.

Levy SA, Lissman BA, Ficke CM. Performance of a *Borrelia burgdorferi* bacterin in borreliosis endemic areas. J Am Vet Med Assoc 1993;202:1834–1838.

Sonenshine DE. Biology of ticks. Vol. 2. New York: Oxford University Press, 1993.

Consulting Editor Karen Helton Rhodes

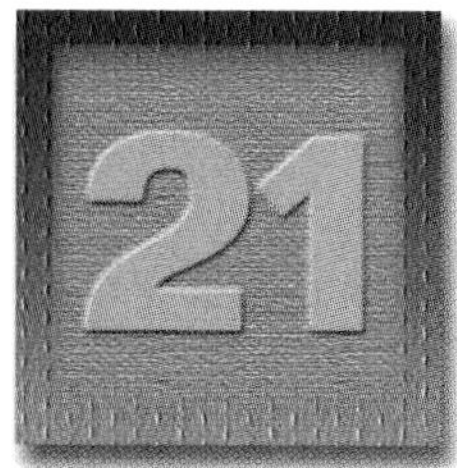

Tick Bite Paralysis

Paul A. Cuddon

Definition/Overview

Flaccid, lower motor neuron paralysis caused by salivary neurotoxins from certain species of female ticks

Etiology/Pathophysiology

- Tick—injects salivary neurotoxins that probably interfere with the depolarization/acetylcholine release mechanism in the presynaptic nerve terminal, leading to reduction in the release of acetylcholine
- *Ixodes holocyclus* tick infestation—neurotoxin depends strongly on temperature; one adult tick is sufficient to cause neurologic signs, but a large larval or nymphal *Ixodes* tick infestation can also induce signs
- Signs—occur 6–9 days after initial tick attachment
- Not all infested animals develop tick paralysis; not all adult female ticks produce the toxin.
- Nervous—peripheral nervous system and the neuromuscular junction most affected by the neurotoxin; cranial nerves can become involved, including the vagal, facial, and trigeminal nerves; sympathetic system also affected
- Respiratory—may see paralysis of the intercostal muscles and diaphragm; caudal brainstem respiratory center may be affected

Signalment/History

Incidence/Prevalence

- North America and Australia—somewhat seasonal (more prevalent in the summer months); in the warmer areas (southern U.S.; northern Australia) may become a year-round problem
- Overall incidence—low in the U.S.; higher in Australia

Geographic Distribution

- U.S.—*Dermacentor variabilis:* wide distribution over the eastern two-thirds of the country and in California and Oregon; *D. andersoni:* from the Cascades to the Rocky Mountains; *Amblyomma americanum:* from Texas and Missouri to the Atlantic Coast; *A. maculatum:* high temperature and humidity of the Atlantic and Gulf of Mexico seaboards
- Australia—limited to the coastal areas of the east; especially associated with areas of bush and scrub

Species

- Australia—dogs and cats
- U.S.—dogs; cats appear to be resistant

Historical Findings

- Patient walked in a wooded area approximately 1 week before onset of signs.
- Onset—gradual; starts with unsteadiness and weakness in the pelvic limbs

Clinical Features

Non-Ixodes Tick

- Once neurologic signs appear, there is rapid ascending lower motor neuron paresis to paralysis.
- Patient becomes recumbent in 1–3 days, with hyporeflexia to areflexia and hypotonia to atonia.
- Pain sensation preserved
- Cranial nerve dysfunction—not a prominent feature; may note facial weakness and reduced jaw tone; sometimes dysphonia and dysphagia early in the course
- Respiratory paralysis—uncommon in the U.S.; may occur in severely affected patients
- Urination and defecation usually normal

Ixodes Tick

- Neurologic signs—much more severe and rapidly progressive; ascending motor weakness can progress to paralysis within a few hours
- Sialosis, megaesophagus, and vomiting or regurgitation characteristic
- Sympathetic nervous system—mydriatic and poorly responsive pupils; hypertension; tachyarrhythmias; high pulmonary capillary hydrostatic pressure; pulmonary edema
- Caudal medullary respiratory center—additive to the peripheral pulmonary changes, causing progressive fall in respiratory rate without a change in tidal volume, resulting in hypoxia, hypercapnia, and respiratory acidosis

- Respiratory muscle paralysis—much more prevalent; dogs and cats progress to dyspnea, cyanosis, and respiratory paralysis within 1–2 days if not treated

Differential Diagnosis

Causes

United States

- *D. variabilis*—common wood tick
- *D. andersoni*—Rocky Mountain wood tick
- *A. americanum*—lone star tick
- *A. maculatum*—Gulf Coast tick

Australia

I. holocyclus—secretes a far more potent neurotoxin than that of the North American species

Diseases

- Botulism
- Acute polyneuropathy
- Coonhound paralysis
- Acute polyradiculoneuritis
- Distal denervating disease
- Generalized (diffuse) or multifocal myelopathy

Diagnostics

Laboratory Tests

Arterial blood gases—severely affected patients; low PaO_2, high $PaCO_2$, and low pH

Imaging

Thoracic radiography (*Ixodes* tick)—megaesophagus

Diagnostic Procedures

- Thoroughly search for a tick—head, neck, body and limbs, ear canals, mouth, rectum, vagina, prepuce, and in between the digits and foot pads; immediately remove tick.
- Electrodiagnostics (electromyogram)—normal insertion activity and an absence of spontaneous myofiber activity (no fibrillations and positive sharp waves); lack of motor unit action potentials; motor nerve stimulation is followed by either a dramatic decrease in amplitude or a complete absence of compound muscle action potentials.

Therapeutics

Inpatient—any neurologic dysfunction suggesting tick paralysis; hospitalize until either a tick is found and removed or appropriate treatment to kill a hidden tick is performed.

- Inpatient supportive care—essential until patient begins to show signs of recovery
- Oxygen cage—hypoventilation and hypoxia
- Artificial ventilation—respiratory failure
- Intravenous fluid therapy—generally not required unless recovery is prolonged
- Keep patient in a quiet environment.
- *Ixodes* tick paralysis—keep patient in a cool, air-conditioned area; toxin is temperature sensitive; avoid activity to prevent increase in body temperature
- Withhold food and water if patient has dysphagia or vomiting/regurgitation.

Drugs of Choice

- U.S.—if the tick cannot be found, dip the patient in an insecticidal bath; often the only treatment needed
- Australia—must neutralize circulating toxin via hyperimmune serum (0.5–1 mg/kg IV), depending on severity of clinical signs; if severe, phenoxybenzamine, an α-adrenergic antagonist (1 mg/kg IV diluted in saline and given slowly over 20 min) appears to be beneficial in relieving the sympathetic effects; acepromazine (0.5–1 mg/kg IV) can be used as an alternative (it has α-adrenergic blocking effects)

Contraindications

- Drugs that interfere with neuromuscular transmission are contraindicated (e.g., tetracyclines, aminoglycosides, and procaine penicillin).
- *Ixodes* tick—atropine contraindicated in the advanced stages of disease or with marked bradycardia

Precautions

Ixodes tick—administer intravenous fluids at a very slow rate to avoid further complications of pulmonary congestion

Comments

Client Education

- Non-*Ixodes* tick—inform client that good nursing care is essential, although the patient's recovery is rapid after removal of ticks
- *Ixodes* tick—warn client that signs often continue to worsen despite tick removal; thus, more aggressive treatment to neutralize the toxin must be undertaken.
- Non-*Ixodes* tick—reassess neurologic status after tick removal at least daily—should see rapid improvement in muscle strength in animals
- *Ixodes* tick—monitor neurologic status and respiratory and cardiovascular functions continuously and intensively even after tick removal, because of the residual effect of neurotoxin
- Vigilantly check for ticks after exposure (at least every 2–3 days); signs do not occur for 4–6 days after tick attachment.
- Weekly insecticidal baths or the use of insecticide-impregnated collars helps.
- Short-term acquired immunity develops after exposure to *Ixodes* neurotoxin.

- No long-term complications if the patient survives the acute effects of the toxin
- Non-*Ixodes* tick—prognosis good to excellent if ticks are removed; recovery occurs in 1–3 days
- *Ixodes* tick—prognosis often guarded; recovery prolonged; death in 1–2 days without treatment
- Although humans can acquire the disease by being bitten by the same ticks (especially in Australia), tick paralysis is not transmitted to humans from affected pets.

Suggested Reading

Braund KG. Clinical syndromes in veterinary neurology. 2nd ed. St. Louis: Mosby, 1994.

Ilkiw JE. Tick paralysis in Australia. In: Kirk RW, ed. Current veterinary therapy VIII. Small animal practice. Philadelphia: Saunders, 1983:691–693.

Malik R, Farrow BRH. Tick paralysis in North America and Australia. Vet Clin North Am 1991;21:157–171.

Author Paul A. Cudden

Consulting Editor Karen Helton Rhodes

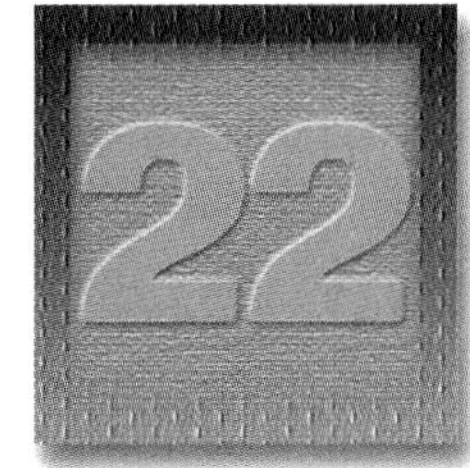

Fleas and Flea Control

Karen A. Kuhl and Jean S. Greek

Definition/Overview

- Flea allergy dermatitis—hypersensitivity reaction to antigens in flea saliva with or without evidence of fleas and flea dirt
- Flea infestation—large number of fleas and a large amount of flea dirt with or without a flea allergy dermatitis

Etiology/Pathophysiology

- Flea bite hypersensitivity (FBH)—caused by a low molecular weight hapten and two high molecular weight allergens that help initiate the allergic reaction
- High molecular weight allergens—increase binding to dermal collagen; when bound, form a complete antigen necessary for eliciting FBH
- Flea saliva—contains histamine-like compounds that irritate skin
- Intermittent exposure favors FBH; continuous exposure is less likely to result in hypersensitivity.
- Both IgE and IgG antiflea antibodies have been noted.
- Immediate and delayed hypersensitivity reactions have been noted.
- Late-phase IgE-mediated response—part of FBH reaction; occurs 3–6 hr after exposure
- Cutaneous basophil hypersensitivity—part of FBH reaction; an infiltration of basophils into the dermis; mediated either by IgE or IgG; subsequent exposures cause the basophils to degranulate; manifests as immediate and delayed hypersensitivity

Signalment/History

- Dogs and cats
- FBH—any breed; most common in atopic breeds
- FBH—rare < 6 months of age; average age range, 3–6 years, but may be seen at any age
- FBH—intermittent exposure to fleas increases the likelihood of development; commonly seen in conjunction with atopy

Historical Findings

- Compulsive biting
- Chewing (corncob nibbling)
- Licking, primarily in the back half of the body but may include the antebrachial regions
- Cats—scratching around the head and neck
- Signs of fleas and flea dirt

Clinical Features

- Depends somewhat on the severity of the reaction and the degree of exposure to fleas (i.e., seasonal vs. year-round)
- Finding fleas and flea dirt is beneficial, although not essential, for the diagnosis of FBH; sensitive animals require a low exposure and tend to overgroom, making identification of the parasites difficult.
- Dogs—lesions concentrated in a triangular area of the caudal-dorsal-lumbosacral region; caudal aspect of the thighs, lower abdomen, inguinal region, and cranial forearms usually involved; primary lesions are papules; secondary lesions (e.g., hyperpigmentation, lichenification, alopecia, and scaling) common in uncontrolled FBH; secondary folliculitis and furunculosis may be seen.
- Cats—several patterns are seen; most common is a miliary crusting dermatitis in a wedge-shaped pattern over the caudal dorsal lumbosacral region and often around the head and neck; other presentations are alopecia of the inguinal region with or without inflammation or eosinophilic plaques and other forms of eosinophilic granuloma complex.
- Exposure to other animals and previous flea treatment should be ascertained.

Differential Diagnosis

- Food allergy
- Atopy
- Sarcoptic mange
- Cheyletiellosis
- Primary keratinization defects

Diagnostics

- Cats—hypereosinophilia may be detected
- Skin scrapings—negative
- Flea combings—fleas or flea dirt, but often nothing is found
- RAST and ELISA—variable accuracy; both false-positive and false-negative results reported
- Diagnosis usually based on historical information and distribution of lesions
- Fleas or flea dirt is supportive but is often quite difficult to find, especially in cats.
- Identification of *Dipylidium caninum* segments is supportive.
- Intradermal allergy testing with flea antigen—reveals positive immediate reactions in 90% of flea-allergic animals; delayed reactions (24–48 hr) may sometimes be observed in allergic animals that show no immediate reaction
- The most accurate test may be response to appropriate treatment.

Biopsy

- Superficial perivascular dermatitis
- Eosinophilic intraepidermal microabscesses—strongly suggest FBH
- Eosinophils as a major cellular component of the dermis—supportive of FBH
- Histopathologic evaluation—cannot accurately differentiate FBH from atopy, food allergy, or other hypersensitivities

Therapeutics

- Corticosteroids—anti-inflammatory dosages for symptomatic relief while the fleas are being controlled
- Antihistamines—symptomatic relief
- Fipronil (GABA antagonist)—monthly spot treatment for cats and dogs and spray treatment for dogs; activity against fleas and ticks; resistant to removal with water; excellent safety and efficacy profile
- Imidacloprid—monthly spot treatment for cats and dogs; excellent safety and efficacy profile
- Systemic treatments—limited benefit because they require a flea bite that has already initiated FBH; may help animals with flea infestation; primarily licensed for use in only dogs; lufenuron, a chitin inhibitor, available as an oral formulation for cats and dogs and as an injection for cats; permethrin available as a spot treatment and reputed to have some repellent activity; imidacloprid (flea adulticide) available as a spot treatment for cats and dogs.
- Sprays—usually contain pyrethrins and pyrethroids (synthetic pyrethrins) with an insect growth regulator or synergist; generally effective $< 48–72$ hr; advantages are low toxicity and repellent activity; disadvantages are frequent applications and expense
- Indoor treatment—fogs and premises sprays; usually contain organophosphates, pyrethrins, and/or insect growth regulators; apply according to manufacturer's directions; treat all areas of the house; can be applied by the owner; advantages are weak chemicals and generally inexpensive; disadvan-

tage is labor intensity; premises sprays concentrate the chemicals in areas that most need treatment

- Professional exterminators—advantages are less labor-intensive, relatively few applications, sometimes guaranteed, disadvantages are strength of chemicals and cost; specific recommendations and guidelines must be followed
- Inert substances—boric acid, diatomaceous earth, and silica aerogel; treat every 6–12 months; follow manufacturer's recommendations; very safe and effective if applied properly
- Outdoor treatment—concentrated in shaded areas; sprays usually contain pyrethroids or organophosphates and an insect growth regulator; powders are usually organophosphates; product containing nematodes (*Steinerma carpocapsae*) is very safe and chemical-free

Precautions

- Insecticidal sprays and dips should not be used on dogs and cats ≤ 3 months, unless otherwise specified on the label.
- Pyrethrin/pyrethroid-type flea products—adverse reactions include depression, hypersalivation, muscle tremors, vomiting, ataxia, dyspnea, and anorexia
- Organophosphates—adverse reactions include hypersalivation, lacrimation, urination, defecation, vomiting, diarrhea, miosis, fever, muscle tremors, seizures, coma, and death
- All pesticides must be applied according to label directions.
- Toxicity—if any signs are noted, the animal should be bathed thoroughly to remove any remaining chemicals and treated appropriately
- Rodents and fish are very sensitive to pyrethrins.

Possible Interactions

- Organophosphate treatments—do not use more than one form at a time.
- Topical organophosphates—avoid in cats, very young animals (< 3 months of age), and sick or debilitated animals
- Straight permethrin sprays or spot-ons—do not use in cats
- Cythioate—contraindicated in heartworm-positive dogs and greyhounds
- Piperonyl butoxide—do not use in concentrations > 1% in cats

Alternative Drugs

- Powders—usually contain organophosphates or carbamates; advantage is high residual effectiveness; disadvantages are dry skin and toxicity; organophosphates and carbamates should be avoided in cats
- Dips, sprays, powders, and foams—dips usually contain organophosphates and synthetic pyrethrins and should not be used more than once per week; follow manufacturer's instructions for safest and best results; after repeated use, these agents can be drying or irritating; newer, safer spot treatments have essentially replaced these products

Comments

- Inform owners that there is no cure for FBH.
- Advise owners that flea-allergic animals often become more sensitive to flea bites as they age.

- Inform owners that controlling exposure to fleas is currently the only means of therapy; hyposensitization has not worked satisfactorily.
- Pruritus—a decrease means the FBH is being controlled
- Fleas and flea dirt—absence is not always a reliable indicator of successful treatment in very sensitive animals
- Year-round warm climates—year-round flea control
- Seasonally warm climates—begin flea control in May or June
- Approximately 80% of atopic dogs are also allergic to flea bites.
- Organophosphates—use with utmost caution in old animals; not recommended for use in very young animals (<3 months)
- In areas of moderate to severe flea infestation, people can be bitten by fleas; usually papular lesions are located on the wrists and ankles.
- Corticosteroids and organophosphates—do not use in pregnant bitches and queens
- Carefully follow the label directions of each individual product to determine its safety.

Suggested Reading

Bevier-Tournay DE. Fleas and flea control. In: Kirk RW, Bonagura JD, eds. Current veterinary therapy X. Philadelphia: Saunders, 1989:586–591.

Griffin CE, Kwochka KW, MacDonald JM. Current veterinary dermatology. St. Louis: Mosby, 1993.

Consulting Editor Karen Helton Rhodes

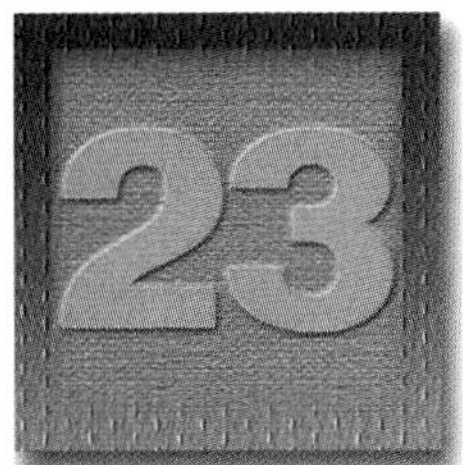

Flea Control Products

John MacDonald

Products That Affect Flea Development

Insect Growth Regulators

Insect growth hormones (insect growth regulators [IGRs] or juvenoids) are natural chemicals in insects that control various stages of the insect's metabolism, morphogenesis, and reproduction. They are important in organ development and maturation and the development and growth of the larvae in general. Maturation and ultimately pupation of flea larvae, however, depend on the absence of natural juvenile hormones that are essential for the earlier growth.

Synthetic compounds produced to mimic natural insect growth hormones represent the class of products called IGRs. Advantages of IGRs include safety, residual activity, and ovicidal/larvacidal effects.

Pyriproxifen (Nylar) is a new-generation IGR currently on the market in a variety of formulations with impressive potency (exceeding both methoprene and fenoxycarb) and requires only very small concentrations for residual effectiveness. It also demonstrates ovicidal activity. Pyriproxifen is stable in ultraviolet light and has longer residual activity without being broken down by the insect. Products on the market containing pyriproxifen (Nylar) include pressurized canisters, foggers, and liquid concentrate for mixture with water for premise application. Several on-the-animal products are available, including a prediluted pump spray for on-the-animal application. A pet collar containing pyriproxifen is labeled for 1 year of activity and is currently available for use in the cat. A systemic formulation of pyriproxifen may be marketed in the future.

Methoprene is still available, but is predominantly sold through non-veterinarian retail outlets. It may be useful for inside application or use on the animal, but it has the disadvantage of being inactivated by ultraviolet light under some conditions. It is also broken down by the natural esterase produced by the flea larvae, limiting its residual activity. It has been formulated as a microencapsulated product and continues to be popular with some pet owners for application on the animal. Veterinarian use of methoprene is limited with more use of pyriproxifen.

Insect Development Inhibitors

Insect development inhibitors (IDIs) are chemicals that interfere with the development of the flea but do not mimic the activity of insect growth hormone as do IGRs. The common IDI that is used is lufenuron, which is categorized as a benzoylphenyl urea. Its activity is the inhibition of synthesis and deposition of chitin. Because normal chitin development is critical for the survival of the insect ova and larvae, lufenuron is very effective on the developing larvae. It has virtually no mammalian toxicity because mammals do not produce chitin, which makes it very safe.

Lufenuron is a lipophilic compound that is stored in body fat and gradually released. It is administered once a month at a dose of 10 mg/kg for dogs and 30 mg/kg for cats, and must be taken with food to obtain adequate absorption. Lufenuron has no adulticidal activity. The major attributes are simplicity of treatment, safety, and effect on flea development. It is available in formulation with a heartworm preventative (milbemycin) and has recently been approved for parenteral administration that provides 6 months of activity from a single injection. One limitation of systemic insect development inhibitors and growth regulators is the time required to disrupt the life cycle in a highly flea-infested area. Another limitation of systemic insect development inhibitors concerns the flea-allergic animal because the product does not reduce an active flea infestation and requires adult fleas to feed, thereby eliciting an allergic response. Systemic products that interfere with the development of pre-adult stages of the flea are often a good "safety net" for the flea-allergic dog, but may not be satisfactory as the only method of control.

Sodium Polyborate

Sodium borate compounds are used exclusively for inside premise application and have a significant effect on ova and larva development. Certain formulations of borate have demonstrated 12 months of residual activity from a single application in a clinical situation. Regular vacuuming may be performed without disrupting the efficacy; however, carpet shampooing may limit the residual activity. Toxicity studies have been conducted with a sodium polyborate compound demonstrating low-risk characterization and minimal toxicity potential. Sodium polyborate compounds are considered very safe and some are labeled for use in schools, food preparation areas, and nursing homes. Sodium polyborate treatment is still an effective method of flea control for the indoors and its greatest attribute is residual activity and safety.

Products For Use On the Animal

Pyrethrins, Pyrethroids, and Organophosphates

Conventional on-the-animal products have included topical parasiticides representing pour-ons and sprays containing pyrethrins, pyrethroids, or in some limited use, organophosphates. These products may be effective in controlling flea infestations but have limited residual activity and have been replaced almost completely by the newer residual products. Pyrethrin/permethrin compounds containing conventional concentrations must be applied every other day to avert an active flea infestation, or weekly at higher concentrations (2% permethrin). Concentrated solutions of permethrin should not be used on cats and only when indicated by label statements. Weekly pour-on parasiticides may also be included in the treatment regimen. Effectiveness of these products is often incomplete and may not sufficiently break the flea life cycle as the exclusive treatment. Premise treatment usually needs to be incorporated in the program to attain adequate control. Some products contain pyriproxifen (an IGR) with the pyrethrin or permethrin, which adds a useful dimension to prevent development of future generations of fleas. The use of a water protectant (Forapearl) has been helpful to extend efficacy, particularly if water exposure is prominent. These products may be helpful as adjunctive therapy but have limitations compared with other on-the-animal products with residual activity.

Organophosphates such as chlorpyrifos or phosmet for use on the animal have nearly been eliminated from routine use by veterinarians, although some are available in other retail outlets (pet stores and feed stores). Some pet owners continue to incorporate them in flea control programs, although organophosphates have limited usefulness because of the availability of other products.

Imidacloprid (Advantage)

Imidacloprid (Advantage) is a chlorinated heterocycle insecticide formerly introduced for crop pest control and structural pest control (termiticide) and now approved for on-the-animal adulticidal flea treatment. The active compound is a member of the class called chloronicotinyl. It is a novel product—with no other similar chemical currently existing—and has only recently been developed for on-the-animal application to control fleas. Imidacloprid binds to the acetylcholine receptor site on the postsynaptic portion of insect nerve cells and prevents transmission of impulses along the insect's nerve, resulting in death. Imidacloprid acts on the nicotinic receptor sites specifically, and because muscarinic receptors are present in mammals, this mode of action is specific for insects. It is prepared as a 9.1% solution and is applied as a spot treatment for dogs and cats, with recommendations of a 28-day reapplication rate. Preliminary data demonstrate both acute and residual adulticidal activity with 98–100% flea kill within 24 hours. Studies have demonstrated 98% flea control for at least 14 days and 96% control for 21 days.

Imidacloprid has shown activity against larvae and has been studied in simulated situations that have shown decreased development of flea populations in the environment when the dog in that habitat had been treated with the product. An umbrella effect has also been demonstrated with young nursing animals whose flea infestation regressed when the parent female was treated. Imidacloprid may be used in animals as young as 6–7 weeks and applied at a frequency of as often as weekly, if necessary. Variation in effectiveness may vary depending on pets habits, water exposure, bathing intervals, and the flea infestation. Concern for efficacy breakdown after bathing or exposure to water has, to some extent, been clarified by limited studies sponsored by the manufacturer that demonstrated no significant effect following short-term water immersion or limited shampoo therapy.

No evidence of toxicity has been observed during safety studies in animals receiving exaggerated dosages and used with other medications. Adverse reactions have not been observed in dogs infected with heartworms. Attributes of imidacloprid include acute flea-killing activity, safety, and residual activity.

Fipronil (Frontline Spray/Top Spot)

Fipronil (Frontline Spray / Top Spot) is a phenylpyrazole that has been available for a short time in the U.S., although it has been in Europe for some time. It interferes with the passage of the chloride ion through the gamma-aminobutyric acid (GABA) regulated chloride channel of invertebrates, disrupting CNS activity. It has very selective neurotoxicity which does not affect mammals. Fipronil also has affinity for sebaceous secretions and, following treatment, is found in hair follicles and sebaceous glands; it is then redistributed to the skin surface for residual insecticidal activity. The extent of efficacy for adulticidal flea control is expected to be 28 days or longer from a single application but may vary depending on geographical location, exposure to water, interval of bathing, and extent of flea infestation.

Fipronil is also acaricidal and is recommended in situations in which there is tick infestation. Regional efficacy may be variable with regards to tick control. Limited anecdotal information has demonstrated some scabicidal effectiveness in clinical cases. The manufacturer has demonstrated 95% control of flea infestation 4 weeks after application. The advantage of fipronil is the long-term on-the-animal adulticidal activity, making it particularly advantageous for flea-allergic dogs in contrast to systemics, which require flea feeding. Because the product is absorbed in the skin and re-released, limited bathing or exposure to water may not significantly alter the activity. Studies sponsored by the manufacturer demonstrate no significant decrease in the 4-week residual effect of fipronil with limited concurrent bathing.

The disadvantage of the fipronil spray formulation is the alcohol base, which may have a drying or irritancy effect—particularly if the skin is inflamed, excoriated, or eroded. Another limitation is the quantity necessary for effective flea control. Precise dosing is essential for maximal efficacy, which may require substantial spray solution for the larger dog, thus increasing expense and labor. Thickly coated animals may have less effective flea control because of inadequate penetration to the skin with the spray. Cats have a shorter duration of activity lasting only 2–3 weeks.

Consulting Editor Karen Helton Rhodes

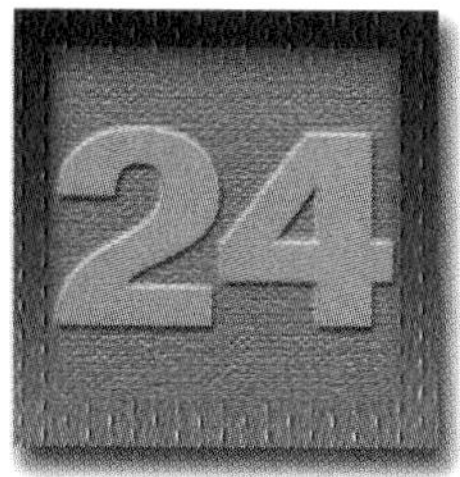

Cheyletiellosis

Alexander H. Werner

Definition/Overview

- A highly contagious parasitic skin disease of dogs, cats, and rabbits, caused by infestation with *Cheyletiella* spp. mites
- Signs of scaling and pruritus can mimic other more common diseases.
- Often referred to as "walking dandruff," because of the large mite size and excessive scaling
- Prevalence varies by geographic region owing to mite susceptibility to common flea-control insecticides.
- Human (zoonotic) lesions can occur.

Etiology/Pathophysiology

- *Cheyletiella yasguri*—dogs (Fig. 24-1)
- *Cheyletiella blakei*—cats
- *Cheyletiella parasitivorax*—rabbits

Signalment/History

- Dogs and cats
- More common in young animals
- Cocker spaniels, poodles, and long-haired cats are frequent asymptomatic carriers.
- Cats may exhibit bizarre behavioral signs or excessive grooming.

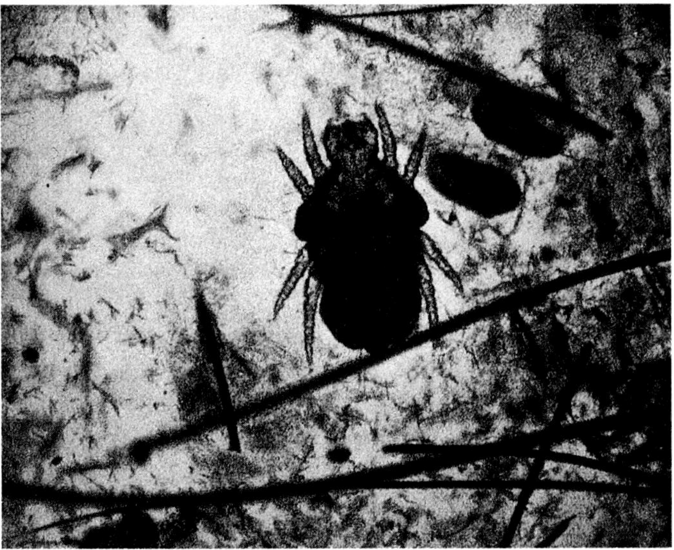

Figure 24-1 *Cheyletiella yasguri* (dog).

- Pruritus—none to severe, depending on the individual's response to infestation
- Infestation may be suspected after lesions in humans have developed.
- Young animals and those in frequent contact with others are most at risk.
- Common sources of infestation—animal shelters, breeders, and grooming establishments

Clinical Features

- Scaling—most important clinical sign; diffuse or plaque-like; most severe in chronically infested and debilitated animals (Fig. 24-2)
- Lesions—dorsal orientation is commonly noted
- Underlying skin irritation may be minimal.
- Cats may exhibit bilaterally symmetrical alopecia.

Differential Diagnosis

- Cheyletiellosis should be considered in every animal that has scaling, with or without pruritus.
- Also consider—seborrhea, flea-allergic dermatitis, *Sarcoptes* spp. mite infestation, atopy, food hypersensitivity, and idiopathic pruritus

Diagnostics

- Examination of epidermal debris—very effective in diagnosing infestation
- Collection of debris—flea combing (most effective), skin scraping, and acetate tape preparation
- *Cheyletiella* mites are large and can be visualized with a simple handheld

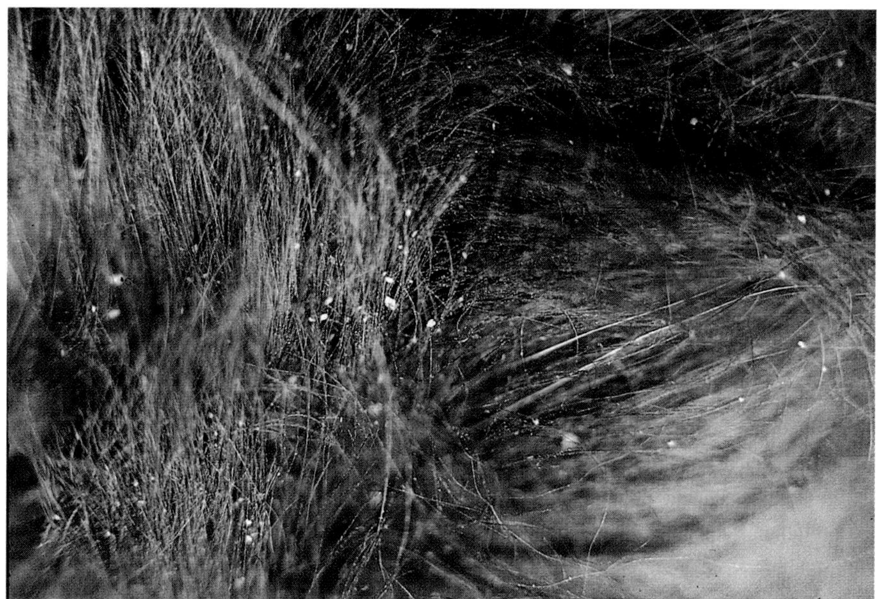

Figure 24-2 Cheyletiellosis in a cat. Note the excessive scaling within the haircoat.

magnifying lens; scales and hair may be examined under low magnification; staining is not necessary.

- Response to insecticide preparations may be required to definitively diagnose suspicious cases in which mites cannot be identified.

Therapeutics

- Must treat all animals in the household
- Clip long coats to facilitate treatment.
- Mainstay—6–8 weekly baths to remove scale, followed by rinses with an insecticide
- Lime-sulfur and pyrethrin rinses—cats, kittens, puppies, and rabbits
- Pyrethrin or organophosphates—dogs
- Routine flea sprays and powders—not always effective
- Environmental treatment with frequent cleanings and insecticide sprays—important for eliminating infestation
- Combs, brushes, and grooming utensils—discard or thoroughly disinfect before reuse
- Zoonotic lesions—self-limiting after eradication of the mites from household animals
- Alternatives (or additions) to topical therapy—amitraz and ivermectin
- Amitraz (Mitaban)—use on dogs (4 rinses at 2-week intervals)
- Ivermectin—highly effective (300 μg/kg SC 3 times at 2-week intervals); dogs, cats, and rabbits > 3 months old; pour-on forms have shown efficacy in cats (500 μg/kg 2 times at 2-week intervals)

Comments

- Ivermectin—not FDA-approved for this use in dogs, cats, or rabbits; client disclosure and consent are paramount before administration; several dog breeds (e.g., collies, shelties, Australian shepherds) have shown increased sensitivity and should not be treated
- Treatment failure necessitates re-evaluation for other causes of pruritus and scaling.
- Reinfestation may indicate contact with an asymptomatic carrier or the presence of an unidentified source of mites (e.g., untreated bedding).
- Zoonotic potential: A pruritic papular rash may develop in areas of contact with the pet.

Suggested Reading

Moriello KA. Cheyletiellosis. In: Griffin CE, Kwochka KW, MacDonald JM, eds. Current veterinary dermatology: the science and art of therapy. St. Louis: Mosby, 1993.

Consulting Editor Karen Helton Rhodes

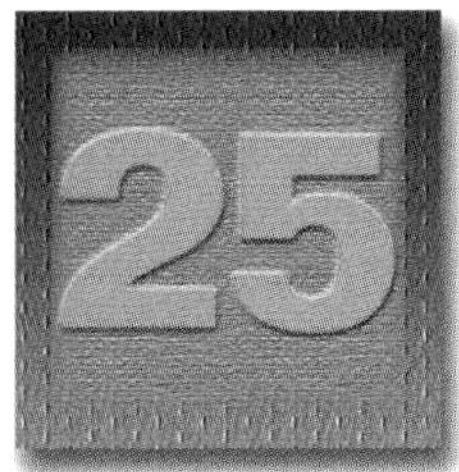

Sarcoptic Mange

Linda Medleau and Keith A. Hnilica

Definition/Overview

- A nonseasonal, intensely pruritic, highly contagious parasitic skin disease of dogs caused by infestation with the mite *Sarcoptes scabiei* var. *canis*

Etiology/Pathophysiology

- Mites burrow through the stratum corneum and cause intense pruritus by mechanical irritation, production of irritating byproducts, and secretion of allergenic substances that produce a hypersensitivity reaction in sensitized dogs.

Signalment/History

- Dogs of all ages and breeds
- Exposure to a carrier dog 2–6 weeks before development of symptoms
- Living outside (roaming dogs)
- Boarded at kennel
- Visits to veterinarian's office
- Visits to groomer
- Residence at animal shelter
- Nonseasonal extremely intense pruritus

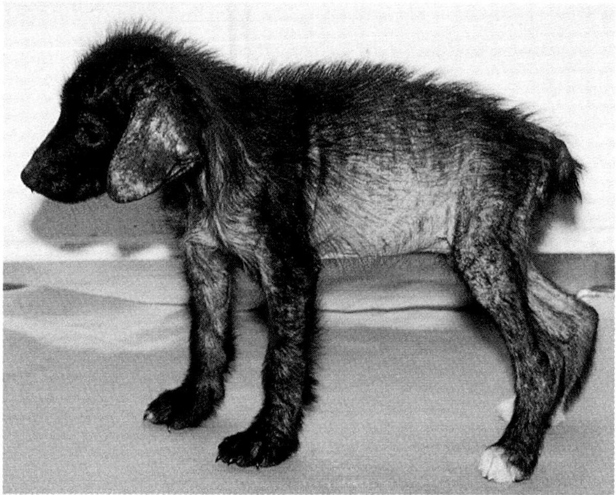

Figure 25-1 Young mixed-breed dog showing the typical total body distribution of cutaneous lesions associated with scabies infestation. Alopecia, erythema, papules, crusts, and scale are evident.

Clinical Features

- Alopecia and erythematous rash—elbows, hocks, ventral abdomen, and chest (Fig. 25-1)
- Lesions on ear margins—vary from barely perceptible scaling to alopecia or crusts; ear canals not affected (Fig. 25-2)
- Chronic—periocular and truncal alopecia; secondary crusts, excoriations, and pyoderma
- Possible peripheral lymphadenopathy
- Frequently bathed dogs—chronic pruritus but no skin lesions

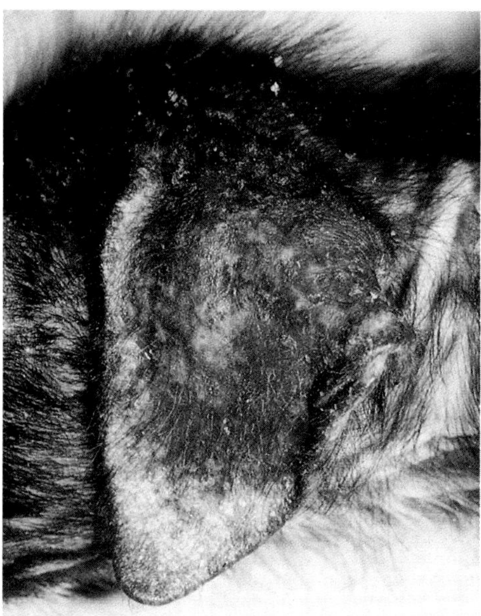

Figure 25-2 Same dog as in Figure 25-1. Classic ear margin lesions consisting of crusts and scale.

- Dogs—often minimal or no response to anti-inflammatory doses of steroids
- Multiple dog households—more than one dog usually show signs

Differential Diagnosis

- Food allergy
- Atopy
- *Malassezia* dermatitis
- Flea-allergic dermatitis
- *Cheyletiella*
- Pyoderma
- Demodicosis
- Contact allergy
- *Pelodera* dermatitis
- Pruritic impetigo

Diagnostics

- ELISA technique—identify *Sarcoptes*-infested dogs; early studies show good results
- Commercial tests not available
- Positive pinnal-pedal reflex—rubbing the ear margin between the thumb and forefinger should induce the dog to scratch with the ipsilateral hind leg; occurs in 75–90% of cases
- Superficial skin scrapings—positive in only 20% of cases (Fig. 25-3)
- Fecal flotation—occasionally reveals mites or ova

Figure 25-3 *Sarcoptes scabiei* mite and ova found on superficial skin scrapings of the ear margin.

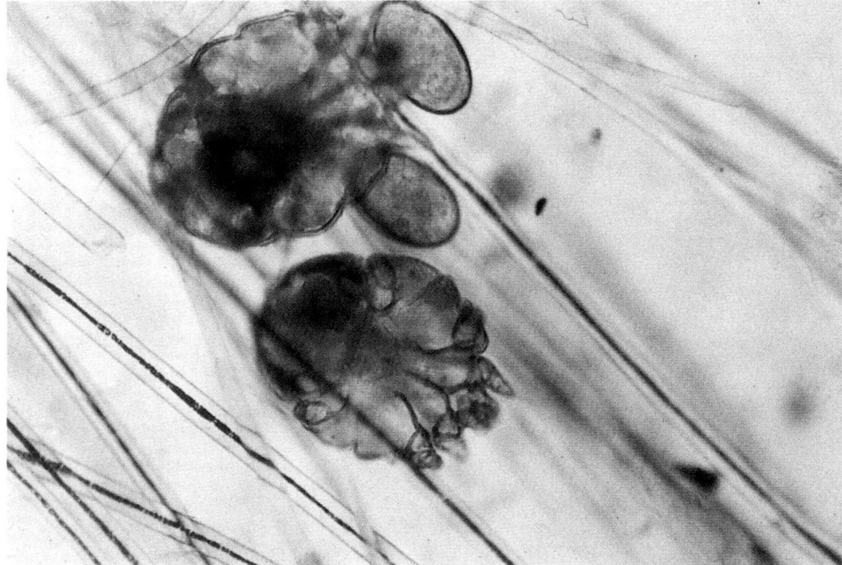

- Favorable response to scabicidal treatment—most common method for tentative diagnosis
- Any dog with nonseasonal pruritus that responds poorly to steroids should be treated with a scabicide (even if skin scrape results are negative) to definitively rule out sarcoptic mange.

Therapeutics

- Scabicidal dips—the entire dog must be treated; treatment failures often linked to owner's reluctance to apply dip to the patient's face and ears; do not let the patient get wet between treatments
- All in-contact dogs—should be treated, even those with no clinical signs; may be asymptomatic carriers
- Thoroughly clean and treat environment; *Sarcoptes* mites can survive for up to 3 weeks.

Drugs

- Ivermectin—highly effective; 0.2–0.4 mg/kg SC or PO every 1–2 weeks for 2–4 treatments; do not use in herding breeds
- Milbemycin (Interceptor)—effective when used at 0.75 mg/kg PO q24h; may be effective at 2 mg/kg PO every week for 3 weeks
- Amitraz (Mitaban) dip—250 ppm; may be effective at every 1–2 weeks for 3 treatments; make sure entire body is covered, including the face and ears
- Whole-body rinse solution—2–3% solution of lime sulfur (LymDip) or organophosphate (Paramite) dip; apply for 5–6 weeks; make sure entire body is covered, including the face and ears
- Topical antiseborrheic therapy in conjunction with scabicidal therapy helps speed clinical resolution of the lesions.
- Systemic antibiotics—may be needed for 21 days or longer to resolve any secondary pyoderma
- Antihistamines or low-dose glucocorticoids (0.5 mg/kg q12h for 1st week of treatment), if mites were identified; may make pruritus diminish more quickly
- Revolution (Pfizer)—topical selamectin; excellent response to one (or two) applications

Comments

- Ivermectin—use with extreme caution in collies, Shetland sheepdogs, old English sheepdogs, Australian shepherds, and their crossbreeds; toxicity is more likely to occur in herding-type breeds
- It can take as long as 4–6 weeks for the intense pruritus and clinical signs to resolve, owing to the hypersensitivity reaction.
- Topical treatments are prone to failure, owing to incomplete application of the treatment solution.
- Reinfection can occur if the contact with infected animals continues.
- Always consider sarcoptic mange as a possible cause of pruritus in allergic dogs that cease to respond to steroid therapy.
- Approximately 30% of dogs with *Sarcoptes* infections will also react to house dust mite antigens.
- People who come in close contact with an affected dog may develop a pruritic, papular rash on their arms, chest, or abdomen; human lesions are usu-

ally transient and should resolve spontaneously after the affected animal has been treated; if the lesions persist, clients should seek advice from their dermatologist.

ABBREVIATION

ELISA = enzyme-linked immunoadsorbent assay

Suggested Reading

De Jaham C, Henry CJ. Treatment of canine sarcoptic mange using milbemycin oxime. Can Vet J 1995;36:42–43.

Griffin CE. Scabies. In: Griffin CE, Kwochka KW, MacDonald JM, eds. Current veterinary dermatology: the science and art of therapy. St. Louis: Mosby, 1993:85–89.

Consulting Editor Karen Helton Rhodes

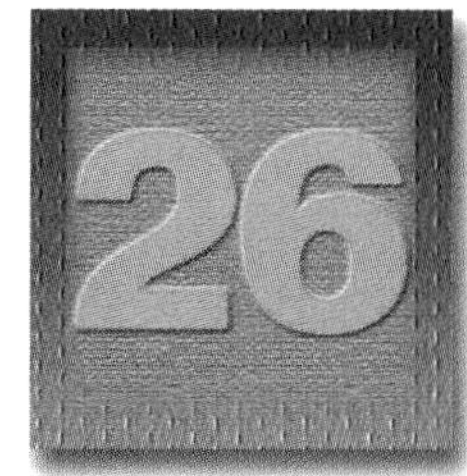

Demodicosis

Karen Helton Rhodes

Definition/Overview

- An inflammatory parasitic disease of dogs and rarely cats that is characterized by an increased number of mites in the hair follicles, which often leads to furunculosis and secondary bacterial infection
- May be localized or generalized in dogs

Etiology/Pathophysiology

Dogs

- *Demodex canis*—a mite; part of the normal fauna of the skin; typically present in small numbers; resides in the hair follicles and sebaceous glands of the skin (Fig. 26-1)
- Pathology develops when numbers exceed that tolerated by the immune system.
- The initial proliferation of mites may be the result of a genetic or immunologic disorder.

Cats

- Poorly understood disorder
- Mites have been identified on the skin and within the otic canal.
- Two species: *D. cati* and an unnamed species

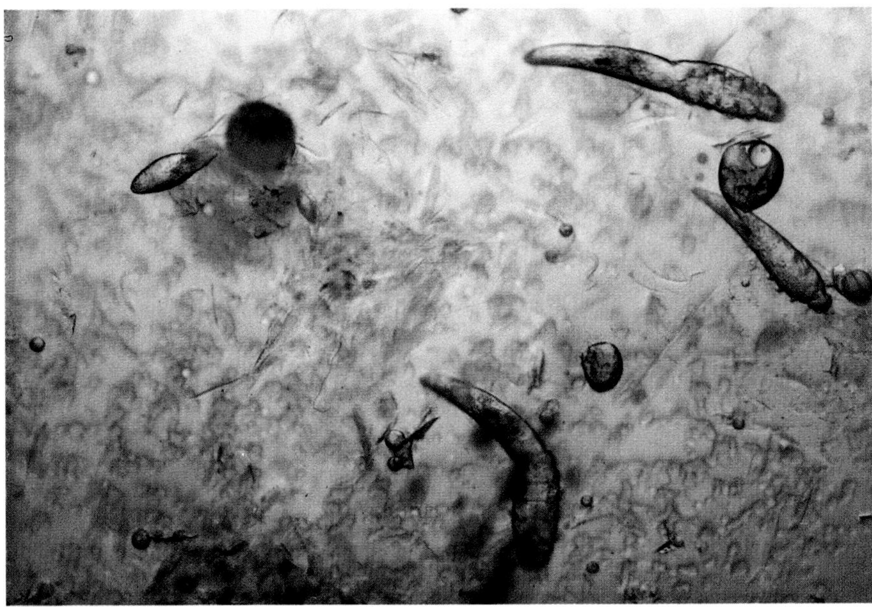

Figure 26-1 *Demodex canis* mites. Skin scraping. Note the different stages of the mite, including an egg.

Dog/Cat

Dead and degenerate *D. canis* mites may be found in noncutaneous sites (e.g., lymph node, intestinal wall, spleen, liver, kidney, urinary bladder, lung, thyroid gland, blood, urine, and feces) and are considered to represent drainage to these areas by blood and/or lymph.

Signalment/History

- Dogs and rarely cats
- Potential increased incidence in Siamese and Burmese cat breeds
- Localized—usually in young dogs; median age 3–6 months
- Generalized—both young and old animals

Dogs

- Exact immunopathologic mechanism unknown
- Studies indicate that dogs with generalized demodicosis have a subnormal percentage of IL-2 receptors on their lymphocytes and subnormal IL-2 production.
- Genetic factors, immunosuppression, and/or metabolic diseases may predispose animal.

Cats

- Often associated with metabolic diseases (e.g., FIV, systemic lupus erythematosus, diabetes mellitus)

- Unnamed species—short and blunted; rarely a marker for metabolic disease; individual reports indicate that it may be transferable from cat to cat within the same household

Clinical Features

Dogs

Localized

- Lesions—usually mild; consist of erythema and a light scale
- Patches—several may be noted; most common site is the face, especially around the perioral and periocular areas; may also be seen on the trunk and legs

Generalized

- Can be widespread from the onset, with multiple poorly circumscribed patches of erythema, alopecia, and scale. (Fig. 26-2)
- As hair follicles become distended with large numbers of mites, secondary bacterial infections are common, often with resultant rupturing of the follicle (furunculosis). (Fig. 26-3)
- With progression, the skin can become severely inflamed, exudative, and granulomatous. (Fig. 26-4)

Cats

- Often characterized by partial to complete multifocal alopecia of the eyelids, periocular region, head, and neck

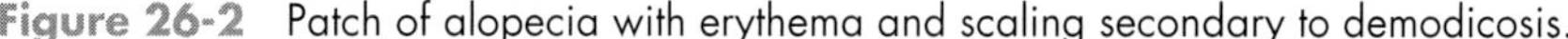

Figure 26-2 Patch of alopecia with erythema and scaling secondary to demodicosis.

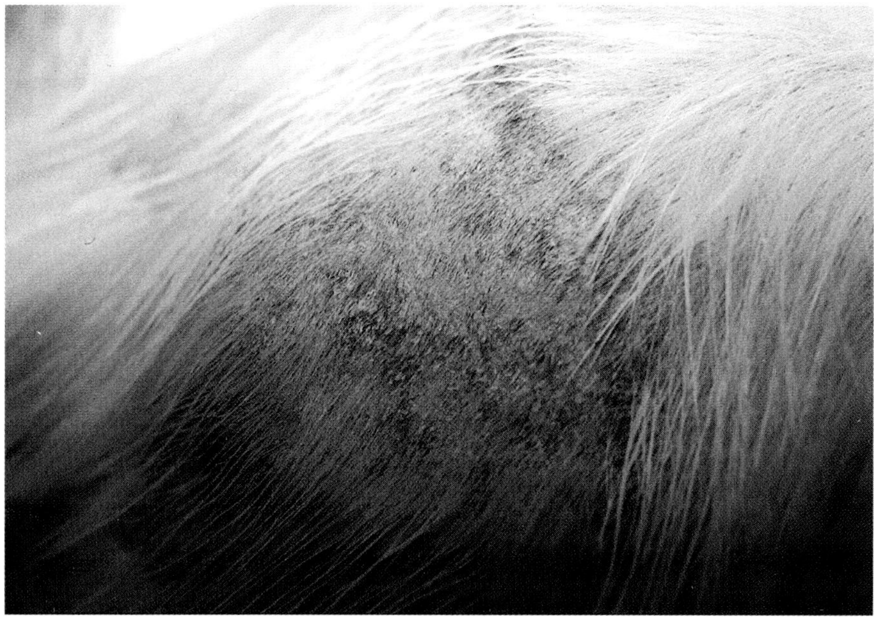

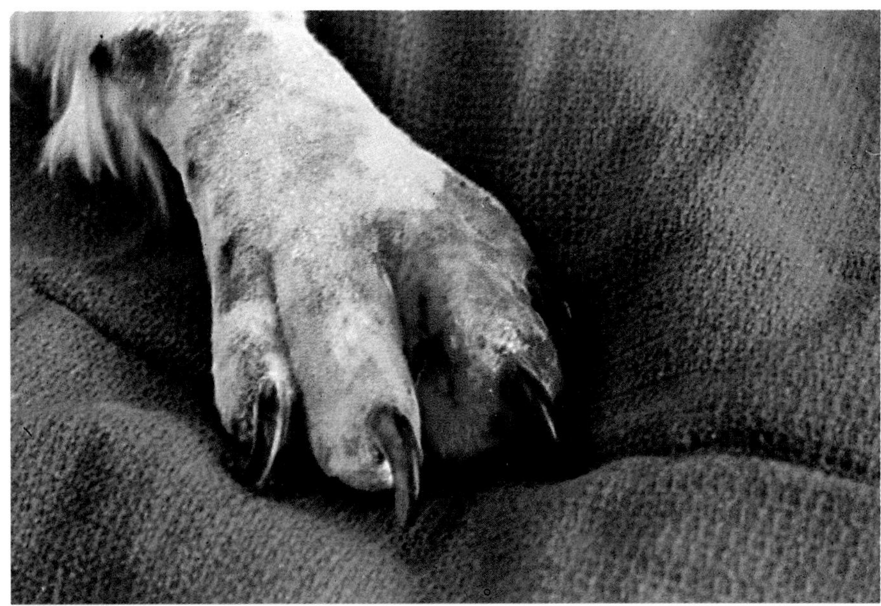

Figure 26-3 Swelling of the digits caused by demodicosis and secondary furunculosis.

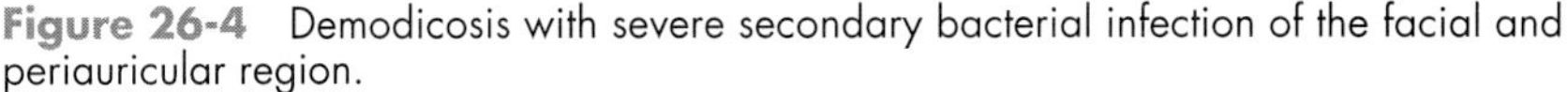

Figure 26-4 Demodicosis with severe secondary bacterial infection of the facial and periauricular region.

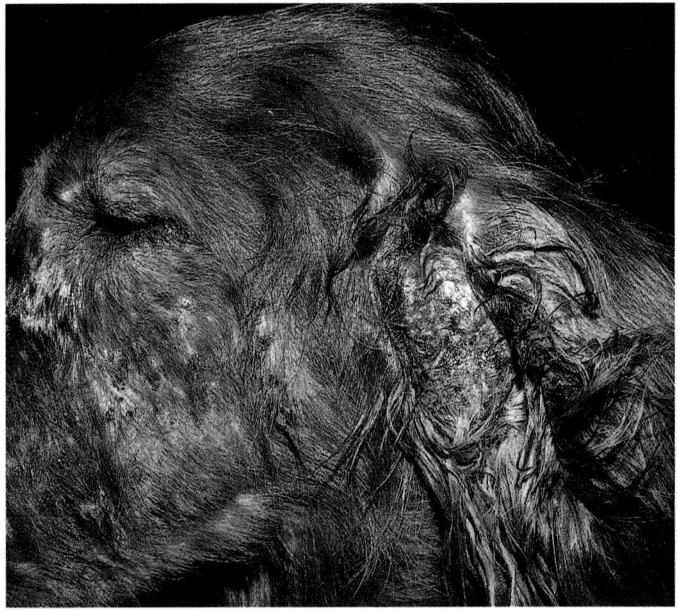

- Lesions—variably pruritic with erythema, scale, and crust; those caused by the unnamed species often quite pruritic
- Ceruminous otitis externa has been reported.

Differential Diagnosis

Dogs

- Bacterial folliculitis/furunculosis
- Dermatophytosis
- Contact dermatitis
- Pemphigus complex
- Dermatomyositis
- Systemic lupus erythematosus

Cats

- Allergic dermatitis
- Scabies

Diagnostics

- May be useful for identifying underlying metabolic diseases in cats
- FeLV and FIV serology—identify underlying metabolic diseases in cats
- Skin scrapings—diagnostic for finding large numbers of mites in the majority of cases
- Cutaneous biopsy—may be needed when lesions are chronic, granulomatous, and fibrotic (especially on the paw)

Therapeutics

- Localized—conservative; most cases (90%) resolve spontaneously with no treatment
- Evaluate the general health status of dogs with either the localized or the generalized form.
- Generalized (adult dog)—frequent management problem; expense and frustration with the chronicity of the problem are issues; many cases are medically controlled, not cured

Drugs

Amitraz (Mitaban; Taktic-EC)

- A formamidine, which inhibits monoamine oxidase and prostaglandin synthesis; an α_2-adrenergic agonist
- Use weekly (the label reads every other week) at 1/2 vial (5 mL)/gal water until resolution of clinical signs and no mites are found on skin scrapings; do not rinse off; let air-dry.
- Treat for 1 month following negative skin scrape.

- Apply a benzoyl peroxide shampoo before application of the dip as a bactericidal therapy and to increase exposure of the mites to the miticide through follicular flushing activity.
- The efficacy is proportional to the frequency of administration and the concentration of the dip.
- May be mixed with mineral oil (3 mL amitraz to 30 mL mineral oil) for application to focal areas, such as pododemodicosis
- Success with the 9% amitraz collar has not been established, although there are positive anecdotal reports.
- Between 11% and 30% of cases will not be cured; may need to try an alternative therapy or control with maintenance dips every 2–8 weeks.

Ivermectin (Ivomec; Eqvalan Liquid)

- A macrocyclic lactone with GABA agonist activity.
- Daily oral administration of 0.3–0.6 mg/kg very effective, even when amitraz fails
- Treat for 60 days beyond negative skin scrapings (average 3–8 months).
- Ivermectin—contraindicated in collies, Shetland sheepdogs, old English sheepdogs, other herding breeds, and crosses with these breeds; sensitive breeds appear to tolerate the acaricidal dosages of milbemycin (see below).

Milbemycin (Interceptor)

- A macrocylic lactone with GABA agonist activity
- Dosage of 1 mg/kg PO q24h cures 50% of cases; 2 mg/kg PO q24h cures 85% of cases.
- Treat for 60 days beyond multiple negative skin scrapings.

Cats

- Exact protocols are not defined.
- Topical lime-sulfur dips or amitraz solutions applied weekly for 4 treatments often lead to good resolution of clinical signs.

Comments

Amitraz

- Most common side effects—somnolence, lethargy, depression, anorexia seen in 30% of patients for 12–36 hr after treatment
- Other side effects—vomiting, diarrhea, pruritus, polyuria, mydriasis, bradycardia, hypoventilation, hypotension, hypothermia, ataxia, ileus, bloat, hyperglycemia, convulsions, death
- The incidence and severity of side effects do not appear to be proportional to the dose or frequency of use.
- Humans can develop dermatitis, headaches, and respiratory difficulty after exposure.
- Yohimbine at 0.11 mg/kg IV is an antidote.

Ivermectin and Milbemycin

- Signs of toxicity—salivation, vomiting, mydriasis, confusion, ataxia, hypersensitivity to sound, weakness, recumbency, coma, and death

Possible Interactions

- Amitraz—may interact with heterocyclic antidepressants, xylazine, benzodiazepines, and macrocyclic lactones
- Ivermectin and milbemycin—cause elevated levels of monoamine neurotransmitter metabolites, which could result in adverse drug interactions with amitraz and benzodiazepines
- Multiple skin scrapings and evidence of clinical resolution are used to monitor progress.
- Avoid breeding animals with generalized form.

Expected Course and Prognosis

- Prognosis (dogs)—depends heavily on genetic, immunologic, and underlying diseases
- Localized—most cases (90%) resolve spontaneously with no treatment; <10% progress to the generalized form
- Adult-onset (dogs)—often severe and refractory to treatment
- Adult-onset—sudden occurrence is often associated with internal disease, malignant neoplasia, and/or immunosuppressive disease; approximately 25% of cases are idiopathic over a follow-up period of 1–2 years

See Also

- Amitraz toxicity
- Ivermectin toxicity

Abbreviations

- FeLV = feline leukemia virus
- FIV = feline immunodeficiency virus
- GABA = γ-aminobutyric acid
- IL = interleukin

Suggested Reading

Scott DW, Miller WH, Griffin CE, eds. Parasitic skin diseases. In: Muller & Kirk's small animal dermatology. 5th ed. Philadelphia: Saunders, 1995:417–432.

Consulting Editor Karen Helton Rhodes

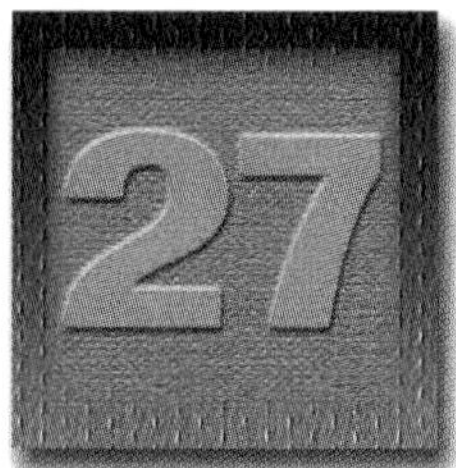

Ear Mites

Karen A. Kuhl and Jean S. Greek

Definition/Overview

Otodectes cynotis mites cause a hypersensitivity reaction that results in intense irritation of the external ear of dogs and cats (Fig. 27-1).

Signalment/History

- Common in young dogs and cats, although it may occur at any age
- No breed or sex predilection

Clinical Features

- Pruritus primarily located around the ears, head, and neck; occasionally generalized
- Thick, red-brown or black crusts—usually seen in the outer ear
- Crusting and scales may occur on the neck, rump, and tail.
- Excoriations on the convex surface of the pinnae often occur, owing to the intense pruritus.

Differential Diagnosis

- Flea bite hypersensitivity
- Pediculosis

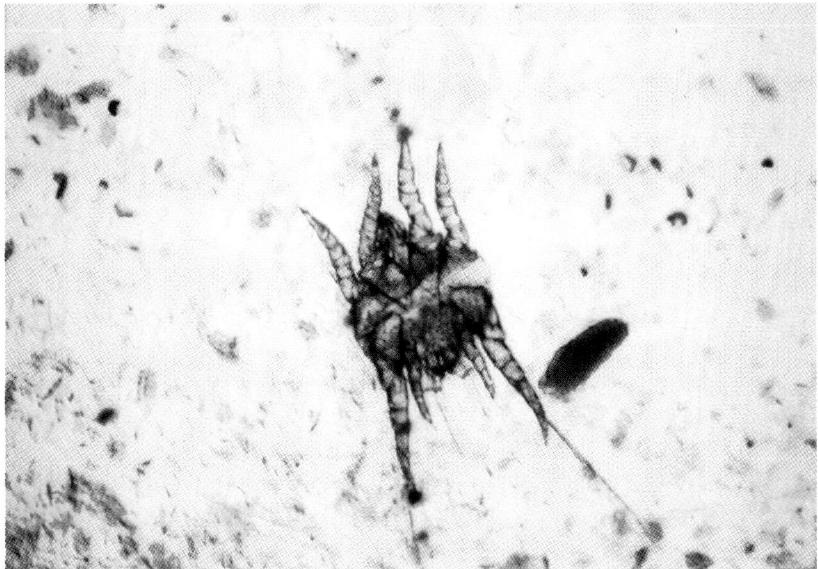

Figure 27-1 *Otodectes* mite from an ear swab.

- Pelodera dermatitis
- Sarcoptic mange
- Chiggers
- Allergic dermatitis

Diagnostics

- Skin scrapings—identify mites, if signs are generalized
- Ear swabs placed in mineral oil—usually a very effective means of identification

Therapeutics

- Very contagious; important to treat all in-contact animals
- Thoroughly clean and treat the environment.
- First clean the ears thoroughly with mineral oil or a commercial ear cleaner to remove debris.
- Rotenone-based products—treat ears twice per week initially; then decrease to weekly; continue for 2 weeks after clinical cure.
- Ivermectin—as an alternative; use systemically or topically; systemic: (bovine 1%) 300 μg/kg SC every 1–2 weeks for approximately 4 treatments was found to be effective; topical: place 500 μg directly in the ears every 1–2 weeks for approximately 5 weeks (associated with a higher incidence of recurrence); topical dosage not approved for use in dogs or cats in the U.S.; dogs with heartworm may exhibit a shock-like reaction, probably owing to dying microfilaria
- Acarexx 0.01% ivermectin otic suspension (Blue Ridge Pharmaceuticals)

- Revolution (Pfizer) topical treatment placed on base of neck
- Amitraz—topical; place 1 mL in 33 mL mineral oil directly into the ear; not approved for this use
- Pyrethrin-based flea spray—treat entire animal weekly for 4–6 weeks if not using systemic ivermectin
- Environment—treat with a flea-type preparation two times, 2–4 weeks apart

Comments

- Ivermectin—do not use in collies, shelties, their crosses, or other herding breeds; use only if absolutely necessary in animals <6 months of age; an increasing number of toxic reactions have been reported in kittens
- Amitraz—reported to cause adverse reactions in cats when used topically for generalized infestations; thus, use with caution
- An ear swab and physical examination should be done 1 month after therapy commences.
- For most patients, prognosis is good.
- Rarely, the infestation will be cleared only to find an underlying allergy that keeps the otitis externa active.
- The mites will also bite humans (rare).

Suggested Reading

Scott DW, Miller WH, Griffin CE. Muller & Kirk's small animal dermatology. 5th ed. Philadelphia: Saunders, 1995.

Consulting Editor Karen Helton Rhodes

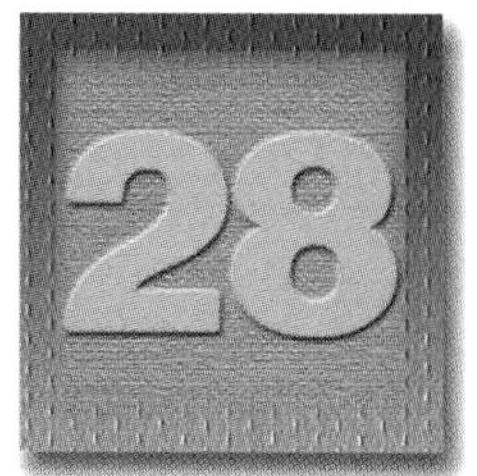

Amitraz Toxicosis

Steven R. Hansen

Definition/Overview

- Amitraz—formamidine acaricide; applied topically to control ticks, mites, and lice
- Amitraz-containing products (for dogs)—formulated as a 19.9% emulsifiable concentrate in 10.6-mL bottles for dilution and application as a topical pour-on and as a 9.0% impregnated 25-in. 27.5-g collar
- Systems affected—nervous; endocrine/metabolic (β cells of the pancreas); gastrointestinal
- Clinical signs—most associated with α_2-adrenoreceptor agonist
- After high-dose oral administration (dogs)—peak plasma concentration reached at approximately 6 hr; elimination half-life as long as 24 hr; metabolites excreted in the urine
- Ingestion of sustained-release-impregnated collars—constant release and continued systemic exposure until collar segments have passed in the stool
- Toxicosis—generally occurs when impregnated collars are ingested, when improperly diluted solutions are applied topically, or when solutions are taken orally
- Idiosyncratic reactions may occur.

Signalment/History

- Thorough history—usually identifies use topically or as a collar
- Dogs—common, owing to more common use

- Cats and other species—rarely reported
- Predilection for old animals
- Develop acutely after exposure
- Ingestion of impregnated collar or pieces of collar
- Inappropriate direct application
- Ingestion of undiluted product
- After application of properly diluted and applied solutions—less common
- Elderly, sick, or debilitated animals—may be predisposed

Clinical Features

- Minor to severe depression
- Weakness
- Ataxia
- Recumbency
- Bradycardia
- Hypothermia
- Vomiting
- Diarrhea
- Polyuria
- Abdominal pain
- Death

Differential Diagnosis

- Recreational and prescription drugs—marijuana; opioids; barbiturates; benzodiazepines; phenothiazines; antihypertensive medications; skeletal muscle relaxants; other depressant drugs or chemicals
- Ivermectins, avermectins, milbemycins—generally very high dose or exceptionally sensitive breed
- Alcohols—ethanol; ethylene glycol (antifreeze); methanol (windshield washer fluid); isopropyl alcohol (rubbing alcohol)
- Tick paralysis, botulism, cranial trauma, diabetes, hyperadrenocorticism, hypothyroidism, severe anemia, cardiac failure, and anaphylactic shock—marked depression or weakness

Diagnostics

- Hyperglycemia—common
- Elevated liver enzymes—uncommon
- Abdominal radiography—may reveal a collar buckle in the gastrointestinal tract
- Identify amitraz on hair or in gastrointestinal contents—analytical methods described; useful only to prove exposure; no data available correlating concentration with clinical signs
- High-dose, prolonged exposure—increased liver weight; slight enlargement of hepatocytes; thinning of the zonae fasciculata and reticularis; slight hyperplasia of the zona glomerulosa of the adrenal glands

Therapeutics

- Inpatient—severely affected patients
- Mild sedation after correctly applied sponge-on solutions—often transient; may require no treatment
- Mild signs after topical application—scrub with a hand dishwashing detergent; rinse with copious amounts of warm water; institute nonspecific supportive therapy (e.g., intravenous fluids, maintenance of normal body temperature, and nutritional support); monitor 1–2 days until improvement is noted
- Ingestion of collar possible—endoscopic retrieval of the collar—removal of large segments from the stomach may be beneficial; usually numerous small pieces are located throughout the gastrointestinal tract, making removal unrealistic

Collar Ingestion, Asymptomatic Patient

- Emetic—3% USP hydrogen peroxide (2.2 mL/kg PO; maximum 45 mL after feeding a moist meal); apomorphine and especially xylazine not recommended Activated charcoal (2 g/kg PO) containing sorbitol as an osmotic cathartic—administer by stomach tube; re-administer every 4 hr until pieces of collar are noted in the stool and the patient is markedly improved.

Marked Depression

- May require pharmacologic reversal of the α_2-adrenergic effects
- Yohimbine (Yobine)—0.11 mg/kg IV, administered slowly; reverses depression and bradycardia within minutes; objective is to keep the patient in a state of low-level depression with normal heart rate, body temperature, and blood glucose concentrations
- Collar ingestions—monitor for recurrence of symptoms; may need additional yohimbine until collar segments appear in the stool
- Atipamezole (Antisedan)—0.05 mg/kg, IM; reported to reverse poisoning within 10 min; repeated as needed; an alternative when yohimbine is unavailable
- Yohimbine and atipamezole—may require initial repeated administration every 4–8 hr, because half-life in dogs is shorter than in other species and elimination half-life of amitraz is longer

Comments

- Yohimbine and atipamezole—excessive administration may result in apprehension, CNS stimulation, and rarely, seizures
- Body temperature, serum glucose, and heart rate—important parameters
- Close observation for recurrence of clinical signs—required for 24–72 hr
- Yohimbine and atipamezole—requires readministration in severe cases, because reversal effects subside before collar segments have passed or before amitraz has been eliminated from the body
- No long-term adverse effects expected
- Elderly, sick, or debilitated animals may take longer to fully recover.

Suggested Reading

Grossman MR. Amitraz toxicosis associated with ingestion of an acaricide collar in a dog. J Am Vet Med Assoc 1993:203:55–57.

Hugnet C, Buronfosse F, Pineau X, et al. Toxicity and kinetics of amitraz in dogs. Am J Vet Res 1996;57:1506–1510.

Author Steven R. Hansen

Consulting Editor Karen Helton Rhodes

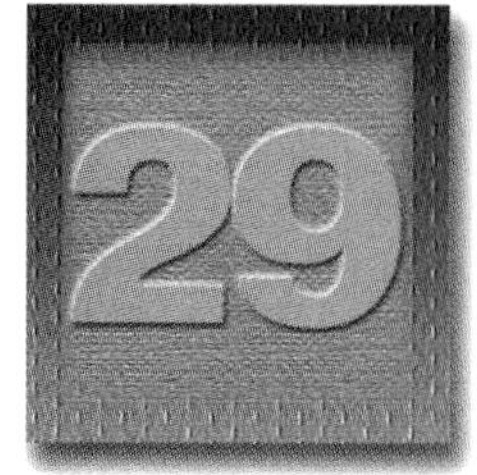

Ivermectin Toxicity

Allan J. Paul

Definition/Overview

- Toxicity—dogs given large extra-label dosages (≥ 10–15 times recommended dosage)

Etiology/Pathophysiology

- Ivermectin—potentiates the release and binding of the neuroinhibitory substance GABA at certain synapses in the CNS; metabolized and excreted by the liver
- Sensitivity—some dogs unusually sensitive; differences may relate to a defect in the blood-brain barrier, higher than normal amounts of unbound ivermectin in the plasma, or an ivermectin-specific blood-brain transport mechanism

Signalment/History

- Collies—most commonly affected; not all are sensitive
- Australian shepherds and old English sheepdogs—common
- May be a genetic component in sensitive animals
- No age or sex predilections

Clinical Features

- Mydriasis
- Depression
- Drooling
- Vomiting
- Ataxia
- Tremors
- Disorientation
- Weakness, recumbency
- Nonresponsiveness
- Blindness
- Bradycardia
- Hypoventilation
- Coma
- Death

Differential Diagnosis

- Overdoses of other ivermectin compounds—milbemycin oxime
- Other toxicants or diseases affecting CNS

Diagnostics

- Arterial blood gases—may reveal high $PaCO_2$ and low PaO_2 caused by respiratory depression and hypoventilation
- Physostigmine—1 mg IV; temporary (30–40-min) return to consciousness or resumed alertness and muscle activity after the administration supports but does not confirm diagnosis; does not speed recovery; not indicated for treatment; glycopyrrolate administered first may prevent severe bradycardia

Therapeutics

- Mainstay—supportive and symptomatic care
- Proper fluid therapy, maintenance of electrolyte balance, nutritional support, and prevention of secondary complications—important goals
- Nutritional support—institute early, preferably within 2–3 days of exposure; severe CNS depression or coma may last for weeks
- Frequent turning of patient, appropriate bedding, physical therapy, attentive nursing care, and other standard treatment measures for a recumbent patient important
- Apply ocular lubricants.
- Mechanical ventilation—may be required with respiratory depression
- No known reversal agent
- Atropine or glycopyrrolate—may be administered as needed to treat bradycardia
- Avoid other drugs that stimulate the GABA receptor—benzodiazepine tranquilizers

Comments

- Prognosis and eventual outcome—depend on individual and breed sensitivity, amount of drug ingested or injected, how rapidly clinical signs develop, response to supportive treatment, and overall health of patient
- Convalescence may be prolonged (several weeks); good supportive care in many seemingly hopeless cases has resulted in complete recovery.

Suggested Reading

Paul AJ, Tranquilli WJ. Ivermectin. In: Kirk RW, ed. Current veterinary therapy X. Philadelphia: Saunders, 1989:140–142.

Author Allan J. Paul

Consulting Editor Karen Helton Rhodes

Organophosphate and Carbamate Toxicity

Steven R. Hansen and Elizabeth A. Curry-Galvin

Definition/Overview

- Results from exposure to organophosphorous compounds or carbamate, which are common active ingredients in household and agricultural insecticide products
- Animal products—organophosphate: chlorpyrifos, coumaphos, cythioate, diazinon, famphur, fenthion, phosmet, and tetrachlorvinphos; carbamate: carbaryl and propoxur
- Agricultural, lawn, and garden products—organophosphate: acephate, chlorpyrifos, diazinon, disulfoton, malathion, parathion, terbufos, and others; carbamate: carbofuran and methomyl

Etiology/Pathophysiology

- Cause nervous system effects by inhibiting cholinesterase, which includes acetylcholinesterase, pseudocholinesterase, and other esterases
- Acetylcholinesterase—normally hydrolyzes the neurotransmitter acetylcholine in nervous tissue, RBCs, and muscle, resulting in termination of nervous transmission
- Pseudocholinesterase—found in plasma, liver, pancreas, and nervous tissue, mainly in cats
- Cholinesterase inhibition—allows acetylcholine accumulation at the postsynaptic receptor; causes stimulation of effector organs; spontaneous reactivation after organophosphorous compound binding is very slow and, once aging occurs, is virtually nonexistent; reversible after carbamate binding

- Nervous system—effects result from overriding stimulation of parasympathetic pathways; may also result from sympathetic stimulation; acetylcholine stimulates nicotinic receptors of the somatic nervous system (skeletal muscle), parasympathetic preganglionic nicotinic and postganglionic muscarinic receptors (cardiac muscle, pupil, blood vessels, smooth muscles in lung and gastrointestinal tract, exocrine glands), and sympathetic preganglionic nicotinic receptors (adrenal and indirectly cardiac muscle, pupil, blood vessels, smooth muscles in lung and gastrointestinal tract, exocrine glands).
- Animals with inherently low cholinesterase activity—more susceptible to cholinesterase depression
- Cholinesterase activity—more easily inhibited in cats than in dogs

Signalment/History

- Cats and small or exceptionally lean dogs—most susceptible
- Lean dogs (e.g., sight hounds and racing breeds) and lean longhair cats—more susceptible to cholinesterase inhibition because of lack of fat; many organophosphorous compounds and metabolites are stored in fat and slowly released into circulation
- Organophosphate-containing dips labeled for dogs only—inappropriately applied to cats
- Young animals—more likely intoxicated owing to lower detoxification capability
- Intact males more susceptible to some organophosphates
- Concurrent exposure to multiple organophosphate- and/or carbamate-containing products
- Exposure to floors that are damp with organophosphorous premise products
- Incorrect dilution of insecticides

Clinical Features

- Parasympathetic stimulation—usually predominates
- Sympathetic stimulation—may result in lack of specific expected signs; may note opposite signs from those expected
- Medical history—often discloses heavy or repeated applications of flea and tick insecticides; evidence of exposure to an agricultural product
- Carbamate insecticides (methomyl and carbofuran)—may cause rapid onset of seizures and respiratory failure; treat aggressively without delay
- Organophosphate insecticides (cats)—chronic anorexia, muscle weakness, and muscle twitching, with or without episodes of acute toxicosis, which may last for days to weeks

Physical Examination Findings

- Hypersalivation
- Vomiting
- Diarrhea
- Miosis
- Bradycardia
- Depression

- Ataxia
- Muscle tremors
- Seizures
- Hyperthermia
- Dyspnea
- Respiratory failure
- Death
- Patient may not exhibit all signs
- Sympathetic stimulation—signs reversed

Differential Diagnosis

- History of exposure, amount of exposure, and clinical signs—should be consistent with toxicosis
- Exposure to other insecticidal products—pyrethrin/pyrethroids (flea and tick); D-limonene (citrus flea and tick); fipronil (flea and tick); imidacloprid (flea)
- Other pesticides—strychnine; fluoroacetate (1080); 4-aminopyridine (avicide); metaldehyde (snail bait); zinc/aluminum phosphide (rodenticide); bromethalin (rodenticide)
- Other toxicants—chocolate; caffeine; cocaine; amphetamine

Diagnostics

Cholinesterase Activity

- Reduced to $< 25\%$ of normal in whole blood, retina, or brain—suggests exposure to a cholinesterase-inhibiting compound
- Test results—must be interpreted in context of the amount of exposure and the clinical signs and the time of their onset
- Use laboratories experienced in handling animal samples.
- Chlorpyrifos—experimentally exposed animals may remain clinically normal with no detectable cholinesterase activity
- Carbamate inhibition—reactivation may occur during sample transport and testing, giving false-negative results
- Detection of insecticides—tissue (e.g., brain, liver, kidney, and fat); stomach contents; gastrointestinal tract; fur or hair; negative results do not rule out toxicosis
- May find pieces of chewed containers in the gastrointestinal tract

Therapeutics

- Outpatient—mild signs from exposure to flea and tick collars and powders; treated by simply removing the collar or brushing excess powder from the coat
- Inpatient—continued salivation, tremors, or dyspnea
- Basis—stabilization; decontamination; antidotal treatment with atropine (and pralidoxime chloride for organophosphate toxicosis); supportive care
- Oxygen—if necessary, until respiration returns to normal

- Fluid therapy—may be needed in anorexic cats
- Bathing (dermal exposure)—use hand dishwashing detergent; rinse with copious amounts of water
- Diazepam (0.05–1.0 mg/kg IV) or phenobarbital (3.0–30 mg/kg IV to effect, low dosage in cats)—controls seizures
- Atropine sulfate—0.2 mg/kg one-quarter IV, remaining SC, as needed; administered immediately; repeated only as needed to control life-threatening clinical signs from muscarinic stimulation
- Pralidoxime chloride (Protopam)—10–15 mg/kg IM, SC q8-12h until recovery; discontinue after three doses if no response; reduces muscle fasciculations; most beneficial against organophosphorous insecticides when started within 24 hr of exposure; even several days after dermal exposure may stimulate anorexic cats (with or without tremors) to resume eating; if refrigerated and wrapped in foil, reconstituted bottles may be successfully used for up to 2 weeks
- Ingestion of liquid insecticidal solution—avoid inducing emesis; risk of aspiration because many solutions contain hydrocarbon solvents
- No clinical signs, liquid solvent not ingested, and very recent ingestion—3% hydrogen peroxide (2.2 mL/kg PO to a maximum of 45 mL) after feeding a moist meal
- Evacuation of the stomach for patient with clinical signs—gastric lavage with the patient intubated, under anesthesia, with a large-bore stomach tube; then administration of activated charcoal (2.0 g/kg PO) containing sorbitol as a cathartic in a water slurry
- Diarrhea—do not administer sorbitol-containing product

CONTRAINDICATIONS

- Phenothiazine tranquilizers may potentiate organophosphate toxicosis.

PRECAUTIONS

- Atropine—avoid overuse; may cause tachycardia, CNS stimulation, seizures, disorientation, drowsiness, and respiratory depression

Comments

CLIENT EDUCATION

- Stress the importance and closely follow insecticide label directions.
- Caution client that cats with chronic anorexia and weakness may need days to weeks of supportive care for full recovery.
- Monitor heart rate, respiration, and fluid and caloric intake.
- Avoid use on sick or debilitated animals.
- Avoid simultaneous use of organophosphate and carbamate products.
- Chronic organophosphate insecticide–induced weakness and anorexia (cats)—may last 2–4 weeks; most patients fully recover with aggressive nursing care
- Acute toxicosis treated promptly—good prognosis

Suggested Reading

Fikes JD. Feline chlorpyrifos toxicosis. In: Kirk RW, Bonagura JD, eds. Current veterinary therapy XI. Philadelphia: Saunders, 1992:188–191.

Fikes JD. Organophosphate and carbamate insecticides. Vet Clin North Am Small Anim Pract 1990;20:353–367.

Authors Steven R. Hansen and Elizabeth A. Curry-Galvin

Consulting Editor Karen Helton Rhodes

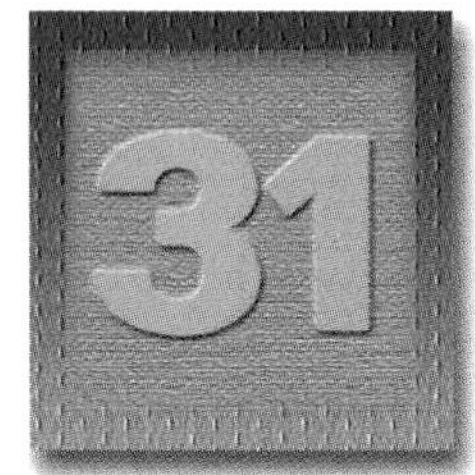

Pyrethrin and Pyrethroid Toxicity

Steven R. Hansen and Elizabeth A. Curry-Galvin

Definition/Overview

- Insecticides
- Pyrethrins—natural; derived from *Chrysanthemum cinerariaefolium* and related plant species
- Pyrethroids—synthetic; include allethrin, cypermethrin, deltamethrin, fenvalerate, fluvalinate, permethrin, phenothrin, and tetramethrin
- Affect the nervous system—reversibly prolong sodium conductance in nerve axons, resulting in repetitive nerve discharges; enhanced effect in hypothermic mammals and cold-blooded animals

Signalment/History

- Adverse reactions occur more frequently in cats; small dogs; and young, old, sick, or debilitated animals.
- Cats—more sensitive; less-efficient metabolic pathways, extensive grooming habits, and long haircoats that can retain large quantities of topically applied product
- Patients with subnormal body temperatures after anesthesia or sedation—predisposed to clinical signs

Clinical Features

- Result from immune-mediated allergic hypersensitivity and anaphylactic reactions, genetic-based idiosyncratic reactions, and neurotoxic reactions; may be challenging to differentiate among these

- Mild—hypersalivation; paw flicking; ear twitching; mild depression; vomiting; diarrhea
- Moderate to serious—protracted vomiting and diarrhea; marked depression; ataxia; muscle tremors (must be differentiated from paw flicking and ear twitching)
- Extreme dermal or oral overdose—may produce seizures or death
- Cats—especially sensitive to concentrated permethrin-containing products labeled for use on dogs; may develop muscle tremors, ataxia, seizures, and death within hours
- Allergic reactions—urticaria; hyperemia; pruritus; anaphylaxis; shock; respiratory distress; (rarely) death
- Idiosyncratic reactions—not allergic; resemble toxic reactions at much lower doses
- Death—thoroughly investigate to rule out predisposing underlying conditions

Differential Diagnosis

- Exposure history (amount and frequency of product usage), type and severity of clinical signs, and onset and duration of clinical signs—must be consistent before a tentative diagnosis can be made
- Organophosphorous compounds, carbamate, or D-limonene toxicosis
- With sudden death—flea bite anemia, cardiomyopathy, or hyperthyroidism
- Anaphylactic and idiosyncratic reactions

Diagnostics

- Pyrethrins—analytical tests for detection in tissues or fluids not generally available
- Pyrethroids—some types can be detected in tissues to confirm exposure
- Cholinesterase activity—not reduced; may rule out exposure to organophosphate or carbamate insecticides

Therapeutics

- Adverse reactions (salivation, paw flicking, and ear twitching)—often mild and self-limiting
- Patient saturated with spray products—dry with a warmed towel; brush
- Continued mild signs—bathe at home with a mild hand dishwashing detergent
- Progression to tremors and ataxia—hospitalize
- Seriously affected patient—fluid support with balanced electrolyte solution recommended
- Symptomatic patient within 1–2 hr of ingestion—gastric lavage with patient under sedation and an endotracheal tube in place; use a large-bore stomach tube; repeat flushing until clear water is seen draining from the stomach tube
- Maintenance of a normal body temperature—critical

- Minor tremors—diazepam (0.05–1.0 mg/kg IV) or phenobarbital (3.0–30 mg/kg IV to effect, low dosage in cats)
- Severe, uncontrollable tremors or seizures—especially for cats exposed to permethrin; methocarbamol (Robaxin-V injectable at 55–220 mg/kg IV not to exceed 330 mg/kg/day; administer one-half dose rapidly IV, wait until the patient begins to relax, continue administration to effect)
- Large ingestion or dermal overdose of a pyrethroid (e.g., permethrin on cats)—activated charcoal (2.0 g/kg PO or by stomach tube) containing sorbitol as a cathartic
- Emetics—rarely warranted; most formulations are rapidly absorbed liquids containing water, various alcohols, or hydrocarbon solvents; do not use with hydrocarbon solvent exposure (potential for aspiration); if indicated, if the patient is asymptomatic, and if it is within 1–2 hr of ingestion: induced with 3% hydrogen peroxide (2.2 mL/kg, maximum 45 mL) after feeding
- Atropine sulfate—not antidotal; avoid; can cause tachycardia, CNS stimulation, disorientation, drowsiness, respiratory depression, and even seizures
- Judiciously avoid hypothermia.

Comments

- Proper application of flea-control products—greatly reduces incidence of adverse reactions; correct dose of most sprays: 1–2 pumps of a typical trigger sprayer per pound body weight
- Reduction of salivation by sensitive cats (sprays)—spray onto a grooming brush; evenly brush through haircoat
- Liquids—term *dip* common; never submerge animal; pour on body; sponge to cover dry areas
- Premise products—do not apply topically unless labeled for such use; after treating house or yard, do not allow animal in the area until product has dried and environment has been ventilated
- Do not apply dog-only products on cats.
- Hypersalivation—may recur for several days after use of flea-control product when patient (especially cat) grooms itself
- Most clinical signs (mild to severe) resolve within 24–72 hr.

Suggested Reading

Hansen SR, Villar D, Buck WB, et al. Pyrethrins and pyrethroids in dogs and cats. Compend Contin Educ Pract Vet 1994;16:707–713.

Authors Steven R. Hansen and Elizabeth A. Curry-Galvin

Consulting Editor Karen Helton-Rhodes

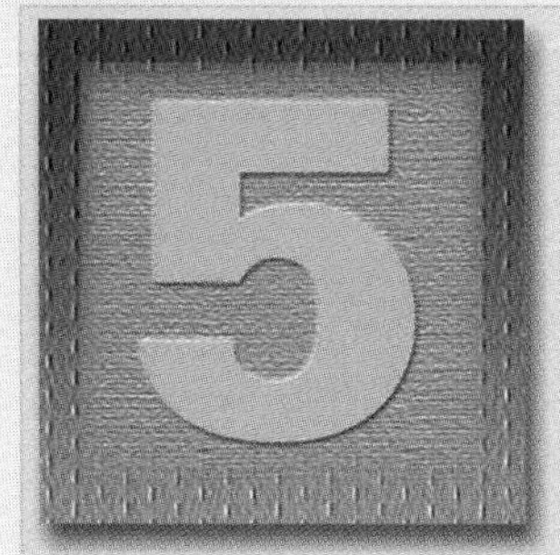

Allergic and Hypersensitivity Dermatitis

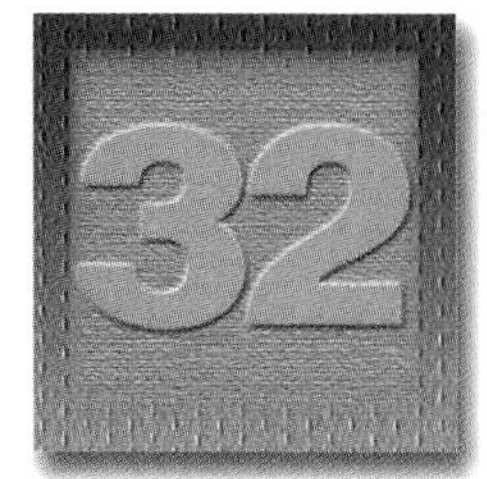

Pruritus

W. Dunbar Gram

Definition/Overview

The sensation that provokes the desire to scratch, rub, chew, or lick; an indicator of inflamed skin

Etiology/Pathophysiology

- A specific end organ has not been found.
- The sensation of itch is conducted by A δ fibers and C fibers of the peripheral nervous system to the dorsal root of the spinal cord.
- The axons, some of which cross over, ascend via the lateral spinothalamic tract and synapse in the caudal thalamus and then to the sensory cortex.
- Other factors can modify the perception of pruritus at this level.

Signalment/History

- Highly variable; depends on the underlying cause
- History—often the most important guide to necessary tests; severe condition, which constantly keeps the patient and owner awake, suggests scabies, flea allergy/infestation, food allergy, or cutaneous yeast infection; all but the latter typically have an acute onset

Clinical Features

- The act of scratching, licking, biting, or chewing
- For some animals, evidence of self-trauma and cutaneous inflammation is necessary to make the diagnosis if the history is incomplete.
- Cats—can be secretive lickers; alopecia without inflammation may be the only sign
- Alopecia—in most cases, a clear history of pruritus is noted; without pruritus, may accompany endocrine diseases; some animals may excessively lick themselves without the owners' knowledge; demodicosis, dermatophytosis, bacterial pyoderma, seborrhea, some cutaneous neoplasms, and unusual diseases (e.g., leishmaniasis) may cause alopecia with varying degrees of inflammation and pruritus

Differential Diagnosis

- Parasitic—fleas, scabies, *Demodex, Otodectes, Notoedres, Cheyletiella,* trombicula, lice, *Pelodera,* endoparasite migration
- Allergic—parasite, atopy, food, contact, drug, bacterial hypersensitivity
- Bacterial/fungal
- Miscellaneous—primary and secondary seborrhea, calcinosis cutis, cutaneous neoplasia, immune-mediated dermatosis; psychogenic diseases and endocrine dermatosis variable
- Uncomplicated atopy—initially very steroid responsive; originally seasonal; often progresses to nonseasonal, pruritic disease with a predilection for the face, feet, ears, forelimbs, axilla, and rump; flea- and food-allergic animals are predisposed to atopy and may show similar signs

Diagnostics

- Skin scrapes, epidermal cytology, and dermatophyte cultures (with microscopic identification)—identify primary or co-existing diseases caused by parasites or other microorganisms
- Wood's lamp—do not use as the sole means of diagnosing or excluding dermatophytosis, owing to false negatives and misinterpretations of fluorescence.

Allergy Testing

- Two methods—skin testing (intradermal skin testing) and blood testing; skin testing is the historical standard and the preferred method; some veterinary dermatologists use both tests
- Skin testing—identify individual allergens; takes into account the important allergy-associated immunoglobulins (IgGd and systemic as well as localized IgE)
- Blood testing—commercial tests for allergies measure only serum IgE, not IgGd; disadvantage, some tests determine groups or mixes of allergens
- Allergy extract—correlate positive reactions with the history; then formulate the immunotherapy solution; contains a mixture of specific allergens, based

on the history, test results, and the veterinarian's (or the laboratory's) clinical experience; concentration may vary with the type of test done and may affect the success rate

Skin Biopsy

- Useful when associated lesions are unusual and an immune-mediated disease is expected or the history and physical findings do not correlate
- Results should be interpreted by a trained veterinary dermatopathologist.

Trial Courses

Canine Scabies

- Can be difficult to diagnose
- Skin scrapes often negative
- Trial course (lime sulfur, ivermectin) often necessary to rule out
- Ivermectin—use caution; associated with idiosyncratic reactions and death

Food Allergy

- Blood and skin tests—not recommended for diagnosis
- Hypoallergenic dietary trial most appropriate test
- Trial—must include only novel food; use a diet that has been confirmed as hypoallergenic through clinical trials; avoid meat-flavored treats and medicines (heartworm preventatives); continue trial until patient improves or for 8–10 weeks; if improvement is noted, reintroduce original diet and monitor for itching for 7–14 days; return of itching may occur within hours; reintroduction of original diet confirms food allergy

Therapeutics

- More than one disease may be contributing to the itching; if treatment for an identified condition does not result in improvement, consider other causes.
- Use of a mechanical restraint (e.g., Elizabethan collar) can help but is seldom feasible in the long term.

Topical Therapy

- Helpful for mild cases
- Localized—sprays, lotions, and creams
- Generalized—shampoos
- Colloidal oatmeal—available in all forms; may be very beneficial; duration of effect usually < 2 days
- Antihistamines—beneficial effect not demonstrated
- Anesthetics—very short duration of effect
- Antibacterial shampoo—controls bacterial infections; some (e.g., benzoyl peroxide or iodine) may exacerbate the condition due to irritant effect
- Lime sulfur—may be antipruritic; has antiparasitic, antibacterial, and antifungal properties; disadvantages are bad odor and staining
- Steroids—most useful topical medication; excessive use causes localized and systemic side effects; hydrocortisone mildest and most common; stronger

drugs (e.g., betamethasone) more effective, more expensive, and cause more side effects; some contain ingredients (e.g., alcohol) that increase irritation

- Sometimes the application of any substance, including water (especially warm water), can worsen itching sensation; cool water is often soothing.

Systemic Therapy

- Three pathways lead to inflammation and itching.
- Steroids—block all three pathways; undesirable side effects; consider drugs that block individual pathways
- Antihistamines—hydroxyzine, diphenhydramine, and chlorpheniramine; block only one pathway
- ω-3 and ω-6 fatty acids—available as powder, liquid, and capsules; help block individual pathways that lead to inflammation; 6–8 weeks until maximum effect is observed; prevent rather than stop inflammation; help control dry or flaky skin
- Psychogenics—can help control itching; amitriptyline (Elavil; a human antidepressant) has rather potent antihistaminic actions in dogs, with side effects similar to antihistamines; doxepin is similar; fluoxetine (Prozac) used with variable success in treating canine lick granuloma (acral lick dermatitis); diazepam (Valium) has been beneficial; reports of acute hepatotoxicity in cats
- The use of nonsteroid drugs is less convenient but diminishes the potential for serious side effects; if not totally effective in controlling clinical signs, they often help reduce the amount of steroids necessary to decrease itching.

Steroids

- Most well-known drug used to control itching
- Significant long-term and not always obvious side effects
- Used wisely, usually safe
- Avoid long-term daily administration of oral corticosteroids (including prednisone or methylprednisolone).
- Avoid long-term daily or alternate-day administration of triamcinolone (Vetalog).
- Short-term use seldom causes serious problems.
- Avoid with a history of pancreatitis, diabetes mellitus, calcinosis cutis, demodicosis, dermatophytosis, and other infectious diseases.
- Immunosuppressive drugs (e.g., azathioprine)—use in extremely rare cases; because of potential profound side effects, reserve for cases in which euthanasia is being considered or when all other treatments have failed.

Comments

- Sometimes the application of anything topically, including water and products containing alcohol, iodine, and benzoyl peroxide, can exacerbate itching; cool water may be soothing.
- Steroids—avoid with infectious causes
- Multiple causes (e.g., flea allergy, inhalant allergy, and pyoderma) common; eradication or control of one cause may not be enough to reduce the condition.

- Food and airborne/inhalant-allergic animals may do well during winter on a hypoallergenic diet; clinical signs may return in the warmer months in association with inhalant allergies.
- Monitor patients receiving chronic steroids every 3–6 months for signs of iatrogenic Cushing disease.
- Client frustration owing to the chronic nature of pruritus
- Skin scrapes and other tests may be initially negative or normal but may later become diagnostic.
- Complications common with chronic steroid use

Suggested Reading

Bevier DE. Long-term management of atopic disease in the dog. In: DeBoer DJ, ed. Vet Clin North Am Small Anim Pract 1995;25:1487–1505.

Consulting Editor Karen Helton Rhodes

Clinical Management of Pruritic Inflammatory Skin Disease

Karen Helton Rhodes

The pruritic patient is a common problem in veterinary medicine. Many of the diseases that promote pruritus are not curable and must therefore be controlled over a long duration of time. An underlying etiology must first be determined before considering long-term antipruritic therapy. Corticosteroids are the most frequently used drugs in veterinary medicine, yet should not be used as a maintenance form of therapy until an etiology has been determined and other medications have been tested.

Canine and feline allergic dermatitis is the hallmark of pruritic inflammatory diseases in veterinary medicine and will be used as the model for the following discussion. The discussed medications are not meant to replace appropriate "diagnostic" procedures (i.e., food elimination diet trials, intradermal skin testing, etc.) but rather to augment the therapeutic management protocol chosen for the individual patient.

Much of the confusion in the management of the pruritic patient stems from the fact that the exact mediator(s) and pathophysiology of pruritus are unknown. Limited information is available in the veterinary literature of pruritus in the dog and cat. Most investigators make the assumption that because antihistamines are not capable of relieving pruritus in a large percentage of animals, proteolytic enzymes must be the primary mediator rather than histamine. Because most proteases are potent histamine releasers, this explanation cannot be entirely correct. Recent attention has focused on the eicosanoids. Because of this confusion, the selection of an appropriate medication is therefore difficult and often depends on therapeutic trials. This "trial and error" method of drug selection is both costly and frustrating for the client.

Proposed Pathophysiology of Pruritus

Various stimuli that cause itching may elicit two distinct responses: *spontaneous* itch (an itch that is localized to the site of the stimulus and persists only briefly after the stimulus is removed) and *pathologic* itch (an itch that is more poorly localized or diffuse). Both itch and pain sensations are the result of the activation of a network of free nerve endings at the dermoepidermal junction. However, these nerve endings alone do not determine itch sensitivity; certain regions of the skin that have a low threshold for pruritus do not have higher numbers of nerve endings compared with less sensitive areas. Itch is considered a primary sensory modality rather than subthreshold pain, as was previously believed. The phenomenon of itchy skin is familiar to all physicians and veterinarians. Whether this form of pruritus relies on specific receptors (unmyelinated slow-conducting C fibers rather than rapid-conducting A fibers) or activation of a facilitating circuit of adjacent neurons following stimulation is unknown.

Influences of the CNS on pruritus have been described as a "gate-control" system. Simultaneous firing of large-diameter myelinated fibers presynaptically inhibits firing of the smaller afferent fibers so that the sensation that they usually evoke is diminished in intensity or even not perceived. Psychological factors are capable of influencing the "gate-control" system. The discovery that opioid pentapeptides (enkephalins) could act as neurotransmitters has led to speculation regarding an additional gating system for pain composed of inhibiting descending fibers. These mediators relieve pain and may subsequently cause pruritus by activating enkephalinergic inhibitory interneurons, modifying the sensation of pain. In addition to the influence on the CNS, these opioids may influence the peripheral nervous system as well by potentiating histamine-induced itch. Enkephalin-like immunoreactivity has been identified in the Merkel cell. Systemic administration of the opiate antagonist naloxone hydrochloride (Narcan) elevates the sensory threshold for itch and causes initial, although unsustained, decrease in pruritus.

Peripheral mediators of pruritus include histamine, proteases, peptides, arachidonic acid products, and serotonin. Histamine in low concentrations induces itch, whereas larger amounts elicit pain. A superficial injection of histamine causes itch, whereas a deep injection causes pain. Histamine receptors are classified as H1 and H2. Via decreased cAMP, H1, but not H2, receptors are involved in histamine-evoked itching. H2 receptors (via increased cAMP) play a regulatory role by acting as a negative feedback system in some species. This histamine-induced pruritus may be initiated via H1 receptors, and also via the activation of other mediators such as substance P or prostaglandins.

Proteases, another class of peripheral mediators, include endogenous (trypsin, chymotrypsin, fibrinolysin, kallikrein) and exogenous (ficin, papain, streptokinase) mediators. The pruritogenic effect of these enzymes is unrelated to their proteolytic activity. Proteases are potent histamine releasers and most likely initiate pruritus via this mechanism. Kallikrein is the only known protease to cause pruritus independent of histamine release. Peptides, such as bradykinin, vasoactive intestinal peptide, neurotensin, secretin, and substance P are potent histamine releasers.

Inflammation of the skin may be associated with the transformation of the cell membrane component arachidonic acid in a number of cell types, including keratinocytes, into a variety of pro-inflammatory fatty acids. These include the prostaglandins, polymorphonuclear chemoattractant monohydroxy fatty acids, and leukotrienes. Prostaglandins, primarily PgE1, amplify pharmacologically induced itching by lowering the threshold of the free nerve ending receptors to the effects of histamine and proteolytic enzymes. Pro-inflammatory mediators also include 12-hydroxyeicosatetraenoic acid, 5-hydroxyeicosatetraenoic acid, and leukotrienes C4, D4, and E4. Serotonin injected intradermally can cause pruritus.

The influence of skin temperature on itch remains unclear. Empirical observations suggest that pruritus is aggravated when the skin is warm (part of the rationale for bathing in lukewarm or cool warm water). Itching may also be influenced by diurnal rhythms of the body, which have been attributed to both diurnal skin temperature fluctuations as well as epinephrine fluctuations. UVA and UVB may influence pruritus by inactivating pruritogens. UVB has also been reported to alter vitamin D metabolism, causing an alteration in ions and thereby less itching.

The immunologic aspects of pruritus are also less than conclusive. Immunologic defects associated with allergic dermatitis in the animal are under investigation. Antipruritic medications may be directed at a specific alteration in the immune system of the patient. Suspected alterations include endothelial cells that abnormally express adhesion molecules, increase in T-helper cells, hyperstimulatory epidermal Langerhans cells, B-cell overproduction of IgE, increased dermal levels of eosinophil-derived MBP, serum IgA alterations, local stimulation of Langerhans cells in the epidermis, increased phosphodiesterase activity, lowered plasma triglyceride levels, and so forth.

This limited knowledge forms the basis behind many of our therapeutic choices to control pruritus in animals. The exact pathomechanism of pruritus and even the specific etiology and pathogenesis of allergic dermatitis are still a mystery.

Proposed Pathophysiology of "Atopic" Skin Disease

1. Percutaneous absorbed allergen (allergen penetration enhanced by epidermal barrier defect)
2. Allergen encounters allergen-specific IgE on Langerhans cells
3. Allergen is trapped by Langerhans cells, processed, and presented to allergen-specific T cells
4. Expansion of allergen-specific Th2 cells, which produce IL3, IL4, IL5, IL6, and IL10
5. An increase in Th2 cells causes an increase in allergen-specific IgE production via IL4 (will also see a proportional decrease in Th1 cells, which are responsible for inhibiting allergen-specific IgE production via alpha-interferon)
6. Therefore, enhanced production of allergen specific IgE by B cells

Drugs Used in Controlling Pruritus

Glucocorticoids

Glucocorticoids are without question the most effective drugs in controlling pruritus.
Anti-inflammatory effects of steroids include the following:

1. Decreased migration of neutrophils into the tissue
2. Inhibited release of inflammatory cytokines from macrophages (IL1, TNF-alpha, prostaglandins)
3. Inhibited phagocytosis by macrophages
4. Inhibited migration of eosinophils into tissue
5. Decreased numbers of lymphocytes in circulation
6. Depressed lymphocyte activation
7. Decreased expression of cytokines from lymphocytes
8. T cells more affected than B cells
9. Improved vascular integrity by antagonism of vasoactive amines
10. Decreased synthesis of inflammatory mediators

11. Inhibited synthesis of cyclo-oxygenase enzyme and inhibition of phospholipase A2, which lowers concentrations of prostaglandins, prostacyclin, thromboxane, and leukotrienes (See Table 33-1 for a comparison of steroid potency.)

PROGESTERONE COMPOUNDS

Ovaban (megastrol acetate) and DepoProvera (medroxyprogesterone acetate) have been used in cats to control pruritus, but should not be used in dogs. The mechanism of action is unclear, but probably produces a potent glucocorticoid-like effect.

Dosage

Begin with 5 mg/cat/day for 1 week, then 2.5 to 5.0 mg/cat every other day for 1 week, then gradually decrease to 5 mg once or twice a week, and finally decrease to 2.5 to 5.0 mg/cat every 7–14 days.

Side effects:

1. PU/PD, adrenal suppression
2. Mood alterations
3. Diabetes mellitus
4. Pyometra
5. Hair coat color change
6. Diarrhea

MEDICATIONS AND SUPPLEMENTS AFFECTING THE BIOSYNTHESIS AND METABOLISM OF ARACHIDONIC ACID (AA)

NSAIDs and Lipoxygenase Inhibitors (affect metabolism of AA)

Nonsteroidal anti-inflammatory drugs such as aspirin appear to have limited use in controlling pruritus. One study reported a 2% success rate when buffered aspirin was administered to dogs at a dosage of 25 mg/kg q8h. NSAIDs block the arachidonic acid cycle by inhibiting the cyclo-oxygenase pathway.

Lipoxygenase inhibitors (e.g., Benoxaprofen) block the lipoxygenase pathway. Very limited use in the dog (5-lipoxygenase inhibitor) produced poor results.

Table 33-1

Comparison of Steroid Potency (Commonly Used Medications)

Drug	Duration of Action	Potency/ Comparative	MC Effects
Hydrocortisone (cortisol)	8–12	1	2
Prednisone/prednisolone	12–36	4	1
Methylprednisolone	12–36	5	½
Triamcinolone	12–36	5	0
Dexamethasone	32–48	25	0
Betamethasone	32–48	25	0

Essential Fatty Acid Metabolites

Essential fatty acid metabolites affect the biosynthesis of arachidonic acid (AA) and can bypass some pathways. Essential fatty acids for the dog are linoleic and linolenic. For the cat, they include linoleic, linolenic, and arachidonic acid sources of fatty acids: GLA (gamma-linolenic acid), an omega-6 fatty acid contained in evening primrose oil); EPA (eicosapentaenoic acid), an omega-3 fatty acid contained in marine fish oil; and ALA (alpha-linolenic acid), an omega-3 fatty acid contained in vegetable oil (soy, canola, linseed). Most essential fatty acid supplements use a combination of EPA and GLA. In theory, increased quantities of EPA and GLA may help decrease pruritus and inflammation by altering the potency and quantity of eicosanoids (PG and LT). EPA can displace AA in cell membrane and when the cells are activated during inflammation, more EPA is metabolized by cyclo-oxygenase and lipoxygenase than is AA. EPA breakdown products are less inflammatory than is AA products.

EPA – prostaglandins of the 3 series and leukotrienes of the 5 series (less inflammatory)

AA – prostaglandin 2, 12-HETE, leukotriene 4 (very inflammatory)

GLA is metabolized to DGLA (dihomo-gamma linolenic acid) which is further metabolized to PGE1 (anti-inflammatory). ALA can be metabolized to EPA.

Clinical trials with EFA supplementation are varied and best used in combination with other medications. Antihistamines may produce a synergistic effect with EFAs.

Side effects:

1. Transient decreased platelet aggregation after 3 months of use (no clinical effects)
2. Increased risk of pancreatitis
3. Fish odor on breath

Antihistamines

Antihistamines are grouped into two classes: H1 receptor antagonists and H2 receptor antagonists. (Table 33-2)

Side effects:

1. Sedation
2. Dry mouth
3. Blurred vision
4. Urinary retention
5. Appetite stimulation

Adverse effects:

1. Seizures and coma from overdose (first generation)
2. Cardiotoxic at high concentrations; ketoconazole may potentiate these effects (second generation) (synergistic effect with corticosteroids and thus allow lowering of the steroid dose needed [30% reduction])

Psychotropic Drugs

Psychotropic drugs are primarily used for obsessive/compulsive disorders (OCD). Many pruritic cases may have a component of OCD. Some of these drugs can also bind to histamine as well as serotonin receptors and are thus powerful antihistamines as well (i.e., amitryptilline). These medications have varied effectiveness and should not be the "first line of defense." Avoid use with monoamine oxidase inhibitors. (Table 33-3)

Table 33-2

Antihistamines: Grouped into two Classes: H1 Receptor Antagonists and H2 Receptor Antagonists

Drug	Dosage	Dog/Cat
H1 Receptor Antagonists (First Generation)		
Chlorpheniramine/	0.25–0.5 mg/kg q8–12h	Dog
Chlor-Trimeton	2–4 mg/cat q12h	Cat
Diphenhydramine/Benadryl	2–4 mg/kg q8–12h	Dog
Hydroxyzine/Atarax	1.0 mg/kg q6–8h	Dog
Trimeprazine/Temaril	0.5 mg/kg q12h	Dog
Clemastine/Tavist	0.05–1.0 mg/kg q12h	Dog
Cyproheptadine/Periactin	1 mg/kg q8–12h	Dog and Cat
Doxepin/Sinequan	2.2 mg/kg q12h	Dog
H1 Receptor Antagonists (Second Generation)†		
Terfenadine/Seldane	5–10 mg/kg q12h	Dog
Astemizole/Hismanal	1 mg/kg q12h	Dog (poor results)
Loratidine/Claritin	5–20 mg/day	Dog
	2.5 mg	Cat
Cetirizine/Zyrtec	5–10 mg/dog	
	5.0 mg/cat	
H2 Receptor Antagonists		
Cimetidine/Tagamet	6–10 mg/kg q8h	Dog (use in combination with Atarax)*

†Less sedating because lack the antimuscarinic properties and do not cross the blood-brain barrier easily.

*H2 receptors are normally used for their antisecretory effects, yet there is some evidence they may be helpful for dermatologic disease. Tagamet and Atarax can be used in combination to treat pruritus. Cometidine or ranitidine may enhance relief from pruritus and wheal formation in refractory cases of urticaria. The H2 receptor antagonists can inhibit metabolism of H1 receptor antagonists if they are coadministered, thus increasing plasma levels of the H1 receptor antagonist.

*Synergistic effect with corticosteroids and thus allow lowering of the steroid dose needed (30% reduction).

Miscellaneous Drugs

Many of the following medications are still in trial and the exact dosage is unknown.

Oxatomide/Mast Cell Stabilizer

- Dosage: 15–30 mg q12h
- Allergic cats (one report from France)

Misoprostol/Prostaglandin E1 Analogue

- Dosage: 6 μg/kg TID
- Dogs

Table 33-3

Psychotropic Drugs Used to Treat Obsessive/Compulsive Disorders

Drug	Dosage	Dog/Cat	Effects
Amitryptilline/ Elavil	1–2 mg/kg/day	Dog and cat	Dry mouth, constipation, urine retention (contraindicated in patients with cardiac disease & seizure history)
Buspirone/ Buspar	2–4 mg/kg q12h	Cat	
Fluoxetine/ Prozac	1–2 mg/kg/day	Dog	Poor success... Anuria
Clomipramine/ Anafranil	1–2 mg/kg/day	Dog	Poor success... Anuria
Diazepam/ Valium	1–2 mg/cat q12–24h	Cat	Idiosyncratic fatal hepatic necrosis
Pentazocine/ Talwin	2.2 mg/kg q12h	Dog	Limited data
Naltrexone/ Trexan	2.2 mg/kg q24h	Dog and cat	Limited data

- Side effects are mild
- PGE1 has been demonstrated to inhibit the late-phase reaction in allergic disease
- Inhibits granulocyte activity, lymphocyte proliferation, and cytokine production (IL1 and TNF-alpha)
- Might prove synergistic with antihistamines, which inhibit the immediate phase
- One study showed excellent efficacy in 61% of cases (18 dogs)

Erythromycin/Antibiotic

- Dosage: 10 mg/kg q8h
- Dog
- Anti-inflammatory properties involve an inhibition of neutrophil chemotaxis
- A mast cell–derived neutrophil chemotactic factor is present in some hypersensitivity disorders and neutrophils are frequently found in the skin of atopics.

Ketoconazole/Antifungal

- Dosage: 10 mg/kg q12h
- Dog
- Used in cases of pruritic yeast dermatitis in the dog (yeast hypersensitivity?)

- Topical ketoconazole has been reported in the human literature to have anti-inflammatory properties similar to those of hydrocortisone.
- Inhibits 5-lipoxygenase activity and all-trans-retinoic acid

TRENTAL/PENTOXIFYLLINE

- Dosage: 10 mg/kg BID
- Best for contact dermatitis, often used with vitamin E

ARAVA

- Dosage: 1–3 mg/kg day
- Variable response
- Need 30 mg/mL trough level

CYCLOSPORINE A/NEORAL

- Dosage: 5 mg/kg/day (minimum of 1 month trial)
- Expensive, variable response
- No food 2 hours before or after administering medication
- May be able to lower dose if used with Ketoconazole at 2.5 mg/kg/day (cyclosporine can be lowered to 2.5 mg/kg/day)
- Side effects: hepatotoxicity

Topicals: Shampoos, Rinses, Lotions, Gels, Sprays, Creams

All systemic medications should be used with topical shampoos to control pruritus. The topical treatment plan is formulated based on the primary diagnosis and is perhaps the *most* important part of the treatment protocol. Owner compliance is extremely important.

Author Karen Helton Rhodes

Hypersensitivity Reaction (Anaphylaxis)

Paul W. Snyder

Definition/Overview

- Acute manifestation of a type I hypersensitivity reaction mediated through the rapid introduction of an antigen into a host having antigen-specific antibodies of the IgE subclass
- The binding of antigen to mast cells sensitized with IgE results in the release of preformed and newly synthesized chemical mediators.
- Anaphylactic reactions may be localized (atopy) or systemic (anaphylactic shock).
- Anaphylaxis not mediated by IgE is designated an anaphylactoid reaction and will not be discussed.

Etiology/Pathophysiology

- First exposure of the patient to a particular antigen (allergen) causes a humoral response and results in production of IgE, which binds to the surface of mast cells; the patient is then considered to be sensitized to that antigen.
- Second exposure to the antigen results in cross-linking of two or more IgE molecules on the cell surface, resulting in mast cell degranulation and activation; release of mast cell granules initiates an anaphylactic reaction.
- Major mast cell–derived mediators include histamine, eosinophilic chemotactic factor, arachidonic acid, metabolites (e.g., prostaglandins, leukotrienes, and thromboxanes), platelet-activating factor, and proteases, which cause an inflammatory response of increased vascular permeability, smooth muscle contraction, inflammatory cell influx, and tissue damage.

- Clinical manifestations depend on the route of antigen exposure, the dose of antigen, and the level of the IgE response.
- Familial basis reported for type I hypersensitivity reaction in dogs

Signalment/History

- Dogs—numerous breeds documented as having a predilection for developing atopy
- Cats—no breeds documented as having predilection for atopy
- Dogs—age of clinical onset ranges from 3 months to several years of age; most affected animals 1–3 years old
- Cats—age of clinical onset ranges from 6 months to 2 years
- Dogs—atopy more common in females
- Cats—no reported sex predilection
- Previous exposure (sensitization) increases the chance of the animal developing a reaction.

Clinical Features

- Initial clinical signs vary depending on the route of exposure to the inciting antigen (allergen).
- Shock—end result of a severe anaphylactic reaction
- Shock organ—dogs, liver; cats, respiratory and gastrointestinal systems
- May be localized to the site of exposure, but may progress to a systemic reaction
- Onset of signs immediate (within minutes)
- Dogs—pruritus, urticaria, vomiting, defecation, and urination
- Cats—intense pruritus about the head, dyspnea, salivation, and vomiting
- Localized cutaneous edema at the site of exposure
- Hepatomegaly in some dogs
- Hyperexcitability possible in early stages
- Depression and collapse terminally

Differential Diagnosis

- Other types of shock
- Trauma
- Depends on the major organ system involved or if reaction is localized; diagnosis can be made largely on the basis of history and clinical signs
- Virtually any agent; those commonly reported include venoms, blood-based products, vaccines, foods, and drugs
- Intradermal skin testing to identify allergens
- Radioallergosorbent test to quantify the concentration of serum IgE specific for a particular antigen
- Lesions vary, depending on severity of reaction, from localized cutaneous edema to severe pulmonary edema (in cats) and visceral pooling of blood (in dogs)

- Other nonspecific findings vary and are characteristic of shock.
- Nonspecific characteristics of localized reactions include edema, vasculitis, and thromboembolism

Therapeutics

- In an acutely affected animal, the reaction is considered a medical emergency requiring hospitalization.
- Elimination of inciting antigen, if possible

Systemic Anaphylaxis

- Goal—emergency life support through the maintenance of an open airway, preventing circulatory collapse, and re-establishing physiologic parameters
- Administer fluids intravenously at shock dosages to counteract hypotension.

Localized Anaphylaxis

- Goal—limit the reaction and prevent progression to a systemic reaction.
- If a food-based allergen is suspected (uncommon), avoid foods associated with hypersensitivity reaction.

Systemic Anaphylaxis

- Epinephrine hydrochloride parenterally (1:1000; 0.01 mL/kg) for shock
- Corticosteroids for shock—prednisolone sodium succinate (10–30 mg/kg IV q8h) or dexamethasone sodium phosphate (6–15 mg/kg IV q12h)
- Atropine sulfate (0.04 mg/kg IM) to counteract bradycardia and hypotension
- Aminophylline (10 mg/kg IM or slowly IV) in severely dyspneic patients

Localized Anaphylaxis

- Diphenhydramine hydrochloride (1–2 mg/kg IV or IM)
- Prednisolone (2 mg/kg PO)
- Epinephrine hydrochloride (0.15 mL SC at site of initiation)
- If shock develops, initiate treatment for a systemic anaphylaxis.

Comments

- Discuss the unpredictable nature of the disease.
- Discuss the need to recognize that the animal has an allergic condition that may require immediate medical care.
- Closely monitor hospitalized patients for 24–48 hr.
- If inciting antigen (allergen) can be identified, eliminate or reduce exposure.
- If localized reaction is treated early, prognosis is good.
- If the animal is in shock on examination, prognosis is guarded to poor.

Suggested Reading

Mueller DL, Noxon JO. Anaphylaxis: pathophysiology and treatment. Compend Contin Educ Pract Vet 1990;12:157–170.

Author Paul W. Snyder

Consulting Editor Karen Helton Rhodes

Atopy

Jon D. Plant and Lloyd M. Reedy

Definition/Overview

Predisposition to become allergic to normally innocuous substances, such as pollens (grasses, weeds, and trees), molds, house dust mites, epithelial allergens, and other environmental allergens

Etiology/Pathophysiology

- Susceptible animals become sensitized to environmental allergens by producing allergen-specific IgE, which binds to receptor sites on cutaneous mast cells; further allergen exposure (inhalation, percutaneous absorption) causes mast cell degranulation, which is a type I immediate hypersensitivity reaction, and results in the release of histamine, proteolytic enzymes, cytokines, chemokines, and many other chemical mediators.
- Non-IgE antibodies (IgGd) and a late-phase reaction (8–12 hr) may also be involved.
- Canine—although there is an inherited predisposition, the mode of inheritance is unknown and other factors may also be important
- Feline—unclear

Signalment/History

- Canine—true incidence unknown; estimated at 3–15% of the canine population; reported to be the second most common allergic skin disease

- Feline—unknown; generally believed to be much lower than that for dogs
- Canine—any breed, including mongrels; because of genetic predisposition, it may be recognized more frequently in certain breeds or families, which can vary geographically
- In the United States (canine)—Boston terriers, Cairn terriers, Dalmatians, English bulldogs, English setters, Irish setters, Lhasa apsos, miniature schnauzers, pugs, Sealyham terriers, Scottish terriers, West Highland white terriers, wire-haired fox terriers, and golden retrievers
- Canine—mean age at onset 1–3 years; range 3 months–6 years; signs may be so mild the first year that they are not noted but are usually progressive and clinically apparent before 3 years of age
- Both sexes are probably affected equally.

Historical Findings

- Facial, pedal, or axillary pruritus
- Early onset
- Family history of atopy
- May be seasonal
- Recurring skin or ear infections
- Temporary response to glucocorticoids
- Symptoms progressively worsen with time.

Clinical Features

- Hallmark sign—pruritus (itching, scratching, rubbing, licking)
- Primary lesions may occur, but most cutaneous changes are believed to be produced by self-induced trauma.
- Areas most commonly affected—interdigital spaces, carpal and tarsal areas, muzzle, periocular region, axillae, groin, and pinnae
- Lesions—vary from none to broken hairs or salivary discoloration to erythema, papular reactions, crusts, alopecia, hyperpigmentation, lichenification, excessively oily or dry seborrhea, and hyperhidrosis (apocrine sweating)
- Secondary bacterial and yeast skin infections (common)
- Chronic relapsing otitis externa
- Conjunctivitis may occur.

Differential Diagnosis

- Food hypersensitivity—may cause identical lesion distribution and physical examination findings but should be nonseasonal; may occur concurrently with atopy; differentiation is made by noting response to hypoallergenic diet
- Flea bite hypersensitivity—most common cause of seasonal pruritus in many geographic regions; may occur concurrently with atopy; differentiation is made by noting lesion distribution, response to flea control, and results of intradermal skin testing
- Sarcoptic mange—often occurs in young or stray dogs; usually causes severe pruritus of the ventral chest, lateral elbows, lateral hocks, and pinnal margins; multiple skin scrapings and/or complete response to a trial of miticidal therapy are indicated to rule out sarcoptic mange

- Secondary pyoderma—usually caused by *Staphylococcus intermedius;* characterized by follicular papules, pustules, crusts, and epidermal collarettes
- Secondary yeast infections—usually caused by *Malassezia pachydermatis*; characterized by erythematous, scaly, crusty, greasy, and very malodorous body folds and intertriginous areas; demonstration of numerous budding yeast organisms by skin cytology and obtaining a favorable response to antifungal therapy are diagnostic
- Contact dermatitis (allergic or irritant)—may cause severe erythema and pruritus of the feet and thinly haired areas of the ventral abdomen; history of exposure to a known contact sensitizer or irritant, response to a change of environment, and patch testing may be diagnostic; thought to be rare in dogs and cats

Diagnostics

- Eosinophilia—rare in dogs without concurrent flea infections; common in cats

Atopy—Identify Causes

- Airborne pollens (grasses, weeds, and trees)
- Mold spores (indoor and outdoor)
- House dust mite
- Animal danders
- Insects (controversial)

Serologic Allergy Tests

- Tests to measure the amount of allergen-specific IgE antibody in the patient's serum are commercially available.
- Advantages over IDST—availability; large areas of hair do not have to be shaved
- Disadvantages—frequent false-positive reactions; limited number of allergens tested; inconsistent assay validation and quality control (may vary with the laboratory used)
- Reliability in cats is unknown.

IDST

- Small amounts of test allergens are injected intradermally and wheal formation is measured.
- Most accurate method of identifying offending allergens for possible avoidance or inclusion in an immunotherapy prescription
- Results are sometimes difficult to interpret in cats owing to the relatively small wheals.
- Skin biopsy—may help rule out other differential diagnoses; results are usually not pathognomonic. Dermatohistopathologic changes—acanthosis, mixed mononuclear superficial perivascular dermatitis, sebaceous gland metaplasia, and secondary superficial pyoderma

Therapeutics

- Essential fatty acid supplementation may be beneficial in some cases.

Immunotherapy (Hyposensitization)

- Administration (usually SC injections) of gradually increasing doses of the causative allergens to affected patients in an attempt to reduce their sensitivity
- Allergens selected—based on allergy test results, patient history, and knowledge of local flora
- Indicated when it is desirable to avoid or reduce the amount of corticosteroids required to control signs, when signs last longer than 4–6 months per year, or when nonsteroidal forms of therapy are ineffective
- Successfully reduces pruritus in 60–80% of dogs and cats
- The response is usually slow, often requiring 3–6 months to up to 1 year.

Corticosteroids

- May be given for short-term relief and to break the itch-scratch cycle
- Should be tapered to the lowest dosage that adequately controls pruritus
- Best choices—prednisone suspension (0.5 to 1.0 mg/kg SC or IM); prednisone or methylprednisolone tablets (0.2 to 0.5 mg/kg PO q48h)
- Repository injectable corticosteroids should be avoided in dogs.
- Cats may require methylprednisolone acetate treatment (4 mg/kg SC or IM).

Antihistamines

- Less effective than are corticosteroids
- Efficacy as a sole treatment is probably in the 10–20% range.
- May act synergistically with essential fatty acid supplements
- Corticosteroid therapy can often be avoided or given at a reduced dosage when used concurrently.
- Dogs—hydroxyzine (1–2 mg/kg PO q8h), chlorpheniramine (0.2–0.4 mg/kg PO q12h), diphenhydramine (2.2 mg/kg PO q8h), and clemastine (0.04–0.10 mg/kg PO q12h)
- Cats—chlorpheniramine (0.5 mg/kg PO q12h); efficacy estimated at 10–50%

Precautions

- Corticosteroids—use judiciously in dogs to avoid iatrogenic hyperglucocorticism and associated problems, aggravation of pyoderma, and induction of demodicosis
- Antihistamines—can produce drowsiness, anorexia, vomiting, diarrhea, and even increased pruritus; use with caution in patients with cardiac arrhythmias
- The antihistamine astemizole has been associated with life-threatening cardiac arrhythmias in humans when administered concomitantly with imidazole antifungal drugs.

Alternative Drugs

- Frequent bathing in cool water with antipruritic shampoos can be beneficial.
- Supplementation with ω-3 and ω-6 fatty acids helps some pruritic patients; some studies have indicated that ω-3 (eicosapentaenoic acid 66 mg/kg/day) may be more effective than ω-6 (linoleic acid 130 mg/kg/day); other studies suggest that a 5:1 ratio of ω-6:ω-3 in the diet is indicated.

- Tricyclic antidepressants (doxepin 1.0–2.0 mg/kg PO q12h; or amitriptyline 1.0–2.0 mg/kg PO q12h) have been given to dogs as antipruritics but their overall effectiveness and mode of action is unclear; not extensively studied in the cat

Comments

- Explain the progressive nature of the condition.
- Inform client that it rarely goes into remission and cannot be cured.
- Inform client that some form of therapy may be necessary for life.
- Examine patient every 2–8 weeks when a new course of therapy is started.
- Monitor pruritus, self-trauma, pyoderma, and possible adverse drug reactions.
- Once an acceptable level of control is achieved, examine patient every 3–12 months.
- CBC, serum chemistry profile, and urinalysis—recommended every 6–12 months for patients on chronic corticosteroid therapy.
- If the offending allergens have been identified through allergy testing, the owner should undertake to reduce the animal's exposure as much as possible.
- Minimizing other sources of pruritus (e.g., fleas, food hypersensitivity, and secondary skin infections) may reduce the level of pruritus enough to be tolerated by the animal.
- Secondary pyoderma and concurrent flea allergy dermatitis are common.
- Not life-threatening unless intractable pruritus results in euthanasia
- If left untreated, the degree of pruritus worsens and the duration of signs lasts longer each year of the animal's life.
- Only rare cases spontaneously resolve.

Abbreviation

IDST = intradermal skin test

Suggested Reading

Reedy LM, Miller WH, Willemse T. Allergic skin diseases of dogs and cats. 2nd ed. Philadelphia: Saunders, 1997.

Authors Jon D. Plant and Lloyd M. Reedy
Consulting Editor Karen Helton Rhodes

FOOD REACTIONS

David Duclos

Definition/Overview

Pruritic, nonseasonal reactions associated with ingestion of one or more substances in the animal's food

Pathophysiology/Etiology

- Pathogenesis not completely understood
- Immediate and delayed reactions to specific ingredients—documented in the veterinary literature; immediate reactions presumed to be type I hypersensitivity reactions; delayed owing to type III or IV
- Food intolerance—nonimmunologic, idiosyncratic reaction; involves metabolic, toxic, or pharmacologic effects of offending ingredients
- Nonimmune (food intolerance) reactions—result of ingestion of foods with high levels of histamine or substances that induce histamine either directly or through histamine-releasing factors
- Food hypersensitivity is the most common term used because it is not easy to distinguish between immunologic and idiosyncratic reactions.
- Immune-mediated reactions—result of the ingestion and subsequent presentation of one or more glycoproteins (allergens) either before or after digestion; sensitization may occur at the gastrointestinal mucosa, after the substance is absorbed, or both.
- It is speculated that, in juvenile animals, intestinal parasites or intestinal infections may cause damage to the intestinal mucosa, resulting in the abnormal absorption of allergens and subsequent sensitization.

Signalment/History

- Approximately 5% of all skin diseases and 10–15% of all allergic diseases in dogs and cats are the result of food hypersensitivity.
- Third-most-common pruritic skin disease in the dog; second-most-common in the cat
- Percentages vary greatly with clinicians and geographic location.
- A wide range of signs that can mimic any of the other hypersensitivity reactions
- Skin/exocrine—pruritus in any location on the body; otitis externa
- Gastrointestinal—vomiting; diarrhea; more frequent bowel movements; flatulence
- Nervous—very rare; seizures have been documented with food hypersensitivity/intolerance
- Nonseasonal pruritus of any body location
- Poor response to anti-inflammatory doses of glucocorticoids suggests food hypersensitivity.

Clinical Features

- *Malassezia* dermatitis, pyoderma, and otitis externa
- Plaques
- Pustules
- Erythema
- Crusts
- Scale
- Self-induced alopecia
- Excoriation
- Lichenification
- Hyperpigmentation
- Urticaria
- Angioedema
- Pyotraumatic dermatitis

Differential Diagnosis

- Flea bite hypersensitivity—usually confined to the caudal half of the body; often seasonal
- Atopy—associated with pruritus on the face, ventrum, and feet; often seasonal; if pruritus first occurs at <6 months or >6 years of age, then food hypersensitivity may be more likely than inhalant allergy
- Drug reactions—history of drug administration before the development of signs and improvement after withdrawal of the suspected drug confirms the diagnosis
- Scabies—pruritus often very specific in the location (ears, elbows, and hocks); mites in skin scrapings and response to specific therapy confirm the diagnosis

Diagnostics

Food Elimination Diet

- Definitive test for food hypersensitivity
- Tailored to the individual patient
- The diet must be restricted to one protein and one carbohydrate to which the animal has had limited or no previous exposure.
- It may take up to 13 weeks for maximum improvement of the clinical signs.
- If the patient is sensitive to one or more foods, noticeable improvement will be seen by the 4th week of the diet.

Challenge and Provocation Diet Trials

- Used if the patient improves on the elimination diet
- Challenge—feed the patient with the original diet; a return of the signs confirms that something in the diet is causing the signs; the challenge period should last until the signs return but no longer than 10 days
- Provoke (provocation diet trial)—if the challenge confirmed the presence of a food hypersensitivity; add single ingredients to the elimination diet; test ingredients include a full range of meats (beef, chicken, fish, pork, lamb), a full range of grains (corn, wheat, soybean, rice), eggs, and dairy products; the provocation period for each ingredient should last up to 10 days or less if signs develop sooner (dogs usually develop signs within 1–2 days); results guide the selection of commercial foods that do not contain the offending substance(s)
- Histopathological findings—variable; common findings suggest hypersensitivity; a secondary pyoderma or *Malassezia* infection may be seen

Therapeutics

- Avoid any food substances that caused the clinical signs to return during the provocation phase of the diagnosis.
- Make sure the client understands the principles involved in each phase of the diagnostic test diets.
- Inform client to eliminate treats, chewable toys, vitamins, and other chewable medications (e.g., heartworm preventative) that may contain ingredients from the patient's previous diet.
- Outdoor pets must be confined to prevent foraging and hunting, which might alter the test diet.
- Provide handouts for clients to take home.
- Advise client that all family members must be aware of the test protocol and must help keep the test diet clean and free of any other food sources.
- Systemic antipruritic drugs—may be useful during the first 2–3 weeks of diet trial to control self-mutilation
- Antibiotics or antifungal medication—useful for secondary pyodermas or *Malassezia* infections
- Antibiotics that are known to have anti-inflammatory effects (e.g., tetracycline, erythromycin, and trimethoprim-potentiated sulfas)

- Glucocorticoids and antihistamines must be discontinued for at least 10–14 days while on the diet trial to allow correct assessment of the animal's response.
- Chewable vitamins and heartworm medications may contain offending food substances.

Comments

- Examine patient and evaluate and document the pruritus and clinical signs every 3–4 weeks.
- Avoid intake of any of the proteins included in the previous diet.
- Treats and chewable toys should be limited to known safe substances (e.g., apples, vegetables).
- Other causes of pruritus (e.g., flea bite hypersensitivity; atopy; and external parasites such as sarcoptic, *Notoedres*, and *Cheyletiella* mites) can mask the response to the food elimination diet trial.
- Prognosis is good, if food ingredients are the only cause of the pruritus and offending ingredients are avoided. Rarely, a dog or cat may develop hypersensitivity to new substances, which may require a new elimination diet trial.
- Any other hypersensitivities (flea or atopy) must also be treated.
- Animals who develop pruritus for the first time at < 6 months or > 6 years of age are more likely to have food hypersensitivity than atopy.

Suggested Reading

Jeffers JG, Shanley KJ. Diagnostic testing of dogs for food hypersensitivity. J Am Vet Med Assoc 1991;198:245–250.

MacDonald JM. Food allergy. In: Griffin CE, Kwochka KW, MacDonald JM, eds. Current Veterinary Dermatology. St. Louis: Mosby, 1993:121.

Rosser EJ. Diagnosis of food allergy in dogs. J Am Vet Med Assoc 1993;203:259.

White SD. Food hypersensitivity in 30 dogs. J Am Vet Med Assoc 1986;188:695–698.

Consulting Editor Karen Helton Rhodes

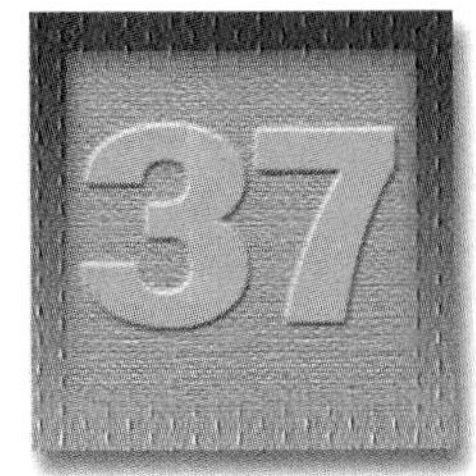

Contact Dermatitis

Alexander H. Werner and Margaret Swartout

Overview/Definition

Irritant contact dermatitis (ICD) and allergic contact dermatitis (ACD)—two rare and distinctly different pathophysiologic syndromes with similar clinical signs

Etiology/Pathophysiology

- *ICD*—results from direct damage to keratinocytes by exposure to a particular compound; damaged keratinocytes induce an inflammatory response directed at the skin
- *ACD*—an immunologic event requiring sensitization, memory, and elicitation: Langerhans cells process antigens that penetrate the skin and present them to naive T cells within lymph nodes; sensitized T cell clones (memory cells) then proliferate and circulate throughout the body; Langerhans cells encounter the antigens again and present them to sensitized T cells, resulting in an immunologic response
- Inflammatory dermatitis—may increase the penetration of antigens through the skin; thus may facilitate ACD
- Reported offending substances—plants, mulch, cedar chips; fabrics, rugs and carpets, plastics, rubber, leather, metal, concrete; soaps, detergents, floor waxes, carpet and litter deodorizers; herbicides, fertilizers, insecticides (including newer topical flea treatments), flea collars; topical preparations and medications

Signalment/History

- Dogs and cats
- ICD—occurs at any age as a direct result of the irritant nature of the offending compound
- ACD—rare in young animals; most animals are chronically exposed to the antigen; extremely rare in cats, except when exposed to D-limonene–containing insecticides
- Predisposed to ACD—German shepherds
- Increased risk for ACD (unsubstantiated)—French poodles, wire-haired fox terriers, Scottish terriers, West Highland white terriers, and golden retrievers

Clinical Features

- Location depends on the way in which the antigen is contacted; commonly limited to glabrous skin and regions frequently in contact with the ground (chin, ventral neck, sternum, ventral abdomen, inguinum, perineum, scrotum, and ventral contact regions of the tail and interdigital areas) (Figs. 37-1, 37-2)
- The thick hair coat of dogs is an effective barrier against contactants.
- In classic cases, extreme erythroderma stops abruptly at the hairline.
- Initially consist of erythema and swelling, leading to papules and plaques; vesicles are uncommon
- Reactions to topical medications (most often otic preparations) are usually localized; generalized reactions, resulting from shampoos or insecticide sprays, are less common.
- Pruritus—moderate to severe; severe is most common

Figure 37-1 Contact dermatitis secondary to exposure from a carpet freshener/deodorizer. Inguinal region primarily affected in this dog.

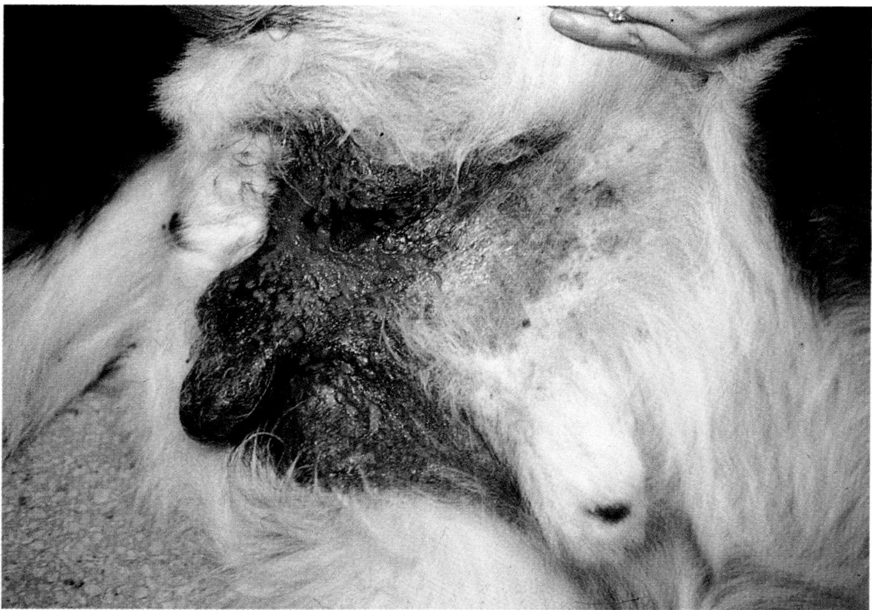

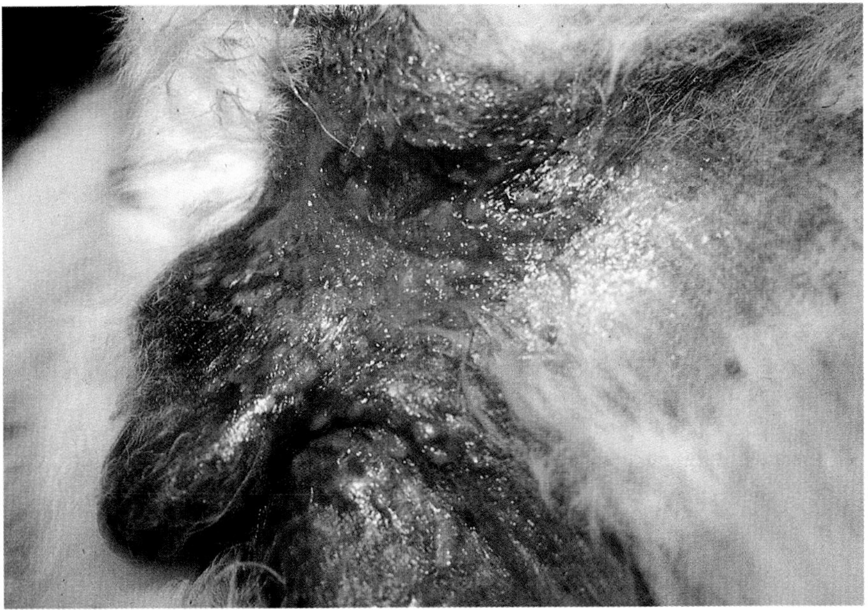

Figure 37-2 Closer view of Figure 37-1. Contact dermatitis.

- A seasonal incidence may indicate that the offending antigen is a plant or outdoor compound.

Differential Diagnosis

- Atopy
- Food allergy
- Drug eruptions
- Parasite hypersensitivity or infestation
- Insect bites
- Pyoderma
- *Malassezia* dermatitis
- Dermatophytosis
- Demodicosis
- Lupus erythematosus
- Seborrheic dermatitis
- Solar dermatitis
- Thermal injuries
- Trauma from rough surfaces

Diagnostics

- Closed-patch testing—sometimes helpful (corticosteroids and NSAIDs must be discontinued 3–6 weeks before testing); use materials directly from the environment or a standard patch test kit for humans (Hermal, Oak Hill, NY) applied to the skin under a bandage for 48 hr

- Best diagnostic test—eliminate contact irritant or antigen; follow with provocative exposure testing
- Bacterial cultures to define secondary pyoderma may be performed, if needed.
- Because the hair coat can protect the skin from contact with antigen, clipping a patch of hair in a nonaffected region should result in development of a local reaction.
- Skin biopsies—intraepidermal vesiculation and spongiosis; superficial dermal edema with perivascular mononuclear cell infiltrate in ICD and ACD; polymorphonuclear cell infiltrate in ICD; leukocyte exocytosis common

Therapeutics

- Eliminate offending substance(s).
- Bathe with hypoallergenic shampoos to remove antigen from the skin.
- Create mechanical barriers, if possible—socks, T-shirts, restriction from environment
- Systemic corticosteroids—prednisone (0.25–0.5 mg/kg PO q24h for 3–5 days; then q48h for 2 weeks)
- Topical corticosteroids for focal lesions
- Recent studies report success in dogs with pentoxifylline (10 mg/kg PO q12h).
- Pentoxifylline—do not administer with alkylating agents, cisplatin, and amphotericin B; cimetidine may increase serum levels of pentoxifylline

Comments

ICD

- Acute condition—may occur after only one exposure; can be manifested within 24 hr of exposure
- Steroids are rarely helpful.
- Lesions resolve 1–2 days after irritant removal.

ACD

- Requires months to years of exposure for the hypersensitivity to develop.
- Re-exposure results in the development of clinical signs 3–5 days following exposure; signs may persist for several weeks.
- Responds well to corticosteroids; but the pruritus returns after discontinuation if the antigenic stimulus has not been removed.
- Hyposensitization is disappointing.
- Prognosis—good if the allergen is identified and removed; poor if the allergen is not identified, which may then require lifelong treatment

Suggested Reading

Walder EJ, Conroy JD. Contact dermatitis in dogs and cats: pathogenesis, histopathology, experimental induction, and case reports. Vet Dermatol 1994;5:149–162.

Consulting Editor Karen Helton Rhodes

Eosinophilic Granuloma Complex

Alexander H. Werner

Definition/Overview

- Cats—often confusing term for three distinct syndromes: eosinophilic plaque, eosinophilic granuloma, and indolent ulcer; grouped primarily owing to their clinical similarities, their frequent concurrent development, and their positive response to corticosteroids
- Dogs—eosinophilic granulomas in dogs (EGD) rare; not part of disease complex; specific differences from cats are listed separately

Etiology/Pathophysiology

- Eosinophilic plaque—hypersensitivity reaction, most often to insects (fleas, mosquitos); less often to food or environmental allergens
- Eosinophilic granuloma—multiple causes, including hypersensitivity and genetic predisposition
- Indolent ulcer—may have both hypersensitivity and genetic causes
- Eosinophil—major infiltrative cell for eosinophilic granuloma and eosinophilic plaque; leukocyte located in greatest numbers in epithelial tissues; most often associated with allergic or parasitic conditions, but has a more general role in the inflammatory reaction
- EGD—may have both a genetic predisposition and a hypersensitivity cause
- Several reports of related affected individuals and a study of disease development in a colony of specific pathogen-free cats indicate that, in at least some individuals, genetic predisposition (perhaps resulting in a heritable dysfunction of eosinophilic regulation) is a significant component of the disease.

Signalment/History

- Restricted to cats—EGC
- Eosinophilic granulomas occur in dogs and other species, but are not considered part of this disease complex.
- EGD—Siberian huskies (76% of cases)
- Eosinophilic plaque—2–6 years of age
- Genetically initiated eosinophilic granuloma—<2 years of age
- Allergic disorder—>2 years of age
- Indolent ulcer—no age predisposition reported
- EGD—usually <3 years of age
- Cats—predilection for females has been reported only for the indolent ulcer
- EGD—males (72% of cases)
- Distinguishing among the syndromes depends on both clinical signs and histopathologic findings.
- Lesions of more than one syndrome may occur simultaneously.
- Lesions of all three syndromes may develop spontaneously and acutely.
- Development of eosinophilic plaques can be preceded by periods of lethargy.
- A seasonal incidence is common.
- Waxing and waning of clinical signs is common in all three syndromes.

Clinical Features

- Eosinophilic plaques—alopecic, erythematous, erosive patches and plaques; usually occur in the inguinal, perineal, lateral thigh, and axillary regions; frequently moist or glistening (Figs. 38-1, 38-2)
- Eosinophilic granulomas—occur in a distinctly linear orientation (linear granuloma) on the caudal thigh, or as individual or coalescing plaques located anywhere on the body; ulcerated with a "cobblestone" or coarse pattern; white or yellow, possibly representing collagen degeneration; lip margin and chin swelling ("pouting"); footpad swelling, pain, and lameness; oral cavity ulcerations (especially on the tongue, palate, and palatine arches); cats with oral lesions may be dysphagic, have halitosis, and may drool. (Fig. 38-3)
- Lesion development may stop spontaneously in some cats, especially with the heritable form of eosinophilic plaque.
- Indolent ulcers—classically raised and indurated ulcerations confined to the upper lips adjacent to the philtrum (Figs. 38-4, 38-5)
- EGD—lesions are ulcerated plaques and masses; dark or orange color

Differential Diagnosis

- Includes the other diseases in the complex
- Unresponsive lesions—exclude pemphigus foliaceus, dermatophytosis and deep fungal infection, demodicosis, pyoderma, and neoplasia (especially metastatic adenocarcinoma and cutaneous lymphosarcoma)

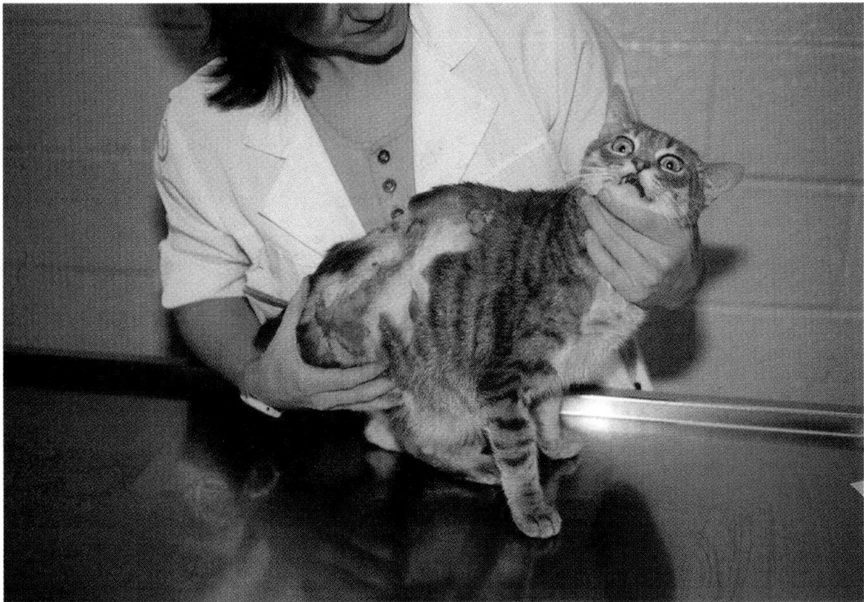

Figure 38-1 Eosinophilic plaque in an adult cat.

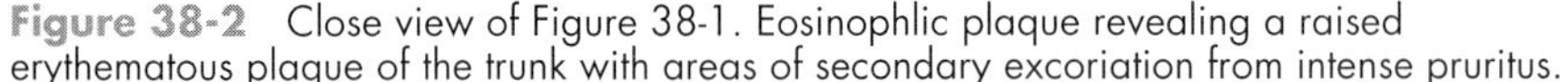

Figure 38-2 Close view of Figure 38-1. Eosinophlic plaque revealing a raised erythematous plaque of the trunk with areas of secondary excoriation from intense pruritus.

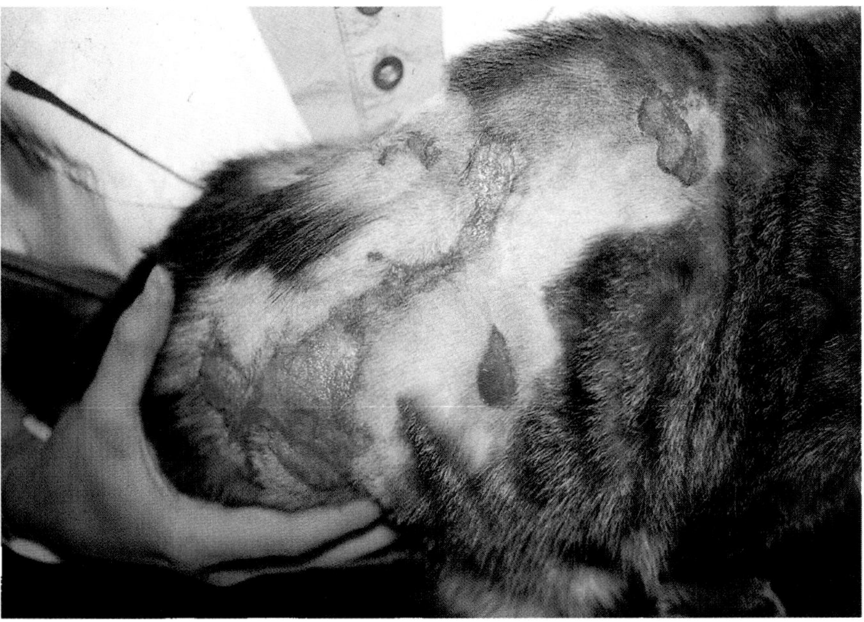

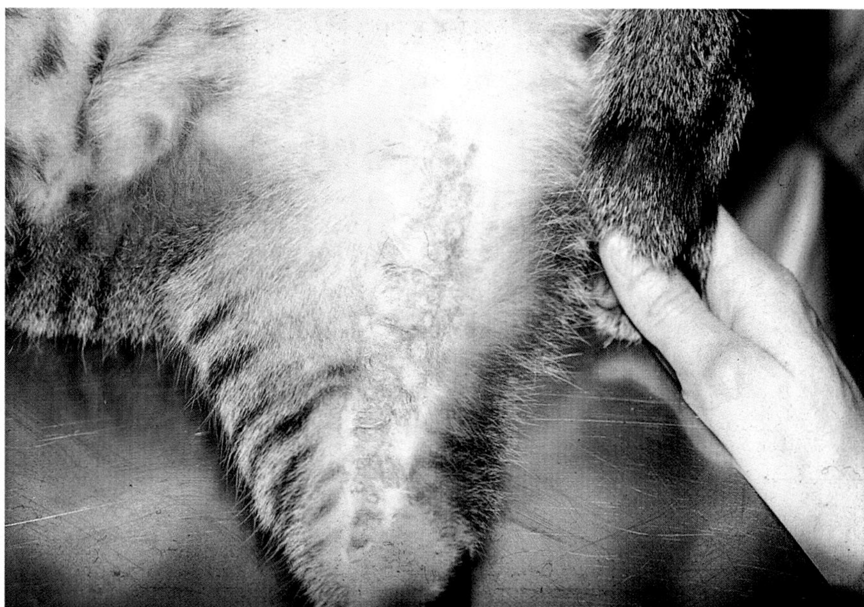

Figure 38-3 Linear granuloma along the caudal aspect of the hindlimb. Note the yellow-pink coloration of the lesions and the ropey raised texture.

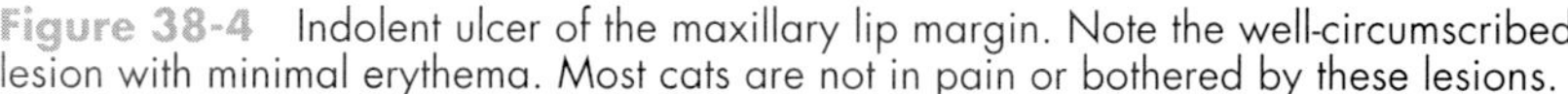

Figure 38-4 Indolent ulcer of the maxillary lip margin. Note the well-circumscribed lesion with minimal erythema. Most cats are not in pain or bothered by these lesions.

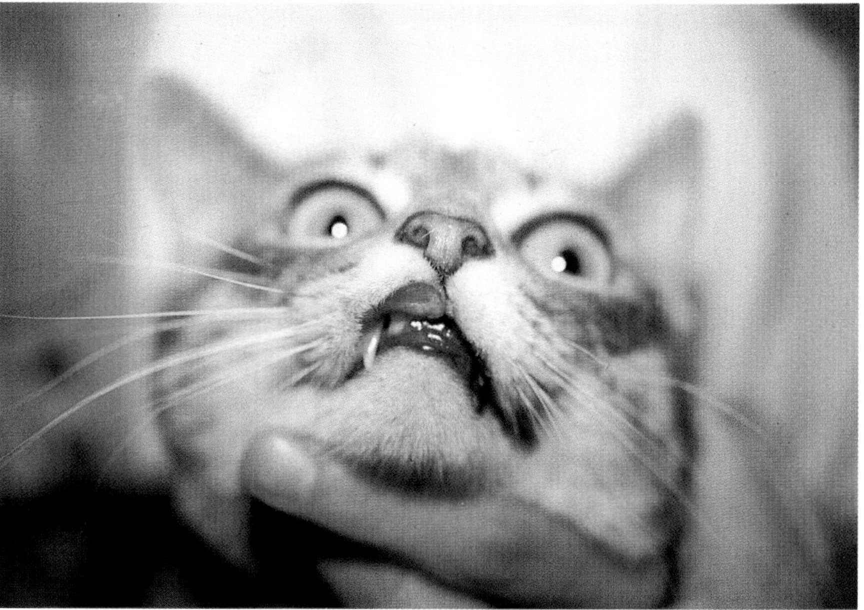

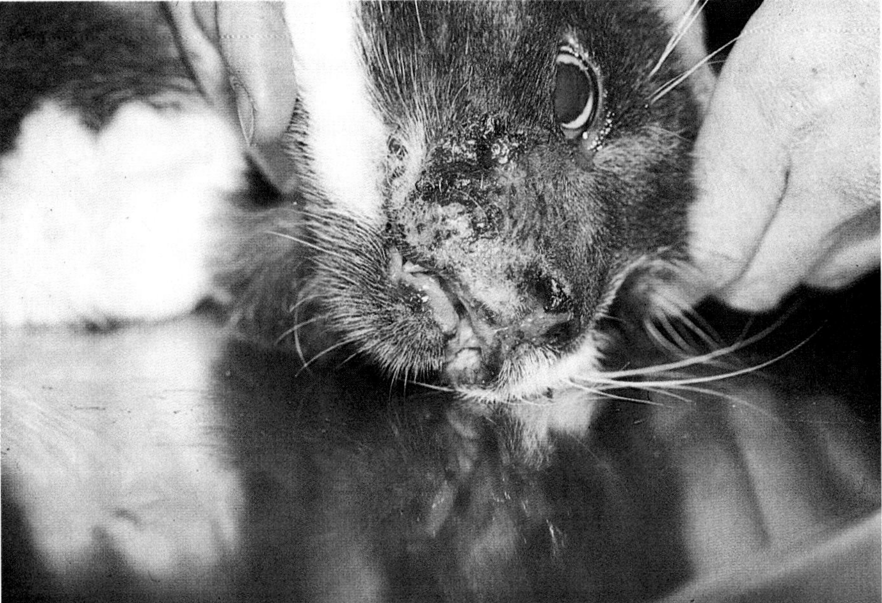

Figure 38-5 Indolent ulcer; severe ulceration with marked remodeling of the tissue. These lesions are often the type that raise concern regarding neoplastic transformation. This cat's tissue was biopsied and the results indicated no evidence of neoplasia.

Diagnostics

- CBC—mild to moderate eosinophilia
- Biochemistry and urinalysis—usually normal
- FeLV and FIV—pruritic diseases have been associated with these viruses
- Impression smears from lesions—large numbers of eosinophils
- Comprehensive flea and insect control—assist in excluding flea or mosquito bite hypersensitivity
- Food-elimination trial—for all cases; feed a protein (e.g., lamb, pork, venison, or rabbit) to which the cat has never been exposed; use exclusively for 8–10 weeks; then reinstitute previous diet and observe for development of new lesions
- Environmental allergy (atopy)—identified by intradermal skin testing (some cases); inject small amounts of dilute allergens intradermally; positive reaction (allergy) is indicated by the development of a hive or wheal at the injection site
- In vitro serum tests—available for identifying allergy-specific serum in cats; tests have not been validated and are not recommended
- Histopathologic diagnosis—required for distinguishing the syndromes
- Biopsy samples from indolent ulcers frequently fail to reveal eosinophils.
- Eosinophilic plaque—severe epidermal and follicular acanthosis with eosinophilic exocytosis and spongiosis; intense eosinophilic dermal infiltrate common; epidermis commonly eroded or ulcerated
- Eosinophilic granuloma—distinct foci of eosinophilic degranulation and collagen degeneration similar to granuloma formation; epidermis may be eroded or ulcerated

- Indolent ulcer—early lesions may be indistinguishable from those of eosinophilic granuloma (eosinophilic infiltration and collagen degeneration); late-stage lesions characterized by fibrosis with perivascular neutrophilic and mononuclear infiltration
- EGD—foci of collagen degeneration with palisading granulomas; eosinophilic and histiocytic infiltration

Therapeutics

- Most patients can be treated as outpatients unless severe oral disease prevents adequate fluid intake.
- Try to identify and eliminate offending allergen(s) before providing medical intervention.
- Hyposensitization of intradermal skin test–positive cats—may be successful in 60–73% of cases; preferable to long-term corticosteroid administration
- Discourage patient from damaging lesions by excessive grooming.

EGC—Cat

- Injectable methylprednisone—20 mg/cat, repeat in 2 weeks (if needed); most common treatment
- Corticosteroids—ongoing treatment with prednisone (3–5 mg/kg q48h) rarely required to control lesions; steroid tachyphylaxis may occur and may be specific to the drug administered; may be useful to change the formulation; other drugs: dexamethasone (0.1–0.2 mg/kg q24–72h) and triamcinolone (0.1–0.2 mg/kg q24–72h); higher induction dosages may be required but should be tapered as quickly as possible
- Combination of oral corticosteroids and selective immunosuppressive agents—for severe lesions; e.g., chlorambucil (0.1–0.2 mg/kg q24–48h)
- Chrysotherapy with aurothioglucose—1 mg/kg IM every 7 days; mixed results
- Cyclophosphamide—1 mg/kg q24h for 4 out of every 7 days; another alternative
- α-interferon—30–60 U daily in cycles of 7 days on, 7 days off; limited success; side effects rare; no specific treatment monitoring required
- Antibiotics—trimethoprim-sulfadiazine (15 mg/kg PO q12h), cephalexin (22 mg/kg PO q12h), or amoxicillin trihydrate-clavulanate (12.5 mg/kg PO q12h); effective in some cases; preferable to long-term corticosteroid administration; response may be the result of the anti-inflammatory activity of these drugs rather than their primary bactericidal properties
- Radiation, surgical excision, and immunomodulation (e.g., levamisole, bacterin injections)—occasional reports of success
- CO_2 laser—newer treatment modality; may offer relief from individual or painful lesions, especially those in the mouth
- Topical—application of potent corticosteroid ointments may help with isolated lesions but is rarely practical
- Megestrol acetate—2.5–5 mg every 2–7 days; can be effective in rare cases; not recommended because of the severity of possible side effects

EGD—Dog

- Oral prednisone—0.5–2.2 mg/kg/day initially; then taper gradually
- Cessation of therapy without recurrence is common.

Comments

- Corticosteroids—baseline and frequent hemograms, serum chemistry profiles, and urinalyses
- Selective immunosuppressant drugs—frequent hemograms (biweekly at first, then monthly or bimonthly as therapy continues) to monitor for bone marrow suppression; routine serum chemistry profiles and urinalyses (monthly at first, then every 3 months) to monitor for complications (renal disease, diabetes mellitus, and urinary tract infection)
- If a primary cause (allergy) can be determined and controlled, lesions should resolve permanently, unless the animal re-encounters the offending allergen.
- Most lesions wax and wane, with or without therapy; thus, an unpredictable schedule of recurrence should be anticipated.
- Drug dosages should be tapered to the lowest possible level (or discontinued, if possible) once the lesions have resolved.

ABBREVIATIONS

EGD = eosinophilic granulomas in dogs

Suggested Reading

Power HT, Ihrke PJ. Selected feline eosinophilic skin diseases (eosinophilic granuloma complex). In: Kunkle G, ed. Feline dermatoses. Vet Cin North Am, Small Anim Pract. Philadelphia: Saunders, 1995.

Rosenkrantz WS. Feline eosinophilic granuloma complex. In: Griffin CE, Kwochka KW, MacDonald JM, eds. Current veterinary dermatology: the science and art of therapy. St. Louis: Mosby, 1993.

Consulting Editor Karen Helton Rhodes

HYPEREOSINOPHILIC SYNDROME

Karen M. Young

Overview/Definition

- Idiopathic persistent eosinophilia caused by sustained overproduction of eosinophils in the bone marrow

Etiology/Pathophysiology

- Hypothesized to be caused by severe reaction to an undefined antigen or dysregulation of immunologic control of eosinophil production
- Multisystemic syndrome with invasion of tissues by eosinophils and subsequent organ damage and dysfunction, leading to death
- Organ damage caused by effects of eosinophil granule products and eosinophil-derived cytokines that are released in the tissues from activated or necrotic cells
- Probably includes a heterogeneous group of disorders
- Common sites of infiltration—gastrointestinal tract (especially intestine and liver), spleen, and lymph nodes (especially mesenteric nodes)
- Less common sites of infiltration—skin, kidney, heart, thyroid, lung, adrenal glands, and pancreas

Signalment/History

- Cats—may occur more frequently in female, middle-aged, domestic shorthair animals than in others

- Dogs—rare and incompletely described
- Lethargy
- Anorexia
- Intermittent vomiting and diarrhea
- Weight loss
- Less frequently—fever, pruritus, and seizures

Clinical Features

- Fever
- Emaciation
- Hepatosplenomegaly
- Thickened (diffuse or segmental) intestine that is nonpainful
- Mesenteric, and possible peripheral, lymphadenopathy
- Mass lesions caused by eosinophilic granulomatous inflammation involving lymph nodes or organs
- Pruritic erythroderma

Differential Diagnosis

- Identifiable causes of eosinophilia—parasitism, hypersensitivity disorder, infectious disease, immune-mediated disease, and neoplasia; with these conditions, eosinophilia is usually limited in degree and remains confined to a specific organ, such as the lungs in feline asthma
- Eosinophilic leukemia—distinction is controversial; differentiating criteria of this leukemia: (1) immature eosinophils seen in higher numbers in the circulation and constitute a higher percentage of the leukocyte differential; (2) anemia more common; (3) myeloid:erythroid ratio in bone marrow is higher (> 10:1) and blast forms are more numerous; (4) tissue infiltrates consist of immature eosinophils and may show a sinusoidal pattern in the liver without fibrosis; (5) in cats, chloroma-like masses in the kidneys reported

Diagnostics

- Leukocytosis with eosinophilia (usually marked), possibly with a left shift in the eosinophil series; eosinophil count range: 3,200–130,000 cells/μL
- Basophilia
- Anemia in some animals
- In animals with organ dysfunction, biochemical abnormalities may be seen.
- Rule out identifiable causes of eosinophilia—fecal flotation, heartworm test, fungal culture, and biopsy to detect neoplasm
- Intestinal mucosal irregularities and thickened intestine seen on radiographic contrast studies
- Bone marrow—hypercellularity, eosinophilic hyperplasia (up to 40% of nucleated cells consist of eosinophils), lack of morphologic abnormalities, and high myeloid:erythroid ratio (mean 7.27:1)
- Biopsy of affected organ or mass

- Spleen—eosinophilic infiltrate in red pulp, sometimes in white pulp
- Gastrointestinal tract—mucosal and submucosal eosinophilic infiltrates in small intestine, sometimes in colon and stomach
- Lymph nodes—reactive hyperplasia and infiltration of cords and sinuses with eosinophils
- Heart—eosinophilic infiltrates in the myocardium and endocardium; fibrosis and thrombus formation
- Less frequently—eosinophilic infiltrates in the skin, liver, lung, pancreas, kidney, adrenal, and thyroid gland

Therapeutics

- Use long-term maintenance therapy to control or reduce the eosinophilia and organ damage.
- Massive tissue infiltration impedes treatment and usually lends a poor prognosis.
- High serum IgE concentration portends a good response to treatment with prednisone and a better prognosis.
- Corticosteroids—prednisolone, 1–3 mg/kg/day initially; then taper to alternate-day administration if eosinophilia is suppressed; if eosinophilia returns, resume higher daily dose.
- Chemotherapeutic agents—try if eosinophilia is steroid resistant, but the paucity of case reports describing these therapies precludes recommending their use
- Hydroxyurea (inhibits DNA synthesis)—administer to reduce the eosinophil count if not normal or near normal after 7–14 days of treatment with steroids; most likely would be used long-term if effective in conjunction with steroids
- Cyclosporine—suppresses production of eosinophilopoietic factors by T cells
- Vincristine and alkylating agents, such as chlorambucil, effective in humans
- Reduce dosage or discontinue drug if bone marrow suppression or thrombocytopenia develops.

Comments

- Aggressive cytotoxic therapy has been deleterious in some human patients.
- Monitor eosinophil count (not always indicative of tissue infiltrates) and myelosuppression if chemotherapeutic drugs are used.
- Monitor clinical signs (e.g., anorexia, lethargy, vomiting, and diarrhea) and any physical abnormalities.

Suggested Reading

Huibregtse BA, Turner JL. Hypereosinophilic syndrome and eosinophilic leukemia: a comparison of 22 hypereosinophilic cats. J Anim Hosp Assoc 1994;30:591–599.

Consulting Editor Karen Helton Rhodes

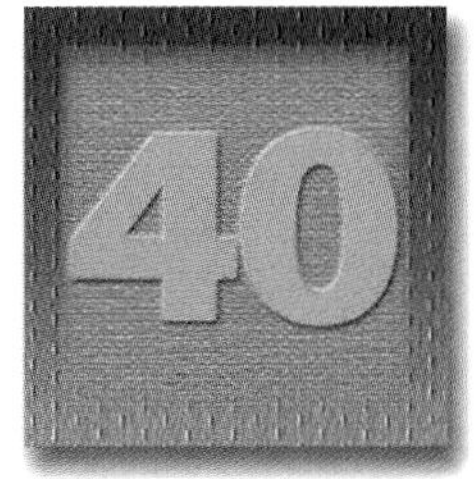

Cutaneous Drug Eruption

Daniel O. Morris

Overview/Definition

- A spectrum of diseases and clinical signs that vary markedly in clinical appearance and pathophysiology
- Likely that many mild drug reactions go unnoticed or unreported; thus, incidence rates for specific drugs are unknown and most of the facts available on drug-specific reactivities have been extrapolated from reports in the human literature

Etiology/Pathophysiology

- Drugs of any type
- Exfoliative erythroderma—most often associated with shampoos and dips
- Can occur after the first dose after weeks to months of administration of the same drug
- Immunologic versus physiologic reaction
- Apoptotic diseases

Signalment/History

- Dogs and cats
- Age, breed, and sex predispositions—unknown
- Some types of drug reactions appear to have a familial basis (e.g., rabies vaccine reactions in dogs have been diagnosed in litter mates).

Clinical Features

- Pruritus—can be activated by a wide variety of compounds; most common symptom of drug eruption in humans
- Macular and papular rashes—commonly accompany pruritus as a nonspecific sign of inflammation
- Exfoliative erythroderma—a diffuse erythematous response caused by vasodilation; often leads to exfoliation (diffuse scaling)
- Urticaria/angioedema—results from an immediate (type I) hypersensitivity; requires prior sensitization; increased vascular permeability leads to fluid leakage into the interstitium
- Hypersensitivity vasculitis—inflammation of cutaneous vasculature; results in poor blood flow and anoxic injury to recipient tissue; in most cases, thought to represent a type III hypersensitivity response
- Erythema multiforme (EM)—macules or plaques expand peripherally and may clear in the center, producing a bull's-eye appearance; multiple shapes/forms can be seen
- Toxic Epidermal Necrolysis (TEN)—extensive necrosis and sloughing of the epidermis in sheets; results in a moist and intensely inflamed skin surface
- Drug-induced pemphigus/pemphigoid—least common drug reaction in animals; can closely mimic the autoimmune (spontaneous) forms of these diseases

Differential Diagnosis

- Pruritus, macular/papular rashes, and urticaria/angioedema—allergic diseases (atopy, food allergy, contact allergy) and reactions to ectoparasites (scabies, flea bite allergy, stinging insects)
- Exfoliative erythroderma—rule out cutaneous T cell lymphoma in old dogs and cats
- Vasculitis—infectious, neoplastic, and autoimmune diseases; many cases of vasculitis are idiopathic
- EM—rule out respiratory infections and internal neoplasms.
- Pemphigus/pemphigoid—consider drug reaction whenever these diseases are diagnosed; however, spontaneously occurring autoimmune disease is much more common

Diagnostics

- When cutaneous vasculitis is suspected or diagnosed—potential for concurrent hepatic, renal, and gastrointestinal disease
- Dogs with vasculitis—rickettsial serology, ANA
- Cats with vasculitis—FIV and FeLV serology
- Bacterial and fungal cultures and sensitivity testing—for vasculitis with pyogranulomatous inflammation
- Skin biopsy for histopathology—mandatory for diagnosis of most drug-induced diseases (vasculitis, EM, TEN, pemphigus/pemphigoid)

Therapeutics

- Discontinue use of the offending drug.
- TEN—intensive supportive care and fluid/nutritional support because of fluid and protein exudation and risk of sepsis
- Corticosteroids—controversial

Comments

- Inpatient—if debilitated
- Outpatient—regular rechecks, depending on physical condition
- Some reactions appear to activate self-perpetuating immune responses.
- Some drug metabolites may persist for days to weeks and provoke a continued response.
- TEN—prognosis poor
- Vasculitis—prognosis guarded when there are systemic complications. Associated with arthropathy, hepatitis, glomerulonephritis, and neuromuscular disorders, among others

Suggested Reading

Scott DW, Miller WH, Griffin GE, eds. In: Muller & Kirk's small animal dermatology. 5th ed. Philadelphia: Saunders, 1995:590–606.

Consulting Editor Karen Helton Rhodes

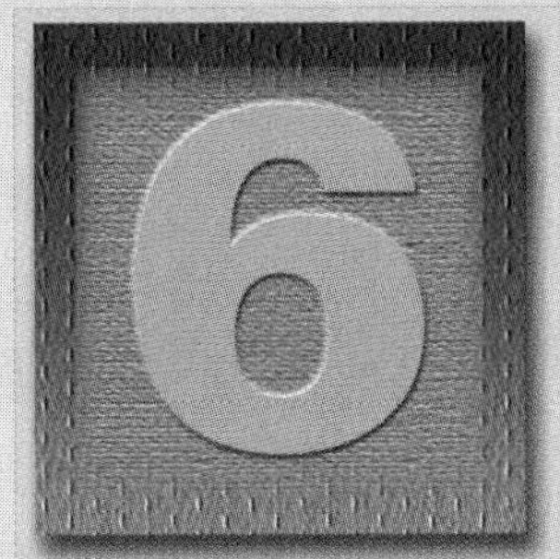

Infectious Dermatoses

Sepsis and Bacteremia

Sharon K. Fooshee

Definition/Overview

- Bacteremia—defined as the presence of bacterial organisms in the bloodstream
- Sepsis—systemic response to bacterial infection (e.g., fever, hypotension)
- Terms are not synonymous, although often used interchangeably

Etiology/Pathophysiology

- Shedding of bacterial organisms into the bloodstream—may occur transiently, intermittently, or continually
- The most critical host response for elimination of bacteremia—provided by mononuclear phagocyte system of the spleen and liver; activation leads to release of numerous cellular mediators (cytokines), some of which are beneficial and others detrimental; may lead to death of the host
- Neutrophils—relatively more important for defense against extravascular infection
- Bacteremia—transient, subclinical event or may escalate to overt sepsis when the immune system is overwhelmed; generally of more pathologic significance when the bloodstream is invaded from venous or lymphatic drainage sites
- With peracute development of septicemia—increased or decreased cardiac output, decreased systemic vascular resistance, and increased vascular permeability; ultimately, refractory hypotension develops, leading to multiorgan failure and death

- Endocarditis—may develop; presence of bacteremia alone is not sufficient for induction; multiple factors involving both the host and the bacterial organism must be favorable for bacterial adherence to heart valves
- Coagulation disorders and thromboembolism
- Kidney and myocardium especially prone to septic embolization
- With chronic bacteremia—antigenic stimulation of the immune system may lead to immune-complex deposition
- Dogs—gram-negative organisms (especially *Escherichia coli*) most common; gram-positive cocci and obligate anaerobes also important; polymicrobial infection reported in about 20% of dogs with positive blood cultures
- Cats—bloodstream pathogens usually gram-negative bacteria from the Enterobacteriaceae family or obligate anaerobes; *Salmonella* most common gram-negative organism cultured
- *Pseudomonas aeruginosa*—uncommon isolate from animal blood cultures

Signalment/History

- Dogs and cats
- No age, sex, or breed predispositions reported
- Large-breed male dogs—predisposed to bacterial endocarditis and discospondylitis
- Development may be acute or may occur in a vague or episodic fashion.
- Variable and may involve multiple organ systems
- May be confused with those of immune-mediated disease
- Clinical—more severe when gram-negative organisms are involved
- Dogs that develop overt sepsis—the earliest signs are usually referable to the gastrointestinal tract
- Cats—respiratory system more commonly involved

Clinical Features

- Intermittent or persistent fever
- Lameness
- Depression
- Tachycardia
- Heart murmur
- Weakness
- Consider other causes of fever, heart murmur, joint or back pain, or hypotension.
- Clinical signs of more chronic bacteremia may be confused with immune-mediated disease.

Diagnostics

- Identify risk factors
- Peracute—pyometra and disruption of the gastrointestinal tract most often associated
- More protracted onset—infections of the skin, upper urinary tract, oral cavity, and prostate

- Hyperadrenocorticism, diabetes mellitus, liver or renal failure, splenectomy, malignancy, and burns—predisposing factors
- Immunodeficient state—chemotherapy, FIV, splenectomy; particular risk
- Glucocorticoids—considered an important risk factor for bacteremia; allows greater multiplication of bacteria in extravascular tissues
- Intravenous catheter—provides rapid venous access for bacteria
- Indwelling urinary catheters—may be a predisposing factor
- Neutrophilic leukocytosis with a left shift and an associated monocytosis—most common hematologic abnormalities
- Neutropenia—may develop
- Hypoalbuminemia and a high ALP (up to two times upper limit of normal)—up to 50% of affected dogs
- Hypoglycemia—about 25% of affected dogs
- With suspected catheter-induced sepsis—submit catheter tip for culture
- Urine culture—may be useful; positive culture does not determine if urinary tract is primary or secondary source of infection
- May identify source of bacteremia (e.g., pyometra) or secondarily infected organs (e.g., discospondylitis)

BLOOD CULTURE

- Indications—any patient that develops fever (or hypothermia), leukocytosis (especially with a left shift), neutropenia, shifting leg lameness, recent-onset or changing heart murmur, or any sign of sepsis that cannot be explained
- Essential for confirming suspected bacteremia and for optimizing management of the patient; one study of critically ill animals reported approximately 75% of cats and 50% of dogs had positive blood cultures.
- Clinical findings—not reliable for discriminating between particular types of bacteria

Guidelines

- Current antimicrobial therapy—does not preclude collection of blood cultures; advise laboratory that patient is receiving antibiotics; steps can be taken to inactivate certain medications
- Anaerobic cultures—special bottles may not be necessary
- Sets (pairs) of samples—inform laboratory that for each submitted pair of bottles, one is for aerobic culture and the other for anaerobic
- Collect at least two (and preferably three) sets of samples—improves chance of obtaining a positive culture and facilitates interpretation of results
- Volume—the greater the volume of collected blood, the better the chances of obtaining positive cultures; often, only a few organisms present per milliliter of blood; 10 mL of blood per culture recommended; may not be possible for cats and small dogs; have an assortment of culture bottles available (including 25, 50, and 100 mL); small bottles useful for small patients for maintaining appropriate blood-to-culture broth ratio
- Timing—for most patients, sufficient to take three cultures over a 24-hr period; for critically ill patients, take three cultures over a 2-hr period

Collection

- Bottles—warm to room temperature; apply alcohol or iodine to the rubber stopper

- Patient—clip hair; thoroughly disinfect skin before venipuncture, to avoid contamination; wipe with 70% alcohol, then apply an iodine-based disinfectant; allow a minimum of 1 min of contact time with the skin
- Withdrawing blood—wearing a sterile glove, palpate the vein; draw blood into a sterile syringe; evacuate all air from the syringe; attach a new needle before inoculating blood into the bottles
- Samples—maintain culture bottles at room temperature for transport to the laboratory

Media

- Commercial multipurpose nutrient broth media—recommended
- A medium that supports growth of both aerobes and anaerobes—ideal
- Often, the laboratory that processes the culture will supply culture bottles.

Interpretation of Results

- Single positive culture—not possible to distinguish true bacteremia from sample contamination
- Two or more positive cultures identified as the same organism desired
- Coagulase-negative staphylococci, α-hemolytic streptococci, and *Acinetobacter*—probably contamination
- *Enterobacteriaceae, Bacteroidaceae, Pseudomonas aeruginosa, Staphylococcus aureus, Staphylococcus intermedius,* β-hemolytic streptococci, and yeasts—nearly always clinically significant bacteremia
- Negative results from two or three successive cultures—generally eliminates bacteremia owing to common pathogens; some less common bacteria may take several weeks to grow

Therapeutics

- Success—requires early identification of the problem and aggressive intervention; careful monitoring essential, because the status of patient may change rapidly
- Hypotension—intravenous fluids; isotonic fluids (e.g., lactated Ringer) at a rate up to 90 mL/kg/hr in dogs and 55 mL/kg/hr in cats; use caution when hypoalbuminemia or increased vascular permeability is a concern
- Volume expanders (e.g., hydroxyethyl starch)—may help maintain oncotic pressure
- With hypoglycemia—may add dextrose to intravenous fluids
- Electrolytes and acid-base balance—correct abnormalities
- Abscesses—locate and drain
- External sources of infection—give appropriate attention to wound care and bandage changes
- Internal sources of infection (e.g., pyometra or disruption of the bowel)—surgical intervention essential
- Nutritional support—provide by assisted feeding or placement of a feeding tube
- Antibiotics—usually selected before culture and sensitivity results are available; empiric therapy acceptable while waiting for results; do not delay treatment

- Antimicrobials—give intravenously; direct therapy to cover all possible bacterial organisms (gram-positive and -negative; aerobic and anaerobic)
- If patient not in shock—a good choice is a first-generation cephalosporin; dogs and cats: administer cefazolin at 40 mg/kg IV as a loading dose; then 20–30 mg/kg IV q6–8h (dogs and cats)
- Aminoglycosides—add to protocol if more aggressive therapy is warranted; administer gentamicin at 2–4 mg/kg IV q8h (dogs and cats)

Comments

- Glucocorticoids and NSAIDs (controversial)—value in treating septic shock; do not improve survival unless given within the first few hours of the onset; may complicate the clinical picture in potentially ischemic organs (e.g., gastrointestinal tract and kidneys)
- Aminoglycosides—use with caution with renal impairment
- Aminoglycoside therapy—monitor renal function
- Blood pressure and ECG—monitor, if indicated
- Gram-negative septicemia—high rate of mortality; death owing to hypotension, electrolyte and acid-base disturbances, and endotoxemic shock
- Suspected discospondylitis (dogs)—may need to screen for *Brucella canis*

See Also

- Abscessation
- Anaerobic Infection
- Endocarditis, Bacterial
- Shock, Septic

Abbreviations

- ALP = alkaline phosphatase
- FIV = feline immunodeficiency virus

Suggested Reading

Dow SW, Jones RL. Bacteremia: pathogenesis and diagnosis. Compend Contin Educ Pract Vet 1989;11:432–444.

Purvis D, Kirby R. Systemic inflammatory response syndrome: septic shock. Vet Clin North Am Small Anim Pract 1994;24:1225–1247.

Consulting Editor Karen Helton Rhodes

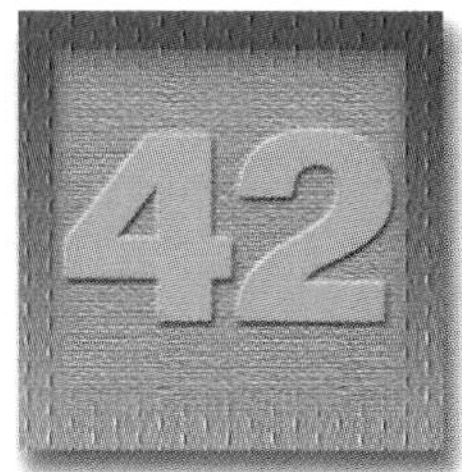

Abscessation

Johnny D. Hoskins

Definition/Overview

An abscess is a localized collection of purulent exudate contained within a cavity.

Etiology/Pathophysiology

- Bacteria are often inoculated under the skin via a puncture wound; the wound surface then seals.
- When bacteria and/or foreign objects persist in the tissue, purulent exudate forms and collects.
- Accumulation of purulent exudate—if not quickly resorbed or discharged to an external surface, stimulates formation of a fibrous capsule; may eventually lead to abscess rupture
- Prolonged delay of evacuation—formation of a fibrous abscess wall; to heal, the cavity must be filled with granulation tissue from which the causative agent may not be totally eliminated; may lead to chronic or intermittent discharge of exudate from a draining sinus tract

Causes

- Foreign objects
- Pyogenic bacteria—*Staphylococcus* spp.; *Escherichia coli;* β-hemolytic *Streptococcus* spp.; *Pseudomonas; Mycoplasma* and *Mycoplasma*-like organisms (L-forms); *Pasteurella multocida; Corynebacterium; Actinomyces* spp.; *Nocardia*

- Obligate anaerobes—*Bacteroides* spp.; *Clostridium* spp.; *Peptostreptococcus; Fusobacterium*

General Comments

- Determined by organ system and/or tissue affected
- Associated with a combination of inflammation (pain, swelling, redness, heat, and loss of function), tissue destruction, and/or organ system dysfunction caused by accumulation of exudate

Signalment/History

- History of traumatic insult or previous infection
- A rapidly appearing painful swelling with or without discharge, if affected area is visible

Clinical Features

- Determined by the organ system or tissue affected
- A discrete mass may be detectable.
- Inflammation and discharge from a fistulous tract may be visible if the abscess is superficial and has ruptured to an external surface.
- A variably sized, painful mass of fluctuant to firm consistency attached to surrounding tissues may be palpable.
- Fever if abscess is not ruptured and draining
- Sepsis occasionally, especially if abscess ruptures internally

Differential Diagnosis

Mass Lesions

- Cyst—less or only transiently painful; slower growing
- Fibrous scar tissue—firm; nonpainful
- Granuloma—less painful; slower growing; generally firmer without fluctuant center
- Hematoma/seroma—variable pain (depends on cause); nonencapsulated; rapid initial growth but slow increase once full size is attained; unattached to surrounding tissues; fluctuant and fluid-filled initially but more firm with organization
- Neoplasia—variable growth; consistent; painful

Draining Tracts

- Mycobacterial disease
- Mycetoma—botryomycosis, actinomycotic mycetoma, eumycotic mycetoma
- Neoplasia
- Phaeohyphomycosis
- Sporotrichosis
- Systemic fungal infection—blastomycosis, coccidioidomycosis, cryptococcosis, histoplasmosis, trichosporosis

Diagnostics

- CBC—normal or neutrophilia with or without regenerative left shift. Neutropenia and degenerative left shift if sepsis present
- Urinalysis and serum chemistry profile—depend on system affected
- Prostatic—pyuria
- Liver and/or pancreatic—high liver enzymes and/or total bilirubin
- Pancreatic (dogs)—high amylase/lipase
- Diabetes mellitus—persistent hyperglycemia and glucosuria
- FeLV and FIV—for cats with recurrent or slow-healing abscesses
- CSF evaluation—increase in cellularity and protein expected with brain abscess
- Adrenal function—evaluate for hyperadrenocorticism
- Radiography—soft tissue density mass in affected area; may reveal foreign body
- Ultrasonography—determine if mass is fluid filled or solid; determine organ system affected; reveal flocculent-appearing fluid characteristic of pus; may reveal foreign object
- Echocardiography—helpful for diagnosis of pericardial abscess
- CT or MRI—helpful for diagnosis of brain abscess

Aspiration

- Reveals a red, white, yellow, or green liquid
- Protein content—> 2.5–3.0 g/dL
- Nucleated cell count—3,000–100,000 (or more) cells/µL; primarily degenerative neutrophils with lesser numbers of macrophages and lymphocytes
- Pyogenic bacteria—may be seen in cells and free within the fluid
- If the causative agent is not readily identified with a Romanovsky-type stain, specimens should be stained with an acid-fast stain to detect mycobacteria or *Nocardia* and PAS stain to detect fungus.

Biopsy

- Sample should contain both normal and abnormal tissue in the same specimen.
- Impression smears—stained and examined
- Tissue—submit for histopathologic examination and culture
- Contact the diagnostic laboratory for specific instructions.

Culture

- Affected tissue and/or exudate—aerobic and anaerobic bacteria and fungus
- Blood and/or urine—isolate bacterium responsible for possible sepsis
- Bacterial sensitivity

Pathologic Findings

- Pus-containing mass lesion accompanied by inflammation
- Palpable—variably firm or fluctuant mass
- Ruptured—may see pus draining directly from the mass or an adjoining tract

- Exudate—large numbers of neutrophils in various stages of degeneration; other inflammatory cells; necrotic tissue
- Surrounding tissue—congested; fibrin; large number of neutrophils; variable number of lymphocytes; plasma cells; macrophages
- Causative agent variably detectable

Therapeutics

- Establish and maintain adequate drainage
- Surgical removal of nidus of infection or foreign object(s) if necessary
- Institution of appropriate antimicrobial therapy
- Apply hot packs to inflamed area as needed.
- Use protective bandaging and/or Elizabethan collars as needed.
- Accumulated exudate—drain abscess; maintain drainage by medical and/or surgical means.
- Sepsis or peritonitis—aggressive fluid therapy and support
- Appropriate débridement and drainage—may need to leave the wound open to an external surface; may need to place surgical drains
- Antimicrobial drugs—effective against the infectious agent; gain access to site of infection
- Broad-spectrum agent—bactericidal and with both aerobic and anaerobic activity; until results of culture and sensitivity are known; dogs and cats: amoxicillin (11–22 mg/kg PO q8–12h); amoxicillin/clavulanic acid (12.5–25 mg/kg PO q12h); clindamycin (5 mg/kg PO q12h); and trimethoprim/sulfadiazine (15 mg/kg PO IM q12h); cats with *Mycoplasma* and L-forms: doxycycline (3–5 mg/kg PO q12h)
- Aggressive antimicrobial therapy—sepsis or peritonitis

Comments

- Monitor for progressive decrease in drainage, resolution of inflammation, and improvement of clinical signs
- Percutaneous abscesses—prevent fighting
- Anal sac abscesses—prevent impaction; consider anal saculectomy for recurrent cases
- Prostatic abscesses—castration possibly helpful
- Mastitis—prevent lactation (spaying)
- Periorbital abscesses—do not allow chewing on foreign object(s)
- Sepsis is complication
- Peritonitis/pleuritis if intra-abdominal or intrathoracic abscess ruptures
- Compromise of organ function
- Delayed evacuation may lead to chronically draining fistulous tracts.
- Minimal for pyogenic bacteria—zoonotic potential
- Mycobacteria and systemic fungal infections carry some potential for zoonosis.

Abbreviations

- CSF = cerebrospinal fluid
- FeLV = feline leukemia virus

- FIV = feline immunodeficiency virus
- PAS = periodic acid-Schiff

Suggested Reading

Birchard SJ, Sherding RG, eds. Saunders manual of small animal practice. Philadelphia: Saunders, 1994.

DeBoer DJ. Nonhealing cutaneous wounds. In: August JR, ed. Consultations in feline internal medicine. Philadelphia: Saunders, 1991:101–106.

McCaw D. Lumps, bumps, masses, and lymphadenopathy. In: Ettinger SJ, Feldman EC, eds. Textbook of veterinary internal medicine. 4th ed. Philadelphia: Saunders, 1995:219–222.

Consulting Editor Karen Helton Rhodes

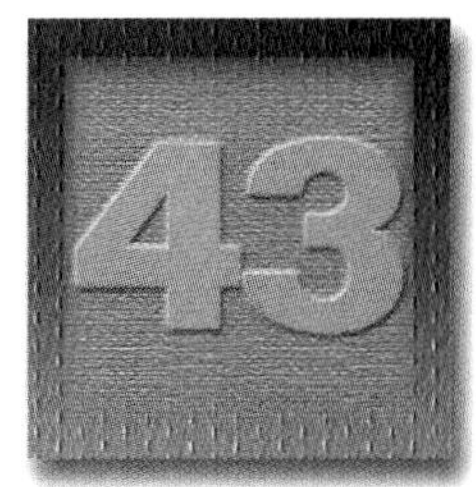

Bacterial Pyoderma: Folliculitis and Furunculosis

Ellen C. Codner and Karen Helton Rhodes

Definition/Overview

Bacterial infection of the skin

Etiology/Pathophysiology

Skin infections occur when the surface integrity of the skin has been broken, the skin has become macerated by chronic exposure to moisture, normal bacterial flora have been altered, circulation has been impaired, or immunocompetency has been compromised.

Causes

- *Staphylococcus intermedius*—most frequent
- *Pasteurella multocida*—an important pathogen in cats
- Deep—may be complicated by gram-negative organisms (e.g., *E. coli, Proteus* spp., *Pseudomonas* spp.)
- Rarely caused by higher bacteria (e.g., *Actinomyces, Nocardia,* mycobacteria, *Actinobacillus*)

Signalment/History

- Dogs—very common
- Cats—uncommon

- Breeds with short coats, skin folds, or pressure calluses
- German shepherds develop a severe, deep pyoderma that may only partially respond to antibiotics and frequently relapses.
- Acute or gradual onset
- Variable pruritus—underlying cause may be pruritic or the staphylococcal infection itself may be pruritic

Clinical Features

- Superficial—usually involves the trunk; extent of lesions may be obscured by the hair coat
- Deep—often affects the chin, bridge of the nose, pressure points, and feet; may be generalized (Figs. 43-1, 43-2)

Lesions

- Papules
- Pustules
- Hemorrhagic bullae
- Crusts
- Epidermal collarettes (Fig. 43-3)
- Circular erythematous or hyperpigmented spots (Fig. 43-4)
- Target lesions
- Alopecia, moth-eaten hair coat
- Scaling
- Lichenification
- Abscesses
- Furunculosis, cellulitis
- Allergy—pruritus usually precedes the rash; pruritus will not resolve with resolution of the pyoderma
- Endocrine problem causing a relapsing pyoderma—consider if pruritus resolves with resolution of the pyoderma; reports of polydipsia, polyuria, pendulous abdomen, lethargy, weight gain, and/or signs of feminization

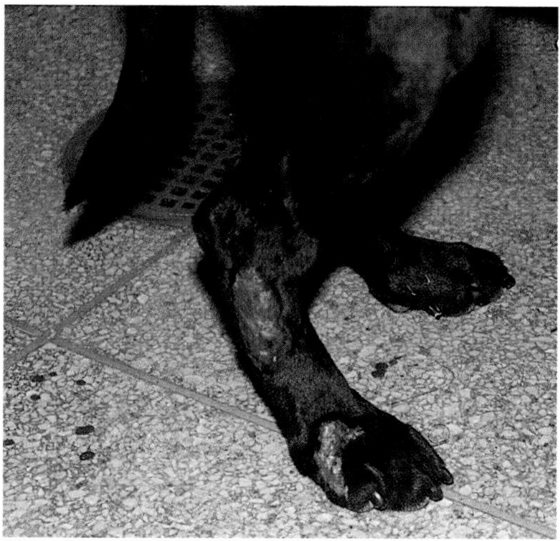

Figure 43-1 Deep pyoderma with lesions predominant on the extremities. Furunculosis and cellulitis.

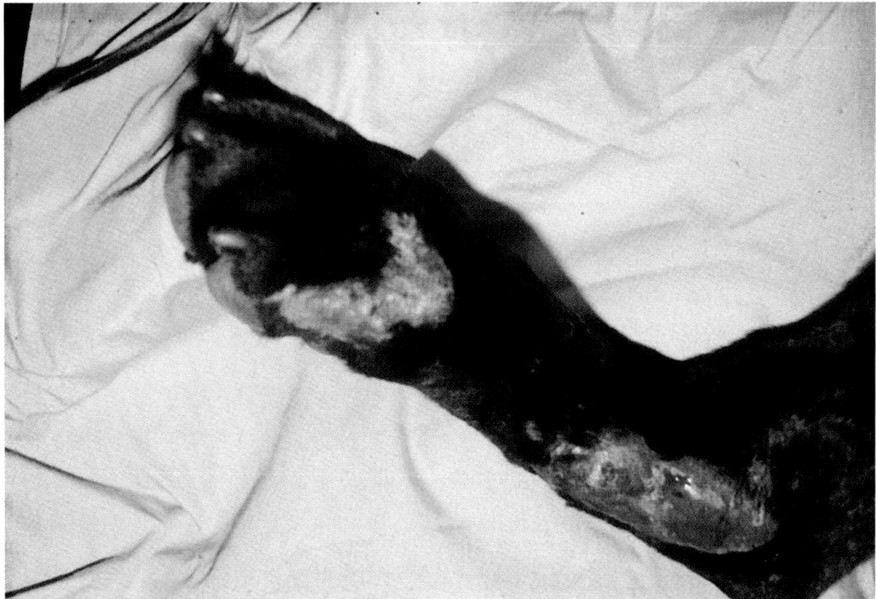

Figure 43-2 Close-up view of deep pyoderma in Figure 43-1.

Figure 43-3 Superficial pyoderma. Note crust with peripheral epidermal collarettes.

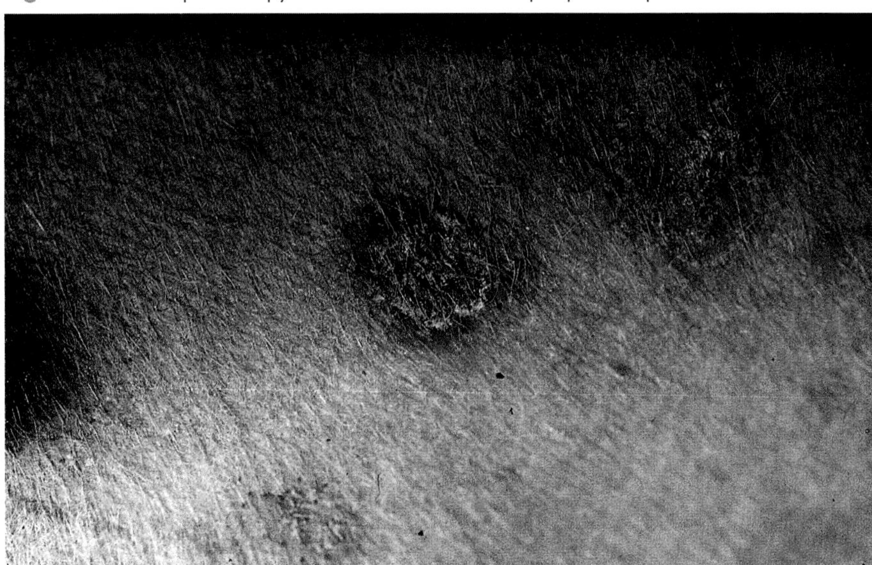

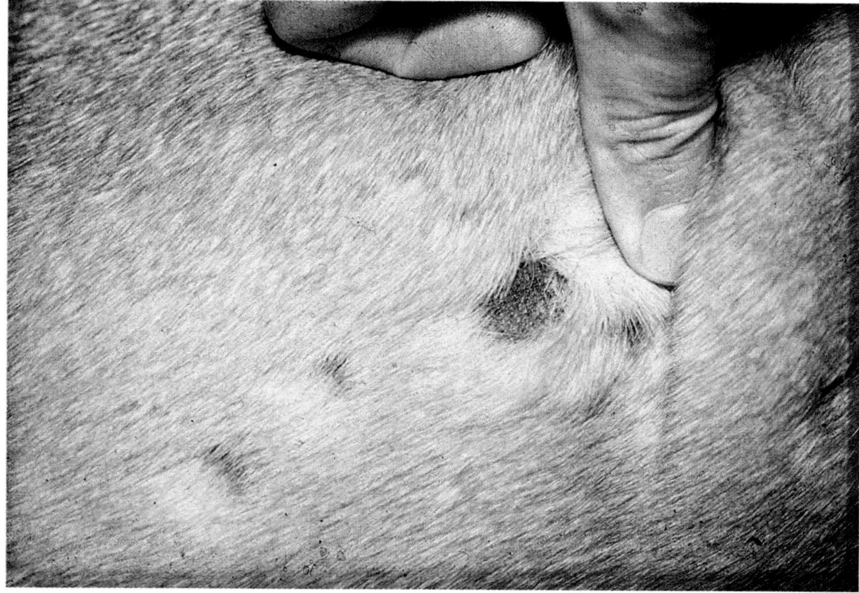

Figure 43-4 Hyperpigmented macule caused by post-inflammatory hyperpigmentation as a resolving stage of superficial pyoderma.

- Flea allergy or atopy—may be seasonal
- Pustular disease—superficial staphylococcal pyoderma; dermatophytosis; demodicosis; pemphigus foliaceus; and subcorneal pustular dermatosis
- Furunculosis—deep staphylococcal pyoderma; higher bacterial infection; demodicosis; dermatophytosis; opportunistic fungal infections; deep fungal infections; panniculitis; and zinc-responsive dermatosis
- Superficial pyoderma in short-coated breeds is often misdiagnosed as urticaria, because of the acute onset of pruritic papules misdiagnosed as hives.

Diagnostics

- Identify risk factors
- Allergy—flea; atopy; food; contact
- Fungal infection—dermatophyte
- Endocrine disease—hypothyroidism; hyperadrenocorticism; sex hormone imbalance
- Immune incompetency—glucocorticoids; young animals
- Seborrhea—acne; schnauzer comedo syndrome
- Conformation—short coat; skin folds
- Trauma—pressure points; grooming; scratching; rooting behavior; irritants
- Foreign body—foxtail; grass awn
- Superficial—normal or may reflect the underlying cause (e.g., anemia owing to hypothyroidism; stress leukogram and high serum alkaline phosphatase owing to Cushing disease; eosinophilia owing to parasitism)
- Generalized, deep—may show leukocytosis with a left shift and hyperglobulinemia; also changes related to the underlying cause

- Skin scrapings, dermatophyte culture, intradermal allergy testing, hypoallergenic food trial, endocrine tests—identify the underlying cause
- Skin biopsy
- Direct smear from intact pustule—neutrophils engulfing bacteria
- Cytology—differentiate pemphigus foliaceus (acantholytic keratinocytes) and deep fungal infections (blastomycosis, cryptococcosis) from pyodermas; tissue grains may identify filamentous organisms characteristic of higher bacteria

Culture

- Usually positive for *S. intermedius*
- Other gram-negative organisms besides staphylococci and higher bacteria may be cultured from deep pyodermas.
- Contents of an intact pustule—most reliable results
- Punch biopsy obtained by sterile technique—if no pustules are noted; more likely to get false-negative results
- Freshly expressed exudate from a draining tract or beneath a crust—may yield the pathogen or a contaminant; least reliable method

Pathologic Findings

- Subcorneal pustules
- Intraepidermal neutrophilic microabscesses
- Perifolliculitis
- Folliculitis
- Furunculosis
- Nodular to diffuse dermatitis
- Panniculitis
- Inflammatory reaction—suppurative or pyogranulomatous
- Tissue grains within pyogranulomas—observed most often with *Staphylococcus, Actinomyces, Actinobacillus,* and *Nocardia*
- Special stains—identify gram-negative bacteria or acid-fast organisms

Therapeutics

- Severe, generalized, deep—may require IV fluids, parenteral antibiotics, or daily whirlpool baths
- Benzoyl peroxide or chlorhexidine shampoos—remove surface debris
- Whirlpool baths—deep pyodermas; remove crusted exudate; encourage drainage
- Hypoallergenic if secondary to food allergy; otherwise a high-quality, well-balanced dog food
- Avoid high-protein, poor-quality "bargain" diets and excessive supplementation.
- Fold pyodermas require surgical correction to prevent recurrence.
- *S. intermedius* isolates—usually susceptible to cephalosporins, cloxacillin, oxacillin, methicillin, amoxicillin-clavulanate, erythromycin, and chloram-

phenicol; somewhat less responsive to lincomycin and trimethoprim-sulfonamide; frequently resistant to amoxicillin, ampicillin, penicillin, tetracycline, and sulfonamides

- Amoxicillin-clavulanate—most isolates of *Staphylococcus* and *P. multocida* susceptible; generally effective for skin infections in cats
- Superficial—initially may be treated empirically with one of the antibiotics listed above
- Recurrent, resistant, or deep—base antibiotic therapy on culture and sensitivity testing
- Multiple organisms with different antibiotic sensitivities—choose antibiotic on basis of staphylococcal susceptibility
- Steroids—will encourage resistance and recurrence even when used concurrently with antibiotics
- Erythromycin, lincomycin, and oxacillin—vomiting; administer with small amount of food
- Gentamicin and kanamycin—renal toxicity usually precludes their prolonged systemic use
- Trimethoprim-sulfa—associated with keratoconjunctivitis sicca, fever, hepatotoxicity, polyarthritis, and hematologic abnormalities; may lead to low thyroid test results
- Chloramphenicol—use with caution in cats; may cause mild, reversible anemia in dogs
- Staphage lysate, staphoid AB, or autogenous bacterins—may improve antibiotic efficacy and decrease recurrence in a small percentage of cases

Comments

- Administer antibiotics for a minimum of 2 weeks beyond clinical cure; this is usually about 1 month for superficial pyodermas, and 2–3+ months for deep pyodermas.
- Routine bathing with benzoyl peroxide or chlorhexidine shampoos—may help prevent recurrences
- Some cases that continue to relapse may be managed with subminimal inhibitory concentrations of antibiotics (long-term/low-dose).
- Padded bedding—may ease pressure-point pyodermas
- Topical benzoyl peroxide gel or mupirocin ointment may be helpful adjunct therapies
- Likely to be recurrent or nonresponsive if underlying cause is not identified and effectively managed
- Impetigo—affects young dogs before puberty; associated with poor husbandry; often requires only topical therapy
- Superficial pustular dermatitis—occurs in kittens; associated with overzealous "mouthing" by the queen
- Pyoderma secondary to atopy—usually begins at 1–3 years of age
- Pyoderma secondary to endocrine disorders—usually begins in middle adulthood

Suggested Reading

Muller GH, Kirk RW, Scott DW. Small animal dermatology. 4th ed. Philadelphia: Saunders, 1989.

Authors Ellen C. Codner and Karen Helton Rhodes
Consulting Editor Karen Helton Rhodes

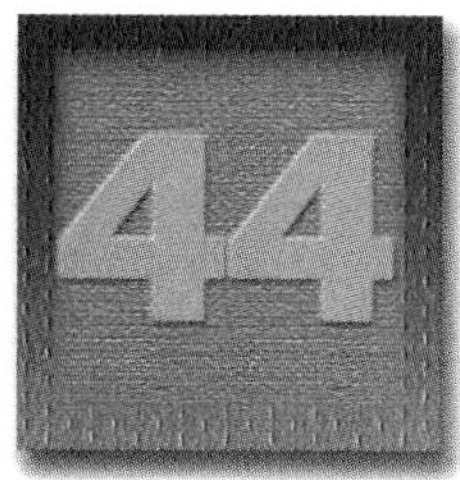

Anaerobic Bacterial Infections

Sharon K. Fooshee

Overview/Definition

Caused by bacteria requiring low oxygen tension

Etiology/Pathophysiology

- Most commonly found genera—*Bacteroides, Fusobacterium, Actinomyces, Clostridium,* and *Peptostreptococcus*
- Individual organisms vary in their potential to withstand oxygen exposure.
- A number of injurious toxins and enzymes may be elaborated by the organisms, leading to extension of the infection into adjacent, healthy tissue.

Signalment/History

- Usually caused by normal flora of the body; a break in protective barriers allows bacterial invasion
- Predisposing factors—bite wounds, dental disease, open fractures, abdominal surgery, and foreign bodies

Clinical Features

- Determined by the body system involved
- Certain areas of the body are more commonly associated with anaerobic infection, perhaps because of proximity to mucosal surfaces.

- It is possible to overlook the potential for anaerobes to be involved in an infectious process, leading to confusion in interpreting culture results and in selecting inappropriate antimicrobials.
- A foul odor associated with a wound or exudative discharge
- Gas in the tissue or associated exudate
- Peritonitis, pyothorax, or pyometra
- Severe dental disease
- Wounds or deep abscesses that do not heal as anticipated

Differential Diagnosis

- Wounds that fail to respond to appropriate medical therapy—aerobic cultures may be negative; suspect anaerobic organisms
- Cats with nonhealing wounds—test for FeLV and FIV
- Middle-aged and old animals—tumor invasion (e.g., in the gastrointestinal tract) may be responsible for establishing infection

Diagnostics

- Neutrophilic leukocytosis and monocytosis common
- Biochemical abnormalities depend on specific organ involvement.
- Appropriate samples—pus (1–2 mL in stoppered syringe) and tissue (minimum 1-g sample)
- Proper handling of samples—minimize exposure to air when collecting and transporting; appropriate transport devices should be on hand before the sample is collected and include screw-top glass vials with media that accept a Culturette swab and syringes evacuated of all air and capped with a rubber stopper.

Therapeutics

- Thoracic drainage—important with pyothorax (see specific chapter)
- Hyperbaric oxygen—some potential use; may be limited in availability

Surgery

- Should not be delayed when anaerobes are suspected
- Generally indicated for all except pyothorax and CNS infections
- Combined with systemic antimicrobial therapy—the best chance of a positive outcome
- Usually indicated when anaerobic organisms complicate pyometra, osteomyelitis, and peritonitis
- Cleanse the wound of toxins and devitalized tissue
- Enhance drainage of pus
- Improve local blood flow
- Increase oxygen tension

Drugs

- Antimicrobial therapy alone—unlikely to be successful; poor drug penetration into exudates

- Antibiotic selection—largely empiric, owing to the difficulty of isolating anaerobes and the delay in return of culture results; cytology and Gram staining of exudates may aid in selecting the initial antibiotic.
- Although most anaerobic infections are polymicrobial, antibiotic therapy targeted against the anaerobes is more likely to be successful than selecting multiple antibiotics because of the symbiotic nature of the infection.
- Penicillin G—considered the antibiotic of choice (except for *Bacteroides* strains)
- Amoxicillin—comparable to penicillin G in spectrum of activity; convenient and accessible; may be useful to combine with clavulanic acid for *Bacteroides*
- Cefoxitin—the only cephalosporin with reliable activity against anaerobes; expensive
- Clindamycin—may be especially useful for respiratory tract infections
- Chloramphenicol—good tissue penetration; but bacteriostatic
- Metronidazole—useful against all clinically significant anaerobes (except *Actinomyces*)
- Aminoglycosides—uniformly ineffective against anaerobes
- Trimethoprim-sulfa combinations—ineffective; poor penetration into purulent exudates

Abbreviations

- FeLV = feline leukemia virus
- FIV = feline immunodeficiency virus

Suggested Reading

Hirsh DC, Jang SS. Anaerobic infections. In: Greene CE, ed. Infectious diseases of the dog and cat. Philadelphia: Saunders, 1998:258–263.

Consulting Editor Karen Helton Rhodes

Mycobacterial Infections

Carol Foil

Overview/Definition

- Mycobacteria—gram-positive, acid-fast, higher bacteria (genus *Mycobacterium*); obligate or sporadic pathogens in humans and animals

Etiology/Pathophysiology

- Tuberculosis—caused by *M. tuberculosis* (humans), *M. bovis* (cattle and some wild mammals), and *M. microti* (voles); dogs and cats exposed to infected primary hosts sporadically infected; disseminated or multi-organ disease caused by obligately parasitic organism; rare in dogs and cats in developed countries
- Leprosy—*M. leprae* (human) and *M. lepraemurium* (murine); cats: well-localized skin infection associated with intracellular acid-fast organism that cannot be cultured by any standard microbiologic methods; causal organism debated
- Subcutaneous or systemic infections (dogs and cats)—*M. abscessus, M. avium, M. chelonae, M. fortuitum, M. phlei, M. smegmatis, M. thermoresistable,* and *M. xenopi;* sporadic infections; usually as the result of traumatic tissue introduction of the organism
- Atypical mycobacteriosis—systemic or localized infection with *Mycobacterium* species not otherwise classified as causing tuberculosis or leprosy; most organisms free-living saprophytes
- Disseminated infection with *M. avium* (dogs and cats)—often classified as tuberculosis, but epidemiologically and therapeutically better classified as an atypical mycobacteriosis

Signalment/History

Tuberculosis

- Cats and dogs of any age
- Bassett hounds and Siamese cats reported as most susceptible; evidence unclear (possible statistical aberration)
- Source of exposure—always an infected typical host
- Dogs—usually exposed from an infected person in the household (*M. tuberculosis*); route is ingestion of expectorated infectious material; aerosol exposure possible; patients most often found in urban areas with Third World immigrants
- Cats—classically exposed by drinking unpasteurized milk of infected cattle (*M. bovis*); much less common now than in the past; may be exposed by predation on infected small mammals (*M. bovis*, or undefined tuberculosis species)

Feline Leprosy

- Adult free-roaming cats and kittens
- Cases sporadically reported in northeastern USA
- Patients often located near seaports and other coastal locales
- History of bite wound—possible
- Exposure—thought to be by predation on infected rodents

Atypical Mycobacteriosis

- Adult cats—subcutaneous
- Adult dogs—occasional report of respiratory or systemic disease; rarely cutaneous

Figure 45-1 Atypical mycobacteriosis. Note the "melting" lesion, which extends throughout the subcutaneous tissue.

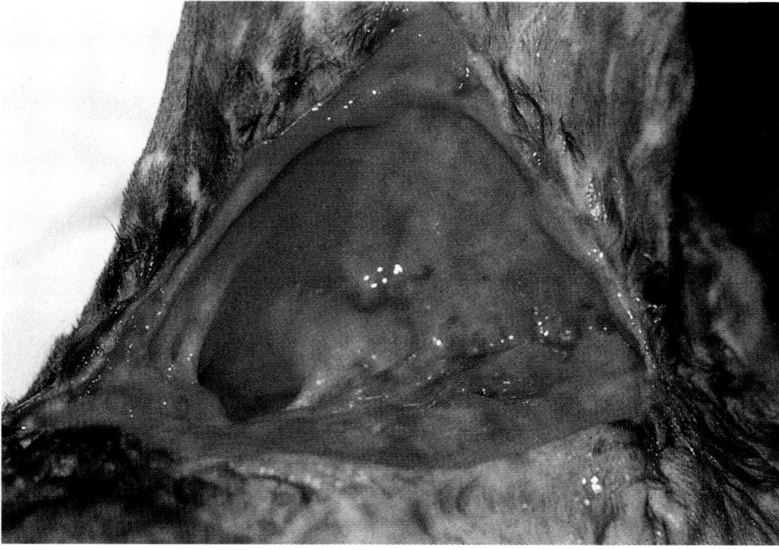

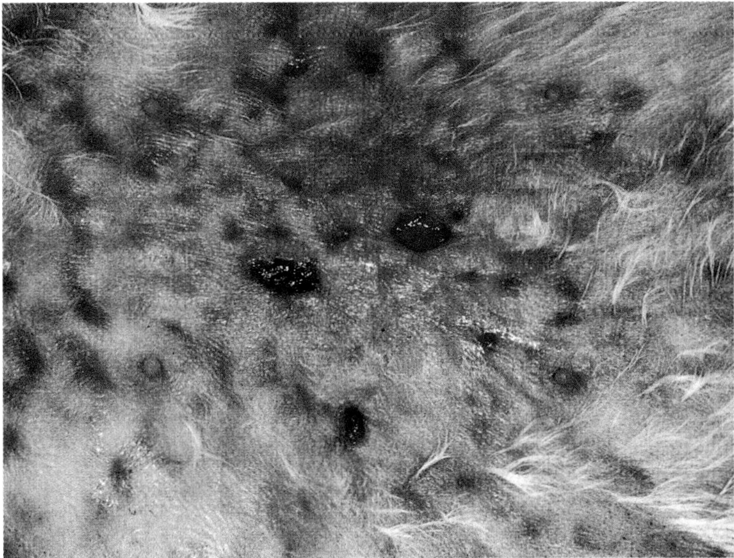

Figure 45-2 Atypical mycobacteriosis. Multifocal ulcerations with satellite lesions.

- Natural habitat of saprophytic species of *Mycobacterium* is a moist environment.
- Trauma and accidental inoculation of the subcutaneous fat may result in infection; history of bite wound possible (subcutaneous disease)
- Fat animals may be more at risk than lean ones.
- Exposure—routes for pulmonary and systemic diseases unknown

Clinical Features

Tuberculosis

- Correlated with route of exposure
- Major sites of involvement—oropharyngeal lymph nodes; cutaneous and subcutaneous tissues of the head and extremities; pulmonary system; gastrointestinal system
- Dogs—respiratory, especially coughing; dyspnea uncommon
- Cats—from contaminated milk: weight loss, chronic diarrhea, and thickened intestines; from predation: cutaneous nodules, ulcers, and draining tracts
- Virtually all dogs and many cats—pharyngeal and cervical lymphadenopathy; retching, ptyalism, or tonsillar abscess; lymph nodes visible or palpably firm, fixed, tender, may ulcerate and drain
- Fever
- Depression
- Partial anorexia and weight loss
- Hypertrophic osteopathy may occur.
- Disseminated disease—body cavity effusion; visceral masses; bone or joint lesions; dermal and subcutaneous masses and ulcers; lymphadenopathy and/or abscesses; CNS signs; and sudden death

Feline Leprosy

- Cutaneous nodules and plaques—single or multiple; usually on head and extremities; may be covered with normal epithelium and hair; may be alopecic or ulcerated and crusted; nonpainful; not attached to underlying structures
- Regional lymphadenopathy may be seen.
- Systemic—none

Atypical Mycobacteriosis

- Cutaneous—traumatic lesion that fails to heal with appropriate therapy; spreads locally in the subcutaneous tissue (panniculitis) (Fig. 45-1), original lesion enlarges, forming a deep ulcer that drains greasy hemorrhagic exudate; surrounding tissue becomes firm; satellite pinpoint ulcers open and drain (Fig. 45-2)
- Cutaneous and subcutaneous—systemic signs rare
- Pulmonary and systemic infections—same as for tuberculosis
- *M. avium*—infection most often disseminated

Differential Diagnosis

The mycobacterial infections have different prognoses, treatment recommendations, and public health consequences but may initially have similar signs, especially cutaneous lesions.

Tuberculosis

- Other mycobacterial infections
- Systemic mycoses
- Lymphosarcoma
- Disseminated mast cell tumor
- Systemic histiocytosis
- Plague
- Disseminated nocardiosis

Feline Leprosy

- Other mycobacterial infections—especially cutaneous tuberculosis
- Plague
- L-form bacterial infection
- *Rhodococcus equi* infection
- Chronic bite wound abscess
- Neoplasia
- Mycetoma
- Dermatophyte pseudomycetoma
- Cytology and biopsy—if acid-fast organisms are identified, consider tuberculosis or cutaneous nocardiosis, both of which can be fastidious and slow growing in culture, leading to the suspicion of unculturable leprosy organism

ATYPICAL MYCOBACTERIOSIS

- Foreign body
- Bacterial abscess
- L-form bacterial infection
- Feline leprosy
- Cutaneous tuberculosis
- *Rhodococcus equi* infection
- Nocardiosis
- Sterile nodular panniculitis
- Deep pyoderma and cellulitis
- Leishmaniasis
- Mast cell tumor
- Sweat gland neoplasia

Diagnostics

- CBC: anemia common in tuberculosis
- Intradermal skin testing with BCG may produce false-positive results
- Radiographs: thoracic, abdominal, or skeletal lesions—suggest granulomatous infectious disease; no specific lesions for mycobacteriosis; pulmonary tuberculosis lesions may become calcified or cavitated
- Based on histopathologic and microbiologic evaluation of biopsy material from affected tissue
- Biopsy specimens—should be uncontaminated by surface bacteria; must incorporate the center of a granulomatous focus
- Smears from affected tissues—for detection with acid-fast bacilli; swabs or aspirations of draining cutaneous lesions or lymph nodes; transtracheal wash; endoscopic brushing; rectal cytology; impression taken at surgical biopsy
- Culture—submit heat-fixed smears and tissue; special media and techniques required; identification of isolates may take several weeks

Pathologic Findings

TUBERCULOSIS

- Granulomas—with prominent necrosis; often poorly demarcated; often surrounded and admixed with other inflammatory cells
- Abundant epithelioid macrophages
- Giant cells uncommon
- Acid-fast bacteria—low numbers detected with ZN acid-fast stain; within epithelioid macrophages
- Lymph nodes—generally obliterated by the pyogranulomatous inflammatory reaction

FELINE LEPROSY

- Lesions—chronic pyogranulomas; lack central necrosis characteristic of tuberculosis
- Organisms—identify by ZN acid-fast stain; usually numerous within epithelioid histiocytes; may be sparse in some chronic lesions

Atypical Mycobacteriosis

- Pyogranulomatous panniculitis
- Dermatitis
- Lesions—typically associated with fat necrosis and extracellular accumulations of lipid; surrounded by a cuff of neutrophils
- Organisms—within the fat vacuoles; identify by H&E stain or modified Fite-Faraco acid-fast stains; typical ZN acid-fast staining technique may wash out fat accumulations and organisms from specimens
- Pulmonary and systemic disease—pyogranulomas; occasional areas of necrosis; no giant cells (as in tuberculosis); organisms usually numerous within macrophages

Therapeutics

- Feline leprosy—cured by surgical excision of lesions
- Subcutaneous atypical mycobacteriosis—may be aided by debulking surgery; benefit of surgery in conjunction with aggressive medical treatment undefined
- Humans—cutaneous lesions have been treated with controlled local heating

Tuberculosis

Primary

- Always use double- or triple-drug oral therapy; never attempt single-drug therapy for any organism.
- Current recommendation—fluoroquinolone (e.g., enrofloxacin), clarithromycin, and rifampin for 6–9 months
- Enrofloxacin, orbifloxacin, and ciprofloxacin—5–15 mg/kg PO q24h
- Rifampin—10–20 mg/kg PO q24h or divided q12h (maximum, 600 mg/day)
- Clarithromycin—5–10 mg/kg PO q24h

Alternatives

- Isoniazid and rifampin—combinations have been used; little is known about their use in cats; one recent report of treatment (cat) with isoniazid, rifampin, and dihydrostreptomycin for 3 months noted weight loss but eventual successful outcome
- Isoniazid—10–20 mg/kg (up to 300 mg total) PO q24h
- Ethambutol—15 mg/kg PO q24h
- Pyrazinamide—instead of ethambutol; 15–40 mg/kg PO q24h
- Dihydrostreptomycin—15 mg/kg IM q24h

Feline Leprosy

- Dapsone—1 mg/kg (up to 50 mg/cat) PO q12h for 2–4 weeks
- Clofazimine—2–8 mg/kg PO q24h for 6 weeks; then every 3–4 days for 1–2 months
- Rifampin—10–20 mg/kg PO q24h or divided q12h

Atypical Mycobacteriosis

- Chemotherapy—may use in vitro sensitivity testing to choose drug
- Antibiotics—macrolides, sulfonamides, tetracyclines, aminoglycosides, and fluoroquinolones generally effective
- Fluoroquinolones and/or clarithromycin—good empirical treatment; same dosages as for tuberculosis; treat for 2–6 months; relapses during course of or after completion of treatment common
- Single-agent therapy has been typically recommended, but double-agent therapy may be warranted owing to poor response over the long term.
- *M. avium*—clofazimine at 2–8 mg/kg PO q24h for 6 weeks; then every 3–4 days for 1–2 months
- Subcutaneous disease (*M. fortuitum*)—topical treatment with a 1:1 solution of 2.27% enrofloxacin in 90% DMSO used successfully in cats; applied 1 mL q12h for a total of 5 mg/kg
- Humans (systemic disease)—ancillary therapy with γ-interferon resulted in resolution of a refractory case

Contraindications/Possible Interactions

- Traditional antituberculosis drugs—be alert for any adverse reactions; experience limited, especially in cats
- Isoniazid—liver toxicity, seizures, neuritis, and drug eruption in humans
- Ethambutol—optic neuritis in humans
- Pyrazinamide—liver toxicity in humans
- Rifampin—anorexia, vomiting, and liver toxicity
- Dapsone—hemolytic anemia, other immune-mediated blood dyscrasias, and liver toxicity
- Clofazimine—orange discoloration of fat, diarrhea and/or weight loss, and hepatic enzyme elevation
- Dihydrostreptomycin—hearing loss and renal damage

Comments

- Antituberculosis and antileprosy drugs—examine at least monthly; monitor for anorexia and weight loss
- Monitor liver enzymes monthly.
- Instruct owners to report cutaneous lesions immediately.
- Clinicians aware of a human tuberculosis case in a household with dogs or cats should counsel owners about the risk of reverse zoonosis.
- Tuberculosis—guarded prognosis, but currently undefined because experience with modern drugs is limited
- Feline leprosy—fair prognosis, especially if lesions are amenable to surgical excision
- Subcutaneous atypical mycobacteriosis—good for survival but guarded for resolution; relapse after cessation of long-term antibiotic therapy occurs in > 40% of cats treated with single-agent therapy
- Pulmonary and disseminated atypical mycobacteriosis—guarded, but may be improved with modern agents and double-drug treatment

ZOONOTIC POTENTIAL

- Tuberculosis—affected domestic pets are possible serious zoonotic threats to owners; public health authorities should be notified of any antemortem or postmortem diagnosis (may be required by law); do not attempt treatment without concurrence of public health authorities
- *M. tuberculosis*—greatest potential for zoonosis, especially with draining cutaneous lesions
- Disease transmission from dogs and cats to humans—very rarely recorded; in recent outbreaks of tuberculosis in cats, no such case was documented

Suggested Reading

Greene CE. Mycobacterial infections. In: Greene CE, ed. Infectious diseases of the dog and cat. Philadelphia: Saunders, 1998:313–325.

Consulting Editor Karen Helton Rhodes

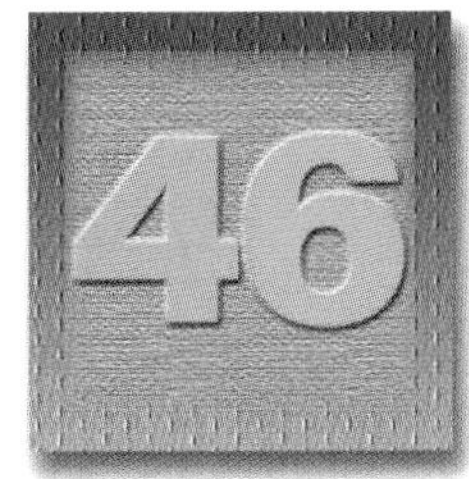

Dermatophilosis

Carol S. Foil

Overview/Definition

- A crusting skin disease in dogs and a nodular subcutaneous and oral disease in cats
- Reported infrequently

Etiology/Pathophysiology

- *Dermatophilus congolensis*—causative agent; gram-positive, branching filamentous bacterium classified as an Actinomycete; common cause of crusting dermatoses in hoofed animals, which causes crusted skin lesions of affected large animals and persists in their environment within crusts and other debris shed from infected hoof stock
- Dogs, cats, and humans can rarely be secondarily infected.

Signalment/History

- Association with farm animals or free-roaming lifestyle often reported
- Cats—episode of trauma; existence of a foreign body; lesions generally chronic; no systemic clinical signs, except when internal organs or large oral lesions develop
- Dogs, cats, and humans can be exposed directly from lesions on large animals or from environmental exposure.

- Infectious stage—requires wetting for activation; probably cannot penetrate intact epithelium, thus antecedent minor trauma or mechanical transmission by biting ectoparasites required
- Deeper infections—presumably acquired by traumatic inoculation of infectious material

Clinical Features

- Dogs—lesions: papular; crusted; mainly on the skin of the trunk or head; circular to coalescent; similar to those in superficial pyoderma caused by *Staphylococcus intermedius;* resemble dermatophilosis in horses (adherent thick, gray-yellow crusts that incorporate hair and leave a circular glistening shallow erosion when removed); pruritus variable
- Cats—subcutaneous, oral, or internal ulcerated and fistulated nodules or abscesses similar to lesions caused by other actinomycetes in this species

Differential Diagnosis

Dogs

- Staphylococcal pyoderma
- Acute moist dermatitis
- Dermatophytosis
- Pemphigus foliaceus
- Keratinization disorder

Cats

- Actinomycosis and nocardiosis
- Atypical mycobacterial granuloma
- Sporotrichosis
- Other subcutaneous fungal infection
- Deep mycotic infection, especially

Cryptococcosis

- Foreign body
- Chronic bite/wound abscess
- Bacterial L-form infection
- *Rhodococcus equi* infection
- Cutaneous or mucosal neoplasm, especially squamous cell carcinoma

Diagnostics

Dogs

- Cytologic examination of crusts—most important procedure; differentiates from more typical bacterial pyodermas
- Organism—distinctive morphology in cytologic and histologic preparations; resembles "railroad tracks" as the bacterium forms chains of small diplococci; chains often branching

- Cytologic diagnosis—from impression smears made of exudate from under crusts or by preparation of minced crusts; mince crusts finely in a drop of water and allow to macerate several minutes; then dry the preparation and stain with any Wright-Giemsa stain
- Histopathologic specimens—from crusts

Cats

- Histopathologic examination—biopsy of ulcerated nodules; procedure of choice
- Cytologic examination—exudate obtained from aspiration or swabbing of a draining tract
- Culture of biopsy specimens—may yield the organism; facilitated if the laboratory is alerted to the possible presence of *Dermatophilus* (aerobic, relatively slow growing, and easily obscured by contamination)
- Culture from crusts—requires the use of special selective medium; generally used to corroborate cytologic findings

Pathologic Findings

- Dogs—crusting and superficial pustular dermatitis; palisading of the crusts with orthokeratotic and parakeratotic hyperkeratosis; organism visualized within the crusts, generally without the use of special bacterial stains
- Cats—pyogranulomatous inflammation; central necrosis; fistulous tract formation; organism visualized near the necrotic center of granulomas, especially with gram stain

Therapeutics

- Dogs—antibacterial shampoo and gentle removal (and disposal) of crusts; shampoo may contain benzoyl peroxide, ethyl lactate, chlorhexidine, or selenium disulfide; one or two applications suffice in most cases
- Cats—for pyogranulomas and abscesses: surgical débridement; exploration for foreign body; establishment of drainage for exudate; maintain effective drainage and postoperative wound care

Drugs

- Penicillin V—10 mg/kg PO q12h for 10–20 days; drug of choice
- Ampicillin—10–20 mg/kg PO q12h for 10–20 days
- Amoxicillin—10–20 mg/kg PO q12h for 10–20 days
- Tetracycline, doxycycline, or minocycline—standard dosage

Comments

- Dogs—re-examine after 2 weeks of treatment to ensure complete resolution of symptoms; give an additional 7 days of systemic therapy
- Cats—monitor biweekly for 1 month after apparent resolution of lesions, depending on their location
- Dogs—excellent prognosis

- Cats—prognosis varies with the location of lesions and extent of surgical débridement; complete resolution can be achieved with timely diagnosis and appropriate surgical and medical therapy
- Veterinarians and animal care workers—very seldom infected, even after traumatic exposure when working with farm animals known to be infected
- Dogs and cats—very unlikely to serve as a source for human infection; caution is warranted for exposure of immunocompromised individuals

Suggested Reading

Greene CE. Dermatophilosis. In: Greene CE, ed. Infectious diseases of the dog and cat. Philadelphia: Saunders, 1998:326–327.

Consulting Editor Karen Helton Rhodes

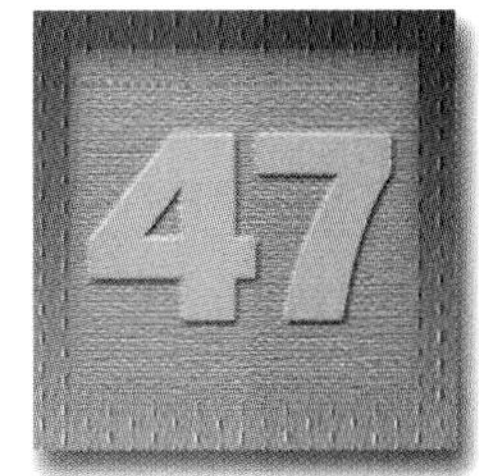

NOCARDIOSIS

Gary D. Norsworthy

Overview/Definition

- An uncommon infection of dogs and cats
- Organism—soil saprophyte; enters body through contamination of wounds or by respiratory inhalation

Etiology/Pathophysiology

- A compromised immune system enhances the likelihood of infection.
- Systems affected—respiratory, skin/exocrine, lymphatic, musculoskeletal, nervous
- *Nocardia asteroides* (dogs and cats)
- *N. brasiliensis* (cats only)
- *Proactinomyces* spp. (rare)

Signalment/History

- Dogs and cats of any breed

Clinical Features

- Depends on the site of infection
- Pleural—pyothorax, resulting in dyspnea, emaciation, and fever

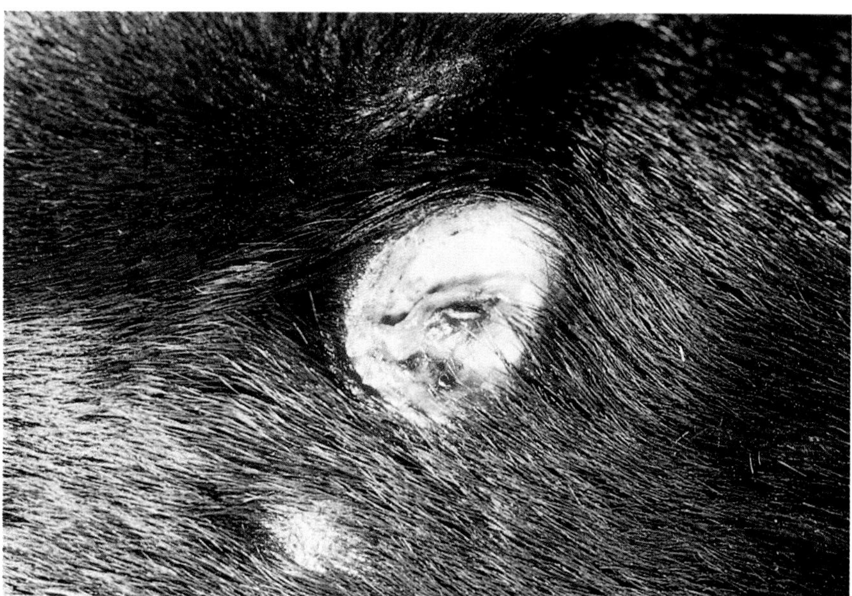

Figure 47-1 Focal nonhealing lesion characteristic of nocardiosis. (Courtesy of Dr. Carol Foil.)

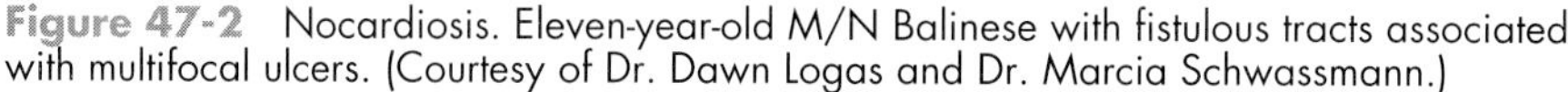

Figure 47-2 Nocardiosis. Eleven-year-old M/N Balinese with fistulous tracts associated with multifocal ulcers. (Courtesy of Dr. Dawn Logas and Dr. Marcia Schwassmann.)

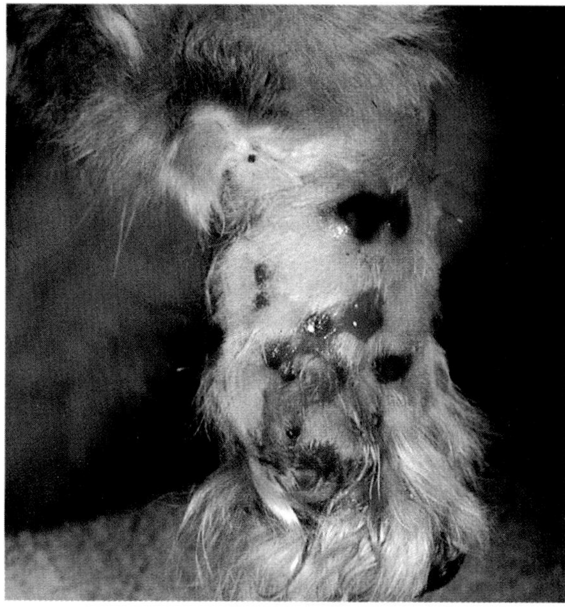

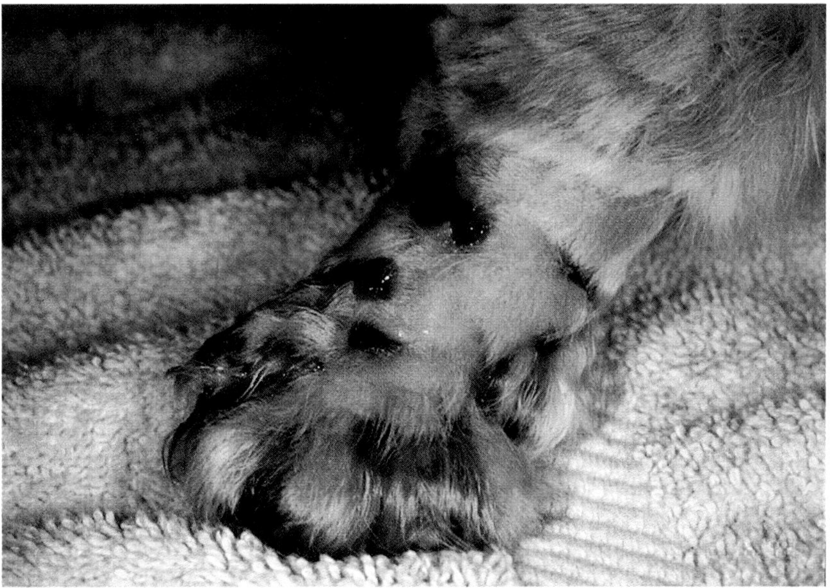

Figure 47-3 Nocardiosis. Close-view of Figure 47-2. (Courtesy of Dr. Dawn Logas and Dr. Marcia Schwassmann.)

- Cutaneous—chronic, nonhealing wounds (Fig. 47-1); often accompanied by fistulous tracts (Figs. 47-2, 47-3); if extended, may result in lymphadenopathy, draining lymph nodes, and osteomyelitis
- Disseminated—most common in young dogs; usually begins in the respiratory tract; lethargy, fever, and weight loss; cyclic fever may be characteristic; CNS may be affected; pleural and/or abdominal effusion may occur

Differential Diagnosis

Cutaneous

- Actinomycosis
- Atypical mycobacteriosis
- Leprosy
- Bite wound abscesses
- Draining tracts resulting from foreign bodies

Pleural

- Bacterial pyothorax
- Thoracic neoplasia
- Chronic diaphragmatic hernia

Disseminated

- Systemic fungal infections
- Feline infectious peritonitis

Diagnostics

- Neutrophilic leukocytosis
- Nonregenerative anemia—with longstanding infections (anemia of chronic disease)
- Chemistries—usually normal; hypergammaglobulinemia may be seen with longstanding infections
- Radiographs—may reveal pleural or peritoneal effusion, pleuropneumonia, or osteomyelitis
- Cytology—thoracentesis or abdominocentesis for samples; stain these or other exudates with Romanowsky, Gram, and modified acid-fast stains for rapid diagnosis; may reveal gram-positive branching filamentous rods and cocci; cannot be distinguished from *Actinomyces* spp.
- Culture—diagnostic; aerobic culturing on Sabouraud medium
- *N. asteroides*—more suppurative pyogranulomatous reaction than with *Actinomyces* spp.
- *N. brasiliensis*—granulomatous reaction with extensive fibrosis
- Although the organism is usually present, it cannot be distinguished histopathologically from *Actinomyces* spp.

Therapeutics

- Pleural or peritoneal effusions and disseminated form—inpatient until clinically stable and effusion removed; fluid therapy for rehydration and maintenance often needed
- Long-term antibiotic therapy and draining fistulous tracts—outpatient
- Diet—encourage consumption by offering foods with appealing tastes and smells; forced enteral feeding for anorectic inpatients essential; orogastric tube feeding preferred
- Surgery—when feasible, surgical drainage should accompany medical therapy; important to place a thoracostomy tube for pleural effusion; attempt surgical drainage and débridement of draining tracts and lymph nodes; take care to identify foreign bodies

Drugs

- Cultured organism—antibiotic sensitivity testing
- No culture or results pending—good first-choice drugs: sulfonamides (e.g., sulfadiazine at 100 mg/kg IV, PO as a loading dose followed by 50 mg/kg IV, PO q12h) and sulfonamide-trimethoprim combinations (30 mg/kg PO q24h)
- Aminoglycosides—gentamicin (3 mg/kg IV, IM, SC q8h); amikacin (6.5 mg/kg IV, IM, SC q8h)
- Tetracyclines—doxycycline (10 mg/kg PO q24h); tetracycline hydrochloride (15–20 mg/kg PO q8h); minocycline (5–12.5 mg/kg PO q12h)
- Erythromycin—10–20 mg/kg PO q8h; or combined with ampicillin (20–40 mg/kg PO q8h) or amoxicillin (6–20 mg/kg PO q8–12h)
- Amoxicillin plus an aminoglycoside—synergistic combination; consider in any serious infection when culturing is not possible or is pending
- Average treatment period is 6 weeks; however, medical treatment should extend several weeks past apparent remission of the disease.

Comments

- Tetracyclines (cats)—may cause fever up to 41.5°C (107°F); discontinue and replace if fever increases during therapy
- Monitor carefully for fever, weight loss, seizures, dyspnea, and lameness the first year after apparently successful therapy because of the potential for bone and CNS involvement.

Suggested Reading

Edwards DF. Actinomycosis and nocardiosis. In: Greene CE, ed. Infectious diseases of the dog and cat. Philadelphia: Saunders, 1998:303–313.

Consulting Editor Karen Helton Rhodes

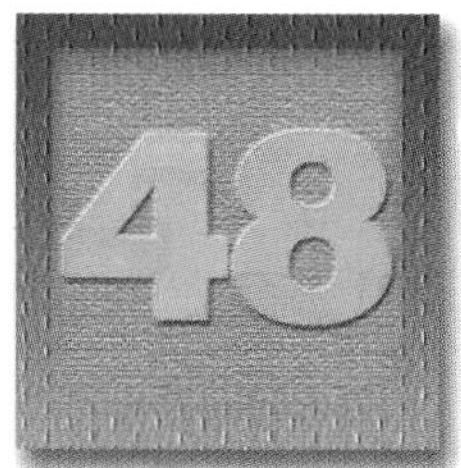

Malassezia Dermatitis

K.V. Mason

Overview/Definition

- *Malassezia pachydermatis* (syn. *Pityrosporum canis*)—yeast; normal commensal of the skin, ears, and mucocutaneous areas; can overgrow and cause dermatitis, cheilitis, and otitis in dogs (Fig. 48-1)
- Yeast numbers in diseased areas are usually excessive, although this is a variable finding.

Etiology/Pathophysiology

- The causes of the transformation from harmless commensal to pathogen are poorly understood but seem related to allergy, seborrheic conditions, and possibly congenital and hormonal factors.
- *Malassezia* dermatitis and *Malassezia*-associated seborrheic dermatitis—common in all geographic regions of the world
- Cats—similar disease, but rare
- High humidity and temperature—may increase the frequency
- Concurrent hypersensitivity disease (particularly atopy, flea allergy, and some food allergy/intolerances) may be a predisposing factor.
- Defects of cornification and seborrheas (especially in young dogs) in predisposed breeds
- Endocrinopathies (especially in old dogs)—suspected to be associated predisposing factors
- Genetic factors—suspected for young onset in predisposed breeds

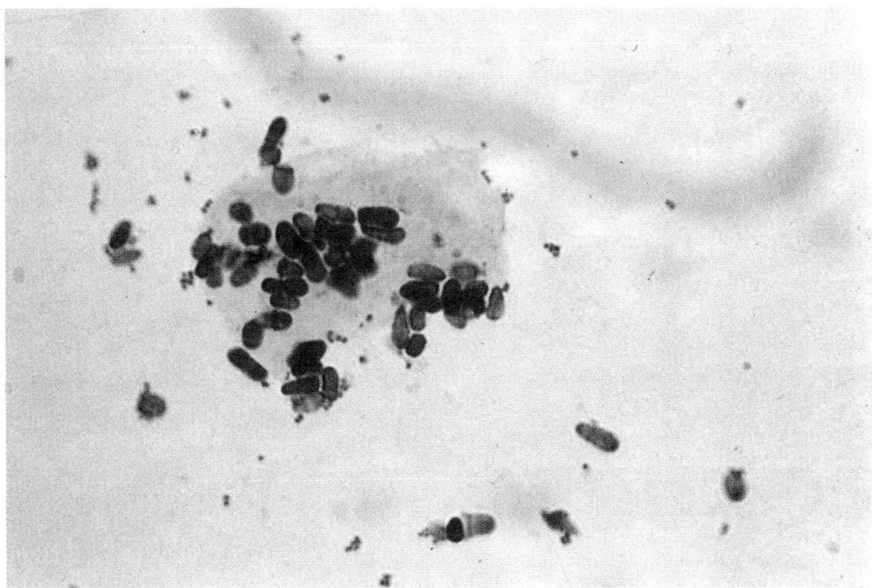

Figure 48-1 Tape preparation ×400 showing *Malassezia* yeasts.

- Concurrent increase in cutaneous *Staphylococcus intermedius* population and resultant pyoderma—confirmed finding; canine seborrheic dermatitis is proposed, in selected cases, to be a result of this combination pathogen overgrowth; treatment of one alone does not result in resolution of all signs, but just unmasks the other; antiyeast treatment alone resolves all signs of *Malassezia* dermatitis
- Idiopathic

Signalment/History

- Any dog breed; however, West Highland white terriers, poodles, basset hounds, cocker spaniels, and dachshunds are predisposed.
- No gender predilection

Clinical Features

- Pruritus—with varying degrees of erythema, alopecia, scale, and greasy malodorous exudation; affects lips, ears, feet, axilla, inguinal area, and ventral neck (Fig. 48-2)
- Hyperpigmentation and lichenification—chronic cases (Fig. 48-3)
- Concurrent black waxy to seborrheic otitis—frequent
- Frenzied facial pruritus—uncommon but characteristic
- Often a history of suspected allergy that worsens and seems to develop resistance to or is resistant to glucocorticoid treatment
- Concurrent pyoderma, hypersensitivities, endocrine, and keratinization disorders (Figs. 48-4, 48-5)

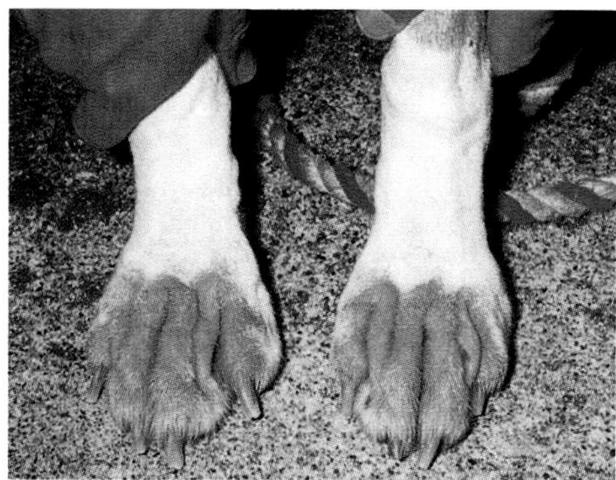

Figure 48-2 Typical *Malassezia* pododermatitis in a Boxer.

Figure 48-3 Typical periocular lesion of *Malassezia* dermatitis.

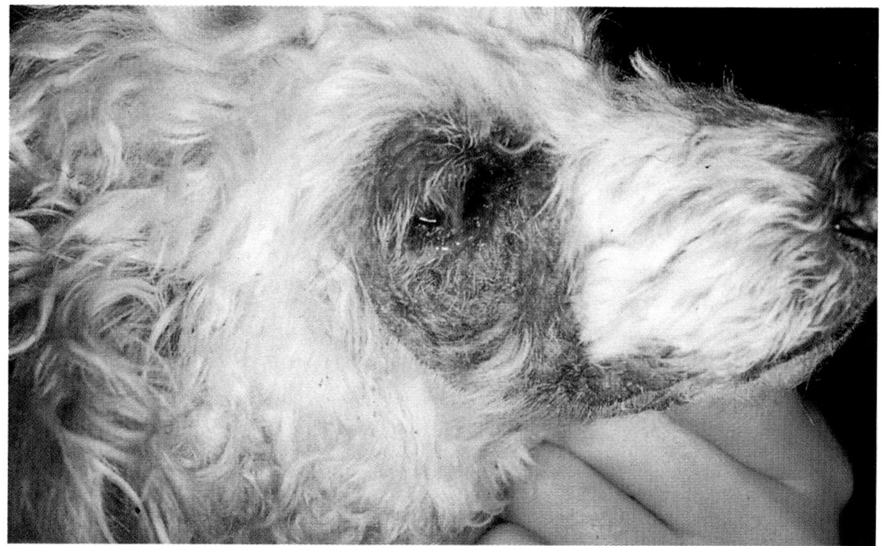

Figure 48-4 Basset hound with *Malassezia*-associated seborrhic dermatitis.

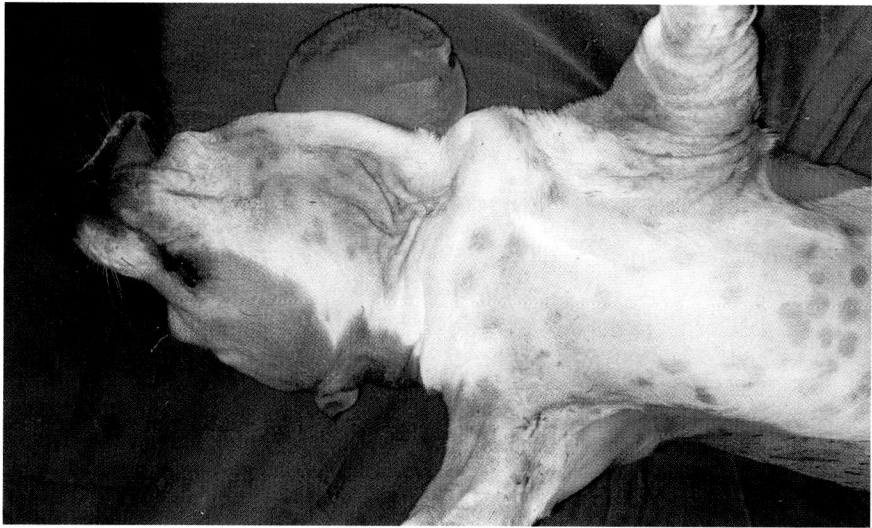

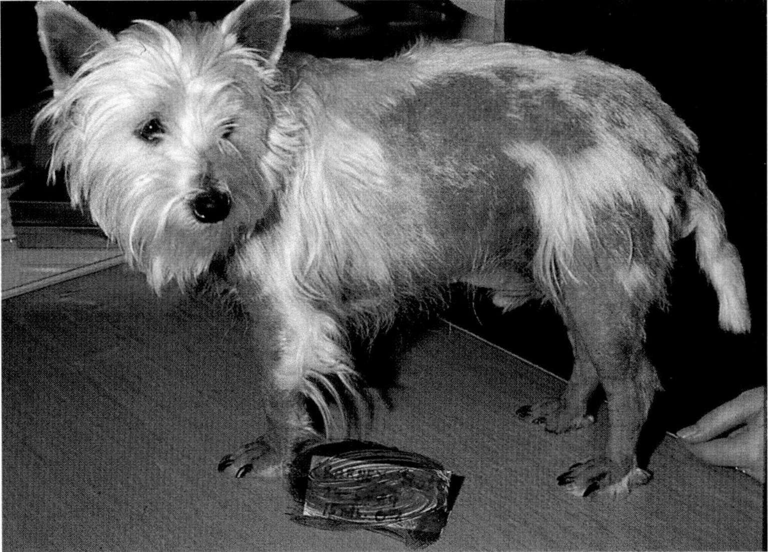

Figure 48-5 West Highland white terrier with *Malassezia*-associated seborrhic dermatitis.

Differential Diagnosis

- Allergic dermatitis, including flea allergy, atopy, and food allergy
- Superficial pyoderma
- Primary and secondary seborrheas
- All associated diseases mentioned above

Diagnostics

- Fungal culture—use contact plates (small agar plates made from bottle lids and filled with Sabouraud agar or preferably modified Dixon agar); press plates onto the affected skin surface; then incubate at 32–37°C for 3–7 days; count the distinctive yellow or buff, round, domed colonies (1–1.5 mm); provides semiqualitative data
- Nonquantitative culture methods—no value, because *Malassezia* is a normal commensal
- Skin cytology—touch, cotton swab, or cellophane tape preparation stained with Diff-Quick; apply stain as a drop directly onto the slide (yeast may wash off during staining); pass a flame under the slide to improve stain penetration and visualization
- Histopathology—valuable if the skin reaction pattern (spongiotic, hyperplastic, superficial, perivascular) is recognized and yeast is seen in the superficial scale; yeast is often lost during collection or processing
- Surface cytology—more reliable; simple, inexpensive, and rapid

Therapeutics

- Goals—confirm diagnosis by associating elimination of signs with reduction in yeast and bacterial numbers

- Identify and treat any predisposing factors or diseases.
- Topical therapy—yeast is principally located in the stratum corneum
- Shampoo treatment—remove scale, exudation, and malodor
- Topical therapies with trial data—(miconazole, selenium sulfides); twice-weekly treatments effective
- Other topical antifungal and antibacterial shampoo treatments may also be of value if given with suitable systemic drugs.
- Alternative combinations—topical keratolytic shampoo treatment with systemic antiyeast and antibacterial drugs
- Localized cases—may respond to creams and lotions containing imidazole compounds
- Ketoconazole—10 mg/kg q24h for 2–4 weeks; widespread or chronic lichenified cases
- Chronic lichenified cases—ketoconazole at 5–10 mg/kg q24h as a short diagnostic for 5–7 days with effective topical antimycotic shampoo treatment; quick response confirms the diagnosis; response can be slow in chronic cases when yeasts are buried deep in epidermal folds
- Topical antimicrobial shampoo—to maintain remission in chronic cases

Comments

- Ketoconazole—rarely may cause hepatic reaction; will mask the signs of hyperadrenocorticism and interfere with adrenal function tests; contraindicated in pregnancy
- Physical examinations and skin cytology findings after 2–4 weeks to monitor therapy
- Treat until only rare organisms can be demonstrated or 7 days after a complete response is achieved.
- Pruritus and odor—usually noticeably improved within 1 week
- Recurrences—common when underlying dermatoses are not well controlled; regular bathing with antifungal-antibacterial shampoo combinations (miconazole plus chlorhexidine) help decrease recurrence

Suggested Reading

Scott DW, Miller WH, Griffin CE. Muller & Kirk's Small Animal Dermatology. 5th ed. Philadelphia: Saunders, 1995.

Consulting Editor Karen Helton Rhodes

Dermatophytosis: Keratinophilic Mycosis

W. Dunbar Gram

Definition/Overview

- A cutaneous fungal infection affecting the cornified regions of hair, nails, and occasionally the superficial layers of the skin
- Most commonly isolated organisms—*Microsporum canis, Trichophyton mentagrophytes,* and *M. gypseum*

Etiology/Pathophysiology

- Exposure to or contact with a dermatophyte does not necessarily result in an infection.
- Infection may not result in clinical signs.
- Dermatophytes—grow in the keratinized layers of hair, nail, and skin; do not thrive in living tissue or persist in the presence of severe inflammation; incubation period: 1–4 weeks
- An affected animal that does not show signs may remain in this inapparent carrier state for a prolonged period of time; some animals never become symptomatic.
- Corticosteroids can modulate inflammation and prolong the infection.
- Cats—*M. canis* is by far the most common agent
- Dogs—*M. canis, M. gypseum,* and *T. mentagrophytes;* incidence of each agent varies geographically
- Reliance on clinical signs and incorrectly interpreted Wood's lamp examination results in overdiagnosis.

Signalment

- Cats—more common in long-haired breeds (Fig. 49-1)
- Clinical signs—more common in young animals
- Although ubiquitous, the incidence is higher in hot and humid regions.
- Lesions may begin as alopecia or a poor hair coat.
- A history of previously confirmed infection or exposure to an infected animal or environment (e.g., a cattery) is a useful but not consistent finding.

Risk Factors

- Immunocompromising disease or immunosuppressive medication
- High population density
- Poor nutrition
- Poor management practices
- Lack of an adequate quarantine period
- Vary from an inapparent carrier state to a patchy or circular alopecia
- Classic circular alopecia—common in cats; often misinterpreted in dogs (Fig. 49-2)
- Scales, erythema, hyperpigmentation, and pruritus—variable (Fig. 49-3)
- Paronychosis, granulomatous lesions, or kerions may occur.

Differential Diagnosis

- Cats—miliary dermatitis and almost any other dermatitis
- Dogs—folliculitis, furunculosis, and most cases of alopecia
- Demodicosis and bacterial skin infection—epidermal collarettes more typical of a bacterial infection; grossly enlarged follicular ostia with furunculosis sug-

Figure 49-1 Persian cat with *M. canis*. This breed is considered predisposed to dermatophytosis. (Courtesy of Dr. Carol Foil.)

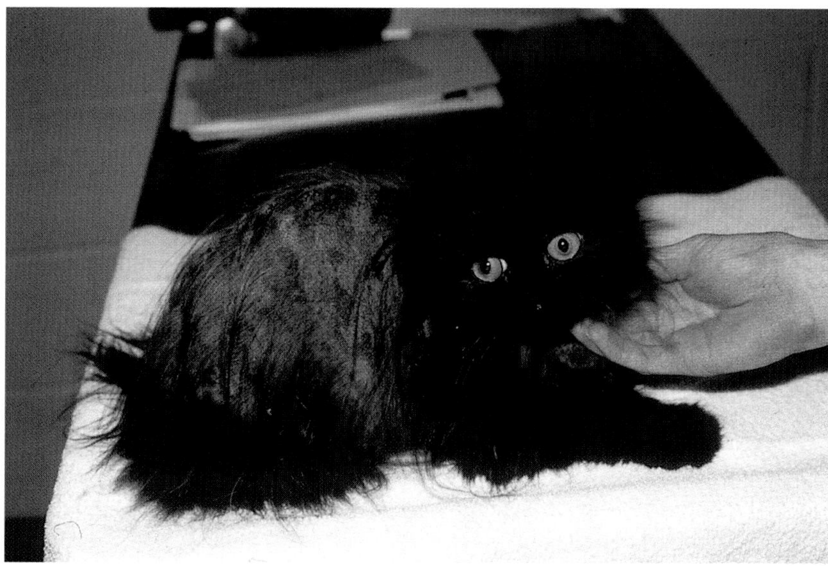

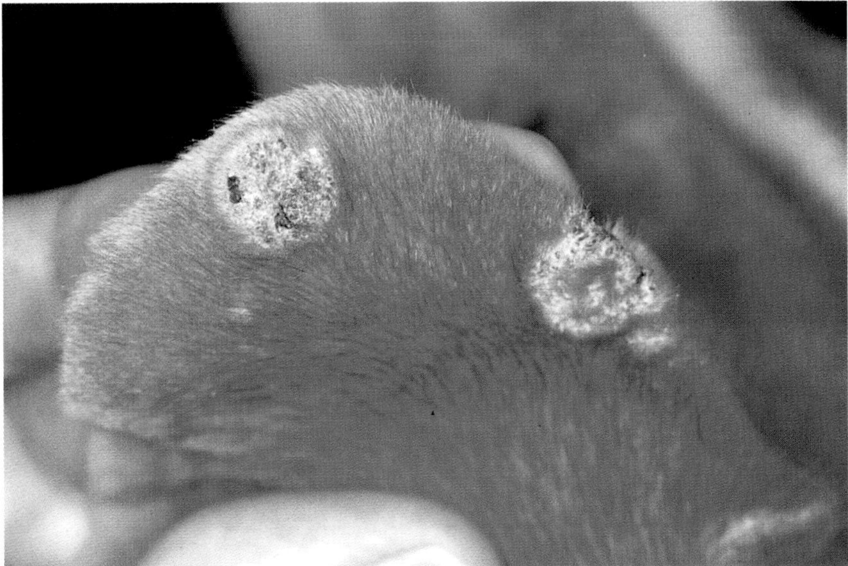

Figure 49-2 Dermatophytosis (*M. canis*) in a dog. Circular patches of alopecia and scale are more characteristic in humans and cats. (Courtesy of Dr. Carol Foil.)

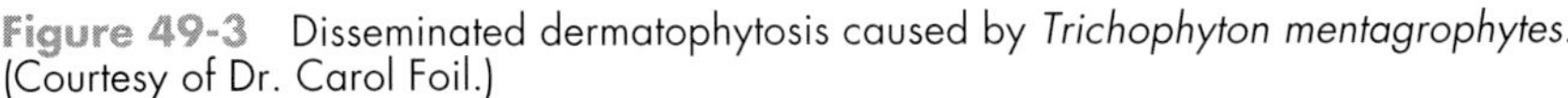

Figure 49-3 Disseminated dermatophytosis caused by *Trichophyton mentagrophytes*. (Courtesy of Dr. Carol Foil.)

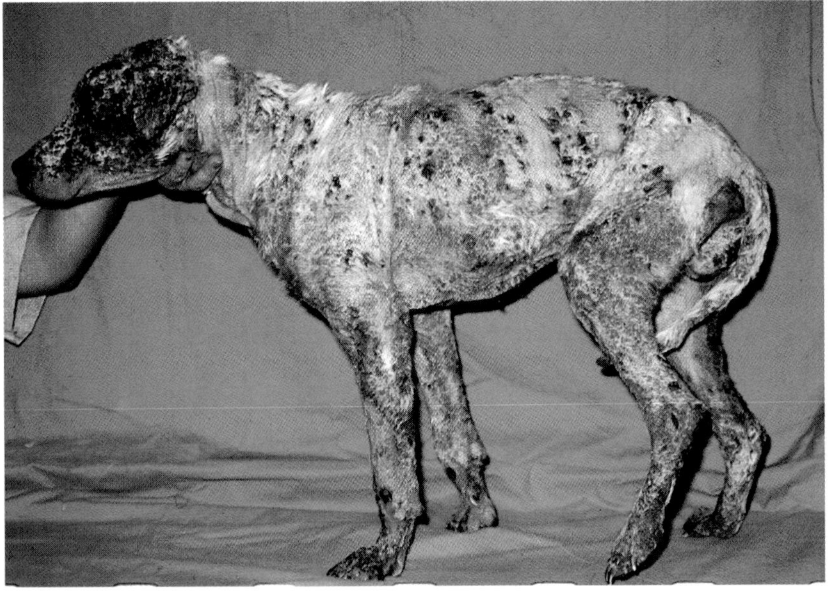

gest demodicosis; these characteristics are not consistent; concurrent bacterial or mite infections can be seen with dermatophytosis; all three diseases can cause focal hyperpigmentation

- Immune-mediated skin diseases—severe inflammation associated with dermatophytosis affecting the face or feet

Diagnostics

- Reliance on clinical signs and incorrectly interpreted Wood's lamp examination results in overdiagnosis.

Fungal Culture with Macroconidia Identification

- Best means of confirming diagnosis
- Hairs that exhibit a positive apple-green fluorescence under Wood's lamp examination are considered ideal candidates for culture.
- Pluck hairs from the periphery of an alopecic area; do not use a random pattern.
- Use a sterile toothbrush to brush the hair coat of an asymptomatic animal to yield better results.
- Test media—change to red when they become alkaline; dermatophytes typically produce this color during the early growing phase of their culture; saprophytes, which also produce this color, do so in the late growing phase; thus, it is important to examine the media daily.
- Microscopic examination of the macroconidia—necessary to confirm pathogenic dermatophyte and to identify genus and species; helps identify source of infection
- Positive culture—indicates existence of a dermatophyte; however, it may have been there only transiently, as commonly occurs when the culture is obtained from the feet, which are likely to come in contact with a geophilic dermatophyte

Microscopic Examination of Hair

- Examination after using a clearing solution can help provide a rapid diagnosis.
- Time-consuming and often produces false-negative results
- Use hairs that fluoresce under Wood's lamp illumination to increase the likelihood of identifying the fungal hyphae associated with the hair shaft.
- Wood's lamp examination—not a very useful screening tool; many pathogenic dermatophytes do not fluoresce; false fluorescence is common; lamp should warm up for a minimum of 5 min and then be exposed to suspicious lesions for up to 5 min; a true positive reaction associated with *M. canis* consists of apple-green fluorescence of the hair shaft; keratin associated with epidermal scales and sebum will often produce a false-positive fluorescence

Skin Biopsy

- Not usually needed
- Can be helpful in confirming true invasion and infection

PATHOLOGIC FINDINGS

- Folliculitis, perifolliculitis, or furunculosis
- Hyperkeratosis
- Intraepidermal pustules
- Pyogranulomatous reaction pattern
- Fungal hyphae may be observed in H&E-stained sections; special stains allow easier visualization of the organism.

Therapeutics

- Consider quarantine owing to the infective and zoonotic nature of the disease.
- A fatty meal improves absorption of griseofulvin.
- An acid meal (add tomato juice) enhances the absorption of ketoconazole.
- Griseofulvin—most widely prescribed systemic drug; microsized formulation: 25–60 mg/kg PO q12h for 4–6 weeks; ultramicrosized formulation: 2.5–5.0 mg/kg PO q12–24h; pediatric suspension: 10–25 mg/kg PO q12h; gastrointestinal upset is the most common side effect; alleviate by reducing the dose or dividing the dose for more frequent administration
- A fatty meal improves absorption of griseofulvin.
- Ketoconazole—not labeled for use in dogs or cats in the U.S.; dose: 10 mg/kg PO q24h or divided twice per day for 3–4 weeks; anorexia is the most common side effect
- An acid meal (add tomato juice) enhances the absorption of ketoconazole.

GRISEOFULVIN PRECAUTIONS

- Bone marrow suppression (anemia, pancytopenia, and neutropenia) can occur as an idiosyncratic reaction or with prolonged therapy.
- Neutropenia—most common fatal reaction in cats; can persist after discontinuation of drug; weekly or biweekly CBC is recommended; can be life-threatening in cats with FIV infection
- Neurologic side effects
- Do not use during the first two trimesters of pregnancy; it is teratogenic.

KETOCONAZOLE PRECAUTIONS

- Hepatopathy has been reported and can be quite severe.
- Inhibits endogenous production of steroidal hormones in dogs

MISCELLANEOUS

- Vaccination—product literature claims are based on clinical signs and Wood's lamp findings; may be useful as an adjuvant to systemic therapy; may be valuable for treating asymptomatic carriers, which can be frustrating to the client and veterinarian and can complicate the diagnosis and management; studies involving dermatophyte cultures as a measure of achieving a cure or prevention are necessary to ensure true efficacy.
- Topical therapy and clipping—once strongly advocated; may help prevent environmental contamination; often associated with an initial exacerbation of signs after the procedures are initiated; lime sulfur (1:16), enilconazole (bottle dilution), and miconazole shampoo are the most effective agents; lime sulfur is odiferous and can stain; enilconazole is not available in the U.S.

Alternative Drugs

Itraconazole—similar to ketoconazole but with fewer side effects; probably more effective; expensive; supplied as 100-mg capsules; dose: 10 mg/kg PO q24h or 5 mg/kg PO q12h

Comments

- Dermatophyte culture is the only means of truly monitoring response to therapy; many animals will clinically improve, but remain culture positive
- Repeat fungal cultures toward the end of the treatment regimen and continue treatment until at least one culture result is negative.
- In resistant cases, the culture may be repeated weekly, using the toothbrush technique; continue treatment until 2–3 consecutive culture results are negative.
- Initiate a quarantine period and obtain dermatophyte cultures of all animals entering the household to prevent reinfection from other animals.
- Consider the possibility of rodents aiding in the spread of the disease.
- Avoid infective soil, if a geophilic dermatophyte is involved.
- Consider using griseofulvin for 10–14 days as a prophylactic treatment of exposed animals.
- Many animals will "self-clear" a dermatophyte infection over a period of a few months.
- Treatment for the disease hastens clinical cure and helps reduce environmental contamination.
- Some infections, particularly in long-haired cats or multianimal situations, can be very persistent.

Client Education

- Inform owner that many short-haired cats in a single-cat environment and many dogs will undergo spontaneous remission.
- Advise that treatment can be both frustrating and expensive, especially in multianimal households or recurrent cases.
- Inform owner that environmental treatment, including fomites, is important, especially in recurrent cases; dilute bleach (1:10) is a practical and relatively effective means of providing environmental decontamination; concentrated bleach and formalin (1%) are more effective at killing spores, but their use is not as practical in many situations; chlorhexidine was ineffective in pilot studies.
- Inform owner that in a multianimal environment or cattery situation, treatment and control can be very complicated; referral to a veterinarian with expertise in this type of situation should be considered.

Suggested Reading

Moriello KA, DeBoer DJ. Dermatophytosis. In: August JR, ed. Consultations in feline internal medicine 2. Philadelphia: Saunders, 1994:219–225.

Scott DW, Miller WH, Griffin CE, eds. Fungal skin diseases. In: Muller & Kirk's Small animal dermatology. 5th ed. Philadelphia: Saunders, 1995:332–350.

Consulting Editor Karen Helton Rhodes

Sporotrichosis

W. Dunbar Gram

Overview/Definition

- A zoonotic fungal disease that may affect the integument or lymphatics or be generalized

Etiology/Pathophysiology

- Caused by the virtually ubiquitous dimorphic fungus *Sporothrix schenckii*, which typically infects via direct inoculation; direct inoculation not a requirement

Signalment/History

- Cats, dogs, and humans
- Dogs—more commonly seen in hunting dogs because of the increased likelihood of puncture wounds associated with thorns or splinters
- Cats—intact male cats that roam outdoors and fight because of the increased likelihood of puncture wounds and acquiring the disease from their opponents
- Animals exposed to soil rich in decaying organic debris appear to be predisposed.
- Puncture wounds associated with foreign bodies provide an increased opportunity for infection in dogs; cat scratches provide a similar opportunity in roaming cats.

- Immunosuppressive disease—risk factor for the disseminated form
- Previous trauma or puncture wound in the affected area—variable finding
- Poor response to previous antibacterial therapy

Clinical Features

- Cutaneous form—dog: associated with numerous nodules, which may drain or crust, typically affecting the head or trunk; cat: lesions often initially appear as wounds or abscesses, mimicking wounds associated with fighting, found on the head, lumbar region, or distal limbs (Fig. 50-1)
- Cutaneolymphatic form—usually an extension of the cutaneous form; spreads via the lymphatics, resulting in new nodules and draining tracts or crusts; lymphadenopathy common
- Disseminated form—associated with the systemic signs of malaise and fever; consider the potential of an underlying immunosuppressive disease as a contributing factor

Differential Diagnosis

- Various bacterial and fungal diseases—consider when symptoms include a nodular granulomatous disease and draining tracts
- Neoplastic conditions
- Parasitic infections (*Demodex* or *Pelodera*)

Diagnostics

- REMEMBER: this is a zoonotic disease and proper precautions should be taken to prevent infection; absence of a break in the skin does not protect against the disease.

Figure 50-1 Sporotrichosis in a cat. Note the ulcerated lesion along the nailbed and footpad. (Courtesy of Dr. Carol Foil.)

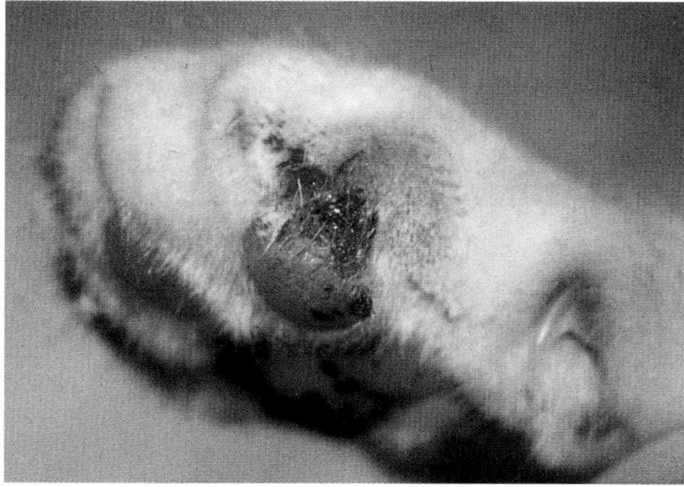

- Cytology of the exudate and staining—cats: often the only test necessary to confirm infection; cigar- to round-shaped yeast may be found intracellularly or free in the exudate; dogs: special fungal stains (PAS or GMS) may aid in the diagnosis; a negative finding does not rule out the disease
- Cultures of the deeply affected tissue—often require surgery to obtain an adequate sample; alert the laboratory that sporotrichosis is a differential diagnosis; secondary bacterial infections common

Therapeutics

- Remember the zoonotic potential when treating patients.
- Sometimes outpatient treatment may be considered.

SSKI-Supersaturated Potassium Iodide

- Treatment of choice—dogs: 40 mg/kg PO q8h with food; cats: 20 mg/kg PO q12h with food
- Continue for 30 days after resolution of the clinical lesions.
- Dogs—if signs of iodism are noted (dry hair coat, excessive scales, nasal or ocular discharge, vomiting, depression, or collapse), discontinue for 1 week; mild symptoms, reinitiate at the same dose; severe or recurrent symptoms, consider other drugs
- Cats—signs of iodism (depression, vomiting, anorexia, twitching, hypothermia, and cardiovascular collapse) are more common; if noted, discontinue; use other drugs

Ketoconazole and Itraconazole

- Shown encouraging results for fungal diseases in cats and dogs
- Dogs—ketoconazole: 15 mg/kg PO q12h, preferably with an acidic meal (e.g., tomato juice), until 1 month after clinical resolution; resolution should occur within approximately 3 months; side effects relatively mild, anorexia most common; acute hepatopathy, pruritus, alopecia, and lightening of the hair color reported
- Cats—ketoconazole: 5–10 mg/kg PO q12–24h, or itraconazole 10 mg/kg/day preferably with an acidic meal until 1 month after clinical resolution; side effects include gastrointestinal disturbances, depression, fever, jaundice, and neurologic signs; may be necessary to alternate drugs

Comments

- Re-evaluate every 2 to 4 weeks for clinical signs and side effects associated with treatment.
- Although difficult, try to determine the source of the original infection to prevent repeat infections.
- Unresponsive to therapy—not unexpected; consider alternative treatment or combined treatment regimens (SSKI and ketoconazole); itraconazole relatively untested but promising
- Zoonotic; proper precautions and client education are of paramount importance

Suggested Reading

Scott DW, Miller WH, Griffin CE. Muller and Kirk's small animal dermatology. 5th ed. Philadelphia: Saunders, 1995.

Consulting Editor Karen Helton Rhodes

Cryptococcosis

Alfred M. Legendre

Definition/Overview

A localized or systemic fungal infection caused by the environmental yeast *Cryptococcus neoformans*

Pathophysiology/Etiology

- *C. neoformans*—grows in bird droppings and decaying vegetation
- Dogs and cats inhale the yeast and a foci of infection is established, usually in the nasal passages; smaller dried, shrunken organisms may reach the terminal airways (uncommon)
- Dissemination—hematogenously from the nasal passages to the brain, eyes, lungs, and other tissues; by extension to the skin of the nose, the eye, retro-orbital tissues, and draining lymph nodes
- Cats—mainly the nose and sinuses; facial skin; nasal planum; nasopharynx; brain; eyes
- Dogs—mainly the head and brain, nasal passages, and sinuses; skin over the nose and sinuses; mucous membranes; draining lymph nodes; eyes; periorbital areas; occasionally lungs and abdominal organs

Signalment/History

- Dogs—rare in U.S.; prevalence 0.00013%
- Cats—7–10 times more common than in dogs

- Some areas of southern California and Australia have an increased incidence.
- Some *Cryptococcus* spp. grow well on eucalyptus trees.
- Dogs—American cocker spaniels, Doberman pinschers, and Labrador retrievers over-represented
- Cats—Siamese at increased risk
- Most common: 2–7 years of age (dogs and cats)
- Dogs—no sex predilection
- Cats—males over-represented
- Cats concurrently infected with FeLV or FIV—higher risk; more extensive disease

Clinical Features

- Lethargy
- Vary depending on organ systems involved

Dogs

- Neurologic—seizures, ataxia, paresis, blindness
- Skin ulceration
- Lymphadenopathy

Cats

- Nasal discharge
- Granulomatous tissue seen at the nares (Fig. 51-1)
- Firm swellings over the bridge of the nose

Physical Examination Findings

- Mild fever—< 50% of patients
- Dogs—anorexia; nasal discharge

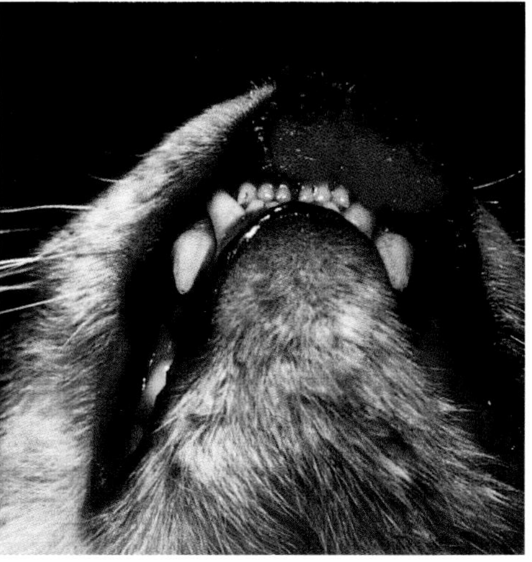

Figure 51-1 Cyptococcosis in the cat. Note the focal ulcerated nodule of the philtrim and lip region as well as the disseminated nodules of the chin area. (Courtesy of Dr. Carol Foil.)

- Cats—increased respiratory noise; ulcerated crusty skin lesions on the head; lymphadenopathy; neurologic; ocular

Differential Diagnosis

Dogs

- Other causes of focal or diffuse neurologic disease—distemper; bacterial meningoencephalitis; brain tumors; rickettsial diseases; granulomatous meningoencephalomyelitis; other fungal diseases
- Nasal lesions, especially at the mucocutaneous junction—considered immune-mediated
- Lymphosarcoma—possible cause of the lymphadenopathy
- With chorioretinitis and optic neuritis—consider other fungal infections, distemper, and neoplasia

Cats

- Nasal lesions—similar to nasal tumors, chronic rhinitis, and chronic sinusitis
- Ulcerative skin changes—may be the result of bacterial infection, fights, or tumor (especially squamous cell carcinoma of the nasal planum)
- Ocular and brain signs—may be attributed to lymphosarcoma, FIV, and toxoplasmosis

Diagnostics

- Mild anemia in some cats
- Eosinophilia occasionally seen
- Chemistries usually normal
- Latex agglutination or ELISA—detect cryptococcal capsular antigen in serum; few false-positive tests; most infected animals have measurable capsular antigen titers; magnitude of titer correlates with extent of infection
- Lateral radiographs of the nasopharynx—cryptococcal granuloma behind the soft palate
- Nasal radiographs (cats)—soft tissue–density material filling the nasal passage; occasional bone destruction of the nasal dorsum
- Thoracic radiographs—not indicated, unless signs of lower respiratory tract disease
- Dogs with neurologic disease—additional procedures: cytologic examination, culture of CSF, and measurement of CSF capsular antigen often make the diagnosis
- Definitive diagnosis—aspirates of the mucoid material in the nasal passages or biopsy of the granulomatous tissue that protrudes from the nares
- Patients with upper respiratory obstruction or severe respiratory noise—granuloma in the nasopharynx; identify by pulling the soft palate forward with a spay hook to expose the mass
- Biopsy—skin lesions of the head; aspirates of involved lymph nodes; usually identifies organisms
- Cultures—confirm the diagnosis; determine drug susceptibility

- Gross lesions—gray, gelatinous mass produced by the polysaccharide capsule; usually found in the nose, sinuses, and nasopharynx of cats
- Neurologic lesions—usually seen in dogs; diffuse or fungal granulomas producing a mass in the brain
- Chorioretinitis with or without retinal detachment or optic neuritis—dogs and cats
- Histologic response—usually pyogranulomatous; inflammatory cell infiltrate may be mild because the polysaccharide capsule interferes with neutrophil migration

Therapeutics

- Neurologic signs—may require inpatient supportive care until stable
- Cats—nasal obstruction influences appetite; encourage patients to eat by offering palatable food
- Patients treated with itraconazole—give medication in fatty food (e.g., canned food) to improve absorption
- Surgical removal of granulomatous masses in the nasopharynx to reduce respiratory difficulties

Drugs of Choice

- Triazole antifungal agents—expensive; itraconazole somewhat economical
- Fluconazole—preferred for ocular or CNS involvement because it is water-soluble and penetrates the nervous system better; cats, 50 mg PO q12h; dogs, 5 mg/kg PO q12h
- Itraconazole—give with a fatty meal to maximize absorption; cats, 10–15 mg/kg PO daily; dogs, 5 mg/kg PO q12h; pellets in the capsule can be mixed with food; no apparent adverse taste
- Flucytosine—100 mg/kg PO divided into 3–4 doses per day; in addition to triazole; helpful when the infection does not respond well

Contraindications

- Avoid steroids

Precautions

- Triazoles—hepatic toxicity; anorexia signals problems; monitor liver enzymes monthly
- Itraconazole—ulcerative dermatitis (differentiate from the skin lesions of cryptococcosis); new skin lesions after the disease is much improved should be considered a drug reaction
- Flucytosine—drug eruptions manifested as depigmentation of lips and nose, ulceration, exudation, and crusting of the skin; bone marrow suppression

Possible Interactions

- Itraconazole—do not give with the antihistamines terfenadine and astemizole or with cisapride

Alternative Drugs

- Amphotericin B (intravenous) and flucytosine—dogs and cats that do not respond to a triazole; monitor BUN closely to avoid permanent renal damage

Comments

- Inform client that this is a chronic disease that requires months of treatment.
- Reassure client that the infection is not zoonotic.
- Monitor liver enzymes monthly in patients receiving a triazole antifungal agent.
- Improvement in clinical signs, resolution of lesions, improvement in well-being, and return of appetite measure the response to treatment.
- Capsular antigen titers—determine response to and duration of treatment; after 2 months of treatment, the titers should decrease substantially if effective; if ineffective, try the other triazole, because organism can become resistant
- The organism is ubiquitous and cannot be avoided.
- Patients with neurologic disease may have seizures and permanent neurologic changes.
- Treatment—anticipated duration 3 months to 1 year; patients with CNS disease require lifelong maintenance
- Cats concurrently infected with FeLV or FIV—may have a worse prognosis
- Capsular antigen titers—measure every 2 months until 6 months after completion of treatment; continue treatment for 2 months after antigen is nondetectable, if possible; if patient maintains low titers for months after all signs of disease have resolved, continue treatment for at least 3 months after reduction in antigen levels and resolution of clinical signs; if titers then rise significantly, resume therapy
- Not considered zoonotic, but possibility of transmission through bite wounds
- Inform client that the organism was acquired from the environment and that he or she could be at increased risk, especially if immunosuppressed.

Suggested Reading

Berthelin CF, Bailey CS, Kass PH, et al. Cryptococcosis of the nervous system in dogs. Part 1, Epidemiologic, clinical and neuropathologic features. Prog Vet Neurol 1994;5:88–97.

Berthelin CF, Legendre AM, Bailey CS, et al. Cryptococcosis of the nervous system in dogs. Part 2, Diagnosis, treatment, monitoring and prognosis. Prog Vet Neurol 1994;5:136–146.

Jacobs GJ, Medleau L, Clavert C, et al. Cryptococcal infection in cats: factors influencing treatment outcome, and results of sequential serum antigen titers in 35 cats. J Vet Intern Med 1997;11:1–4.

Malik R, Dill-Macky E, Maring P, et al. Cryptococcosis in dogs: a retrospective study of 20 consecutive cases. J Med Vet Mycol 1995;33:291–297.

Malik R, Martin P, Wigney DI, et al. Nasopharyngeal cryptococcosis. Aust Vet J 1997;75:483–488.

Malik R, Wigney DI, Muir DB, et al. Cryptococcosis in cats: clinical and mycological assessment of 29 cases and evaluation of treatment using orally administered fluconazole. J Med Vet Mycol 1992;30:133–144.

Medleau L, Jacobs GJ, Marks A. Itraconazole for the treatment of cryptococcosis in cats. J Vet Intern Med 1995;9:39–42.

Consulting Editor Karen Helton Rhodes

Coccidioidomycosis: Systemic Mycosis

Nita Kay Gulbas

Definition/Overview

A systemic mycosis caused by the inhalation of infective arthroconidia of the soil-borne fungus *Coccidioides immitis*

Etiology/Pathophysiology

- Inhalation of infective arthroconidia is the primary route of infection. Fever, lethargy, inappetence, coughing, and joint pain or stiffness may be noticed. Dissemination may occur within 10 days of exposure, resulting in signs related to the organ system involved. Asymptomatic infections may occur, and most animals develop immunity without onset of clinical signs. The majority of animals become solidly immune after initial infection.
- Skin lesions are usually associated with dissemination, but penetrating wounds have rarely been associated with skin lesions.
- Fewer than 10 inhaled arthrospores are sufficient to cause disease in susceptible animals. "Susceptible" refers to the animals in which extrapulmonary dissemination occurs. Signs of dissemination may not be evident for several months after the initial infection.
- Respiratory—the site of initial infection
- Extrapulmonary spread may occur to long bones and joints, eyes, skin, liver, kidneys, CNS, cardiovascular system (pericardium and myocardium), and testes.
- *Coccidioides immitis* grows several inches deep in the soil, where it survives high ambient temperatures and low moisture. After a period of rainfall, the

organism returns to the soil surface where it sporulates, releasing many arthroconidia that are disseminated by wind and dust storms.
- Aggressive nosing about in soil and underbrush may expose susceptible animals to large doses of the fungus in contaminated soil.
- Dust storms after the rainy season; increased incidences are noted after earthquakes
- Land development where much earth disruption occurs may lead to increased exposure.

Signalment/History

- An uncommon disease, even in endemic areas. It occurs more commonly in dogs, and rarely in cats.
- *Coccidioides immitis* is found in the southwestern United States in the geographic Lower Sonoran life zone. It is more common in southern California, Arizona, and southwest Texas and is less prevalent in New Mexico, Nevada, and Utah.
- Most patients are young animals < 4 years of age.

Historical Findings

- Anorexia
- Coughing
- Fever unresponsive to antibiotics
- Lameness
- Weakness, paraparesis, back and neck pain
- Seizures
- Visual changes
- Weight loss

Clinical Features

Dogs

- Coughing
- Dyspnea
- Fever

Signs with Disseminated Disease

- Bone swelling, joint enlargement and lameness
- Cachexia
- Lethargy
- Lymphadenomegaly
- Neurologic dysfunction caused by dissemination to both the central and peripheral CNS
- Skin ulcers and draining tracts
- Uveitis, keratitis

Cats

- Cachexia
- Draining skin lesions

- Dyspnea
- Lameness caused by bone involvement
- Uveitis

Differential Diagnosis

- Pulmonary lesions may resemble those of other systemic mycoses (e.g., histoplasmosis, blastomycosis).
- Lymphadenomegaly may be seen in lymphosarcoma, other systemic mycoses, and localized bacterial infections.
- Bone lesions may resemble those caused by primary or metastatic bone tumors or bacterial osteomyelitis.
- Skin lesions must be differentiated from routine abscesses or other bacterial disease processes.

Diagnostics

- Hemogram—mild nonregenerative anemia, neutrophilic leukocytosis, monocytosis
- Serum chemistry profile—hyperglobulinemia, hypoalbuminemia, azotemia with renal involvement
- Urinalysis—low urine specific gravity and proteinuria with inflammatory glomerulonephritis
- Serologic tests for antibody to C. *immitis* by a laboratory proficient in handling the tests may provide a presumptive diagnosis and aid in monitoring response to therapy.
- Radiography of lung (interstitial infiltrates) and bone (osteolysis) lesions may aid in diagnosis.
- Microscopic identification of the large spherule form of C. *immitis* in lesion or biopsy material is the definitive method of diagnosis. Lymph node aspirates and impression smears of skin lesions or draining exudate may, in some patients, yield organisms.
- Caution should be used if culturing draining lesions suspected of being infected with C. *immitis*, as the mycelial form is highly contagious.
- Biopsy of infected tissue often is preferred to avoid false-negative results. Tissues involved, however, are not readily accessible and serologic testing is a more logical approach.

Pathologic Findings

- Granulomatous, suppurative or pyogranulomatous inflammation present in many tissues.
- Presence of the characteristic spherule forms in affected tissues. In some patients, the numbers of spherules present may be small.

Therapeutics

- Generally treated as outpatients. Patients treated with amphotericin B, however, will require hospitalization several times a week during their treatment period. Concurrent clinical symptoms (e.g., seizures, pain, coughing) should be treated appropriately.

- Restrict activity until clinical signs begin to subside.
- Feed a high-quality palatable diet to maintain body weight.
- The necessity and expense of long-term therapy of a serious illness with the possibility of treatment failure should be reviewed. In addition, the client should be made aware of the possible side effects of the drugs used.
- In cases of focal granulomatous organ involvement (e.g. consolidated pulmonary lung lobe, eye, kidney) surgical removal of the affected organ may be indicated.

Drugs of Choice

Coccidioidomycosis is considered the most severe and life-threatening of the systemic mycoses. Treatment of disseminated disease requires at least 1 year of aggressive antifungal therapy.

Dogs

- Several oral medications in the azole family of drugs are currently available for the treatment of coccidioidomycoses.
- Ketoconazole (KTZ) is dosed at 5–10 mg/kg PO q12h. The medication may be given with food, and there is some belief that co-administration of high doses of vitamin C may improve the absorption of the drug. Treatment should be continued for 1 year.
- Itraconazole (ITZ) is dosed at 5 mg/kg PO q12h. The drug is administered similarly as KTZ. It has been reported to have a higher penetration rate than ketoconazole, but a better clinical response has not been observed.
- Fluconazole (FCZ) is dosed at 5 mg/kg PO q12h and has been noted to greatly increase the success of treatment, especially in neurologic infections. The drug is extremely expensive, and the client should be prepared for the expense. After extended use, the frequency of dosing in some cases may be lowered to once a day.
- Amphotericin B (AMB) is less commonly recommended because of the high risk of renal damage with amphotericin B and the availability of effective oral medications. Amphotericin B can be administered at a dosage of 0.5 mg/kg IV 3 times a week, for a total cumulative dosage of 8–10 mg/kg. It is given IV either as a slow infusion (in dogs that are gravely ill) or as a rapid bolus (in fairly healthy dogs). For slow infusion, add AMB to 250–500 mL of 5% dextrose solution and administer as a drip over a period of 4–6 hours. For a rapid bolus, add AMB to 30 mL of 5% dextrose solution and administer over a period of 5 minutes through a butterfly catheter. To lessen the adverse renal effects of AMB, give 0.9% NaCl (2 mL/kg/hr) for several hours before initiating AMB therapy.
- A combination of AMB and KTZ may be used in dogs that have not responded to either drug alone or have exhibited significant toxicity. It is not clear that combination therapy is any more effective than single drug therapy in the treatment of coccidioidomycoses. For combination chemotherapy, administer AMB as described to a total cumulative dosage of 4–6 mg/kg, together with KTZ at 10 mg/kg PO divided daily for at least 8–12 months.

Cats

- Any of the following azoles may be used in cats:

  Ketoconazole 50 mg total dose PO q12h

Itraconazole 25–50 mg total dose PO q12h
Fluconazole 25–50 mg total dose PO q12h

- Alternatively, AMB can be administered by rapid IV bolus at a dosage of 0.25 mg/kg, 3 times a week, for a total cumulative dosage of 4 mg/kg. This can then be followed by long-term KTZ therapy, depending on the clinical response.

Contraindications/Precautions

- Drugs metabolized primarily by the liver should not be administered along with ketoconazole.
- Drugs metabolized primarily by the kidneys should not be administered along with AMB.
- Side effects of azoles include inappetence, vomiting, and hepatotoxicity. The drugs may be stopped until signs abate, and restarted at a lower dose that may be slowly increased to the recommended dose if the animal is able to tolerate the drug. The newer azoles (ITZ and FCZ) have fewer side effects.
- Side effects of AMB therapy can be severe and include renal dysfunction, fever, inappetence, vomiting, and phlebitis.

Comments

Patient Monitoring

- Serologic titers should be monitored every 2–3 months. Animals should be treated until their titers fall to less than 1:2. Animals displaying poor response to therapy should have a 2–4 hour post pill drug level measured to assure adequate absorption of the drug.
- BUN and urinalysis should be monitored in all animals treated with AMB. Treatment should be temporarily discontinued if the BUN rises above 50 mg/dL or granular casts are noted in the urine.

Prevention/Avoidance

- No vaccine is available for dogs or cats.
- Contaminated soil in endemic areas should be avoided, particularly during dust storms after the rainy season.

Possible Complications

- Pulmonary disease resulting in severe coughing may temporarily worsen after therapy has begun owing to inflammation in the lungs. Low-dose short-term oral prednisone and cough suppressants may be required to alleviate the respiratory signs.
- Hepatotoxicity may result from KTZ therapy.
- Nephrotoxicity may result from AMB therapy.

Expected Course and Prognosis

- The prognosis is guarded to grave. Many dogs will improve following oral therapy; however, relapses may be seen, especially if therapy is shortened. The overall recovery rate has been estimated at 60%, but some report a 90% response to fluconazole therapy.
- The prognosis for cats is not well documented, but rapid dissemination requiring long-term therapy should be anticipated.

- Serologic testing every 3–4 months after completion of therapy is recommended to monitor the possibility of relapse.
- Spontaneous recovery from disseminated coccidioidomycosis without treatment is extremely rare.

Zoonotic Potential

The spherule form of the fungus, as found in animal tissues, is not directly transmissible to people or other animals. Under certain rare circumstances, however, there could be reversion to growth of the infective mold form of the fungus on or within bandages placed over a draining lesion or in contaminated bedding. Draining lesions can lead to contamination of the environment with arthrospores. Care should be exercised whenever handling an infected draining lesion. Special precautions should be recommended to households where the owners may be immunosuppressed.

Pregnancy

- KTZ should be used in pregnant animals only if the potential benefit justifies the potential risk to offspring.
- Teratogenic effects of AMB have not been identified.

Suggested Reading

Armstrong PJ, DiBartola SP. Canine coccidioidomycosis: a literature review and report of eight cases. J Am Anim Hosp Assoc 1983;19:937–945.

Greene RT. Coccidioidomycosis. In: Greene CE, ed. Infectious diseases of the dog and cat. 2nd ed. Philadelphia: Saunders, 1998:391–398.

Legendre AM. Coccidioidomycosis. In: Sherding RG, ed. The cat: diseases and clinical management. 2nd ed. New York: Churchill Livingstone, 1994:561–562.

Stevens DA. Coccidioidomycosis. N Engl J Med 1995;332:1077–1082.

Consulting Editor Karen Helton Rhodes

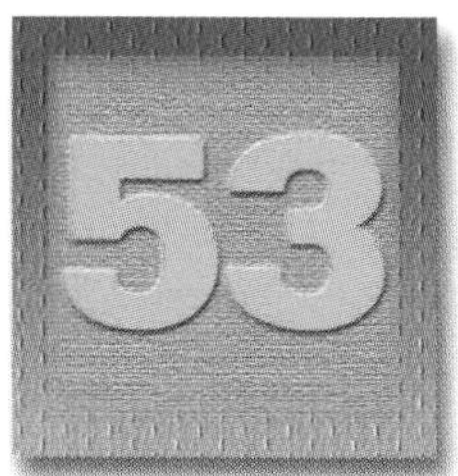

BLASTOMYCOSIS: SYSTEMIC MYCOSIS

Alfred M. Legendre

Definition/Overview

A systemic, mycotic infection caused by the soil organism *Blastomyces dermatitidis*

Etiology/Pathophysiology

- A small spore (conidia) is shed from the mycelial phase of the organism growing in the soil and inhaled, entering the terminal airway.
- At body temperature, the spore becomes a yeast, which initiates the infection in the lungs.
- From this focus of mycotic pneumonia, the yeast disseminates hematogenously throughout the body.
- The immune response to the invading organism produces a pyogranulomatous infiltrate to control the organism.
- The result is organ dysfunction.
- Respiratory—85% of affected dogs have lung disease
- Eyes, skin, lymphatic system, and bones—commonly affected
- Brain, testes, prostate, mammary gland, nasal cavity, gums, and vulva—less commonly affected

Signalment/History

- No genetic predisposition identified
- Depends on environmental and soil conditions that favor growth of *Blastomyces*

- Some areas of Wisconsin—incidence in dogs reaches 1,420/100,000 annually
- Wet environment—fosters growth of the fungus; banks of rivers, streams, and lakes or in swamps; most affected dogs live within 400 m of water
- Exposure to recently excavated areas
- Most common along the Mississippi, Ohio, and Tennessee River basins
- Large breed dogs weighing ≤ 25 kg, especially sporting breeds; may reflect exposure rather than susceptibility
- Dogs—most common 2–4 years of age; uncommon after 7 years of age
- Cats—young to middle-aged
- Dogs—males predominant sex

Historical Findings

- Weight loss
- Depressed appetite
- Cough and dyspnea
- Eye inflammation and discharge
- Lameness
- Draining skin lesions (Figs. 53-1, 53-2)

Clinical Features

Dogs

- Fever up to 104.0°F (40°C)—approximately 50% of patients
- Harsh, dry lung sounds associated with increased respiratory effort—common

Figure 53-1 Focal ulcerated and draining skin lesions of the facial region in this dog owing to blastomycosis. (Courtesy of Dr. Carol Foil.)

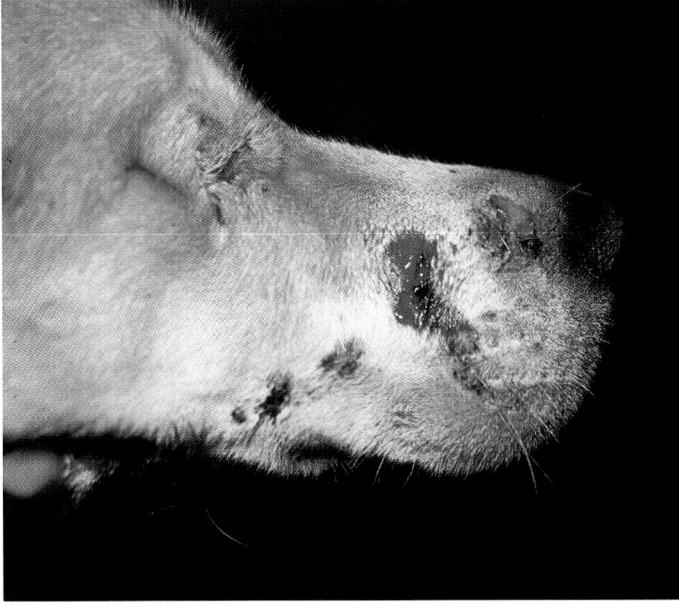

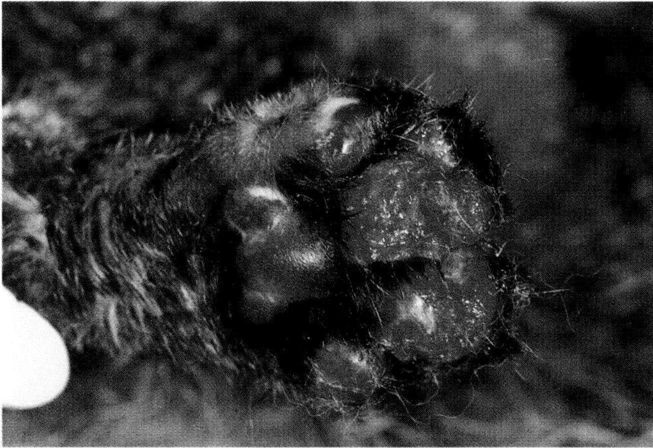

Figure 53-2 Severe ulceration of the foot pad in the cat owing to blastomycosis. (Courtesy of Dr. Carol Foil.)

- Generalized or regional lymphadenopathy with or without skin lesions
- Uveitis with or without secondary glaucoma and conjunctivitis, ocular exudates, and corneal edema
- Lameness—common owing to fungal osteomyelitis
- Testicular enlargement and prostatomegaly—occasionally seen

Cats

- Increased respiratory effort
- Granulomatous skin lesions

Differential Diagnosis

- Respiratory signs—bacterial pneumonia, neoplasia, heart failure, or other fungal infection
- Lymph node enlargement—similar to lymphosarcoma
- The combination of respiratory disease with eye, bone, and skin involvement in a young dog suggests the diagnosis.

Diagnostics

- CBC changes reflect mild to moderate inflammation.
- High serum globulin with borderline low albumin concentrations in dogs with chronic infections
- Hypercalcemia in some dogs secondary to the granulomatous changes
- *Blastomyces* yeasts can be found in the urine of dogs with prostatic involvement.
- AGID—useful for making a diagnosis if organisms cannot be found on cytology or histopathology; positive test strongly supports diagnosis, with a specificity of > 90% negative tests common in dogs with early infection

RADIOGRAPHS

- Lungs—essential for diagnosis and prognosis
- Generalized interstitial to nodular infiltrate
- Tracheobronchial lymphadenopathy—common
- Changes—inconsistent with bacterial pneumonia; may resemble metastatic tumors, especially hemangiosarcoma
- Focal bone lesions—lytic and proliferative; can be mistaken for osteosarcoma

CYTOLOGY/HISTOPATHOLOGY

- Cytology of lymph node aspirates, tracheal wash fluid, or impression smears of draining skin lesions—best method for diagnosis
- Histopathology of bone biopsies or enucleated blind eyes—identify the organism
- Organisms—usually plentiful in the tissues; may be scarce in tracheal washes if there is no productive cough

PATHOLOGIC FINDINGS

- Lesions—pyogranulomatous with many thick-walled, budding yeasts; occasionally very fibrous with few organisms found
- Lungs with large amounts of inflammatory infiltrate do not collapse when the chest is opened.
- Special fungal stains—facilitate finding the organisms

Therapeutics

- Severely dyspneic dogs—require an oxygen cage for a minimum of 1 week before lung improvement is sufficient for comfort in room air; many have worsening of lung disease during the first few days of treatment, owing to an increase in the inflammatory response after the *Blastomyces* organisms die and release their contents.
- Patients with respiratory compromise must be restricted.
- Removal of an abscessed lung lobe may be required when medical treatment cannot resolve the infection.

DRUGS OF CHOICE

Itraconazole

- Dogs—5 mg/kg PO q12h with a fat-rich meal, such as canned dog food, for the first 3 days to achieve a therapeutic blood concentration as soon as possible; then reduce to one a day
- Cats—5 mg/kg PO q12h; open the 100-mg capsules containing pellets and mix with palatable food
- Treat for a minimum of 60 days or for 1 month after all signs of disease have disappeared.

ALTERNATIVE DRUGS

- Amphotericin B—0.5 mg/kg IV every other day in dogs that cannot take oral medication or that do not respond to itraconazole (see Histoplasmosis); use the lipid complex for dogs with renal dysfunction that cannot take itraconazole
- Ketoconazole—10 mg/kg PO q12h; cheaper alternative to itraconazole; lower response rate and higher recurrence rate

CONTRAINDICATIONS/PRECAUTIONS

- Corticosteroids—usually contraindicated because the anti-inflammatory effects allow uninhibited proliferation of the organisms; patients with previous steroid therapy require a longer duration of treatment; for dogs with life-threatening dyspnea, dexamethasone (0.2 mg/kg daily) may be lifesaving when given in conjunction with itraconazole treatment; discontinue steroids as soon as possible

Itraconazole Toxicity

- Anorexia—most common sign; attributed to liver toxicity; monitor serum ALT monthly for duration of treatment or when anorexia occurs; temporarily discontinue drug for patients with anorexia and ALT activities > 200; after appetite improves, restart at half the previously used dose
- Ulcerative dermatitis—seen in some dogs; the result of vasculitis; dose-related condition; temporarily discontinue drug; when ulcers have resolved, restart at half the previously used dose
- For humans, itraconazole is contraindicated with terfenadine and cisapride.

Comments

- Serum chemistry—monthly to monitor for hepatic toxicity or if anorexia develops
- No teratogenic effects of itraconazole at therapeutic doses in rats and mice; embryotoxicity found at high doses; no dog or cat studies; one dog started on itraconazole halfway through her pregnancy delivered a normal litter.

THORACIC RADIOGRAPHS

- Determine duration of treatment.
- Considerable permanent changes in the lungs after the infection has resolved may occur, making determination of persistent active disease difficult.
- At 60 days of treatment—if active lung disease is seen, continue treatment for 30 days
- At 90 days of treatment—if the same as day 60, changes are residual effects of inactive disease; if better than day 60, continue treatment for 30 days; if worse than day 60, continue treatment for 30 days more, then re-radiograph
- At 120 days of treatment—re-radiograph. If worse, continue treatment for further 30 days and then re-radiograph. If inactive disease, continue treatment for 30 more days and then stop.

PREVENTION/AVOIDANCE

- Location of environmental growth of *Blastomyces* organisms unknown; thus difficult to avoid exposure; restricting exposure to lakes and streams could be done but is not very practical.
- Dogs that recover from the infection are probably immune to reinfection.

EXPECTED COURSE AND PROGNOSIS

- Death—25% of dogs die during the first week of treatment; early diagnosis improves chance of survival.
- Severity of lung involvement and invasion into the brain affect prognosis.

- Recurrence—about 20% of dogs; usually within 3–6 months after completion of treatment, even with 60–90 days of treatment; may occur up to 15 months after treatment; a second course of itraconazole treatment will cure most patients; drug resistance to itraconazole has not been observed

Zoonotic Potential

- Not spread from animals to people, except through bite wounds; inoculation of organisms from dog bites has occurred.
- Avoid cuts during necropsy of infected dogs and avoid needle sticks when aspirating lesions.
- Warn clients that blastomycosis is acquired from an environmental source and that they may have been exposed at the same time as the patient; common source exposure has been documented in duck and coon hunters; the incidence in dogs is 10 times that in humans.
- Encourage clients with respiratory and skin lesions to inform their physicians that they may have been exposed to blastomycosis.

Suggested Reading

Krawiec DR, McKiernan BC, Twardock AR, et al. Use of amphotericin B lipid complex for treatment of blastomycosis in dogs. J Am Vet Med Assoc 1996;209:2073–2075.

Legendre AM, Rohrbach BW, Toal RL, et al. Treatment of blastomycosis with itraconazole in 112 dogs. J Vet Intern Med 1996;10:365–371.

Legendre AM. Blastomycosis. In: Greene CE, ed., Infectious diseases of the dog and cat. Philadelphia: Saunders, 1998:371–377.

Consulting Editor Karen Helton Rhodes

Leishmaniasis: Protozoan Dermatosis

Stephen C. Barr

Overview/Definition

- Protozoan—genus *Leishmania;* causes two types of disease: cutaneous and visceral
- Organ systems affected—cutaneous: skin, hepatobiliary, spleen, kidneys, eyes, and joints; visceral: hemorrhagic diathesis
- Affected dogs in the U.S. invariably acquired infection in another country.

Etiology/Pathophysiology

- *L. donovani infantum*—Mediterranean basin, Portugal, and Spain; sporadic cases in Switzerland, northern France, and the Netherlands
- *L. donovani* complex or *L. braziliensis*—endemic areas of South and Central America and southern Mexico
- Endemic cases in dogs (Oklahoma and Ohio) and cats (Texas) have been reported in the U.S., although the disease is not considered endemic here.
- Sandfly vectors—transmit flagellated parasites into the skin of a host
- Cats—often localizes in skin
- Dogs—invariably spreads throughout the body to most organs; renal failure is the most common cause of death
- Incubation period—1 month to several years

Signalment/History

- Dogs—virtually all develop visceral, or systemic, disease; 90% also have cutaneous involvement; no sex or breed predilection

- Cats—cutaneous disease (rare); no sex or breed predilection
- Travel to endemic regions (usually the Mediterranean), where dogs are exposed to infected sandflies
- Transfusion from infected animals can occur.

Clinical Features

Visceral

- Exercise intolerance
- Severe weight loss and anorexia
- Diarrhea, vomiting, epistaxis, and melena—less common
- Dogs—lymphadenopathy; cutaneous lesions; emaciation; signs of renal failure (polyuria, polydipsia, vomiting) possible; neuralgia, polyarthritis, polymyositis, osteolytic lesions, and proliferative periostitis rare; about one-third of patients have fever and splenomegaly

Cutaneous

- Hyperkeratosis—most prominent finding excessive epidermal scale with thickening, depigmentation, and chapping of the muzzle and footpads (Figs. 54-1, 54-2)
- Hair coat—dry; brittle; hair loss
- Dogs—intradermal nodules and ulcers may be seen; abnormally long or brittle nails are a specific finding in some patients
- Cats—cutaneous nodules usually develop

Differential Diagnosis

- Visceral—mycoses (blastomycosis, histoplasmosis); systemic lupus erythematosus; metastatic neoplasia; distemper; vasculitis

Figure 54-1 Leishmaniasis. Focal alopecia with diffuse hyperkeratosis. (Courtesy of Dr. Carol Foil.)

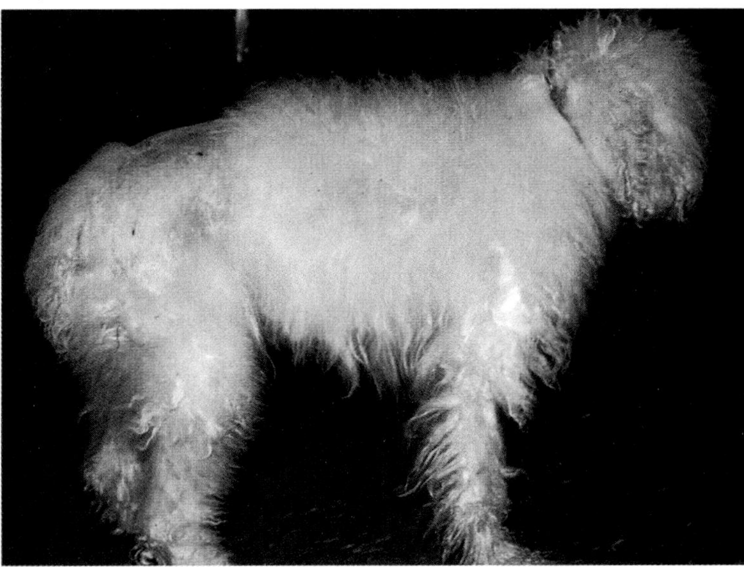

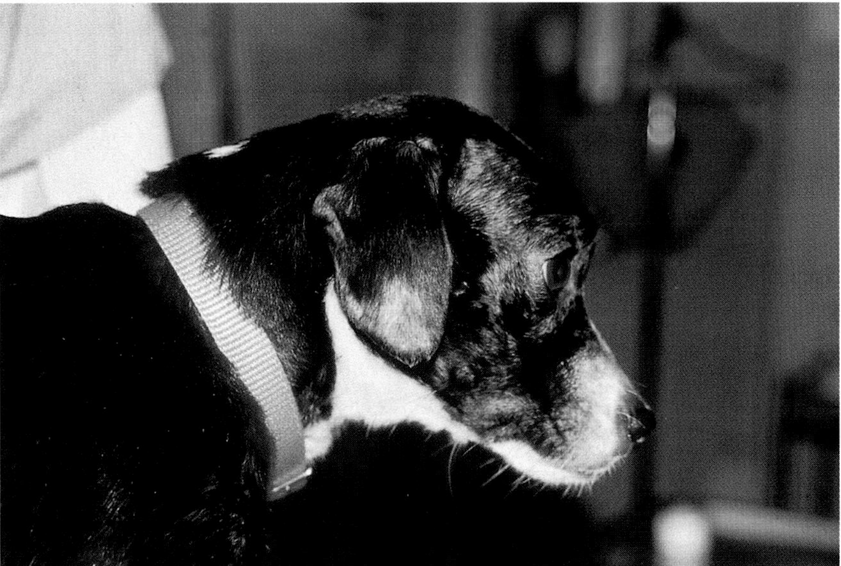

Figure 54-2 Alopecia with multifocal nodules in the dog—associated with leishmaniasis. (Courtesy of Dr. Carol Foil.)

- Cutaneous—other causes of hyperkeratosis: primary idiopathic seborrhea and nutritional dermatoses (vitamin A responsive, zinc responsive); idiopathic nasodigital hyperkeratosis, lichenoid-psoriasiform dermatosis, epidermal dysplasia, and schnauzer comedo syndrome are rare and breed-specific
- Skin biopsy—hyperkeratotic and nodular lesions; existence of organisms confirms diagnosis
- Hyperglobulinemia—differentiate from chronic ehrlichiosis and multiple myeloma

Diagnostics

- Hyperproteinemia with hyperglobulinemia—100% of cases
- Hypoalbuminemia—95% of cases
- Proteinuria—85% of cases
- High liver enzyme activity—55% of cases
- Thrombocytopenia—50% of cases
- Azotemia—45% of cases
- Leukopenia with lymphopenia—20% of cases
- Coombs, antinuclear antibody, and lupus erythematosus cell tests—sometimes positive
- Serologic diagnosis available
- Cultures—skin, spleen, bone marrow, or lymph node biopsies or aspirates; by the Centers for Disease Control and Prevention
- Cytology and histopathology—identify intracellular organisms in biopsies or aspirate specimens (listed above)

Pathologic Findings

- Cell infiltration (mainly histiocytes and macrophages) and characteristic intracellular amastigote forms—identified in many tissues: skin, lymph nodes, liver, spleen, and kidney
- Mucosal ulcerations—stomach, intestine, and colon, occasionally found

Therapeutics

- Emaciated, chronically infected animals—consider euthanasia; prognosis very poor
- Diet—high-quality protein; special for renal insufficiency, if necessary
- Cats—single dermal nodule lesions are best surgically removed
- Advise client of potential zoonotic transmission of organisms in lesions to humans.
- Inform client that organisms will never be eliminated, and relapse, requiring treatment, is inevitable.

Drugs

- Sodium stibogluconate—available from the Centers for Disease Control and Prevention; 30–50 mg/kg IV or SC q24h for 3–4 weeks
- Meglumine antimonate—100 mg/kg IV or SC q24h for 3–4 weeks
- Allopurinol—very efficacious in treating one dog; 7 mg/kg PO q8h for 3 months
- γ-interferon given with antimonials—good success in humans

Contraindications/Precautions

- Seriously ill dogs—start antimonial drugs at lower doses
- Renal insufficiency—treat before giving antimonial drugs; prognosis depends on renal function at the onset of treatment

Comments

- Treatment efficacy—monitor by clinical improvement and identification of organisms in repeat biopsies
- Relapses—a few months to a year after therapy; recheck at least every 2 months after completion of treatment
- Prognosis for a cure—very guarded; antimonial therapy gives dogs some quality of life

Suggested Reading

Slappendel RJ, Ferner L. Leishmaniasis. In: Greene CE, ed. Infectious diseases of the dog and cat. Philadelphia: Saunders, 1998:450–458.

Consulting Editor Karen Helton Rhodes

Feline Calicivirus

Fred W. Scott

Definition/Overview

A common viral respiratory disease of domestic and exotic cats characterized by upper respiratory signs, oral ulceration, pneumonia, and occasionally arthritis

Etiology/Pathophysiology

- Rapid cytolysis of infected cells with resulting tissue pathology and clinical disease
- A small, nonenveloped single-stranded RNA virus; numerous strains exist in nature, with varying degrees of antigenic cross-reactivity; more than one serotype; relatively stable and resistant to many disinfectants.
- Respiratory—rhinitis; interstitial pneumonia; ulceration of the tip of the nose
- Ophthalmic—acute serous conjunctivitis without keratitis or corneal ulcers
- Musculoskeletal—acute arthritis
- Gastrointestinal—ulceration of the tongue common; occasional ulceration of the hard palate and lips; infection occurs in intestines; usually no clinical disease

Signalment/History

- Persistent infection common
- Clinical disease—common in multicat facilities and breeding catteries
- Routine vaccination—reduced incidence of clinical disease; has not decreased the prevalence of the virus

- Concurrent infections with other pathogens (e.g., FHV-1 or FPV)
- Poor ventilation
- Young kittens > 6 weeks old—most common
- Cats of any age may show clinical disease.

Clinical Features

- May present as an upper respiratory infection with eye and nose involvement, as an ulcerative disease primarily of the mouth, as pneumonia, as an acute arthritis, or any combination of these (Fig. 55-1)
- Sudden onset
- Anorexia
- Ocular or nasal discharge, usually with little or no sneezing
- Ulcers on the tongue, hard palate, lips, tip of nose, or around claws
- Dyspnea from pneumonia
- Acute, painful lameness
- Generally alert and in good condition
- Fever
- Ulcers may occur without other signs.

Differential Diagnosis

- Feline viral rhinotracheitis
- Chlamydiosis
- *Bordetella bronchiseptica*

Figure 55-1 Calicivirus infection in the cat. Note the erythema and erosions along the periocular and facial region. (Courtesy of Dr. Joe Taboada.)

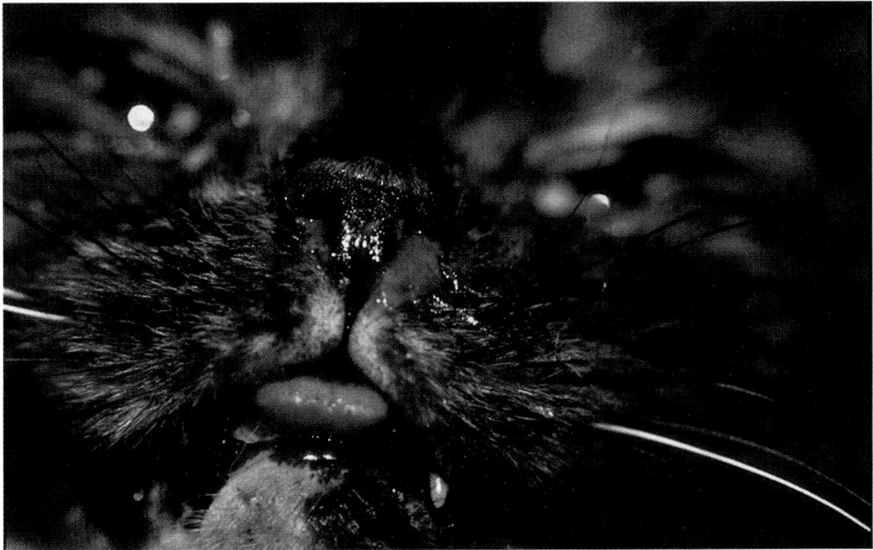

Diagnostics

- Serologic testing on paired serum samples—detect a rise in neutralizing antibody titers against the virus
- Radiographs of the lungs—a consolidation of lung tissue in cats with pneumonia
- Cell cultures to isolating the virus—oral pharynx; lung tissue; feces; blood; secretions from the nose and conjunctiva
- Immunofluorescent assays of lung tissue—viral antigen

Pathologic Findings

- Gross—upper respiratory infection; ocular and nasal discharge; pneumonia with consolidation of large portions of individual lung lobes; possible ulcerations on the tongue, lips, and hard palate
- Histopathologic—interstitial pneumonia of large portions of individual lung lobes; ulcerations on epithelium of the tongue, lips, and hard palate; mild inflammatory reactions in the nose and conjunctiva

Therapeutics

- Outpatient, unless severe pneumonia occurs
- Clean eyes and nose as indicated.
- Provide soft foods.
- Oxygen—with severe pneumonia
- Patients should be restricted from contact with other cats to prevent transmission of the disease.
- Soft foods—if ulcerations restrict eating
- Discuss the need for proper vaccination and the need to modify the vaccination protocol in breeding catteries to include kittens before they become infected (often at 6–8 weeks of age) from a carrier queen.
- No specific antiviral drugs that are effective
- Broad-spectrum antibiotics—usually indicated (e.g., amoxicillin at 22 mg/kg PO q12h)
- Secondary bacterial infections of affected cats are not nearly as important as with FHV-1 infections.
- Antibiotic eye ointments—to reduce secondary bacterial infections of the conjunctiva
- Appropriate pain medication—for transient arthritis pain

Comments

Patient Monitoring

- Monitor for sudden development of dyspnea associated with pneumonia.
- No specific laboratory tests

Prevention/Avoidance

- All cats should be vaccinated at the same time they are vaccinated against FHV-1; routine vaccination with either MLV or inactivated vaccines should be done at 8–10 weeks of age and repeated 3–4 weeks later.

- Breeding catteries—respiratory disease is a problem; vaccinate kittens at an earlier age, either with an additional vaccination at 4–5 weeks of age or with intranasal administration at 10–14 days of age; follow-up vaccinations at 6, 10, and 14 weeks of age
- Annual vaccines recommended; immunity undoubtedly lasts > 1 year
- American Association of Feline Practitioners—classifies FHV, FPV, and calicivirus as core vaccines; recommends vaccination of all cats with these three agents on the initial visit, after 12 weeks of age, and 1 year later; boosters for calicivirus should be given every 3 years
- Vaccination will not eliminate infection in a subsequent exposure but will prevent clinical disease caused by most strains.

Possible Complications

- Interstitial pneumonia—most serious complication; can be life-threatening
- Secondary bacterial infections of the lungs or upper airways
- Oral ulcers and the acute arthritis usually heal without complications.

Expected Course and Prognosis

- Clinical disease—usually appears 3–4 days after exposure
- Once neutralizing antibodies appear, about 7 days after exposure, recovery is usually rapid.
- Prognosis excellent, unless severe pneumonia develops
- Recovered cats—persistently infected for long periods; will continuously shed small quantities of virus in oral secretions
- Affected cats may also be concurrently infected with FHV-1, especially in multicat and breeding facilities.

Suggested Reading

Barr MC, Olsen CW, Scott FW. Feline viral diseases. In: Ettinger SJ, Feldman EC, eds. Veterinary internal medicine. 4th ed. Philadelphia: Saunders, 1995:409–439.

Elston T, Rodan I, Flemming D, et al. 1998 report of the American Association of Feline Practitioners and Academy of Feline Medicine Advisory Panel on feline vaccines. J Am Vet Med Assoc 1998;212:227–241.

Ford RB, Levy JK. Infectious diseases of the respiratory tract. In: Sherding RG, ed. The cat: diseases and clinical management. New York: Churchill Livingstone, 1994:489–500.

Ford RB. Role of infectious agents in respiratory disease. Vet Clin North Am Sm Anim Pract 1993;23:17–35.

Pedersen NC. Feline calicivirus infection. In: Pratt PW, ed. Feline infectious diseases. Goleta, CA: American Veterinary, 1988:61–67.

Consulting Editor Karen Helton Rhodes

Feline Pox Virus Infection

J. Paul Woods

Overview/Definition

- Rare orthopoxvirus that affects cats and causes a papular, crusted, and ulcerative dermatitis

Etiology/Pathophysiology

- Member of the genus *Orthopoxvirus,* family Poxviridae
- Enveloped DNA virus, resistant to drying (viable for years) but readily inactivated by most disinfectants
- Geographically limited to Eurasia
- Relatively common

Signalment/History

- Cats—domestic and exotic
- No age, sex, or breed predisposition
- Reservoir host—wild rodents
- Infection thought to be acquired during hunting; most common in young adults and active hunters, often from rural environment
- Lesions—often develop at the site of a bite wound (presumably inflicted by the prey animal carrying the virus)
- Most cases occur in autumn, when small wild mammals are at maximum population and most active.

- Severe cutaneous and systemic signs with poor prognosis are frequently associated with immunosuppression (iatrogenic or co-infection with FeLV or FIV).
- Cat-to-cat transmission—rare; causes only subclinical infection
- Skin lesions—multiple, circular; dominant feature; usually develop on head, neck, or forelimbs
- Primary lesions—crusted papules, plaques, nodules, crateriform ulcers, or areas of cellulitis or abscesses
- Secondary lesions—erythematous nodules that ulcerate and crust; often widespread; develop after 1–3 weeks
- Pruritus variable
- Systemic—20% of cases; anorexia; lethargy; pyrexia; vomiting; diarrhea; oculonasal discharge; conjunctivitis; pneumonia

Differential Diagnosis

- Bacterial and fungal infections
- Eosinophilic granuloma complex
- Neoplasia—particularly mast cell tumor; lymphosarcoma
- Miliary dermatitis

Diagnostics

- Serologic testing—demonstrate rising titers; hemagglutination inhibition, virus neutralizing, complement fixation, or ELISA; titers may remain high for months or years
- Virus isolation from scab material—definitive diagnosis; 90% positive
- Electron microscopy of extracts of scab, biopsy, or exudate—rapid presumptive diagnosis; 70% positive
- Skin biopsy—characteristic histologic changes of epidermal hyperplasia and hypertrophy; multilocular vesicle and ulceration; large eosinophilic intracytoplasmic inclusion bodies

Therapeutics

- No specific treatment
- Supportive (antibiotics, fluids) when necessary
- Elizabethan collar—to prevent self-induced damage
- Antibiotics—prevent secondary infections
- Immunosuppressive agents (e.g., glucocorticoids and megestrol acetate)—absolutely contraindicated because they can induce fatal systemic disease

Comments

- Natural reservoir host is possibly small rodents; cats infected incidentally
- Vaccines—none available; vaccinia virus may be considered for valuable zoo collections, but its effects in nondomestic cats have not been investigated
- Most cats recover spontaneously in 1–2 months.

- Healing may be delayed by secondary bacterial skin infection.
- Prognosis is poor with severe respiratory or pulmonary involvement.
- Rare human pox virus infections have been linked to contact with infected cats with skin lesions; use basic hygiene precautions (disposable gloves) when handling infected cats.
- May cause painful skin lesions and severe systemic illness, particularly in the very young or elderly, people with a pre-existing skin condition, and the immunodeficient.

Suggested Reading

Gaskell RM, Bennett M. Feline poxvirus infection. In: Chandler EA, Gaskell CJ, Gaskell RM, eds. Feline medicine and therapeutics. Oxford, UK: Blackwell Scientific, 1994:515–520.

Consulting Editor Karen Helton Rhodes

Canine Papillomatosis

Suzette M. LeClerc and Edward G. Clark

Overview/Definition

- Papillomaviruses (PVs)—group of nonenveloped, double-stranded DNA viruses that induce proliferative cutaneous tumors in cats and dogs and mucosal tumors in dogs; each is host and fairly site-specific, with characteristic clinical and microscopic changes in infected tissues
- Tumors—papillomas, warts, or verrucae; generally benign; spontaneously regress; rarely may undergo conversion to SCC
- Lesions—often multiple, well demarcated, and exophytic; sometimes hyperkeratotic plaques or with papules; may be deeply pigmented (black or brown), pink, tan, or white

Etiology/Pathophysiology

- Infection—inoculation through breaks in the epidermis or mucosal epithelium; iatrogenic transmission through use of contaminated instruments possible

Signalment/History

Dogs

- At least five types of PV may infect dogs.
- Oral and ocular papillomas—generally seen in young animals (6 months to 4 years); however, any age may be affected

- Cutaneous papillomas—any age
- Miniature schnauzers and pugs—pigmented sessile papillomas generally manifest before 5 years of age

Cats

- Feline papillomatosis and Bowen's disease—old animals (7 years and up)
- PV-induced lesions have been identified in kittens.
- No breed predisposition
- *Cutaneous* (dogs and cats)—immunosuppression (acquired, congenital, or iatrogenic from use of corticosteroids) facilitates all types of PV infection; defects in cell-mediated immunity thought to have a permissive effect on the persistence of PV-induced lesions

Historical Findings

- Dysphagia
- Ptyalism
- Reluctance to eat
- Halitosis—dogs with oral papillomas

Clinical Features

Dogs

- True cutaneous papillomas—rare; lesion is an exophytic, often pedunculated, papilliferous growth consisting of multiple fronds of epithelium; may be found anywhere on the body; rarely exceed 1 cm in diameter (Fig. 57-1)
- Venereal warts—affect the lower genital tract; probably caused by a novel PV

Figure 57-1 Young beagle with oral papillomas and a single cutaneous papilloma at the mucocutaneous junction of the eyelid. (Courtesy of K. Isakow.)

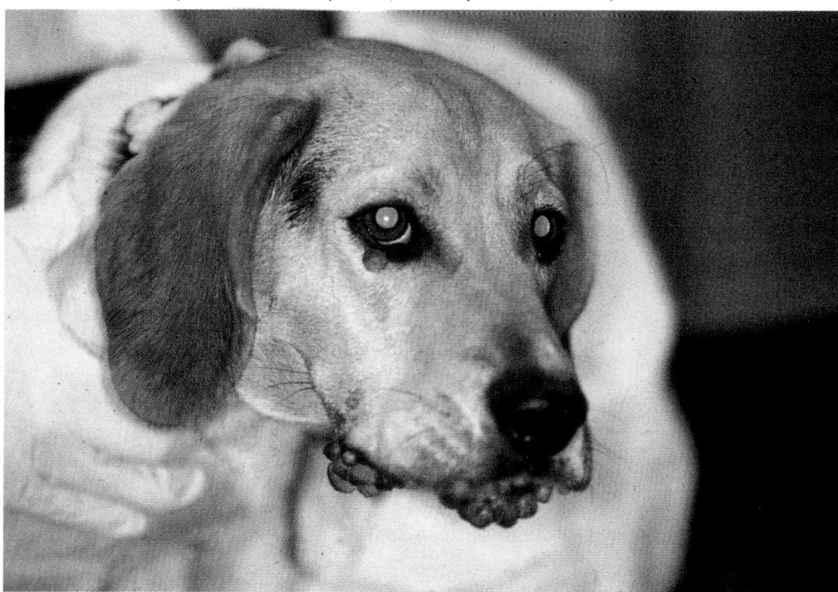

- Cutaneous inverted papillomas—rare; caused by a unique PV; lesions: generally found on the ventral trunk and abdomen, 1–2 cm in diameter, raised and firm, small pore opening to the skin surface
- Familial form—rare; pugs and miniature schnauzers; up to 80 scaly, black plaques scattered on the ventral neck, trunk, and medial aspects of limbs (pigmented epidermal nevi and lentiginosis profusa)

Oral

- Multiple tumors (as many as 100) on the mucocutaneous junctions around the mouth, lips, tongue, palate, epiglottis, and upper esophagus and on the mucosa of the oropharynx
- Early papillomas—discrete, pale, smooth elevations of the mucosa; proceed to develop a filiform to cauliflower-like appearance
- Lesions—may bleed and be ulcerated owing to trauma from teeth
- Halitosis and discharge from the mouth—with secondary bacterial infection of traumatized lesions
- Respiratory distress—rare; multiple tumors may obstruct the airway
- The canine oral PV is believed to be the cause of some eyelid, corneal, and conjunctival papillomas.

CATS

- Exophytic papillomas—exceedingly rare
- Cutaneous—multifocal to coalescing plaques of epidermal hyperplasia that may be pigmented or waxy and white
- Lesions—persistent; may progress to SCC (Bowen's disease or multicentric SCC in situ) (Fig. 57-2)
- SCC in situ lesions—well demarcated; deeply pigmented; erythematous; crusted; occasionally ulcerated; may progress to invasive SCC

Figure 57-2 Multiple lesions of Bowen's disease (feline cutaneous squamous cell carcinoma in situ) and squamous cell carcinoma in an aged cat. (Courtesy of C. Sousa.)

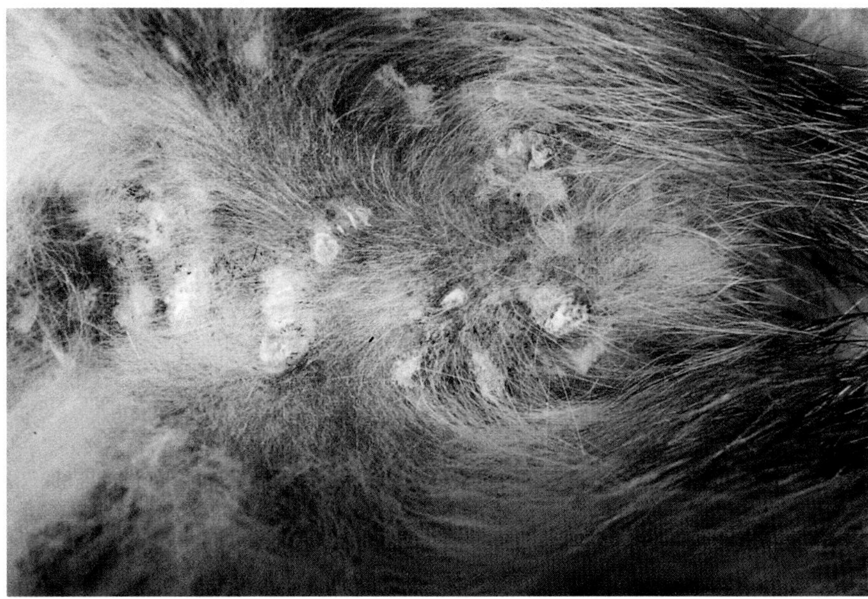

Differential Diagnosis

Dogs

- Oral cavity and oropharynx—fibromatous epulis; transmissible venereal tumor; if ulcerated, SCC
- Cutaneous—sebaceous hyperplasias; cutaneous tags
- Pigmented—melanomas
- Inverted—intracutaneous cornifying epitheliomas

Cats

- Multiple sessile, hyperkeratotic lesions—eosinophilic granulomas or plaques; actinic keratosis; cutaneous lesions of FeLV; multicentric SCC in situ; SCC

Diagnostics

- Oral papillomatosis—gross appearance and physical examination findings generally provide the diagnosis; biopsy of one or two lesions may be used for confirmation
- Histopathology—generally required for cutaneous, venereal, and some ocular papillomas
- Immunohistochemistry—avidin-biotin complex method to detect PV group-related antigens; dogs: helps make the diagnosis; cats: recommended for confirmation of diagnosis

Therapeutics

- Oral—self-limiting; lesions generally regress spontaneously
- Surgery to remove oral tumors (excision, cryosurgery, or electrosurgery)—airway is being occluded; patient is unable to eat comfortably; aesthetic reasons
- Systemic corticosteroids—withdraw if severe or persistent oral or cutaneous disease reoccurs
- Persistent disease (dogs)—may treat with autovaccination; use heat-inactivated autogenous vaccine
- Cats—no efficacious therapy for chronic PV-induced skin lesions; SCC in situ lesions may respond to ^{90}Sr plesiotherapy

Comments

- Monitor lesions carefully to detect signs (ulceration, purulent exudation, and rapid growth) of malignant transformation to SCC.
- Separate dogs with oral papillomatosis from susceptible animals.
- Commercial kennels with outbreaks of oral papillomatosis—may use autogenous vaccines
- Live canine oral PV vaccine—reported to induce hyperplastic epithelial tumors and SCC at vaccination sites; latency period 11–34 months
- Dogs—prognosis usually good; incubation period 1–8 weeks; regression usually occurs at 1–5 months; lesions may persist for 24 months or more

- Cats—long-term prognosis for chronic papillomatosis and Bowen's disease uncertain

Abbreviations

- FeLV = feline leukemia virus
- SCC = squamous cell carcinoma

Suggested Reading

Sundberg JP. Papillomaviruses. In: Castro AE, Heuscele WP, eds. Veterinary diagnostic virology. St. Louis: Mosby, 1992:148–150.

Consulting Editor Karen Helton Rhodes

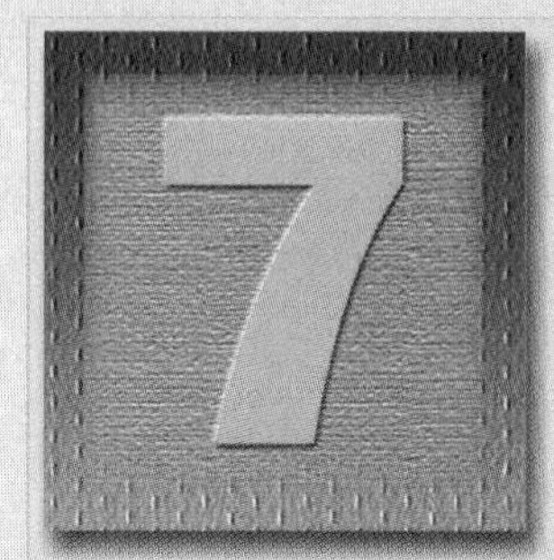

Endocrine Dermatoses

HYPOTHYROIDISM

John W. Tyler

Definition/Overview

- Clinical condition that results from inadequate production and release of tetraiodothyronine (levothyroxine, T_4) and triiodothyronine (liothyronine, T_3) by the thyroid gland
- Characterized by a generalized decrease in cellular metabolic activity

Etiology/Pathophysiology

ACQUIRED HYPOTHYROIDISM

- In dogs, primary acquired hypothyroidism is the most common (>95% of cases) type.
- Caused by lymphocytic thyroiditis (50%) or idiopathic thyroid atrophy (50%)
- Lymphocytic thyroiditis is thought to be immune mediated (cellular and humoral).
- Circulating autoantibodies to thyroglobulin, T_3, or T_4 are usually present, but these autoantibodies can also be found in a variable percentage (13–40%) of normal, euthyroid dogs.
- Rarely, primary hypothyroidism is caused by neoplastic (primary or metastatic) destruction of the thyroid gland or dietary iodine deficiency.
- Rare in cats and is most commonly seen following bilateral thyroidectomy or radioactive iodine therapy; it is often transitory and frequently does not require therapy.

- Accessory thyroid tissue in the neck or thoracic cavity usually undergoes hyperplasia and produces physiologic amounts of thyroid hormones.
- Acquired secondary hypothyroidism is very uncommon in dogs and cats; it is caused by pituitary dysfunction or destruction, leading to decreased thyrotropin (thyroid-stimulating hormone, TSH) production.
- Thyrotropin is the pituitary hormone responsible for stimulating thyroid hormone synthesis and secretion.
- Increased circulating levels of glucocorticoids (endogenous or exogenous) can transitorily suppress TSH secretion by anterior pituitary thyrotropes; this leads to decreased blood levels of T_4 and free T_4.
- Thyrotrope secretion of TSH normalizes when blood glucocorticosteroid levels return to normal.
- Tertiary hypothyroidism caused by decreased thyrotropin-releasing hormone (TRH) production by the hypothalamus has not been documented in dogs or cats.

Congenital Hypothyroidism

- Congenital hypothyroidism is very rare in both dogs and cats.
- Reported causes of primary congenital hypothyroidism in dogs and cats include thyroid agenesis or dysgenesis, dyshormonogenesis, and iodine deficiency.
- Secondary congenital hypothyroidism is most commonly observed in German shepherd dogs with a panhypopituitarism caused by a cystic Rathke's pouch.
- A congenital deficiency in pituitary TSH production was reported in a family of giant schnauzers.

Systems Affected

- Endocrine/metabolic
- Skin/exocrine
- Behavioral
- Neuromuscular
- Reproductive
- Gastrointestinal
- Ophthalmic
- Cardiovascular
- Nervous

Signalment/History

- No known genetic basis for the inheritance of primary hypothyroidism in canines.
- Familial lymphocytic thyroiditis has been reported in individual colonies of borzois, beagles, and Great Danes.
- Primary hypothyroidism is the most common endocrinopathy of dogs; the reported prevalence of hypothyroidism in dogs is 1:156–1:500.
- Hypothyroidism is rare in cats.
- Primary acquired hypothyroidism is more common in medium to large-sized dogs.

- Breeds reported to be predisposed to developing primary acquired hypothyroidism include the golden retriever, Doberman pinscher, Irish setter, Great Dane, Airedale terrier, Old English sheepdog, dachshund, miniature schnauzer, cocker spaniel, poodle, and boxer.
- Most common in middle-aged dogs (4–10 years)
- No definitive sex predilection has been identified; however, castrated male dogs and spayed female dogs appear to be at increased risk.
- Neutering may slightly increase risk of developing primary hypothyroidism.
- Bilateral thyroidectomy may result in hypothyroidism.

Historical Findings

- Most common—lethargy, inactivity, mental dullness, weight gain, hair loss or excessive shedding, lack of hair regrowth following clipping, dry or lusterless haircoat, excessive scaling, hyperpigmentation, recurrent skin infections, and cold intolerance
- Uncommon—generalized weakness, incoordination, head tilt, facial paralysis, seizures, and infertility
- Clinical signs develop slowly and are progressive.

Clinical Features

Dermatologic

- Bilaterally symmetric truncal alopecia that spares the head and extremities—common
- Alopecia is usually nonpruritic unless a secondary pyoderma or other pruritic dermatitis is also present.
- Hairs epilate easily; the haircoat is often dry and lusterless. (Fig. 58-1)

Figure 58-1 Hypothyroidism. Note the dry and dull haircoat. The hair epilates easily—rubbing of the collar has caused alopecia.

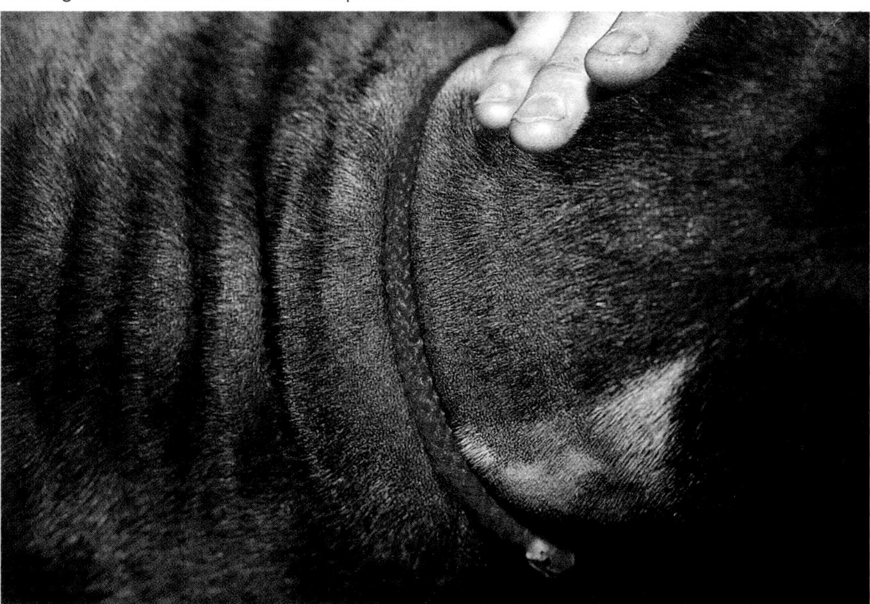

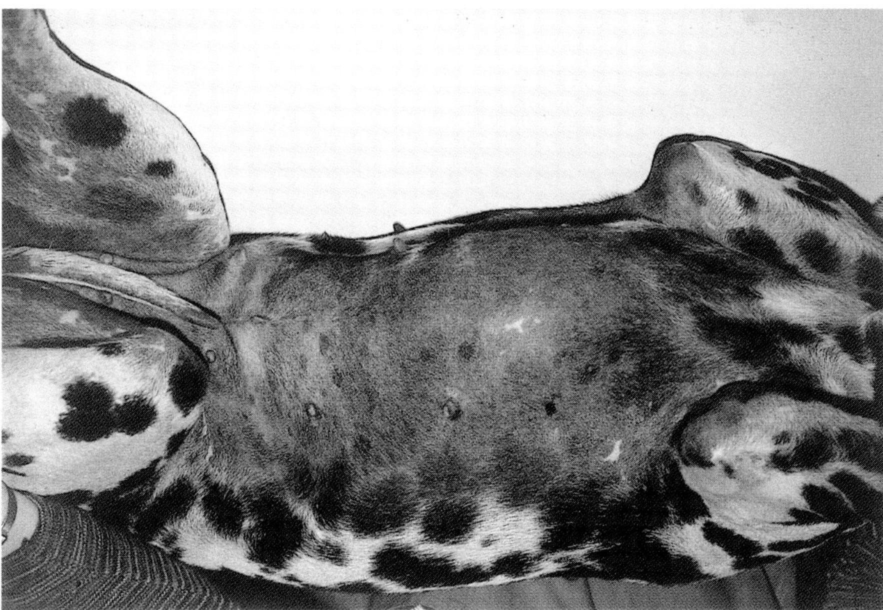

Figure 58-2 Hypothyroidism. Alopecia of the ventrum with secondary hyperpigmentation.

- Alopecia often initially involves the flank area, base of the ears, tail (rat tail) and friction areas (axillae, ventrum of thorax, abdomen and neck, and under the collar).
- Early in the disease course, alopecia may be multifocal and asymmetric; alopecic lesion may have irregular margins.
- Hyperpigmentation and increased thickness of the epidermis are common, particularly in friction areas. (Fig. 58-2)
- Seborrhea—common; can be generalized, multifocal, or localized
- A secondary superficial pyoderma occurs frequently; deep pyoderma is less common.
- Dermal accumulation of mucopolysaccharides can lead to nonpitting edema (myxedema), particularly in the facial area; this produces the classic "tragic" expression associated with hypothyroidism.

Metabolic

- Lethargy, mental dullness
- Weight gain
- Mild hypothermia

Reproductive

- Infertility and prolonged anestrus in females
- Inappropriate galactorrhea in sexually intact bitches

Neuromuscular—Uncommon

- A peripheral neuropathy (localized or generalized) involving lower motor neurons occasionally occurs in hypothyroid dogs.
- Generalized weakness is the most common clinical sign; dogs may have a stiff, stilted gait. Other neurologic findings may include proprioceptive deficits, hyporeflexia, head tilt, facial paralysis/paresis, and ataxia.

- A secondary myopathy characterized by denervation atrophy is usually present in dogs with hypothyroid polyneuropathy.
- Some hypothyroid dogs develop a generalized myopathy without concurrent neurologic involvement; these dogs present for generalized weakness.
- Seizures secondary to marked cerebral atherosclerosis have been rarely reported in hypothyroid dogs with marked hyperlipidemia.
- Laryngeal paralysis, megaesophagus, and Horner's syndrome have been associated with hypothyroidism, but definitive proof of a causal relationship is lacking.

Ophthalmic

- Corneal lipid deposits
- Lipemia retinalis

Felines—Rare

- Unkempt appearance, matting of hair, nonpruritic seborrhea sicca, pinnal alopecia
- Lethargy
- Obesity

Congenital Hypothyroidism—Cretinism

- Mental dullness/retardation, lethargy, inactivity
- Disproportionate dwarfism (large, broad head with short neck and limbs), shortened mandible, protruding tongue, delayed dental eruption
- Constipation/obstipation—particularly in cats
- Hypothermia
- Retention of puppy coat, progressive truncal alopecia (dogs)

Differential Diagnosis

- Dermatologic abnormalities are frequently the predominant clinical abnormality in dogs with hypothyroidism.
- Consider endocrine causes of alopecia (e.g., hyperadrenocorticism, sex hormone–related dermatopathies, growth hormone–responsive dermatosis, and adrenal sex hormone abnormalities).
- If fasting hyperlipidemia (the most common laboratory abnormality in hypothyroid dogs) must rule out diabetes mellitus, hyperadrenocorticism, nephrotic syndrome, acute pancreatitis, biliary obstruction, and primary lipid metabolism abnormalities.

Diagnostics

- Hypercholesterolemia—observed in up to 80% of hypothyroid dogs
- Hypertriglyceridemia and gross lipemia—less common
- Mild, normochromic, normocytic, nonregenerative anemia—up to 50% of hypothyroid dogs
- Mildly elevated serum creatine kinase levels are intermittently identified.
- Do endocrine testing in dogs with clinical signs or laboratory abnormalities suggesting hypothyroidism.

- Routine endocrine testing of sick dogs for hypothyroidism is unnecessary if they do not show signs consistent with hypothyroidism.

Basal Serum Thyroid Hormone Concentrations

- Basal serum T_4 levels in the midnormal to high-normal range rule out a diagnosis of hypothyroidism; further endocrine testing is not indicated.
- A subnormal T_4 concentration is compatible with, but not diagnostic for, hypothyroidism.
- Subnormal T_4 levels can be seen in healthy, euthyroid dogs.
- Serum T_4 levels often drop below normal in dogs with nonthyroidal illness (sick euthyroid syndrome); these animals are not hypothyroid and do not require thyroid hormone supplementation.
- Basal serum T_3 levels are not an accurate means for evaluating thyroid function; one study found normal serum T_3 levels in 74% of hypothyroid dogs; serum T_3 levels can be subnormal in healthy, euthyroid dogs and in euthyroid dogs with nonthyroidal illness.
- Markedly elevated T_4 or T_3 levels in dogs indicate the presence of thyroid hormone autoantibodies; these autoantibodies can cause false elevations or, much less commonly, false decreases in T_4 or T_3 concentrations determined by radioimmunoassay.
- Determination of serum free T_4 (FT_4) levels by equilibrium dialysis is a sensitive and specific way to evaluate a patient for hypothyroidism.
- Low FT_4 concentrations in a patient with compatible clinical signs and low total T_4 levels strongly indicate hypothyroidism; however, FT_4 levels are low in up to 25% of euthyroid dogs with hyperadrenocorticism.
- Severe nonthyroidal illness may suppress FT_4 levels in some euthyroid dogs.
- Determination of serum FT_3 levels is noncontributory to diagnosing hypothyroidism.

Endogenous Thyrotropin (TSH) Concentrations

- Thyrotropin concentrations are increased in most dogs with primary hypothyroidism, but 18–38% of dogs with confirmed hypothyroidism have normal serum TSH levels.
- Elevated TSH levels have been reported in up to 14% of euthyroid dogs with nonthyroidal illness.
- High TSH levels combined with low T_4 or FT_4 concentrations strongly indicate hypothyroidism.

Autoantibodies to Thyroid Hormones and Thyroglobulin (Tg)

- Autoantibodies to Tg and to a lesser extent T_3 and T_4 occur frequently in dogs with hypothyroidism and are consistent with a diagnosis of lymphocytic thyroiditis; these autoantibodies can also occur in healthy, euthyroid dogs.
- Autoantibodies to Tg were found in up to 43% of dogs with nonthyroidal endocrine diseases.
- Healthy dogs with normal T_4 concentrations and autoantibodies to Tg, T_3, or T_4 may be at increased risk for developing hypothyroidism, but this is not proven.

TSH Stimulation Test

- Considered the gold standard for diagnosing clinical hypothyroidism
- Administer exogenous TSH to the patient and determine pre- and poststimulation serum T_4 concentrations.

- In hypothyroid dogs, the T_4 concentration following TSH administration does not rise into the normal reference range and frequently does not exceed the pre-TSH stimulation T_4 concentration.
- T_4 levels increase beyond the upper limit of the normal reference range following TSH stimulation of healthy, euthyroid dogs.
- Dogs with moderate or severe nonthyroidal illness, early primary hypothyroidism, or early secondary or tertiary hypothyroidism may show a muted response to TSH administration.
- T_4 concentrations increase but frequently not above the normal reference range.
- Reevaluate these animals in 3–4 months or following resolution of their nonthyroidal disease, if they still have clinical signs compatible with hypothyroidism.
- Because of the difficulty and expense of obtaining TSH, TSH stimulation testing is not commonly done in private practice; similar diagnostic information can be obtained by evaluating baseline serum T_4, FT_4, and endogenous TSH concentrations.

TRH Stimulation Testing

- Exogenous TRH is administered IV; pre- and poststimulation T_4 or TSH concentrations are measured.
- In euthyroid dogs, both T_4 and TSH concentrations increase above baseline values.
- In hypothyroid dogs, T_4 concentration does not increase significantly over the baseline T_4 value.
- Changes in T_4 concentration in healthy, euthyroid dogs are small and variable, making it difficult to differentiate normal dogs from hypothyroid dogs.
- Thyrotropin levels also increase in dogs with primary hypothyroidism, but the percentage increase over baseline concentrations is less than in euthyroid dogs.
- TRH stimulation testing is not recommended for diagnosing hypothyroidism; better tests are available; evaluating TSH concentrations following TRH administration can differentiate primary hypothyroidism from central hypothyroidism.

Radiography

- Epiphyseal dysgenesis, delayed epiphyseal ossification, and shortened vertebral bodies are present in patients with congenital hypothyroidism; these patients frequently develop radiographic signs of degenerative joint disease as adults.
- Megacolon is a common radiographic finding in cats with congenital hypothyroidism.

Echocardiography

- Indices of left ventricular systolic function are commonly abnormal; these changes are usually not clinically significant unless the dog has concurrent primary heart disease.
- *Electrocardiography*—low-amplitude R waves are commonly observed, bradycardia less frequently

Pathologic Findings

- Lymphocytic thyroiditis is characterized by a diffuse infiltration of lymphocytes and plasma cells into the thyroid parenchyma, with eventual destruction of the gland.

- Idiopathic thyroid atrophy is characterized by parenchymal atrophy and replacement with adipose and connective tissue.
- Epidermal and dermal abnormalities are common.
- Dermatohistopathologic abnormalities commonly seen with hypothyroidism include orthokeratotic hyperkeratosis, sebaceous gland atrophy, epidermal hyperplasia, follicular atrophy, myxedema, and vacuolation of the erector pili muscles.

Therapeutics

- Reduced-fat diet until body weight is satisfactory and T_4 concentrations are normal
- Dogs with primary hypothyroidism respond well to treatment with oral synthetic levothyroxine (L-thyroxine).
- The appropriate dosage for L-thyroxine varies between individuals because of differences in gastrointestinal (GI) absorption and hormone metabolism; possible after patient has responded to therapy and T_4 levels have normalized.
- Treatment is lifelong.
- Most clinical and laboratory abnormalities resolve over a few weeks to a few months.
- Occasionally, dermatologic abnormalities worsen transiently during the first month of therapy.

Drugs of Choice

- Levothyroxine is the treatment of choice.
- The starting dosage is 0.02–0.04 mg/kg/day or 0.5 $mg/m^2/day$ divided BID.
- Adjust dosage on the basis of serum T_4 concentration and clinical response to therapy; initially, use a veterinary name brand product.
- If the patient responds to therapy, once-daily therapy can be tried; however, some patients require continued BID therapy.
- Different brands of L-thyroxine frequently have different GI absorption kinetics; the dosage may change if the brand is changed.

Precautions/Interactions

- The initial dosage of L-thyroxine may need to be decreased in animals with concurrent heart failure, diabetes mellitus, renal failure, liver disease, or hypoadrenocorticism.
- The initial dosage of L-thyroxine is 25% of the standard daily dosage.
- Slowly increase the dosage over 2–4 months until the appropriate dosage is obtained; this allows the patient to adjust slowly to the increased basal metabolic rate.
- Start glucocorticoid replacement therapy prior to L-thyroxine therapy in hypothyroid animals with concurrent hypoadrenocorticism.
- Glucocorticoids, phenytoin, salicylates, androgens, and furosemide may enhance the metabolism of L-thyroxine by inhibiting serum protein binding.
- Sucralfate and aluminum hydroxide can inhibit GI absorption.

Alternative Drugs

- Therapy with synthetic liothyronine (T_3) is not indicated or recommended in the vast majority of hypothyroid dogs.

- Liothyronine therapy is only indicated if a dog fails to achieve a normal serum T_4 concentration following appropriate therapy with at least two different brands of L-thyroxine.
- This probably indicates a lack of intestinal absorption; liothyronine is almost completely absorbed from the gut.
- The initial dosage is 4–6 mg/kg PO TID; final dosage is based on clinical response and on serum T_3 levels in the normal range; some patients can be maintained on BID therapy.

Comments

- Mental alertness and activity levels usually increase within 1–2 weeks after initiation of therapy.
- Dermatologic abnormalities slowly resolve over 1–4 months, as do neurologic deficits that are secondary to hypothyroidism.
- Reproductive abnormalities resolve more slowly.
- If significant clinical improvement does not occur within 3 months of initiation of therapy, with serum T_4 levels in the normal range, the diagnosis of hypothyroidism may be incorrect.
- Check serum T_4 levels after 1 month of therapy.
- Determine peak serum T_4 concentrations 4–8 hr after L-thyroxine administration.
- Serum T_4 concentrations should be in the normal range or mildly increased.
- Patients on once-daily therapy that do not respond to therapy and have a normal or high peak T_4 concentration should have their pre-pill T_4 concentration (trough T_4) assessed; if the trough T_4 concentration is low, twice-daily therapy is indicated.
- Following initial normalization of serum T_4 values, check them yearly, or sooner if clinical signs of hypothyroidism or thyrotoxicosis develop.
- Recheck serum T_4 concentrations 1 month after any change in dosage or brand of L-thyroxine being administered.
- Prolonged administration of an inappropriately high dosage of L-thyroxine can cause iatrogenic hyperthyroidism.
- Clinical signs of thyrotoxicosis include panting, polyphagia, weight loss, polyuria/polydipsia, anxiety, and diarrhea.
- Keep peak serum T_4 concentrations at or below 7.5 mg/dL.
- Dogs treated for acquired primary hypothyroidism have an excellent prognosis; life expectancy is normal.
- Patients with acquired central hypothyroidism may have a poor prognosis if condition is secondary to a tumor or destructive process affecting the pituitary or hypothalamus.
- Primary hypothyroidism has been reported to occur concurrently with primary hypoadrenocorticism and/or insulin-dependent diabetes mellitus in a small number of animals.

Abbreviations

- T_4 = L-thyroxine, tetraiodothyronine
- T_3 = liothyronine, triiodothyronine
- FT_4 = free T_4
- FT_3 = free T_3

- TSH = thyroid-stimulating hormone, thyrotropin
- TRH = thyrotropin-releasing hormone

Suggested Reading

Chastain CB, Panciera DL. Hypothyroid diseases. In: Ettinger SJ, Feldman EC, eds. Textbook of veterinary internal medicine. 4th ed. Philadelphia: WB Saunders, 1995: 1487–1501.

Panciera DL. Hypothyroidism in dogs: 66 cases (1987–1992). J Am Vet Med Assoc 1994;204:761–767.

Peterson ME, Melian C, Nichols R. Measurement of serum total thyroxine, triiodothyronine, free thyroxine and thyrotropin concentrations for diagnosis of hypothyroidism in dog. J Am Vet Med Assoc 1997;211:1396–1402.

Consulting Editor Karen Helton Rhodes

Hyperadrenocorticism (Cushing Disease)

Peter P. Kintzer

Definition/Overview

- Spontaneous hyperadrenocorticism (HAC) is a disorder caused by excessive production of cortisol by the adrenal cortex.
- Iatrogenic HAC results from excessive exogenous administration of glucocorticoids.
- In either instance, clinical signs are a result of the deleterious effects of the elevated circulating cortisol concentrations on multiple organ systems.

Etiology/Pathophysiology

- Some 85–90% of cases of naturally occurring HAC are caused by bilateral adrenocortical hyperplasia resulting from pituitary corticotroph tumors or hyperplasia oversecreting ACTH.
- In the remaining 10–15% of cases, cortisol-secreting adrenocortical neoplasia is present; approximately one-half of these tumors are malignant.
- Iatrogenic HAC results from excessive exogenous administration of glucocorticoids.
- HAC is a multisystemic disorder—the degree to which each system is involved varies considerably; in some patients, signs referable to one system may predominate; others have several systems involved to a comparable degree
- Signs referable to the urinary tract or skin often predominate.

Signalment/History

Considered one of the most common endocrine disorders in dogs; rare in cats

- Dogs—poodles, dachshunds, Boston terriers, boxers, and beagles are reportedly at increased risk
- Cats—no apparent predilection
- No predilection for pituitary-dependent hyperadrenocorticism (PDH) in dogs; two-thirds to three-quarters are female.
- No apparent predilection in cats
- HAC is generally a disorder of middle-aged to old animals; PDH can be seen in dogs as young as 1 year.

Clinical Features

- Severity may vary greatly, depending on the duration and severity of cortisol excess.
- In some cases, the physical presence of the neoplastic process (pituitary or adrenal) contributes.
- Polyuria and polydipsia
- Polyphagia
- Pendulous abdomen
- Hepatomegaly
- Hair loss (Fig. 59-1)
- Lethargy
- Muscle weakness
- Anestrus
- Obesity

Figure 59-1 Hyperadrenocorticism. Note the trunkal alopecia with hyperpigmentation.

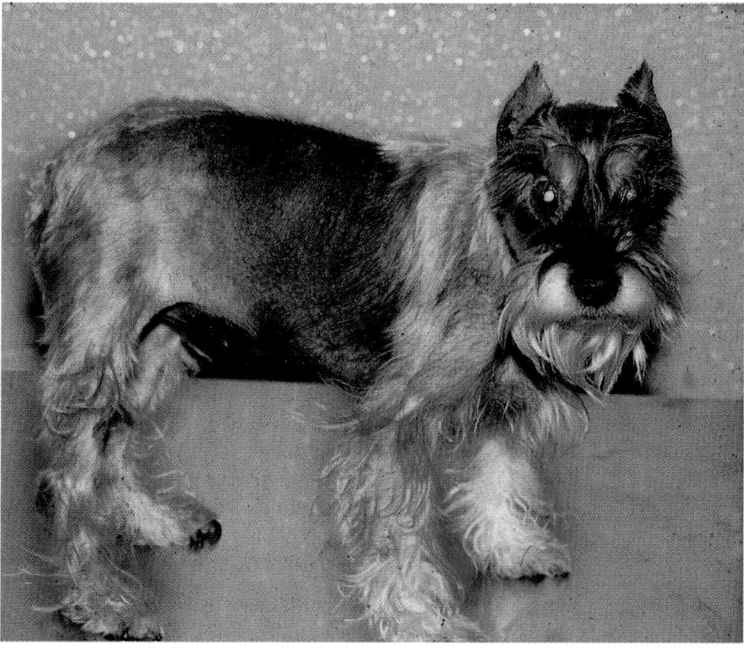

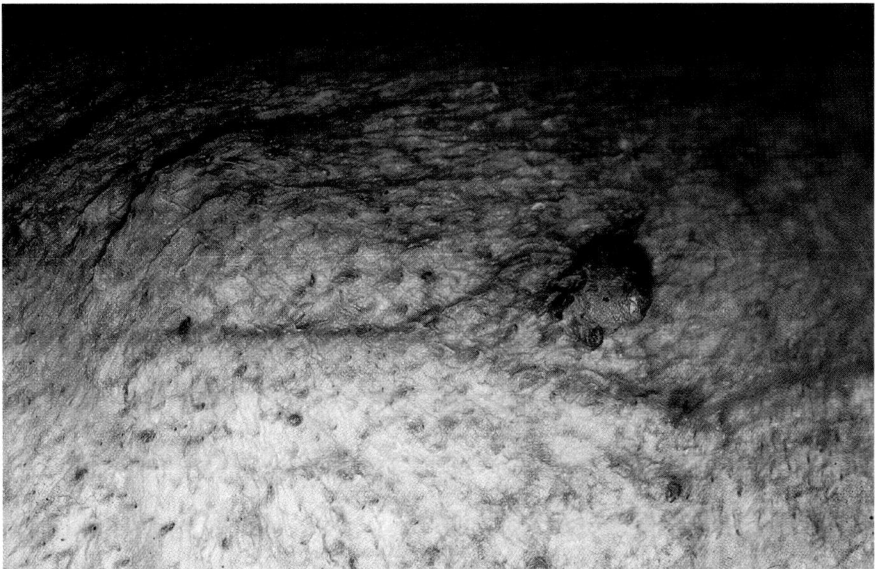

Figure 59-2 Hyperadrenocorticism. Markedly atrophic skin of the ventral abdomen revealing prominent vessels and comedones.

- Muscle atrophy
- Comedones (Fig. 59-2)
- Increased panting
- Testicular atrophy
- Hyperpigmentation
- Calcinosis cutis (Fig. 59-3)

Figure 59-3 Hyperadrenocorticism. Early calcinosis cutis. Note the yellow-pink coloration of the papules. They will palpate as firm "gritty" lesions in many cases and may become quite extensive and severe.

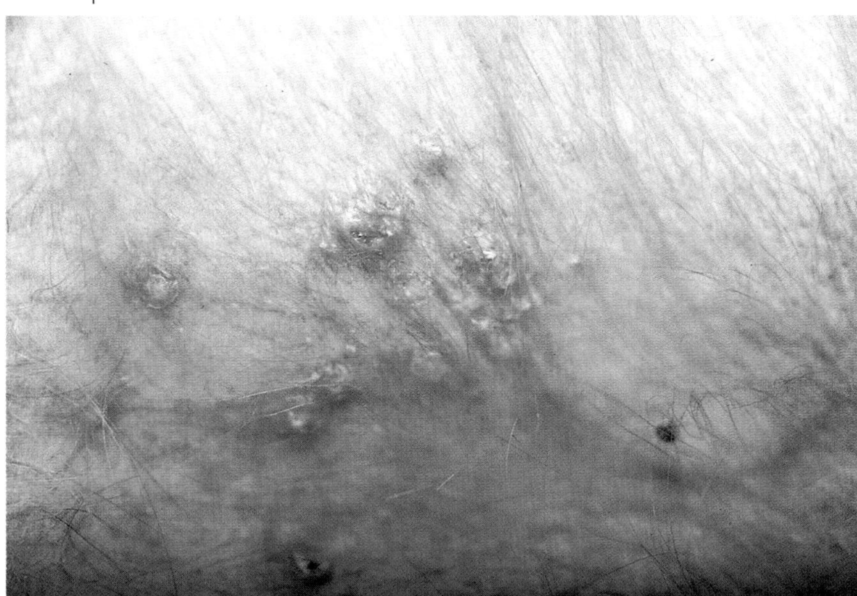

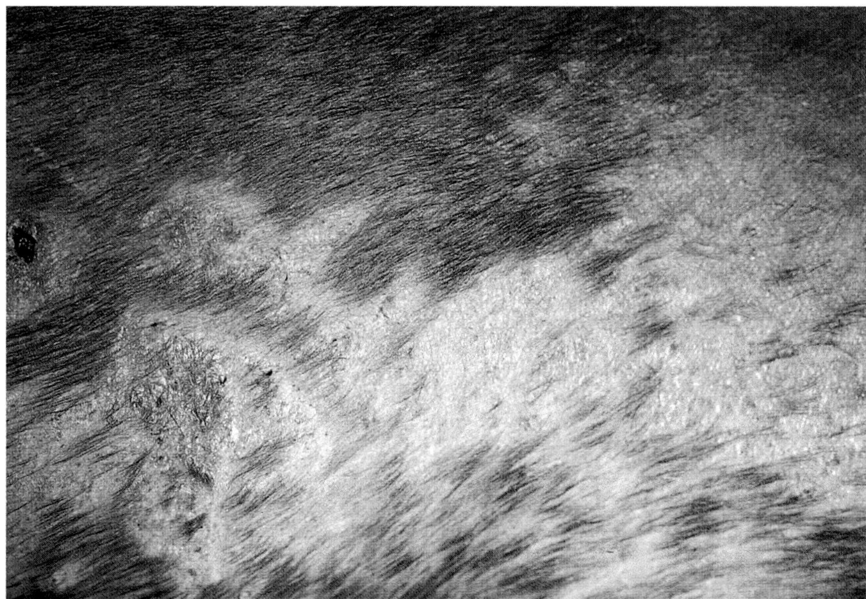

Figure 59-4 Secondary pyoderma associated with hyperadrenocorticism. Often recurrent and persistent.

- Facial nerve palsy
- Atrophic skin
- Secondary pyoderma (Fig. 59-4)

Differential Diagnosis

- Depends on the clinical and laboratory abnormalities displayed
- Hypothyroidism
- Sex hormone dermatoses
- Acromegaly
- Diabetes mellitus
- Hepatopathies
- Renal disease
- Other causes of polyuria/polydipsia

Diagnostics

- Hemogram may show eosinopenia, lymphopenia, leukocytosis, and erythrocytosis.
- Serum chemistry may show elevated alkaline phosphatase, liver enzymes, cholesterol, glucose, and total CO_2.
- Urinalysis may reveal decreased specific gravity, proteinuria, hematuria, pyuria, or bacteriuria.
- Diagnosing HAC—ACTH response test, low-dose dexamethasone suppression test (0.015 mg/kg dexamethasone [Azium] in dogs; 0.1 mg/kg in cats); urinary cortisol:creatinine ratio (negative result virtually excludes HAC; a

positive result must be confirmed with blood test); be cognizant of the effects of nonadrenal illness on these tests (false-positive results)

- Differentiating PDH from AT—high-dose dexamethasone suppression (Current Veterinary Therapy Isone, Azium), plasma ACTH level, CRH response test
- Abdominal radiographs may differentiate PDH from AT, demonstrating mineralization in one-third of AT; chest radiographs are indicated in AT to check for metastases.
- Ultrasonography, CT, and MR—useful for differentiating PDH from AT and for staging AT
- CT and MR—often useful for demonstrating macroadenomas
- PDH—gross examination reveals normal-sized pituitary to pituitary macroadenoma and bilateral adrenocortical enlargement
- Microscopically, see pituitary adenoma or corticotroph hyperplasia of pars distalis or pars intermedia and adrenocortical hyperplasia
- AT—gross examination reveals variable-sized adrenal mass, atrophy of contralateral gland (rarely, bilateral tumors), and metastasis in some patients with adrenal carcinoma
- Microscopically, see adrenocortical adenoma or carcinoma

Therapeutics

Diet

- Usually no need to alter; appropriate reducing or high-fiber diet if concurrent diabetes mellitus

Surgical Considerations

- Hypophysectomy—described, but generally not recommended for treatment of PDH in dogs or cats because of the difficulty of the procedure and the need for intensive monitoring and lifelong hormonal supplementation
- Bilateral adrenalectomy, likewise, is a demanding procedure not generally used for the treatment of PDH in dogs; cats seem to tolerate the surgery somewhat better than dogs; given the appropriate personnel and facilities, it is one of the treatments of choice for feline PDH.
- Surgery is probably the treatment of choice for adrenocortical adenomas and small carcinomas unless the patient is a poor surgical risk or the client refuses surgery.
- Medical control of adrenal-dependent hyperadrenocorticism with ketoconazole is recommended prior to surgery, if possible.

Drugs of Choice

- Mitotane (*o,p′*-DDD) remains the drug of choice for medical management of both PDH and AT in dogs.
- PDH—give an initial loading dose of 40–50 mg/kg/day until both basal and post-ACTH cortisol levels are in the normal resting range (1–5 μg/dL); then 50 mg/kg/week divided; dosage adjustments are based on ACTH response testing (maintain basal and post-ACTH cortisol levels between 1 and 5 μg/dL); if relapse occurs, as indicated by cortisol levels outside the normal resting range, reload for 5–7 days and increase weekly maintenance dose by approximately 50%; give prednisone (0.2 mg/kg/day) during initial and subsequent loading periods

- AT—use mitotane (goal is low-to-undetectable basal and post-ACTH cortisol levels) or administer mitotane at highest tolerated dosage; give prednisone at 0.2 mg/kg/day
- *l*-Deprenyl (selegiline hydrochloride; Anipryl, Deprenyl Animal Health, Inc., Topeka, KN)—may be used as an alternative treatment for PDH; decreases pituitary ACTH secretion by increasing dopaminergic tone to the hypothalamic-pituitary axis, thus decreasing serum cortisol concentrations; indicated only for the treatment of uncomplicated PDH; not recommended for treatment of PDH in dogs with concurrent illnesses such as diabetes mellitus; cannot be used to treat cortisol-secreting adrenocortical neoplasia; initiate therapy with 1 mg/kg daily and increase to 2 mg/kg/day after 2 months if the response is inadequate; if this dose is also ineffective, give alternative therapy
- The multicenter trial performed by Deprenyl Animal Health, Inc. reported that 75–80% of dogs had a good response to therapy as assessed by resolution of clinical signs and monthly low-dose dexamethasone suppression testing; other investigators reported lower efficacy rates (50% or less in some studies); further independent clinical trials are necessary to assess the efficacy of this medication in controlling PDH; adverse effects such as anorexia, lethargy, vomiting, and diarrhea are uncommon (<5% of dogs) and usually mild; disadvantages include the need for lifelong daily administration and the expense of the medication.
- Ketoconazole (10 mg/kg BID initially; up to 20 mg/kg BID in some dogs)—indicated for dogs unable to tolerate mitotane at doses necessary to control HAC and preoperative control of HAC in dogs with AT scheduled for adrenalectomy; may be useful for palliation of clinical signs of HAC in dogs with AT; over one-third of dogs reportedly fail to respond adequately to the drug; adverse effects include anorexia, vomiting, diarrhea, lethargy, and an idiosyncratic hepatopathy
- Feline HAC—the drug of choice for medical management is controversial; further studies are needed; mitotane (50 mg/kg/day then 50 mg/kg/week divided, dosage adjustments based on ACTH response testing) or metyrapone (65 mg/kg BID to TID, dosage adjustments based on ACTH response testing) should be considered; *l*-deprenyl is a newly described alternative for therapy for canine PDH, but its use has not been described in cats with HAC; a short-term safety study in normal cats revealed no significant adverse effects

Precautions

- Side effects of mitotane—not uncommon; mild in most dogs; include lethargy, weakness, anorexia, vomiting, diarrhea, ataxia, and iatrogenic hypoadrenocorticism
- Side effects are more common in dogs with AT given high doses of mitotane.
- Side effects of ketoconazole—seem to be less common; include anorexia, vomiting, diarrhea, and transient liver enzyme elevation
- Side effects of *l*-deprenyl are uncommon.

Alternative Drugs

- Consider radiation therapy for animals with pituitary macroadenomas.
- ACTH levels may take several months to decrease; control HAC with above drugs in the interim.

Comments

Patient Monitoring

- Response to therapy—use periodic ACTH response testing (see references); test after the initial 7–10 days of mitotane or ketoconazole therapy to ensure adequate response, then at 1, 3, and 6 months of maintenance mitotane therapy and every 6–12 months thereafter; adequacy of any necessary mitotane reloading period is checked with an ACTH response test before higher maintenance mitotane dose initiated; depending on the problem, clinical signs resolve within several days to months of appropriate therapy; current label recommendations are to evaluate the efficacy of *l*-deprenyl therapy solely on the basis of resolution of clinical signs of HAC; the ACTH stimulation test is not indicated for assessing the response to treatment
- Some clinicians choose to do low-dose dexamethasone suppression tests every 4–6 weeks to evaluate for normalization (or improvement) of the pituitary-adrenal axis.

Expected Course/Prognosis

- Untreated HAC—generally a progressive disorder with a poor prognosis
- Treated PDH—usually a good prognosis; the average survival time for a dog with PDH treated with mitotane is 2 years; at least 10% survive 4 years; dogs living longer than 6 months tend to die of causes unrelated to their HAC
- Macroadenomas and neurologic signs—poor to grave prognosis
- Adrenal adenomas—usually a good to excellent prognosis; small carcinomas (not metastasized) have a fair to good prognosis
- Large carcinomas and AT with widespread metastasis—generally a poor to fair prognosis, but impressive responses to high doses of mitotane are occasionally seen

Associated Conditions

Neurologic signs in dogs with large pituitary tumors; glucose intolerance or concurrent diabetes mellitus; pulmonary thromboembolism; increased incidence of urinary tract and skin infections; hypertension; proteinuria/glomerulopathy

Abbreviations

- AT = adrenal tumor
- CRH = corticotropin-releasing hormone
- HAC = hyperadrenocorticism
- PDH = pituitary-dependent hyperadrenocorticism

Suggested Reading

Bruyette DS, Ruehl WW, Entrikent, et al: Management of canine hyperadrenocorticism with l-deprenyl (Anipryl). Vet Clin North Am 1997;27(2):273–286.

Duesberg C, Peterson ME. Adrenal disorders in cats. Vet Clin North Am 1997;27(2):321–348.

Guptill L, Scott-Moncrieff JC, Widmer WR. Diagnosis of canine hyperadrenocorticism. Vet Clin North Am 1997;27(2):215–236.

Kintzer PP, Peterson ME. Mitotane treatment of cortisol secreting adrenocortical neoplasia: 32 cases (1980–1992). J Am Vet Med Assoc 1994;205:54–61.

Kintzer PP, Peterson ME. Mitotane therapy of canine hyperadrenocorticism. In: Kirk RW, Bonagura JD, eds. Current veterinary therapy XII. Philadelphia: Saunders, 1995:

Kintzer PP, Peterson ME. Diagnosis and management of canine cortisol-secreting adrenal tumors. Vet Clin North Am 1997;27(2):299–308.

Peterson ME. Hyperadrenocorticism. In: Kirk RW, ed. Current veterinary therapy IX. Philadelphia: Saunders, 1986;27(2):255–272.

Peterson ME, Kintzer PP. Medical therapy of pituitary-dependent hyperadrenocorticism: mitotane. Vet Clin North Am 1997;27(2):255–272.

Consulting Editor Karen Helton Rhodes

Growth Hormone–Responsive Dermatoses

Margaret S. Swartout

Definition/Overview

- Uncommon dermatoses resulting from a growth hormone deficiency or dermatoses responding to growth hormone therapy
- Pituitary dwarfism—the result of a primary growth hormone deficiency
- Adult-onset growth hormone–responsive dermatosis—a clinical syndrome that responds to growth hormone therapy; patients may be strictly growth hormone-deficient; may have one or more of a plethora of hormonal abnormalities, including possible imbalances of adrenal sex hormones

Etiology/Pathophysiology

Pituitary Dwarfism

- *Pituitary dwarfism*—mediated by an autosomal recessive trait, which results in a developmental abnormality of the pituitary and lack of growth hormone production

Adult-Onset

- *Adult-onset*—unknown; breed predisposition suggests a hereditary influence; pituitary neoplasia has been suggested
- Although an absolute growth hormone deficiency may be noted, other causes may lead to a similar clinical syndrome that responds to growth hormone supplementation (e.g., castration-responsive dermatosis, congenital adrenal hyperplasia-like syndrome).

Signalment/History

Pituitary dwarfism

- Most commonly seen in German shepherds; also reported in spitzes, toy pinschers, and Carnelian bear dogs; noted at 2–3 months of age
- Adult-onset—reported in the chow chows, Pomeranians, poodles, keeshonds, Samoyeds, and American water spaniels; generally noted at 1–2 years of age; primarily affects males, although seen in both sexes (neutered and intact) and at all ages
- Patients appear normal at birth; by 2–3 months bilaterally symmetric alopecia begins to be apparent; trunk, neck, and caudal thighs severely affected
- Primary hair growth over face and distal extremities only; retained puppy coat is easily epilated.
- Skin—thin, hypotonic, scaly, and hyperpigmented; comedones noted

Adult-Onset Growth Hormone–Responsive Dermatoses

- Alopecia—bilaterally symmetric; involves trunk, neck, caudomedial thighs, tail, ventral abdomen, perineum, and pinnae; the head and legs are spared (Fig. 60-1)
- Primary hairs are lost first; then loss of secondary hairs in the affected areas; hair readily epilates; tufts of regrowth at trauma or biopsy sites
- Skin—thin and hyperpigmented; secondary seborrhea and pyoderma uncommon

Figure 60-1 This young adult male poodle was found to have low blood growth hormone concentrations before and after a xylazine stimulation test. The owners declined treatment.

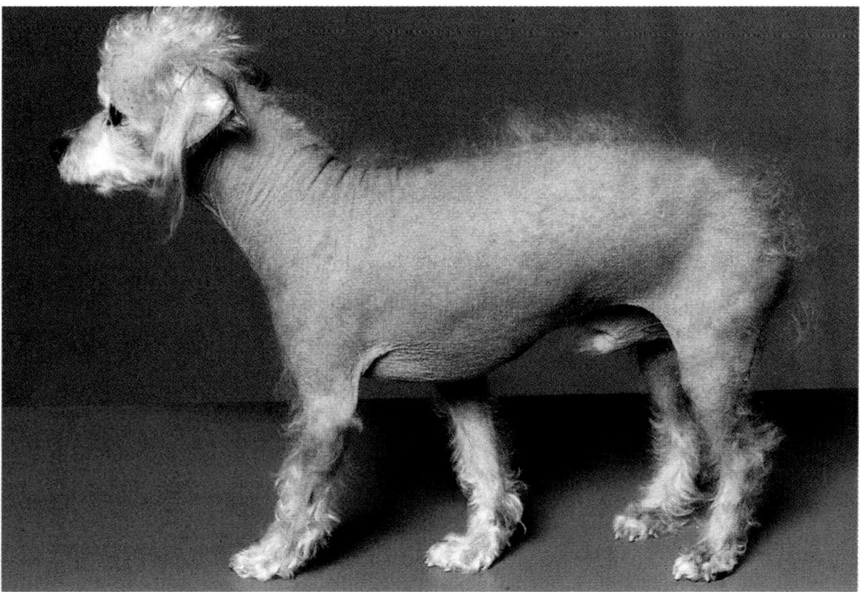

Differential Diagnosis

- *Pituitary dwarfism*—hypothyroidism, malnutrition, and metabolic disorders
- *Adult-onset*—hypothyroidism, hyperadrenocorticism, castration-responsive dermatosis, cyclic flank alopecia, estrogen/testosterone-responsive dermatosis, follicular dysplasia, and congenital adrenal hyperplasia-like syndrome (Fig. 60-2)

Diagnostics

- Growth hormone–stimulation test—dubious value; not currently available
- Somatomedin C (insulin-like growth factor 1)—growth hormone dependent; concentrations parallel body size; release may be impaired by glucocorticoids and estrogens; an indirect assay of growth hormone levels; expected to be low in growth hormone–deficient states (performed at Michigan State University Animal Health Diagnostic Laboratory, Lansing, MI)
- Pituitary dwarfism—low thyroid-stimulating hormone, ACTH, gonadotropin-releasing hormone, and human chorionic gonadotropin response test results
- Insulin response test—may aid diagnosis; causes severe hypoglycemia
- Adrenal reproductive hormone testing—ACTH-stimulation test with evaluation of adrenocortical hormones and their precursors (performed at the University of Tennessee College of Veterinary Medicine Endocrinology Laboratory, Nashville, TN)

Figure 60-2 This young adult neutered male Pomeranian was diagnosed with the congenital adrenal hyperplasia-like syndrome when an ACTH-stimulation test was performed that showed elevation of adrenocortical sex hormones pre- and post-stimulation. Low-dose dexamethasone suppression testing and the ACTH-stimulation test showed normal cortisol indices. Treatment with Lysodren was successful.

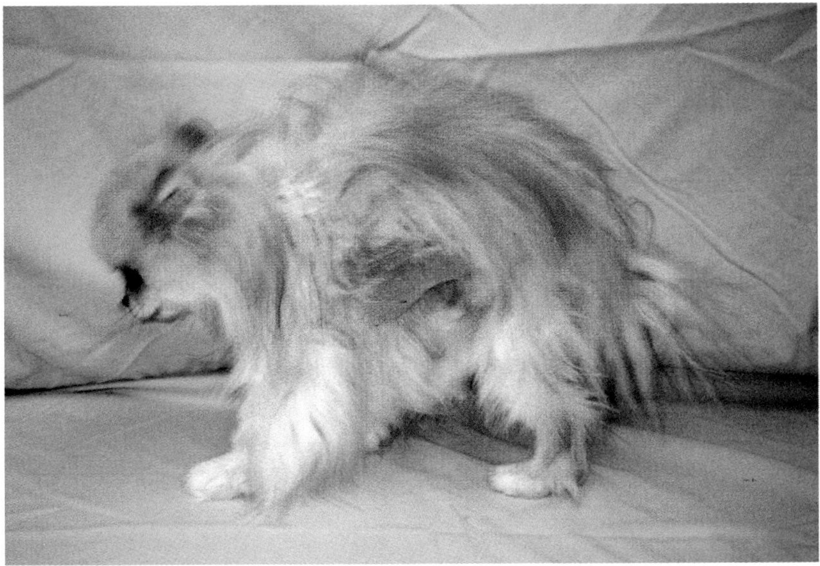

- Skin biopsy—general endocrinopathy; orthokeratotic hyperkeratosis; epidermal atrophy; follicular keratosis, dilation, and atrophy; telogenization of hair follicles; atrophy of sebaceous glands; amounts and sizes of dermal elastin fibers are small; castration-responsive or growth hormone–responsive dermatoses (dogs)—hypereosinophilic tricholemmal keratinization of hair follicles ("flame follicles")

Therapeutics

- L-Thyroxine—0.02 mg/kg PO q12h for a 6-week trial; recommended if the baseline total T_4 is low or low normal
- o,p′-DDD (Lysodren)—15–25 mg/kg PO q24h for 2–7 days; an ACTH-stimulation test to evaluate the response should demonstrate suppression of the baseline cortisol to a low-normal range; poststimulation range is 30–50 ng/mL (3.0–5.0 μg/dL); conduct ACTH-stimulation testing quarterly
- Methyltestosterone—1 mg/kg (maximum dose, 30 mg/dog) PO q48h for a maximum of 3 months; after hair regrowth, maintain at 1 mg/kg (maximum dose, 30 mg/dog) PO every 4–7 days
- Bovine, porcine, or synthetic human growth hormone—0.15 IU/kg SC twice weekly for 6 weeks; may repeat if no response within 3 months
- Intact male dogs—neuter to rule out castration-responsive dermatosis

Comments

- Growth hormones—monitor blood glucose before each treatment; growth hormone is diabetogenic
- Methyltestosterone—cholangiohepatitis, seborrhea, and behavioral changes; monitor liver enzymes and clinical status
- If post-ACTH stimulation blood cortisols are too low, evaluate serum electrolytes to determine the need for mineralocorticoid treatment.
- Growth hormone therapy—anaphylaxis with repeated dosing; diabetes mellitus (transient or permanent)
- Pituitary dwarfism—hair regrowth will begin within 4–8 weeks of beginning therapy and lasts 6 months to 2 years; retreatment is usually necessary
- Adult-onset—hair regrowth is usually observed in 2–12 weeks after therapy and lasts 6 months to 3 years; retreatment is often necessary
- o,p′-DDD—gives a good prognosis for hair regrowth if imbalance of adrenal sex hormone concentrations is suspected; may be a transient increase in epilation, but hair regrowth may be noted 4–12 weeks after beginning therapy
- Signs are confined to the skin, so treatment is not mandatory; owners may decline therapy because of the possible side effects.

Suggested Reading

Schmeitzel LP. Sex hormone-related and growth hormone-related alopecias. Vet Clin North Am Small Anim Pract 1990;20:1579–1601.

Consulting Editor Karen Helton Rhodes

Sex Hormone–Responsive Dermatoses

Margaret S. Swartout

Definition/Overview

Uncommon alopecias and dermatoses suspected to result from an imbalance of sex hormones; often defined on the basis of stimulatory response to sex hormone

Signalment/History

Estrogen-Responsive—Females (Ovarian Imbalance II)

- Possible deficiency or imbalance of estrogen; serum estradiol concentrations may be normal
- Inadequate production of adrenal sex hormones
- Cutaneous defect in the sex hormone receptor/metabolism system
- Rare in dogs
- Extremely rare in cats
- Predisposed breeds—dachshunds and boxers
- Primarily seen in young adults
- May occur after ovariohysterectomy in noncycling, intact females
- Occasionally seen during pseudopregnancy
- Variant—cyclical flank alopecia and hyperpigmentation; noted in Airedales, boxers, and English bulldogs; may worsen in winter

Hyperestrogenism—Females (Ovarian Imbalance I)

- Estrogen excess or imbalance (Fig. 61-1) to cystic ovaries, ovarian tumors (rare), or exogenous estrogen overdose

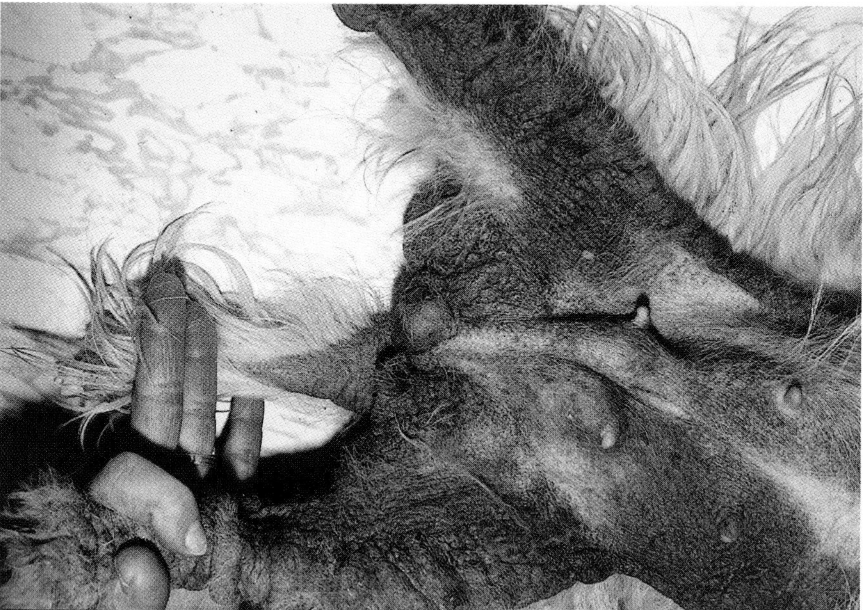

Figure 61-1 Hyperestrogenism (ovarian imbalance type I). Note the hyperpigmentation and prominent mammary gland development.

- Abnormal peripheral conversion of sex hormones
- Ectopic production of sex hormones
- Animals with normal serum estrogen concentrations may have increased numbers of estrogen receptors in the skin.
- Rare in dogs
- Extremely rare in cats
- English bulldogs may be predisposed to cystic ovaries.
- Generally, middle-aged and old intact female dogs

Hyperestrogenism—Male Dogs with Testicular Tumors

- Estrogen excess (or rarely hyperprogesteronism) owing to Sertoli cell tumor (most common), seminoma, or interstitial cell tumor (rarely) (Fig. 61-2)
- Cryptorchidism predisposes animals to the formation of testicular tumors.
- Intact males; usually middle-aged or older
- Predisposed breeds—boxers, Shetland sheepdogs, Weimaraners, German shepherds, Cairn terriers, Pekingese, and collies
- Associated with male pseudohermaphrodism in miniature schnauzers

Hyperandrogenism Associated with Testicular Tumors

Androgen-producing testicular tumors (especially interstitial cell tumors) in intact male dogs

Idiopathic Male Feminizing Syndrome

- Undetermined
- Serum sex hormone concentrations normal

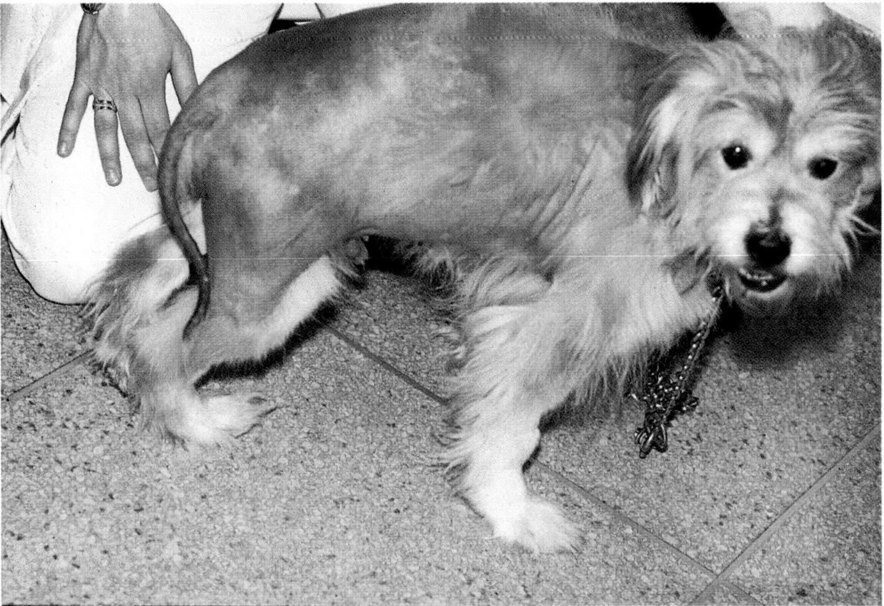

Figure 61-2 Sertoli cell tumor. Note the alopecia of the trunk and tail ("rat tail").

- Blockage of androgen receptors in the skin may prevent attachment of testosterone.
- Intact, middle-aged male dogs

Testosterone-Responsive—Males

- Rare
- Old castrated male dogs
- Afghan hounds over-represented
- Extremely rare in cats
- Suspected hypoandrogenism or a possible defect in the skin sex hormone–receptor system

Castration Responsive

- Intact males with normal testicles
- Estradiol, testosterone, and progesterone—variably high, low, or normal
- Onset 1–4 years or older
- Predisposed breeds—chow chows, Samoyeds, keeshonds, Pomeranians, huskies, malamutes, and miniature poodles

Adrenal Sex Hormone Imbalance (Adrenal Hyperplasia-like Syndrome)

- Adrenal enzyme (21-hydroxylase) deficiency resulting in excessive adrenal androgen or progesterone secretion
- Males and females, intact or neutered
- Onset 1–5 years of age
- Pomeranians predisposed

Clinical Features

- Alopecia—localized alopecia more common than generalized; initially involves the perineum, ventrum, thighs, and cervical areas; later involves the caudodorsal back and flank; flank alopecia may be the first or only sign in some patients with hyperestrogenism and may be seasonal in some spayed females
- Fur—may be soft or dry and brittle
- Nipples, mammary glands, vulva, prepuce, testicles, ovaries, and prostate—often abnormal
- Secondary seborrhea, pruritus, pyoderma, comedones, ceruminous otitis externa, and hyperpigmentation—variable
- Tail gland hyperplasia and perianal gland hyperplasia with macular melanosis—dogs with testicular tumors
- Urinary incontinence—estrogen- and testosterone-responsive conditions

Differential Diagnosis

- Hypothyroidism and hyperadrenocorticism—critical to rule out first; these diseases generally cause truncal alopecia first
- REMEMBER: sex hormones can change the affinity of binding proteins, so that the baseline total T_4 can be normal or above normal in dogs with hyperandrogenemia or hypoestrogenemia.
- Growth hormone–responsive/adrenal hyperplasia dermatosis
- Follicular dysplasia
- Dachshunds—pattern baldness
- Keratinization disorders
- Allergic skin disease

Diagnostics

- Bone marrow hypoplasia or aplasia are noted occasionally in states of estrogen excess, owing to testicular tumors in male and hyperestrogenism in female dogs.
- Serum estrogen/estradiol concentrations—sometimes high (30–40% of patients) with hyperestrogenism of female dogs, hyperestrogenism in male dogs with testicular tumors, and castration-responsive dermatosis; rarely helpful in estrogen-responsive dermatosis, because serum estradiol 17β concentrations in spayed females are similar to those in intact females
- Serum testosterone and progesterone—sometimes elevated in animals with castration-responsive dermatosis; occasionally elevated with hyperestrogenism (ovarian imbalance) in female dogs
- Serum sex hormone concentrations—often normal; treat according to the suspected diagnosis based on clinical signs, by ruling out other disorders, and by noting the response to therapy

Combined ACTH Stimulation and Adrenal Reproductive Hormone Test

- Obtain plasma and serum before injection; administer ACTH (cosyntropin 0.5 IU/kg IV or ACTH gel 0.22 USP U/kg IM); obtain plasma and serum 1 hr later (and a 2-hr sample if ACTH gel is used).

- Partial deficiency of 21-hydroxylase enzyme results in accumulation of steroid precursors (e.g., progesterone, 17-hydroxyprogesterone, androstenedione, and DHEAS), resulting in dermatosis of Pomeranians and other breeds; clinically similar to growth hormone–responsive dermatosis

GnRH (Cystorelin) Response Test

- Demonstrates response of gonads to stimulation
- Especially useful when basal hormones are normal
- Determine baseline serum estradiol, testosterone, and progesterone before injection; administer GnRH (0.22 mg/kg IV); obtain serum samples 1–2 hr later; determine levels of the three sex hormones; values vary with lab.
- Radiography, ultrasonography, and laparoscopy—detect cystic ovaries, ovarian tumors, testicular tumors (scrotal and abdominal), sublumbar lymphadenopathy, and possible thoracic metastases of malignant tumors
- Preputial cytology—may demonstrate cornification of cells (similar to bitch in estrus) in advanced patients with testicular feminizing tumors

Pathologic Findings

- General endocrinopathy findings (see above)—all syndromes, except hyperandrogenism owing to testicular tumors
- Perivascular dermatitis—may be seen in pruritic animals (male feminizing syndrome, hyperestrogenism of female dogs)
- Sebaceous glands—relatively spared in estrogen-responsive dermatosis of female dogs and in testosterone-responsive dermatosis of male dogs
- Hair follicles—hypereosinophilic tricholemmal keratinization ("flame follicles") may be seen with castration-responsive dermatosis

Therapeutics

- Cryptorchid animals—do not breed (prevention and avoidance of problems); neuter when young
- Exploratory laparotomy—diagnosis and treatment (e.g., ovariohysterectomy and castration) for ovarian cysts and tumors and abdominal testicular tumors
- Castration—castration-responsive dermatosis and scrotal testicular tumors
- Discontinue excessive exogenous estrogen administration.

Estrogen-Responsive Dermatosis

- Spayed females—DES at 0.02 mg/kg (maximum, 1 mg) PO q24h for 14–21 days; stop for 1 week; repeat cycle until hair regrowth; then give 2–3 times weekly to maintain hair coat; discontinue during estrus and resume maintenance when estrus subsides; if no response, try methyltestosterone (see below) or milbolerone (at 30 μg [dogs <11 kg] or 50 μg [dogs 11–23 kg]) until hair regrowth and then taper to maintenance
- Intact females—DES (5 mg PO q24h) until bloody discharge; if no response after 7 days, double the dose; give until proestrus day 2 (maximum, 14 days total) until sanguineous vaginal discharge and vulvar edema are noted; then for 2 days more; then LH (5 mg IM) on day 5 of proestrus; then FSH on days 9 and 11 of proestrus

- Alternative treatment—FSH (0.75 mg/kg IM daily) until signs of estrus appear

Testosterone Responsive (Males)/Some Estrogen Responsive (Female Dogs)

- Methyltestosterone—0.5–1.0 mg/kg (maximum, 30 mg) PO q48h until response; may take 1–3 months; after hair regrowth is complete, 2–3 times/week for maintenance
- Respositol testosterone (2 mg/kg [maximum, 30 mg IM every 1–4 months) as needed to maintain normal hair coat

Hyperestrogenism—Female Dogs

- Consider o,p′-DDD (Lysodren) or L-deprenyl.
- Alternative treatments—GnRH or hCG
- Tamoxifen—may be useful

Other Conditions

- Castration-responsive alopecia—may respond to hCG (50 IU/kg IM twice weekly for 6 weeks) or testosterone (see above) if castration is not possible
- Adrenal 21-hydroxylase enzyme deficiency—o,p′-DDD (Lysodren) if adrenal sex hormones are high; beginning dose 15–25 mg/kg PO q24h for 7 days; maintenance doses (15–25 mg/kg PO every 5–14 days) titrated to maintain post-ACTH-stimulation cortisol within the baseline range

General Treatment

- Topical antiseborrheic therapy—conditions with associated keratinization defects and comedones
- Antibiotics—associated pyodermas
- Prednisone—for pruritus if infections and bone marrow suppression have been ruled out; 0.5 mg/kg PO q12h for 5–7 days; then 0.5 mg q24h for 5–7 days; then 0.5 mg/kg q48h for 7 days

Comments

Patient Monitoring

- DES supplementation—CBC for bone marrow hypoplasia or aplasia every 2 weeks for the first month; then every 3–6 months
- Testosterone supplementation—serum biochemistry with an emphasis on liver enzymes every 3–4 weeks for the first 3 months; then every 4–6 months
- o,p′-DDD—electrolytes with ACTH-stimulation testing every 3 months

Possible Complications

- Estrogen—bone marrow hypoplasia (uncommon); aplasia (uncommon); signs of estrus (rare)
- methyltestosterone—cholangiohepatitis (rare); behavior changes (uncommon); seborrhea oleosa

- o,p′-DDD—potential toxicities (e.g., vomiting, diarrhea, collapse, and iatrogenic hypoadrenocorticism)
- Tamoxifen—vulva swelling; discontinue until signs of estrus are gone

Expected Course and Prognosis

- Estrogen responsive—regrowth of hair may take about 3 months and may be transient
- Female hyperestrogenism—improvement should occur within 3–6 months after ovariohysterectomy
- Estrogen- and androgen-secreting tumors—resolution of signs noted within 3–6 months of castration; bone marrow aplasia associated with hyperestrogenism usually does not respond to castration, and the prognosis for recovery is grave; relapse after a positive response to castration may indicate metastasis, and if confirmed, the prognosis is poor
- Castration responsive—response noted 2–4 months after castration
- Testosterone therapy—may result in hair regrowth in 4–12 weeks
- Adrenal sex hormone imbalance—response seen 4–12 weeks after adrenal hyperplasia therapy with o,p'-DDD

Abbreviations

- DES = diethylstilbestrol
- DHEAS = dehydroepiandrosterone sulfate
- FSH = follicle-stimulating hormone
- GnRH = gonadotropin-releasing hormone
- hCG = human chorionic gonadotropin
- LH = luteinizing hormone
- o,p′-DDD = 1,1-(o,p'-dichlorodiphenyl)-2,2-dichloroethane

Suggested Reading

Schmeitzel LP. Sex hormone-related and growth hormone-related alopecias. Vet Clin North Am Small Anim Pract 1990;20:1579–1601.

Consulting Editor Karen Helton Rhodes

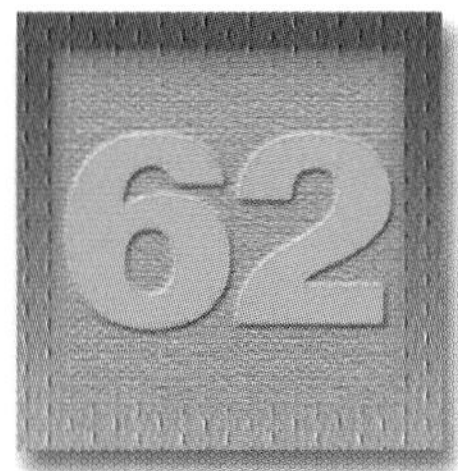

Steroid Hepatopathy

Keith P. Richter

Definition/Overview

Reversible vacuolar change in hepatocytes in dogs, associated with glucocorticoid treatment, hyperadrenocorticism (iatrogenic or spontaneous), or chronic illnesses in other organ systems; typified by high ALP activity without signs of hepatic insufficiency

Etiology/Pathophysiology

- Glucocorticoids—cause reversible glycogen accumulation in hepatocytes within 2–3 days after administration; injectable and reposital forms usually induce more severe changes than do oral forms; topical, ocular, cutaneous, and aural administration may also produce an effect
- Cell swelling—leads to parenchymal enlargement and hepatomegaly
- Response (dogs)—marked individual variation related to the type, route, dosage, duration of treatment, and individual sensitivity; may develop even with low-dose, short-term oral medication
- May develop with systemic diseases not related to glucocorticoid exposure or hyperadrenocorticism
- Association with significant nonhepatobiliary health problems that involve inflammation—suggests a relationship with stress (endogenous glucocorticoid release) or acute-phase reactants

Causes

- Glucocorticoid administration
- Hyperadrenocorticism

- Other adrenal gland hyperfunction—overproduction of sex hormones
- Systemic diseases associated with an acute-phase response or stress—severe dental disease; inflammatory bowel disease; chronic pancreatitis; systemic neoplasia (especially lymphoma); chronic infections (urinary tract, skin); hypothyroidism; inborn errors of lipid metabolism (lipid and glycogen accumulate in hepatocytes)

Signalment/History

- Dogs—common; occurs in up to 33% of patients undergoing liver biopsy; many patients identified through laboratory and imaging studies. Cats—extremely rare; usually hepatic lipidosis
- Breeds predisposed to hyperadrenocorticism (dachshunds, poodles, beagles, boxers, Boston terriers) and hyperlipidemia
- Middle-aged to old dogs—when caused by spontaneous hyperadrenocorticism (>75% older than 9 years); when caused by chronic inflammation or neoplasia
- Dogs of any age—iatrogenic disease subsequent to glucocorticoid administration
- Young dogs—idiopathic hyperlipidemia

Risk Factors

- Pharmacologic doses of glucocorticoids
- Breeds at risk for hyperadrenocorticism
- Spontaneous hyperadrenocorticism—pituitary-dependent or functional adrenal mass
- Other systemic conditions—see Causes
- Breeds at risk for hyperlipidemia—schnauzers, shelties, beagles

Clinical Features

- Often related to multisystemic effects of glucocorticoids or another systemic illness causing stress
- Rarely note signs of hepatic disease or failure
- Glucocorticoid excess—polydipsia and polyuria; polyphagia; endocrine alopecia; abdominal distention; muscle weakness; panting; lethargy
- Other causes—depend on the affected system
- Hepatomegaly
- Relate to glucocorticoid excess or the underlying disease; depend on severity and duration
- Adrenal overproduction of sex hormones—endocrine alopecia with hyperpigmentation

Differential Diagnosis

- Most other diffuse hepatopathies (especially those causing hepatomegaly and high serum hepatic enzyme activities)—passive congestion; neoplasia (primary or metastatic to the liver); inflammatory disease; anticonvulsant hepatopathy; hepatocellular swelling associated with diabetes mellitus (lipid vacuolation)

- Distinguishing features—normal serum total bilirubin concentration; normal to mild abnormalities in hepatic function tests (total serum bile acids concentrations); homogenous hyperechoic liver on ultrasonography; characteristic morphologic findings on hepatic fine-needle aspiration and biopsy
- If laboratory and clinical signs are compatible with the disorder and another underlying cause is not evident or the patient is symptomatic for hyperadrenocorticism, assess the pituitary–adrenal axis.
- Thorough physical assessment—essential; strong association with chronic illness

Diagnostics

CBC

- Depends on underlying disease
- Nonregenerative anemia—chronic inflammatory disease or hypothyroidism
- Relative polycythemia—hyperadrenocorticism
- Stress leukogram—hyperadrenocorticism; treatment with glucocorticoids; stress of other illness
- Thrombocytosis—hyperadrenocorticism

Biochemistry

- ALP and GGT—markedly high serum activities; GGT activity usually parallels that of ALP and cannot differentiate from other disorders
- ALT and AST—moderate increase
- Serum albumin and total bilirubin—usually normal; high bilirubin is unusual and indicates another hepatobiliary or hemolytic disease process
- Hypercholesterolemia—hyperadrenocorticism; some inborn errors of lipid metabolism; hypothyroidism; pancreatitis
- Total serum bile acids—may be normal or slightly to moderately high (up to ~75 μmol/L)
- Ammonia tolerance test—usually normal
- ALP glucocorticoid isoenzyme—always high in dogs with hyperadrenocorticism; also high in affected dogs without associated hyperadrenocorticism; sensitive for ruling out hyperadrenocorticism but cannot differentiate causes
- Pituitary–adrenal axis—evaluated with ACTH-response test or dexamethasone-suppression tests; document and differentiate types of hyperadrenocorticism
- High urine cortisol:creatinine ratio—suggests hyperadrenocorticism; less reliable than ACTH-response test or LDDST (spurious increases may occur in stressed patients)
- ACTH-stimulation test—blunted in patients receiving glucocorticoids
- Thyroid testing—rule out hypothyroidism

Imaging

- Abdominal radiography—reveals hepatomegaly and other underlying conditions
- Thoracic radiography—evaluated for lymphadenopathy or metastatic disease when hyperadrenocorticism is not noted; provides evidence of other primary disease process

- Abdominal ultrasonography—reveals hepatomegaly and diffuse or multifocal hyperechoic hepatic parenchyma; with multifocal disease, may observe a nodular-like pattern; may disclose evidence of underlying primary visceral disease, mesenteric lymphadenopathy, and adrenal size (often enlarged in stressed dogs)

Diagnostic Procedures

- Hepatic aspiration cytology—23- or 25-gauge, 2.5–3.75-cm (1–1.5-in) needle; may aspirate diffusely enlarged liver without ultrasonography; aspirate representative regions with multifocal echogenic pattern, sampling tissue with different echogenicity
- Hepatic biopsy—verify vacuolar change; exclude primary hepatic disease if other systemic diagnoses have not been made; method: ultrasound-guided needle, laparoscopy, or laparotomy
- Cytologic evaluation—may note inflammatory infiltrates, neoplasia, and obvious vacuolar or rarefied appearance of hepatocellular cytosol; expect bile in hepatocytes and canalicular casts between hepatocytes with severe disease
- Tissue evaluation—with suspected suppuration, initiate microbial culture (aerobic and anaerobic bacterial; fungal, if appropriate); special stains: PAS with and without amylase to discern glycogen
- Coagulation assessment—PT, APTT, ACT, fibrinogen, PIVKA, and mucosal bleeding time; indicated before liver biopsy

Pathologic Findings

- Gross—variable; normal liver; mild to moderate hepatomegaly; mild surface irregularity; loss of normal lobular pattern
- Microscopic—abnormalities usually pathognomonic; marked vacuolization and ballooning of hepatocytes in a centrilobular or diffuse distribution; mild hepatic necrosis; extramedullary hematopoiesis; small focal aggregates of neutrophils

Therapeutics

- Hyperlipidemia and pancreatitis—fat restriction
- Adrenocortical masses may be resected
- Pituitary-dependent hyperadrenocorticism—usually treated medically once diagnosis is confirmed; o,p′-DDD (mitotane, Lysodren), ketoconazole, or L-deprenyl
- Management of causal inflammatory conditions that may require immunosuppressive or anti-inflammatory medications—use very low dosages of glucocorticoids combined with other medications (see Alternative Drugs)
- Neoplasia—tumor resection and/or chemotherapy
- Dental disease—antibiotic therapy; appropriate dental procedures
- Pyelonephritis, chronic *Staphylococcus intermedius* dermatitis, or other infectious disorder—long-term antimicrobial treatment based on results of microbial culture and sensitivity tests
- Hypothyroidism—supplemental thyroxin
- Metronidazole, azathioprine, chlorambucil, and cyclophosphamide—may be considered for patients with immune-mediated disorders managed with glucocorticoids

Comments

Precautions

- Glucocorticoids—use caution when administering glucocorticoids to all patients; use an alternate-day protocol to reduce the severity of the disorder and the influence on the pituitary–adrenal axis; use caution when administering to dogs with inborn errors of lipid metabolism (schnauzers are at greatest risk of developing severe disease)

Patient Monitoring

- Hepatomegaly—abdominal palpation and radiography
- Normalizing enzymes—biochemistry
- Hyperadrenocorticism—ACTH-stimulation test to assess treatment efficacy
- Neoplasia—repeat physical examinations and imaging studies
- Control of infection—repeating cultures (e.g., urine)
- Hyperlipidemia—plasma lipemia, triglycerides, and cholesterol

Prevention/Avoidance

- Limit administration of glucocorticoids to confirmed conditions requiring anti-inflammatory or immunosuppressive therapy.
- Use alternate-day therapy and titrate to the lowest effective dose to minimize risk.

Prognosis

- Some patients do not develop disorder even with chronic glucocorticoid therapy.
- Some patients develop very high serum enzymes and disorder persisting for weeks even after short-term glucocorticoid therapy.
- The laboratory and hepatic morphologic abnormalities are completely reversible.

Associated Conditions

- Spontaneous hyperadrenocorticism—pituitary- or adrenal-dependent
- Diabetes mellitus
- Pulmonary thromboembolism
- Urinary tract infections
- Myopathy
- Neuropathy
- Hyperlipidemia
- Inflammatory bowel disease
- Dental disease
- Hypothyroidism
- Neoplasia
- Chronic pancreatitis

Abbreviations

- ACT = activated clotting time
- ALP = alkaline phosphatase
- ALT = alanine aminotransferase

- APTT = activated partial thromboplastin time
- AST = aspartate aminotransferase
- GGT = gamma-glutamyl-transferase
- LDDST = low-dose dexamethasone-suppression test
- PIVKA = proteins invoked by vitamin K absence or antagonism
- PT = prothrombin time

Suggested Reading

Center SA. Hepatic lipidosis, glucocorticoid hepatopathy, vacuolar hepatopathy, storage disorders, amyloidosis, and iron toxicity. In Guilford GW, Center, SA, Strombeck DR, et al., eds. Small animal gastroenterology. Philadelphia: Saunders, 1996:766–801.

Consulting Editor Karen Helton Rhodes

Feline Skin Fragility Syndrome

Karen Helton Rhodes

Definition/Overview

- A disorder of multifactorial causes characterized by extremely fragile skin
- Tends to occur in old cats that may have concurrent hyperadrenocorticism, diabetes mellitus, or excessive use of megestrol acetate or other progestational compounds
- A small number of cats have had no biochemical alterations.

Etiology/Pathophysiology

- Hyperadrenocorticism—pituitary or adrenal dependent
- Iatrogenic—secondary to excessive corticosteroid or progestational drug use
- Diabetes mellitus—rare, unless associated with hyperadrenocorticism
- Possibly idiopathic

Signalment/History

- Naturally occurring disease tends to be recognized in old cats.
- Iatrogenic cases have no age predilection.
- No breed or sex predilection
- Gradual onset of clinical signs
- Progressive alopecia (not always present) (Fig. 63-1)
- Often associated with weight loss, lusterless coat, poor appetite, and lack of energy

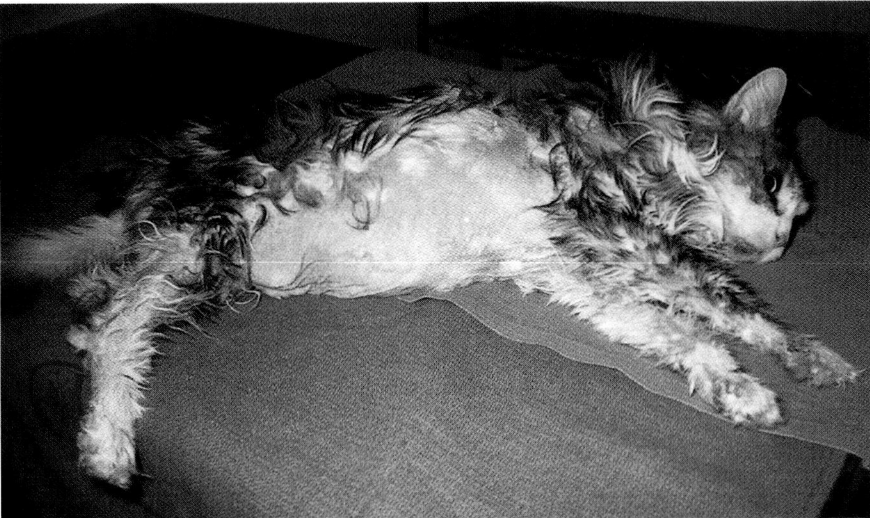

Figure 63-1 Feline hyperadrenocorticism. Truncal alopecia.

Clinical Features

- The skin becomes markedly thin and tears with normal handling. (Figs. 63-2, 63-3)
- The skin rarely bleeds upon tearing.
- Multiple lacerations (both old and new) may be noted on close examination.
- Partial to complete alopecia of the truncal region may be noted. (Fig. 63-4)
- Sometimes associated with rat tail, pinnal folding, pot-belly appearance

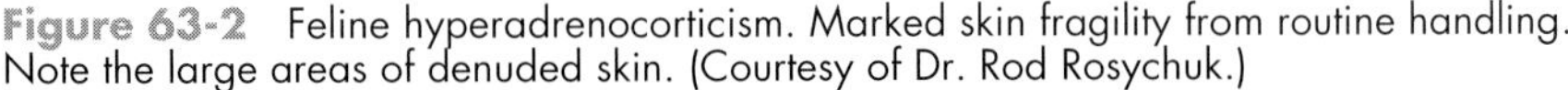

Figure 63-2 Feline hyperadrenocorticism. Marked skin fragility from routine handling. Note the large areas of denuded skin. (Courtesy of Dr. Rod Rosychuk.)

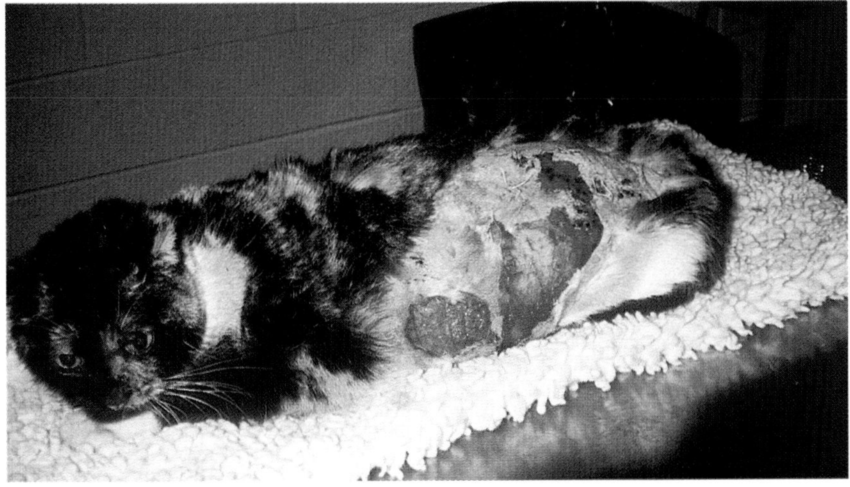

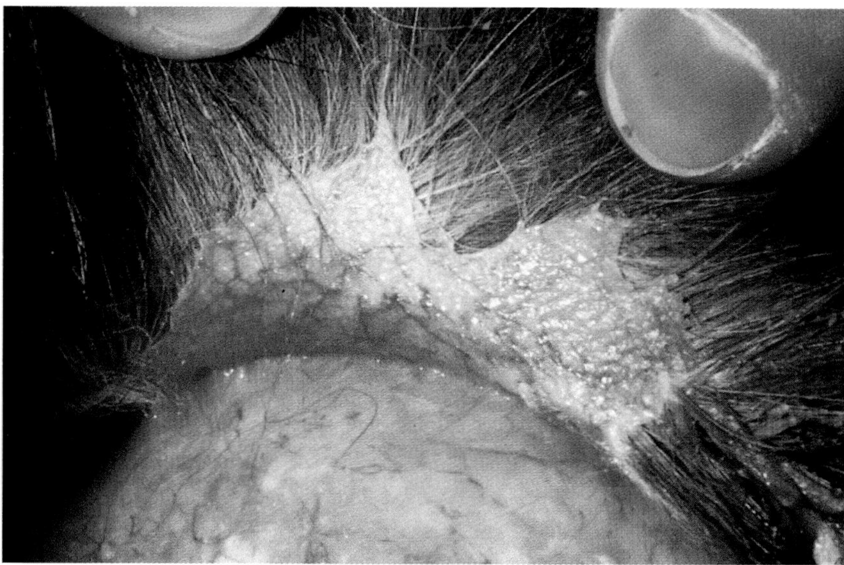

Figure 63-3 Close-up view of Figure 63-2. The skin easily degloves with minimal pain or hemorrhage. Suturing of these lesions is often futile. (Courtesy of Dr. Rod Rosychuk.)

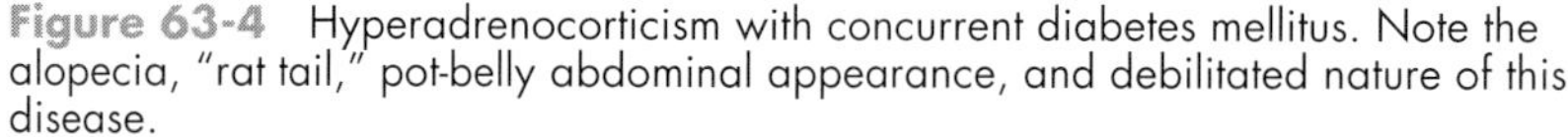

Figure 63-4 Hyperadrenocorticism with concurrent diabetes mellitus. Note the alopecia, "rat tail," pot-belly abdominal appearance, and debilitated nature of this disease.

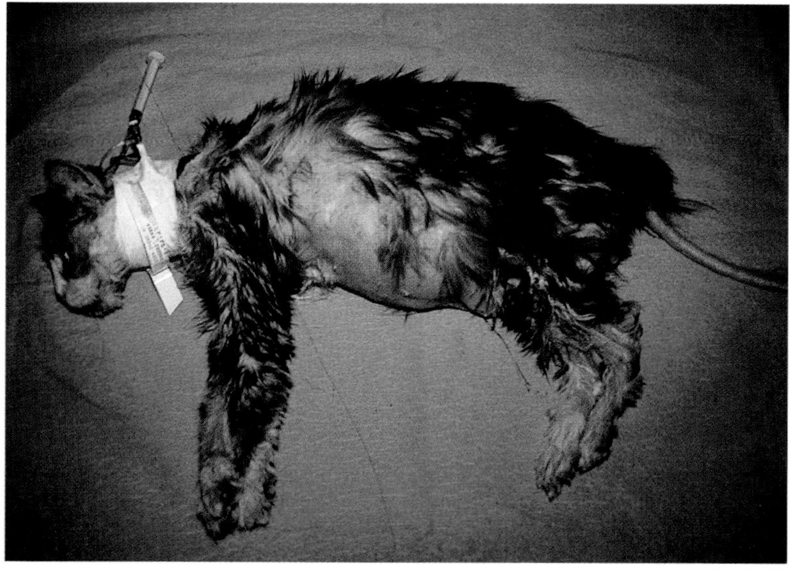

Differential Diagnosis

- Cutaneous asthenia
- Feline paraneoplastic syndrome—pancreatic neoplasia, hepatic lipidosis, cholangiocarcinoma
- Progestogen administration

Diagnostics

- Approximately 80% of cats with hyperadrenocorticism have concurrent diabetes mellitus (hyperglycemia, glucosuria).
- ACTH-stimulation test—70% of cats with hyperadrenocorticism have an exaggerated response.
- LDDST—15–20% of normal cats may fail to decrease cortisol levels; typically unsuppressed with hyperadrenocorticism and nonadrenal illness
- HDDST—normal cats show decreases in cortisol concentrations; typically decreased with nonadrenal illnesses; considered by many clinicians to be the best screening test for hyperadrenocorticism; unreliable for discriminating between adrenal tumors and pituitary-dependent causes of hyperadrenocorticism, because both conditions fail to show suppression
- Endogenous ACTH levels—normal range for most labs is 20–100 pg/mL.
- Abdominal ultrasonography—adrenal masses are often small until end-stage disease.
- CT and MR imaging—small pituitary tumors may be difficult to visualize; MR imaging may be more successful
- Histopathology—suggestive, not diagnostic; epidermis and dermis are thin; attenuated collagen fibers are evident

Therapeutics

- Underlying metabolic disease should be ruled out.
- Many patients are debilitated and require supportive care.
- Surgical correction of the lacerations—not helpful because the tissue cannot withstand any pressure from the sutures
- Hyperadrenocorticism—adrenalectomy is the preferred treatment.
- Cobalt-60 radiation therapy—variable success in the treatment of pituitary tumors
- Medical management—may be useful for preparing patient for surgery and for minimizing postoperative complications (e.g., infections and poor wound healing)
- No known effective medical therapy for feline hyperadrenocorticism
- o,p′-DDD (mitotane)—12.5–50 mg/kg PO q12h; response has been equivocal; side effects include anorexia, vomiting, and diarrhea
- Ketoconazole (nizoral)—10–15 mg/kg PO q12h; variable response
- Metyrapone—65 mg/kg PO q12h; clinical improvement noted more often with this drug than with others

Comments

- Hyperadrenocorticism—closely monitor diabetic cat; adjust insulin to prevent hypoglycemia when the cortisol levels fall
- Patients are often quite debilitated, making any form of treatment risky; close monitoring is required in all cases.
- Prognosis—grave

Suggested Reading

Gross TL, Ihrke PJ, Walder EJ. Veterinary dermatopathology. Philadelphia: Mosby, 1992.

Helton Rhodes K. Cutaneous manifestations of hyperadrenocorticism. In: August JR, ed. Consultations in feline internal medicine. Philadelphia: Saunders, 1997:191–198.

Author Karen Helton Rhodes

Contributing Editor Karen Helton Rhodes

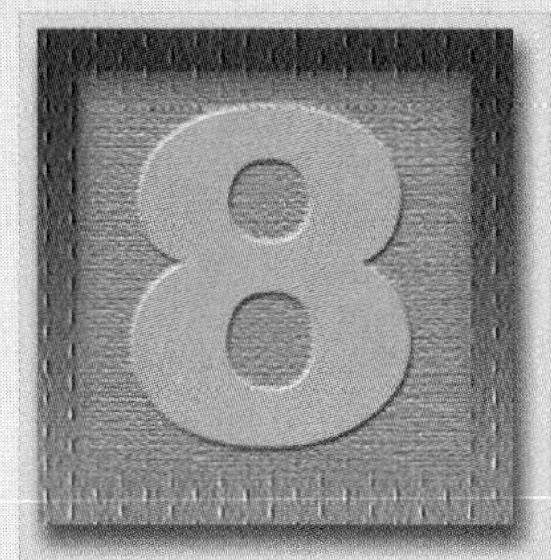

Immunologic/ Autoimmune Disorders

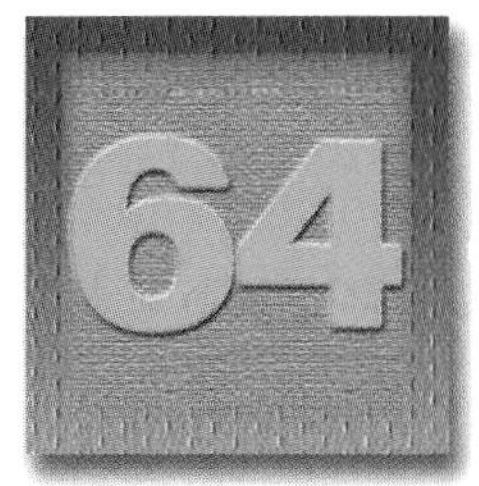

Pemphigus

Margaret S. Swartout

Definition/Overview

- A group of autoimmune dermatoses characterized by varying degrees of ulceration, crusting, and pustule and vesicle formation
- Affects the skin and sometimes mucous membranes

Etiology/Pathophysiology

- Tissue-bound autoantibody directed at interepidermal cell antigen is deposited within the intercellular spaces, causing epidermal cell separation and cell rounding (acantholysis).
- Severity of ulceration and disease—related to depth of autoantibody deposition within the skin
- Types—foliaceus, vulgaris, erythematosus, and vegetans
- Foliaceus—autoantibody deposition in the superficial layers of the epidermis
- Vulgaris—lesions more severe; mediated by autoantibody deposition just above the basement membrane zone; results in deeper ulcer formation

Signalment/History

- Uncommon group of diseases
- Foliaceus—most common type
- Erythematosus—relatively common; may be a more benign variant of pemphigus foliaceus or may be a crossover syndrome of pemphigus and lupus erythematosus

- Vulgaris—second most common type; the most severe form
- Vegetans—rarest type; possibly a relatively benign variant of pemphigus vulgaris
- Foliaceus, erythematosus, and vulgaris—dogs and cats
- Vegetans—dogs only
- Foliaceus—akitas, bearded collies, chow chows, dachshunds, Doberman pinschers, Finnish spitzes, Newfoundlands, and schipperkes
- Erythematosus—collies, German shepherds, and Shetland sheepdogs
- Usually middle-aged to old animals

Clinical Features

P. Foliaceus

- Scales, crust, pustules, epidermal collarettes, erosions, erythema, alopecia, and footpad hyperkeratosis with fissuring
- Occasional vesicles are transient.
- Common involvement—head, ears, and footpads; often becomes generalized (Fig. 64-1)
- Mucosal and mucocutaneous lesions uncommon
- Cats—nipple and nailbed involvement common
- Sometimes lymphadenopathy, edema, depression, fever, and lameness (if footpads involved); however, patients are often in good health (Figs. 64-2, 64-3).
- Variable pain and pruritus
- Secondary bacterial infection possible

P. Erythematosus

- As for pemphigus foliaceus
- Lesions usually confined to head, face, and footpads
- Mucocutaneous depigmentation more common than with other forms (Fig. 64-4).

Figure 64-1 This mature spayed female dog demonstrated ear, periocular, and nasal crusting associated with Pemphigus foliaceus.

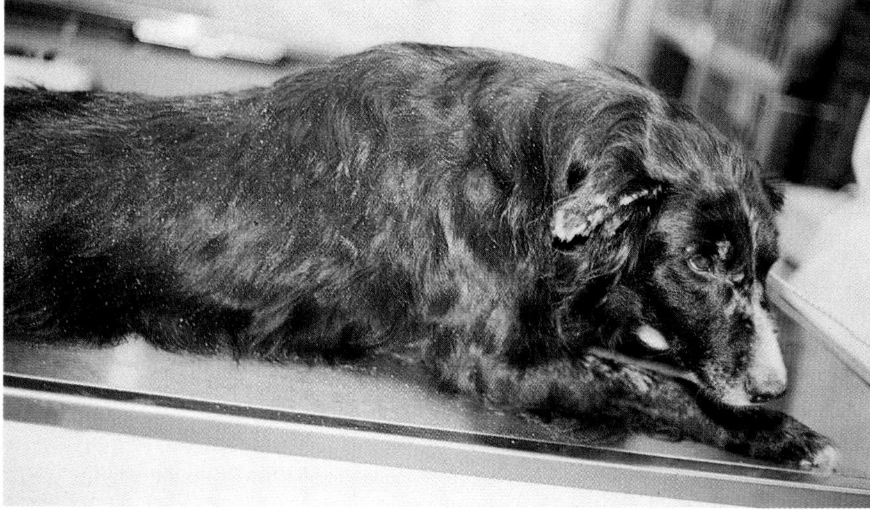

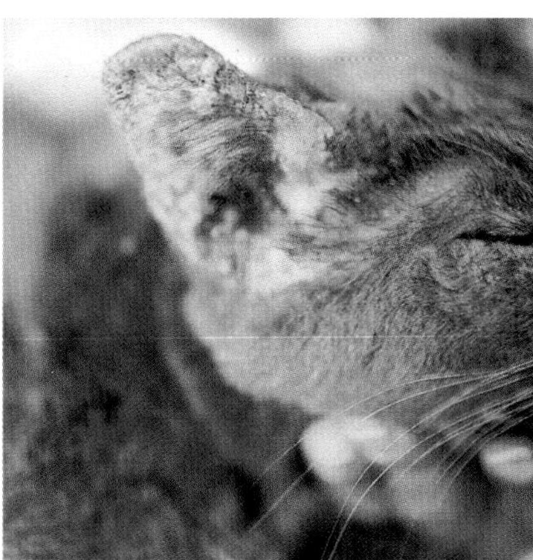

Figure 64-2 Ear crusting and erosion was severe and this neutered male cat was febrile (104°F) at the time of biopsy for histopathology and immunofluorescence; a diagnosis of Pemphigus foliaceus was obtained.

Figure 64-3 Feline Pemphigus foliaceus patients often have sterile pustule-like lesions of the footpads (white spots on dark grey footpads of this cat).

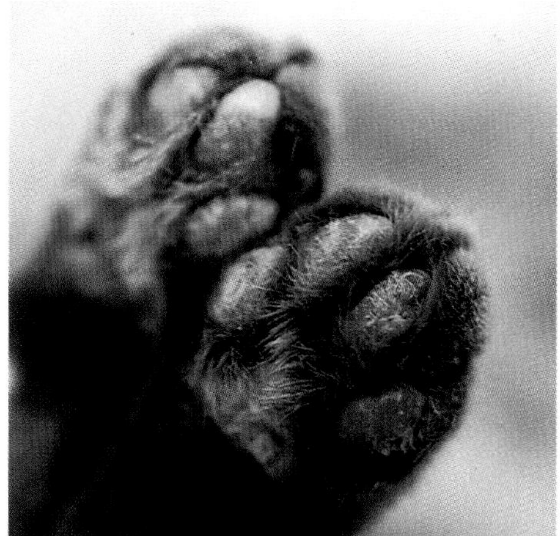

Figure 64-4 Pemphigus erythematosus was manifested in this middle-aged female dog by mucocutaneous ulceration.

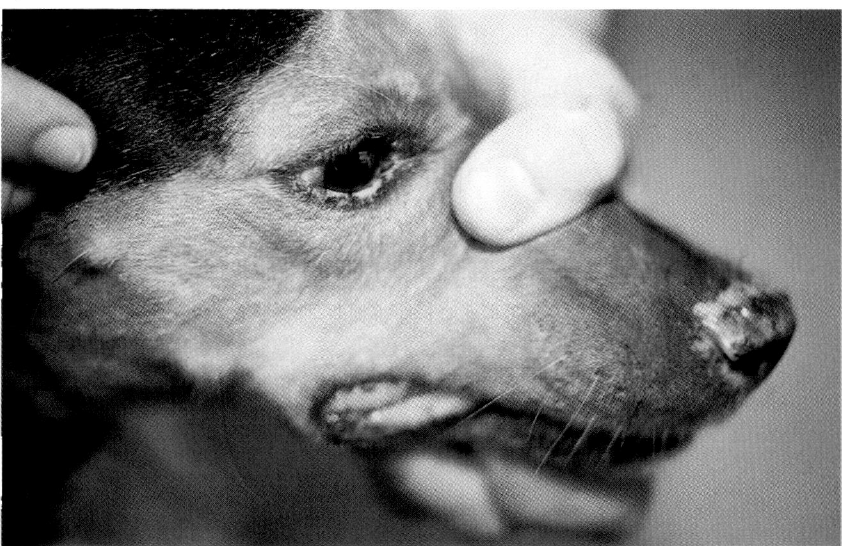

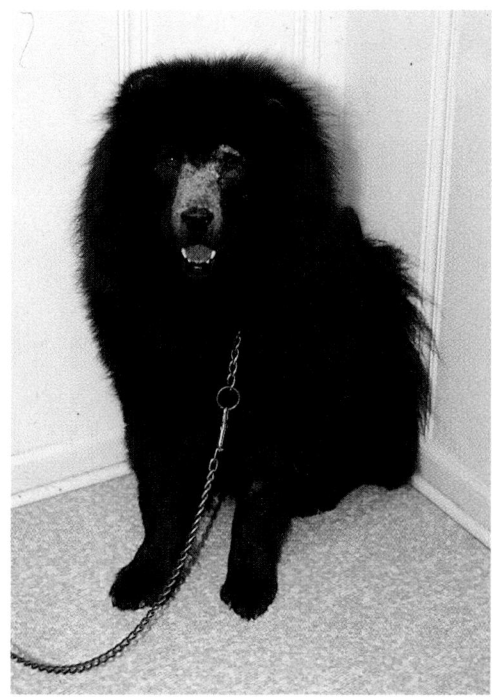

Figure 64-5 This mature intact male chow was in a lot of pain because of severe facial crusting from Pemphigus vulgaris.

P. VULGARIS

- Ulcerative lesions, erosions, epidermal collarettes, blisters, and crusts (Fig. 64-5)
- More severe than Pemphigus foliaceus and erythematosus
- Affects mucous membranes, mucocutaneous junctions, and skin; may become generalized
- Oral ulceration frequent
- Axillae and groin areas often involved
- Positive Nikolsky sign (new or extended erosive lesion created when lateral pressure is applied to the skin near an existing lesion)
- Variable pruritus and pain
- Anorexia, depression, and fever
- Secondary bacterial infections common

P. VEGETANS

- Pustule groups become eruptive papillomatous lesions and vegetative masses that ooze.
- Oral involvement has not been noted.
- No systemic illness

Differential Diagnosis

FOLIACEUS

- Bacterial folliculitis
- Dermatophytosis
- Demodicosis

- Candidiasis
- Keratinization disorders
- Lupus erythematosus
- Pemphigus erythematosus
- Subcorneal pustular dermatosis
- Drug eruption
- Zinc-responsive dermatitis
- Dermatomyositis
- Tyrosinemia
- Mycosis fungoides
- Lymphoreticular malignancies
- Metabolic epidermal necrosis
- Sterile eosinophilic pustulosis
- Linear IgA dermatosis

P. Erythematosus

- Pemphigus foliaceus
- Systemic lupus erythematosus
- Discoid lupus erythematosus
- Nasal pyoderma
- Demodicosis
- Dermatophytosis
- Epidermolysis bullosa simplex
- Uveodermatologic syndrome

P. Vulgaris

- Bullous pemphigoid
- Systemic lupus erythematosus
- Toxic epidermal necrolysis
- Drug eruption
- Mycosis fungoides
- Lymphoreticular neoplasia
- Ulcerative stomatitis causes
- Erythema multiforme

P. Vegetans

- Pemphigus vulgaris
- Bacterial folliculitis
- Pemphigus foliaceus
- Lichenoid dermatoses
- Cutaneous neoplasia

Diagnostics

- Leukocytosis and hyperglobulinemia sometimes noted
- Antinuclear antibody—may be weakly positive in Pemphigus erythematosus only

- Cytology of aspirates or impression smears of pustules or crusts—acantholytic cells and neutrophils
- Bacteriologic culture—identify secondary bacterial infections

Pathologic Findings

- Biopsies of lesional or perilesional skin—acantholysis and intraepidermal clefting; microabscess or pustule formation; surface acantholytic keratinocytes
- Location of epidermal lesions—varies with disease; pemphigus foliaceous and erythematosus have subcorneal or intragranular clefting and acantholysis; Pemphigus vulgaris and vegetans have suprabasilar clefting
- Immunopathology of biopsied skin via immunofluorescent antibody assays or immunohistochemical testing—may demonstrate positive staining in the intercellular spaces in 50–90% of cases; results can be affected by concurrent or previous corticosteroid (or other immunosuppressive drug) administration; indirect immunofluorescence usually negative; Pemphigus erythematosus may demonstrate staining of basement membranes and intercellular spaces

Therapeutics

- Initial inpatient supportive therapy for severely affected patients
- Outpatient treatment with initial frequent hospital visits (every 1–3 weeks); taper to every 1–3 months that remission is achieved and the patient is on maintenance medical regime.
- Low-fat diet—to avoid pancreatitis predisposed by corticosteroids and (possibly) azathioprine therapy
- Advise client that the patient should avoid the sun, because UV light may exacerbate lesions.

Drugs

Pemphigus Vulgaris and Foliaceus

Corticosteroids

- Prednisone or prednisolone—1.1–2.2 mg/kg/day PO divided q12h to initiate control
- Minimum maintenance—0.5 mg/kg PO q48h
- Taper dosage at 2–4 week intervals by 5–10 mg per week.

Cytotoxic Agents

- More than half of patients require the addition of other immunomodulating drugs.
- Generally work synergistically with prednisone, allowing reduction in dose and side effects of the corticosteroid
- Azathioprine—2.2 mg/kg PO q24h, then q48h (dogs); infrequently used in cats, owing to potential for marked bone marrow suppression; feline dose 1 mg/kg q24–48h
- Chlorambucil—0.2 mg/kg daily; best choice for cats
- Cyclophosphamide—50 mg/m^2 PO BSA q48h (dogs)
- Cyclosporine—15–27 mg/kg daily PO; limited application
- Dapsone—1 mg/kg PO q8h; then as needed (dogs); limited application

Chrysotherapy

- Often used in conjunction with prednisone
- Aurothioglucose—administer a test dose of 1 mg IM (animals <25 kg) or 5 mg IM (animals >25 kg) 1st week; 2 mg IM (animals <25 kg) or 10 mg IM (animals >25 kg) 2nd week; then 1 mg/kg IM weekly until a clinical response is noted (generally a lag phase of 6–8 weeks); then 1 mg/kg IM every 2–4 weeks for maintenance
- Auranofin—0.1–0.2 mg/kg PO q12–24h

Pemphigus Erythematosus and Vegetans

- Oral prednisone or prednisolone—1.1 mg/kg PO q24h; then q48h; then to the lowest maintenance dose possible; may be stopped when in remission
- Topical steroids may be sufficient in mild cases.

PRECAUTIONS

- Corticosteroids—polyuria, polydipsia, polyphagia, temperament changes, diabetes mellitus, pancreatitis, and hepatotoxicity
- Azathioprine—pancreatitis
- Cytotoxic drugs—leukopenia, thrombocytopenia, nephrotoxicity, and hepatotoxicity
- Chrysotherapy—leukopenia, thrombocytopenia, nephrotoxicity, dermatitis, stomatitis, and allergic reactions
- Cyclophosphamide—hemorrhagic cystitis
- Immunosuppression—can predispose animal to *Demodex,* cutaneous and systemic bacterial and fungal infection

Alternative Corticosteroids

- Use instead of prednisone if undesirable side effects or poor response occur.
- Methylprednisolone—0.8–1.5 mg/kg PO q12h; for patients that tolerate prednisone poorly
- Triamcinolone—0.2–0.3 mg/kg PO q12h; then 0.05–0.1 mg/kg q48–72h
- Glucocorticoid pulse therapy—11 mg/kg IV methylprednisolone sodium succinate for 3 consecutive days to induce remission; limited application

Topical Steroids

- Hydrocortisone cream
- More potent topical corticosteroids—0.1% betamethasone valerate, fluocinolone acetonide, or 0.1% triamcinonide; q12h; then q24–48h

Miscellaneous

Tetracycline and niacinamide—500 mg PO q8h (dogs >10 kg); half doses for dogs <10 kg; limited application

Comments

- Monitor response to therapy.
- Monitor for medication side effects—routine hematology and serum biochemistry, especially patients on high doses of corticosteroids, cytotoxic

drugs, or chrysotherapy; check every 1–3 weeks; then every 1–3 months when in remission

Pemphigus Vulgaris and Foliaceus

- Therapy with corticosteroids and cytotoxic drugs needed
- Patients may require medication for life.
- Monitoring necessary
- Side effects of medications may affect quality of life.
- May be fatal if untreated (especially pemphigus vulgaris)
- Secondary infections cause morbidity and possible mortality (especially pemphigus vulgaris).

Pemphigus Erythematosus and Vegetans

- Relatively benign and self-limiting
- Oral corticosteroids may eventually be tapered to low maintenance doses; may be stopped in some patients
- Dermatosis develops if untreated; systemic symptoms rare
- Prognosis fair

Suggested Reading

Ackerman LJ. Immune-mediated skin diseases. In: Morgan RV, ed. Handbook of small animal practice. 3rd ed. Philadelphia: Saunders, 1997:941–943.

Angarano DW. Autoimmune dermatosis. In: Nesbitt GH, ed. Contemporary issues in small animal practice: dermatology. New York: Churchill Livingstone, 1987:79–94.

Rosenkrantz WS. Pemphigus foliaceous. In: Griffin CE, Knochka KW, MacDonald JM, et al., eds. Current veterinary dermatology. St. Louis: Mosby, 1993:141–148.

Consulting Editor Karen Helton Rhodes

Bullous Pemphigoid

Margaret S. Swartout

Definition/Overview

- Very rare, autoimmune vesiculobullous severe ulcerative dermatosis of the skin and/or oral mucosa in dogs
- Forms—bullous (commonly identified) and chronic (rare)

Etiology/Pathophysiology

- Deposit of an autoantibody ("pemphigoid antibody") directed against the antigen at the basement membrane zone of skin and mucosa; results in blister formation below the epidermis
- Sunlight may exacerbate lesions.

Signalment/History

- Breed predilection—collies, Shetland sheepdogs, and (possibly) Doberman pinschers
- No age or sex predisposition

Clinical Features

Bullous

- Cutaneous lesions—transient blisters, crusts, epidermal collarettes, and ulcerations (Fig. 65-1)

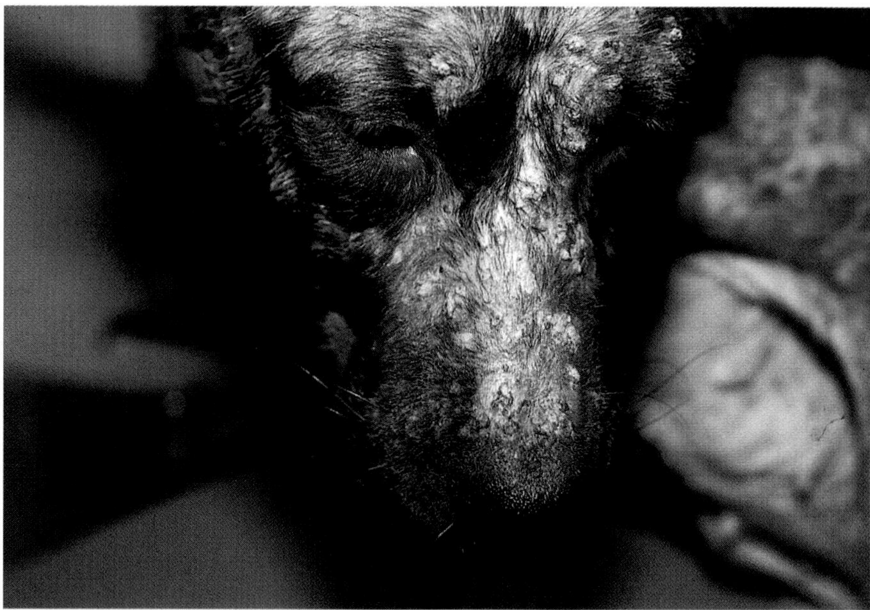

Figure 65-1 Bullous pemphigoid. Note the multifocal bullae and crusts on the bridge of the nose and periocular region in this dog.

- Widespread distribution—mucous membranes, head, neck, axillae, ventral abdomen, groin, and feet (nailbed involvement or footpad ulceration); oral cavity and skin of the axillae and groin most frequently involved
- Onset often acute with severe signs
- Severely affected dogs—anorexia, depression, and pyrexia

Figure 65-2 Chronic Bullous pemphigoid with lesions concentrated at the mucocutaneous junction of the planum nasale and the bridge of the nose.

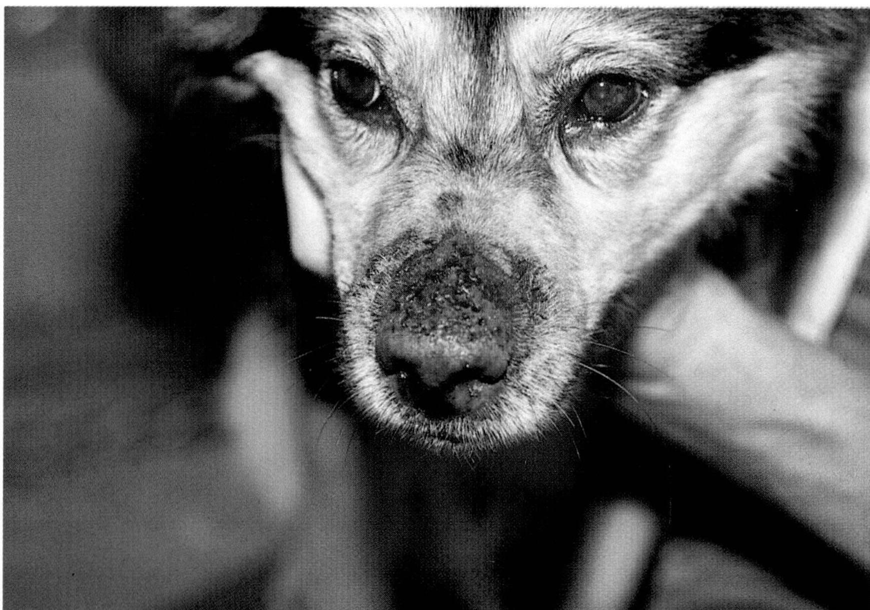

- Pain and pruritus variable
- Signs similar to pemphigus vulgaris

Chronic Pemphigoid

- Clinically benign
- Lesions—confined to the axillae, groin, or isolated mucocutaneous areas (Fig. 65-2)
- Slow and chronic course

Differential Diagnosis

- Pemphigus vulgaris
- Systemic lupus erythematosus
- Erythema multiforme
- Toxic epidermal necrolysis
- Drug eruption
- Mycosis fungoides
- Lymphoreticular neoplasia
- Hidradenitis suppurativa
- Ulcerative stomatitis

Diagnostics

- Leukocytosis, neutrophilia, mild nonregenerative anemia, hypoalbuminemia, and hyperglobulinemia may be seen.
- Antinuclear antibody titer normal
- Lupus erythematosus test negative
- Biopsies of lesions—subepidermal vesicle formation with inflammatory infiltrates of granulocytes and mononuclear cells; no acantholysis
- Direct immunofluorescence usually negative if positive, dermoepidermal junction pattern
- Bacteriologic culture—identification and drug sensitivity of secondary bacteria

Therapeutics

- Supportive inpatient care if serious systemic signs or secondary infections occur
- Subsequent outpatient treatment; frequent hospital rechecks and monitoring every 1–4 weeks
- Low-fat diet—avoids pancreatitis secondary to corticosteroid and possible azathioprine therapy
- Avoid sunlight—UV light may exacerbate lesions

Bullous

- Immunosuppressive agents
- Antibiotics for common secondary bacterial infections

- Gentle soaks/cleansing with antibacterial shampoos or povidone iodine and water

Chronic

- Immunosuppressive therapy
- Topical or intralesional corticosteroids

Drugs

Corticosteroids

- Prednisone or prednisolone—1.1–3.3 mg/kg PO q12h
- Higher doses are probably necessary, but side effects are likely and need to be monitored.

Cytotoxic Agents

- Required by many patients to achieve control, owing to intolerable side effects of high-dose corticosteroids or failure to achieve or maintain remission with corticosteroids alone
- Work synergistically with corticosteroids to reduce side effects
- Azathioprine—2.2 mg/kg PO q24h; then q48h
- Chlorambucil—0.1 mg/kg PO q24h; then q48h
- Cyclophosphamide—50 mg/m^2 BSA q48h
- 6-Mercaptopurine—2.2 mg/kg PO q24h; then q48h
- Dapsone—1 mg/kg PO q8h; then as needed; rarely used

Chrysotherapy with Prednisone

- Aurothioglucose—administer a test dose of 1 mg IM (animals < 25 kg) or 5 mg IM (animals > 25 kg) 1st week; 2 mg IM (animals < 25 kg) or 10 mg IM (animals > 25 kg) 2nd week; then 1 mg/kg IM weekly until a clinical response is noted (usually a lag phase of 6–8 weeks); then 1 mg/kg IM every 2–4 weeks for maintenance
- Auranofin—0.1–0.2 mg/kg PO q12–24h

Contraindications/Possible Interactions

- Corticosteroids—polyuria, polydipsia, polyphagia, temperament changes, hepatotoxicity
- Corticosteroid and azathioprine—pancreatitis
- Cytotoxic drugs—leukopenia, thrombocytopenia, nephrotoxicity, hepatotoxicity
- Chrysotherapy—nephrotoxicity, dermatitis, stomatitis, and allergic reactions
- Cyclophosphamide—hemorrhagic cystitis
- Immunosuppression—may predispose patient to *Demodex,* cutaneous and systemic fungal and bacterial infections

Comments

- Monitor often for signs of immunosuppression or progression of disease and medication side effects (reported, hematologic studies, and serum biochemistry).

Bullous

- May be fatal if untreated
- Treatment must be aggressive; side effects may affect quality of life.
- Lifelong treatment and monitoring of side effects are usually necessary.
- Secondary infections cause morbidity and possible mortality.
- Some patients may not respond to therapy.

Chronic

- Fair prognosis
- Mild, chronic disease treated with relatively low doses of systemic glucocorticoids; some patients can be treated with topical glucocorticoids alone.

Suggested Reading

Scott DW, Miller WH, Griffin CE. Bullous pemphigoid. In: Muller & Kirk's small animal dermatology. 5th ed. Philadelphia: Saunders, 1995:573–578.

Consulting Editor Karen Helton Rhodes

Discoid Lupus Erythematosus

Wayne S. Rosenkrantz

Definition/Overview

- Considered to be a benign variant of SLE
- Its comparative nature to the human form is controversial.
- One of the most common immune-mediated skin diseases
- Predominantly involves the planum nasale, face, ears, and mucous membranes; rarely other areas

Etiology/Pathophysiology

- Exact mechanism undetermined
- Genetic predisposition likely
- Suspected causes—drug reactions, viral initiation, and UV light exposure
- Seasonal exacerbations—associated with increased photoperiod and UV radiation
- UV exposure is a major concern.
- Antigen/antibody deposition at the dermal-epidermal junction

Signalment/History

- Predominantly in dogs; rarely in cats
- Predominant breeds—collies, German shepherds, Siberian huskies, Shetland sheepdogs, Alaskan malamutes, chow chows, and their crosses
- No age predilection

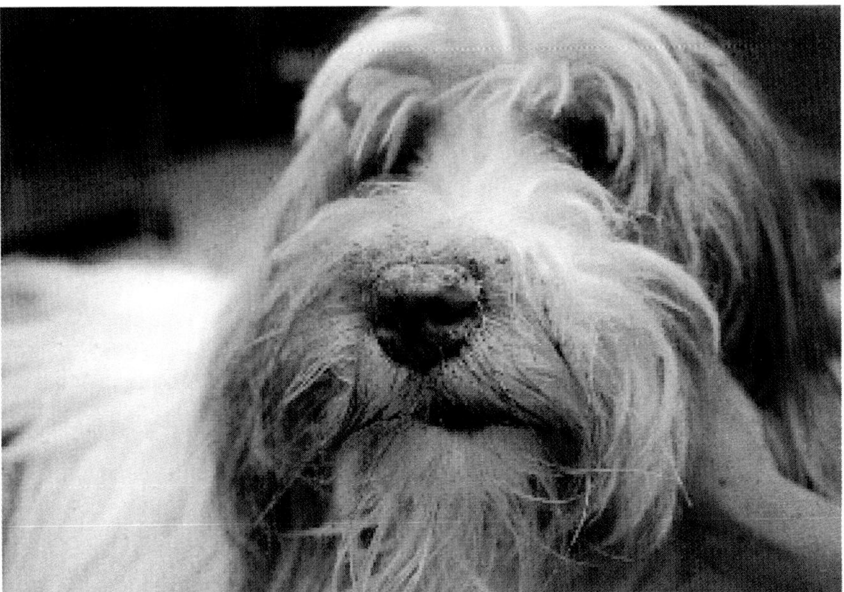

Figure 66-1 Discoid lupus erythematosus. Note the depigmentation of the planum nasale.

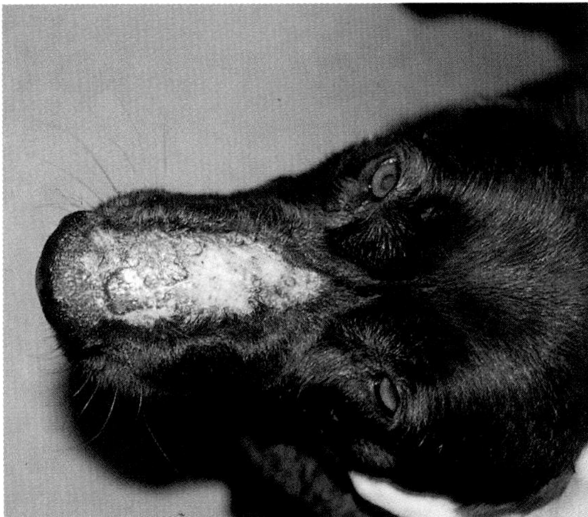

Figure 66-2 DLE. Note the extensive alopecia and scarring evident in this case.

Clinical Features

- Usually starts with depigmentation of planum nasale and/or lips (Fig. 66-1)
- Depigmentation progresses to erosions and ulcerations.
- Tissue loss and scarring can occur (Fig. 66-2).
- May also involve pinnae and periocular region; rarely feet and genitalia

Differential Diagnosis

- Other immune-mediated diseases—Pemphigus foliaceus, Pemphigus erythematosus, SLE, and uveodermatologic syndrome

- Drug reactions, erythema multiforme, and toxic epidermal necrolysis—nasal and facial lesions
- Dermatomyositis—affects some of the same predisposed breeds (collies and Shetland sheepdogs)
- Nasal pyoderma and nasal dermatophytosis—infectious conditions; can mimic discoid lupus erythematosus
- Insect hypersensitivity—one form creates a nasal inflammatory disease
- Contact allergy
- Zinc-responsive dermatosis
- Metabolic epidermal necrosis
- T cell epidermotropic lymphoma—may start on the planum and rostral aspect of the muzzle and lips
- Squamous cell carcinoma—may affect the planum; may occur at a slightly higher incidence in chronic discoid lupus lesions
- Idiopathic leukoderma leukotrichia (vitiligo)—may cause depigmentation of the tissue and hair without concurrent inflammation

Diagnostics

- ANA, LE preparation, and Coombs tests—usually normal or negative
- Biopsies of nonulcerated, slate-gray depigmented lesions—often characterized by interface lichenoid dermatitis with pigment incontinence and variable degrees of dermal mucin
- Immunopathologic examination of nonulcerated samples preserved in Michel's solution—may reveal positive basal laminal fluorescence

Therapeutics

Drugs

- Tetracycline and niacinamide—250 mg each PO q8h for dogs <10 kg; 500 mg PO q8h for larger dogs
- Vitamin E—10–20 IU/kg PO q12h; may help reduce inflammation
- Topical corticosteroids—initially, a potent fluorinated product (e.g., 0.1% amcinonide) q24h for 14 days; then q48–72h for 28 days; if in remission switch to less-potent product (e.g., 0.5% or 2.5% hydrocortisone)
- Prednisone—consider for severe or nonresponsive cases; 2–3 mg/kg daily either solely or in combination with azathioprine 2 mg/kg PO on alternate days; taper prednisone to 0.5–1 mg/kg PO q48h for long-term maintenance

Comments

- Recheck 14 days after initiating treatment for clinical response.
- CBC and biochemistry—every 3–6 months if using topical or oral corticosteroids for control
- CBC and platelet counts—every 2 weeks for the first 3–4 months; then every 3–6 months while on azathioprine
- Avoid using affected animals for breeding.
- May be disfiguring

- May create a source of trauma-induced bleeding
- Avoid direct solar exposure and use waterproof sunblocks with an SPF > 15.

Possible Complications

- Scarring
- Secondary pyoderma
- Bleeding
- Disfigurement

Expected Course and Prognosis

- Progressive but not usually life-threatening if left untreated
- With proper treatment, expect remission in most cases.
- The need for chronic immunosuppressive therapy suggests a more guarded prognosis, but remissions are common with more aggressive therapy.

Abbreviations

- ANA = antinuclear antibody
- LE = lupus erythematosus
- SLE = systemic lupus erythematosus

Suggested Reading

Rosenkrantz WS. Discoid lupus erythematosus: current veterinary dermatology. St. Loius: Mosby, 1993.

Consulting Editor Karen Helton Rhodes

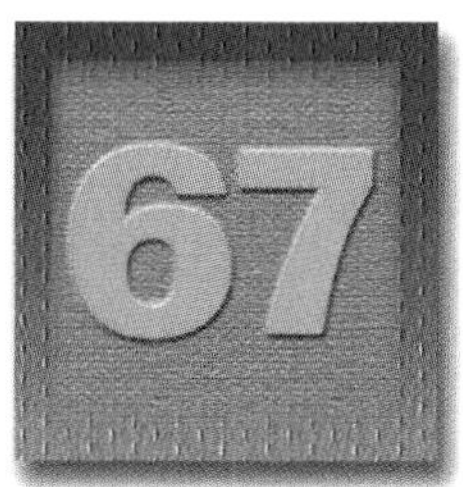

Systemic Lupus Erythematosus

Harm HogenEsch

Definition/Overview

A multisystem autoimmune disease characterized by the formation of autoantibodies against a wide array of self-antigens and circulating immune complexes

Etiology/Pathophysiology

- Cause unknown
- An immunoregulatory defect causes the production of autoantibodies to non-organ-specific nuclear and cytoplasmic antigens and to organ-specific antigens.
- Immune complexes are formed and deposited in the glomerular basement membrane, synovial membrane, skin, blood vessels, and other sites.
- Tissue injury—caused by activation of complement by immune complexes and infiltration of inflammatory cells and by a direct cytotoxic effect of autoantibodies against membrane-bound antigens
- Clinical manifestations depend on the localization of the immune complexes and the specificity of the autoantibodies.

Systems Affected

- Musculoskeletal—deposition of immune complexes in the synovial membranes
- Skin/Exocrine—deposition of immune complexes in the skin
- Renal/Urologic—deposition of immune complexes in the glomeruli

- Hemic/Lymph/Immune—autoantibodies against RBCs, leukocytes, or platelets
- Other organ systems—if there is deposition of immune complexes or autoantibodies

Signalment/History

- Hereditary in a colony of German shepherds
- Linked to the major histocompatibility complex allele DLA-A7
- Mean age 6 years, but can occur at any age
- The onset can be acute or insidious.
- Depend on the site of immune complex deposition and specificity of the autoantibodies
- Waxing and waning course with clinical manifestations often changing over time
- Lethargy
- Anorexia
- Shifting leg lameness
- Skin lesions
- Altered behavior

Clinical Features

- Joints may be swollen and painful.
- Symmetric or focal cutaneous lesions—characterized by erythema, scaling, ulceration, and alopecia; mucocutaneous and oral lesions common (Figs. 67-1, 67-2, 67-3)
- Fever
- Lymphadenopathy and hepatosplenomegaly

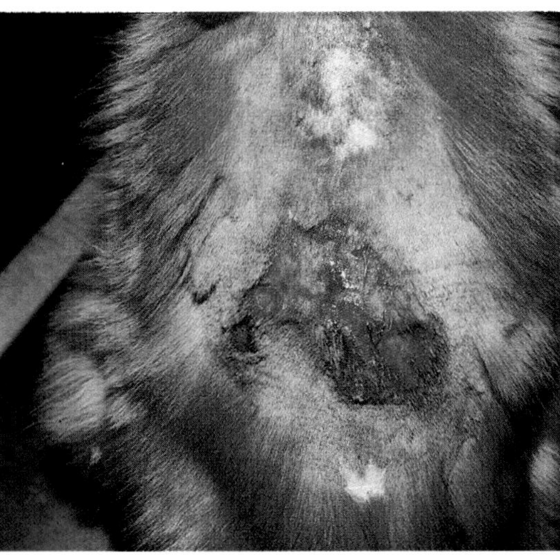

Figure 67-1 Systemic lupus erythematosus. Focal area of ulceration of the dorsum of this cat. There were no other lesions other than intermittent fever of greater than 104°F.

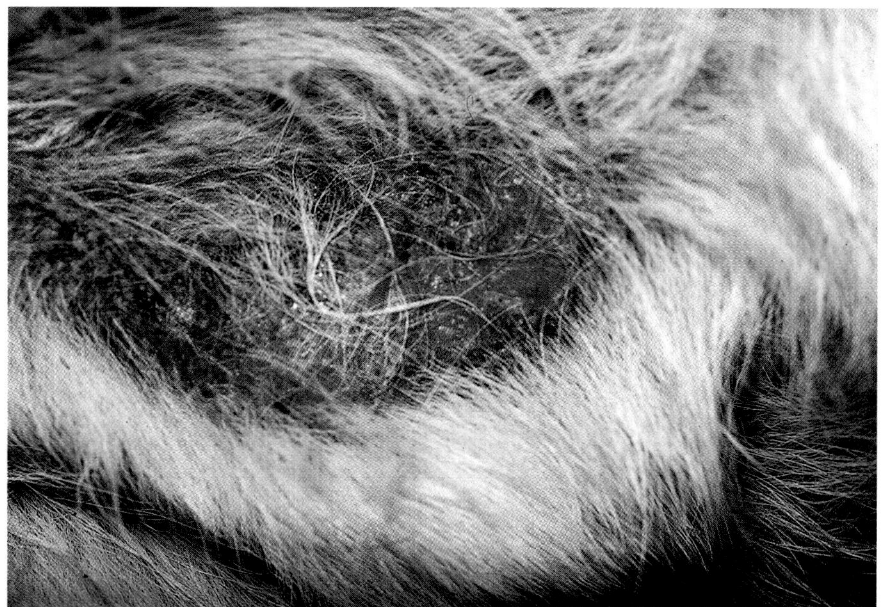

Figure 67-2 SLE in a dog. Focal ulceration over a pressure-point area.

Figure 67-3 SLE. Oral mucosal and lingual ulcerations are extensive in this case.

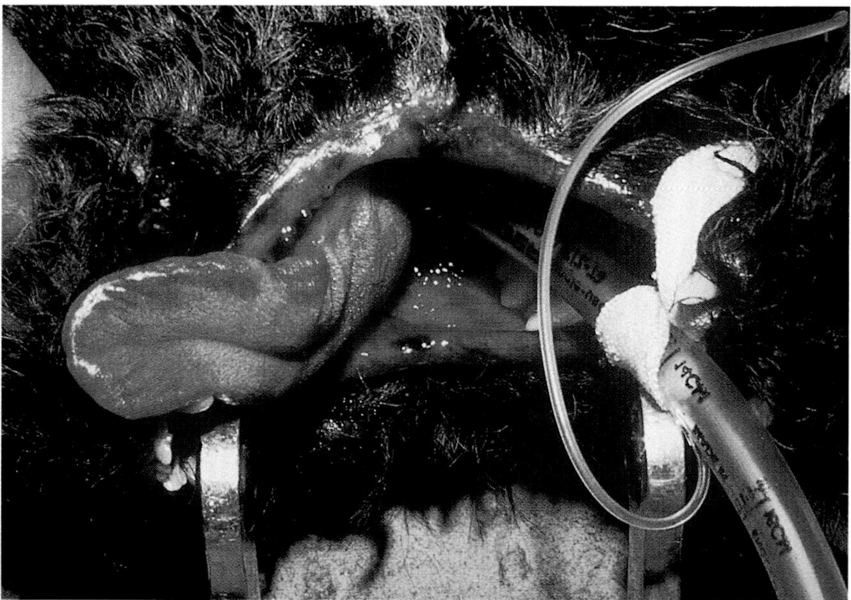

- Arrhythmias, heart murmurs, and pleural friction rubs (i.e., associated with myocarditis, pericarditis, or pleuritis)
- Muscle wasting

Differential Diagnosis

- Neoplastic disease—may be associated with circulating immune complexes; patient may have similar signs as SLE.
- Important to rule out infectious disease, because SLE is treated with immunosuppressive drugs.

Diagnostics

- Definitive diagnosis—positive ANA or LE cell test (or both) and two major signs or one major and two minor signs
- Probable diagnosis—positive ANA or LE cell test (or both) and one major or two minor signs
- Major signs—polyarthritis, proteinuria, dermatitis, hemolytic anemia, leukopenia, thrombocytopenia, and polymyositis
- Minor signs—fever of unknown origin, oral ulcers, peripheral lymphadenopathy, pleuritis, pericarditis, myocarditis, depression, and seizures
- *CBC*—anemia, leukopenia, and thrombocytopenia; leukocytosis (i.e., monocytosis and neutrophilia) resulting from chronic inflammation
- *Anemia*—moderate and nonregenerative (e.g., anemia of chronic disease) or severe and regenerative (e.g., hemolytic)
- *Biochemical analysis*—results vary widely, depending on the organ(s) affected
- *High urine protein:urine creatinine ratio* (>1) indicates true proteinuria that may be caused by glomerulonephritis.
- Patients with hemolytic anemia may have bilirubinuria.
- *Serum electrophoresis*—usually shows high concentration of β- and γ-globulins
- *ANA test*—a sensitive assay; positive results support diagnosis of SLE; false-positive results associated with some infectious diseases (e.g., leishmaniasis and subacute bacterial endocarditis in dogs; FeLV, cholangiohepatitis, and treatment with propylthiouracil in cats)
- *LE test*—positive result supports diagnosis of SLE; less sensitive than the ANA test and cumbersome to perform
- *Direct antiglobulin test* (Coombs test)—positive in patients with immune-mediated hemolytic anemia
- *Radiography* of affected joints reveals nonerosive arthritis, unlike the erosive lesions of rheumatoid arthritis.
- *Arthrocentesis* in patients with lameness or swollen joints; high cell count, with nondegenerate neutrophils and monocytes and low viscosity is a characteristic finding.
- *Bacterial culture* of synovial fluid is negative.
- *Skin biopsy* in patients with skin lesions; save specimen in 10% buffered formalin (for histopathologic examination) and Michel's solution (for immunofluorescence testing).

- *Bone marrow biopsy* in patients with nonregenerative anemia reveals excess iron deposition (anemia of chronic disease).

Pathologic Findings

- Nonerosive polyarthritis with infiltration of synovial membrane by neutrophils and lymphocytes; no pannus formation
- Membranous or membranoproliferative glomerulonephritis
- Mononuclear interface dermatitis with hydropic degeneration of keratinocytes and eosinophilic round bodies representing apoptotic basal keratinocytes
- Vasculitis of dermal blood vessels and panniculitis in some patients
- Immunofluorescence—deposition of immune complexes along the basement membrane of the dermal-epidermal junction
- Vasculitis may be seen in any organ, especially myocardium, pericardium, and meninges.
- Reactive lymphoid hyperplasia in the lymph nodes and spleen

Therapeutics

- Hospitalization may be necessary for initial management (e.g., in a patient with hemolytic crisis); outpatient management is usually possible.
- During episodes of acute polyarthritis, enforced rest is indicated.
- Dietary protein restriction recommended in animals with severe renal disease caused by glomerulonephritis

Drugs

- Goal of treatment—to control the abnormal immune response and to reduce the inflammation
- Corticosteroids—target both objectives; basis of treatment (prednisone, 1–2 mg/kg PO q12h)
- Cytotoxic immunosuppressive drug—add when prednisone fails to improve the condition or when the patient is steroid intolerant; reduce prednisone to 0.5–1 mg/kg PO q12h; use azathioprine (dogs, 2 mg/kg PO q24h), cyclophosphamide (dogs, 50 mg/m^2 PO for 4 consecutive days, then 3 days off, repeat weekly), or chlorambucil (dogs, 2–3 mg/m^2 PO; cats, 1.5 mg/m^2 PO)
- Reduce immunosuppressant drug dosage to lowest possible once remission is achieved.
- For painful joints—aspirin (dogs, 10–25 mg/kg PO q12h; cats, 10–40 mg/kg PO q72h) or carprofen (dogs, 2.2 mg/kg PO q12h)

Contraindications/Precautions

Aspirin should not be given to patients with thrombocytopenia or gastrointestinal ulcers.

- Cats are susceptible to azathioprine toxicity; this drug should be used with caution, if at all (dosage, 1 mg/cat PO q48h).
- Cyclophosphamide can induce hemorrhagic cystitis and bone marrow suppression.
- Treatment with immunosuppressive drugs increases the risk of severe infection.

Alternative Drugs

Cyclosporine (5–10 mg/kg PO q12h) may be tried in refractory patients; use with caution and withdraw if side effects occur (e.g., gastritis, lymphocytoid dermatitis, papillomatosis, and gingival hyperplasia).

Comments

- Weekly physical examination
- CBC and biochemical analysis to monitor side effects of the immunosuppressive drugs, initially weekly
- ANA remains high during remission and is not useful for monitoring the disease.
- Do not breed affected animals.
- Renal failure and nephrotic syndrome secondary to glomerulonephritis a concern
- Prognosis guarded to poor
- The presence of hemolytic anemia and glomerulonephritis and the development of bacterial infection warrant a poor prognosis.

Abbreviations

- ANA = antinuclear antibody
- FeLV = feline leukemia virus
- LE = lupus erythematosus

Suggested Reading

Lewis RM, Picut CA. Veterinary clinical immunology. Philadelphia: Lea & Febiger, 1989.

Halliwell REW, Gorman NT. Veterinary clinical immunology. Philadelphia: Saunders, 1989.

Pedersen NC, Barlough JE. Systemic lupus erythematosus in the cat. Feline Pract 1991;19:5–13.

Consulting Editor Karen Helton Rhodes

Panniculitis

Kevin Shanley

Definition/Overview

- An inflammation of the subcutaneous fat tissue
- Uncommon in dogs and cats
- Multiple causes
- Single or multiple subcutaneous nodules or draining tracts
- Usually involves the trunk
- The lipocyte (fat cell) is susceptible to trauma, ischemic disease, and inflammation from adjacent tissues.
- Histology—divided into lobular (involves the fat lobules), septal (involves the interlobular connective tissue septa), and diffuse (involves both lobular and interlobular septa) types
- Diffuse most common in dogs
- Septal most common in cats

Etiology/Pathophysiology

- Infectious—bacterial, fungal, atypical mycobacteria, infectious embolism
- Immune-mediated—lupus panniculitis, erythema nodosum
- Idiopathic—sterile nodular panniculitis
- Trauma
- Neoplastic—multicentric mast cell tumors, cutaneous lymphosarcoma, pancreatic panniculitis

- Foreign bodies
- Postinjection—corticosteroids, vaccines, other subcutaneous injections

Signalment/History

- No age, sex, or breed predilection
- Sterile nodular panniculitis—dachshunds are predisposed; collies and miniature poodles are at risk; can occur in any breed

Clinical Features

- Lesions—usually occur over the trunk; most dogs have a single nodular lesion over the ventral or lateral trunk; may become cystic and develop draining tracts; may be painful before and just after rupturing; ulcerations often heal with crusting and scarring
- Early cases of single or multifocal disease—nodules are freely movable underneath the skin; skin overlying the nodule is usually normal but may become erythematous or (less often) brown or yellow
- Nodules—vary from a few millimeters to several centimeters in diameter; may be firm and well circumscribed or soft and poorly defined; as they enlarge and develop, may fix to the deep dermis (thus, the overlying skin is not freely movable)
- Involved fat may necrose. (Fig. 68-1)
- Exudate—usually a small amount of oil discharge; yellow-brown to bloody
- Multiple lesions (dogs and cats)—systemic signs common (e.g., anorexia, pyrexia, lethargy, and depression) (Figs. 68-2, 68-3)

Figure 68-1 Idiopathic sterile nodular panniculitis. Note the large ulcerative area on the dorsum of the dog characterized by a greasy exudate indicating fat necrosis.

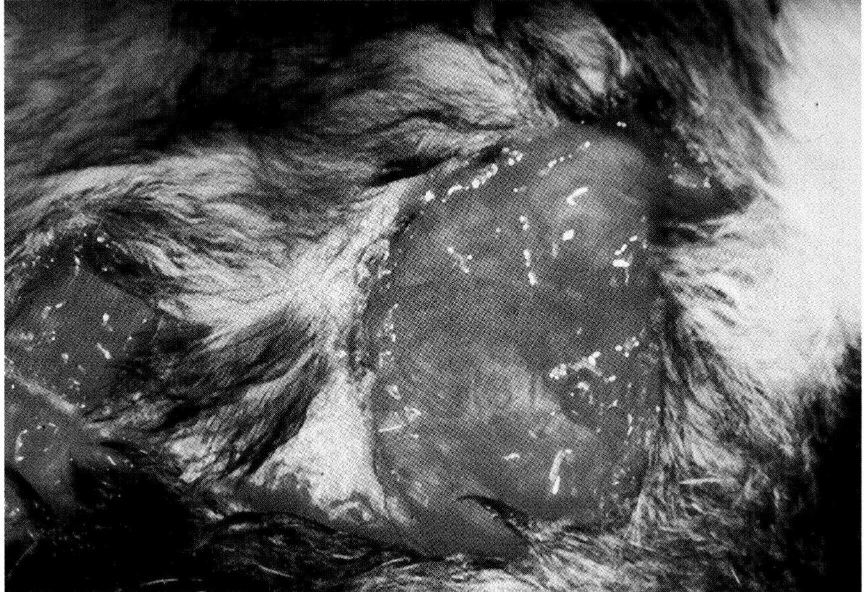

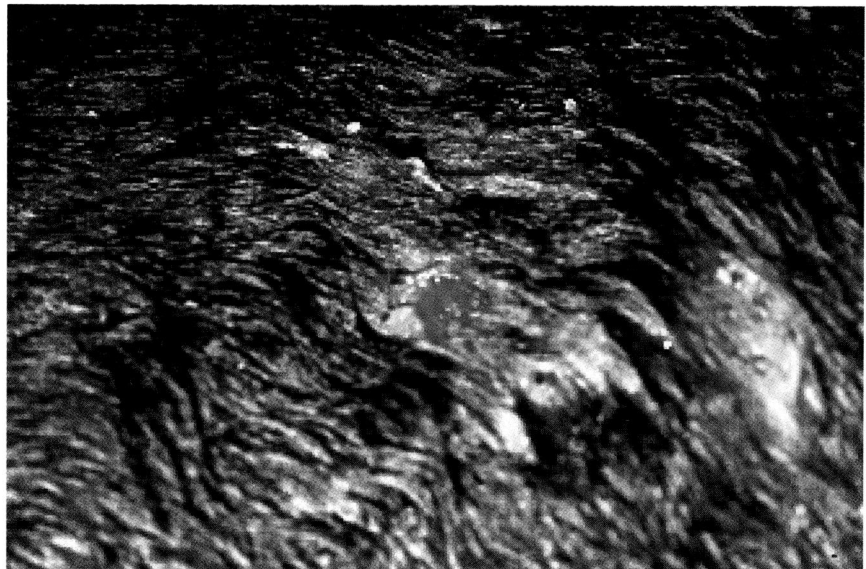

Figure 68-2 Sterile nodular panniculitis. Multifocal lesions before clipping the hair in the affected area (trunk). This dog was febrile and anorexic.

Figure 68-3 Panniculitis. Same dog in Figure 68-2 after the area was clipped. Note the abrupt demarcation between lesional and nonlesional skin.

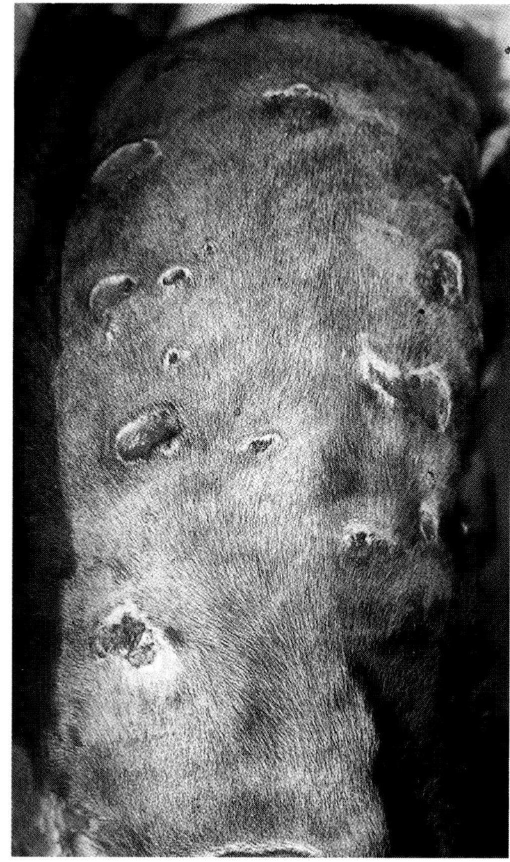

Differential Diagnosis

Deep Pyoderma

- More common than panniculitis
- More likely over pressure points
- May have associated lesions of superficial pyoderma (e.g., papules, pustules, and epidermal collarettes)
- Aspirates and impression smears—marked numbers of neutrophils with variable numbers of mononuclear cells and bacteria
- Culture/sensitivity and biopsies—confirm diagnosis

Cutaneous Cysts

- Usually nonpainful
- Well-demarcated
- Usually no inflammation
- Aspirates—amorphous debris; no inflammatory cells
- Biopsies—confirm diagnosis

Cutaneous Neoplasia

- Lipomas—soft; usually well demarcated
- No inflammation or draining tracts
- Aspirates—lipocytes; no inflammatory cells
- Biopsies—confirm diagnosis

Mast Cell Tumors/Cutaneous Lymphosarcoma/Pancreatic Panniculitis

- Multifocal
- May affect the head, legs, and mucous membranes
- Often erythematous
- Variable presentations
- Aspirates—often suggestive
- Biopsies—confirm diagnosis

Sterile Nodular Panniculitis

- A diagnosis made by ruling out other causes of panniculitis
- Biopsies, cultures, and other diagnostic tests—as indicated by the clinical presentation

Diagnostics

- Occasional regenerative left shift or eosinophilia
- Mild leukocytosis
- Mild normochromic, normocytic nonregenerative anemia
- Antinuclear antibody
- Direct immunofluorescence testing
- Serum protein electrophoresis
- Serum lipase/amylase levels

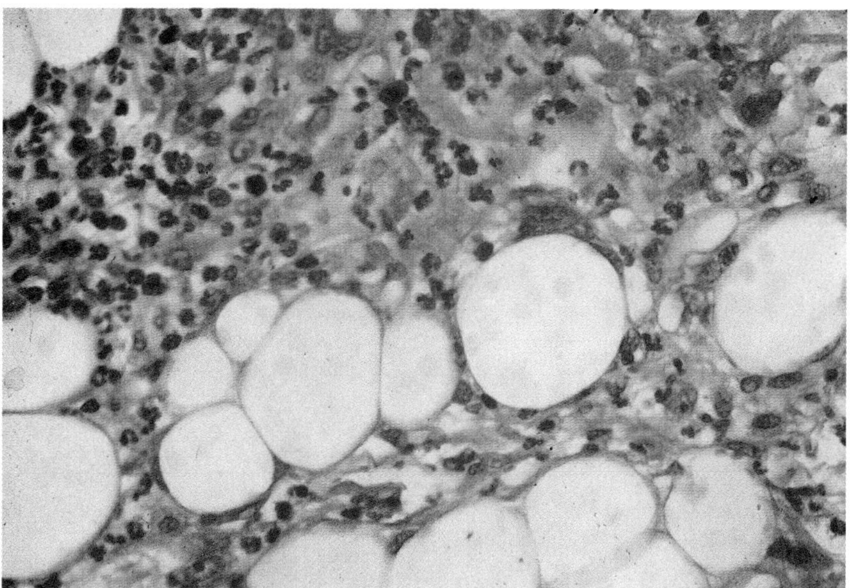

Figure 68-4 Histopathologic panniculitis. Note the massive influx of inflammatory cells around the fat lobules.

- Ultrasound—pancreatitis may be a contributing factor (rare)
- Bacterial culture and sensitivity testing—necessary for identifying primary or secondary bacteria
- Fungal and atypical mycobacteria culture
- Biopsies—negative cultures help diagnose sterile nodular panniculitis
- Special stains of histologic samples—help identify causative agent
- Surgical excisional biopsies—much more accurate than punch biopsy specimens in most cases; punch biopsies do not provide a deep enough sample to make the diagnosis
- Histologic lesions—required to make a diagnosis of panniculitis; determine septal, lobular, or diffuse inflammatory infiltrate by neutrophils, histiocytes, plasma cells, lymphocytes, eosinophils, or multinucleated giant cells; identify necrosis, fibrosis, or vasculitis (Fig. 68-4)

Therapeutics

- Single lesions—cured with surgical excision
- Multiple lesions—require systemic medications
- Positive culture results require appropriate antifungal, antibacterial, or antimycobacterial treatment.
- Sterile nodular panniculitis—systemic treatment with steroids; prednisone (2.2 mg/kg daily) until lesions completely regress (36 weeks); after remission, gradually taper dosage over 2 weeks; occasionally may need slower taper to minimize chance of recurrence; many patients cured; some patients need low-dose alternate-day treatment to maintain remission
- Oral vitamin E—may control mild cases

- Oral potassium iodide or azathioprine (1 mg/kg daily)—alternatives when steroids are contraindicated
- Immunosuppressive agents (i.e. azathioprine)

Comments

- Monitor CBC, platelet count, chemistry profile, and urinalysis if immune-suppressing agents or long-term glucocorticosteroids are used.
- Infectious cases may require long-term therapy with high doses of medications.
- Sterile idiopathic nodular panniculitis often responds quite rapidly to high doses of corticosteroids. Young animals have a more rapid recovery than older animals, which may require a maintenance protocol.

Suggested Reading

Scott DW, Miller WH, Griffin CE. Muller and Kirk's Small animal dermatology. 5th ed. Philadelphia: Saunders, 1995.

Author Kevin Shanley
Consulting Editor Karen Helton Rhodes

Vasculitis

Karen A. Kuhl and Jean S. Greek

Definition/Overview

- An inflammation of blood vessels with a neutrophilic (leukocytoclastic/non-leukocytoclastic), lymphocytic, rarely eosinophilic, granulomatous, or mixed cell types
- Pathomechanisms—type III (immune complex) and type I (immediate) reactions
- Endothelial damage by infectious agent, parasite infestation, endotoxin, or immune complex deposition initiates local inflammation, neutrophil accumulation, and complement activation. Neutrophils release lysosomal enzymes leading to necrosis of vessel wall, thrombosis, and hemorrhage. In humans and dogs with polyarteritis nodosa, intimal proliferation and vessel wall degeneration and necrosis predominate and lead to hemorrhage, thrombosis, and necrosis of involved vessels and adjacent tissues in most patients.
- Nondermal vasculitis (e.g., renal, hepatic, and serosal surfaces of body cavities) may be the mechanism leading to development of clinically apparent signs of systemic disease (e.g., polyarthritis and proteinuria) without causing obvious external lesions.

Signalment/History

- Any age, breed, or sex may be affected.
- Dachshunds and rottweilers may be predisposed.
- Varies depending on cause

- Provocative drug exposure (e.g., penicillin, sulfonamides, streptomycin, and hydralazine) given to sensitized animal
- Exposure to ticks
- Dirofilariasis

Clinical Features

- Palpable purpura
- Hemorrhagic bullae
- Necrosis and "punched-out" ulcers (Figs. 69-1, 69-2)

Figure 69-1 Severe vasculitis secondary to staphylococcal hypersensitivity. Note the "punched-out" areas of ulceration.

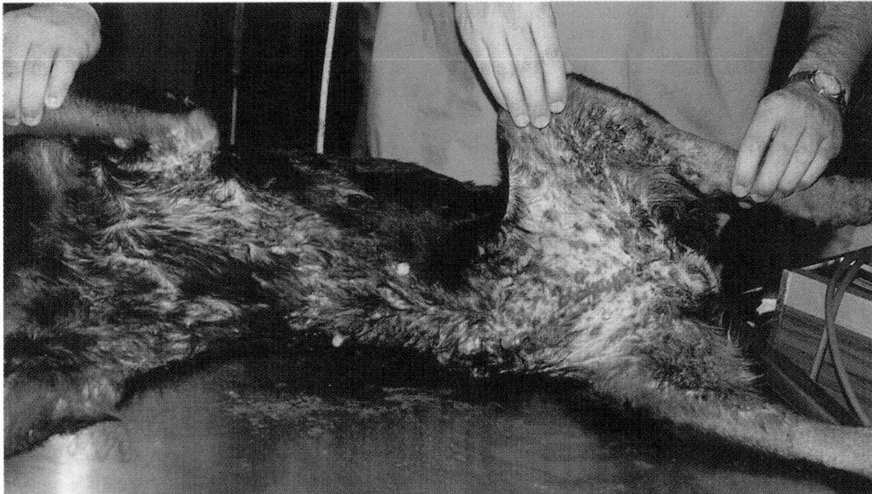

Figure 69-2 Close-up view of Figure 69-1.

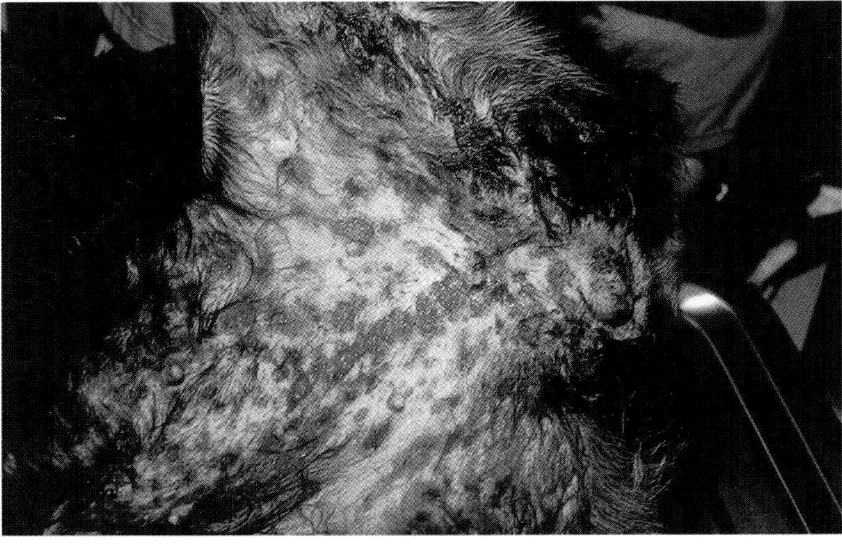

- Affects the extremities (paws, pinnae, lips, tail, and oral mucosa) and may be painful
- Anorexia, depression, pyrexia, pitting edema of the extremities, polyarthropathy, and myopathy—depend on the underlying cause
- Systemic signs reflecting organ involvement (e.g., hepatic, renal, and CNS)
- Systemic signs of illness (e.g., lethargy, lymphadenopathy, pyrexia, vague signs of pain, and weight loss)
- Cutaneous lesions of polyarteritis nodosa (subcutaneous nodules—less common in dogs than in people)
- Signs associated with underlying infectious or immune-related disease (e.g., thrombocytopenia and polyarthropathy)

Causes & Risk Factors

- Systemic lupus erythematosus
- Cold agglutinin disease
- Frostbite
- Disseminated intravascular coagulopathy
- Lymphoreticular neoplasia
- Drug reactions (Fig. 69-3)
- Postvaccine reaction
- Spider bites
- Immune-mediated disease
- Erythema nodosum–like panniculitis
- Rheumatoid arthritis

Figure 69-3 Vasculitis caused by drug eruption. Note both confluent areas of necrosis and target-type lesions.

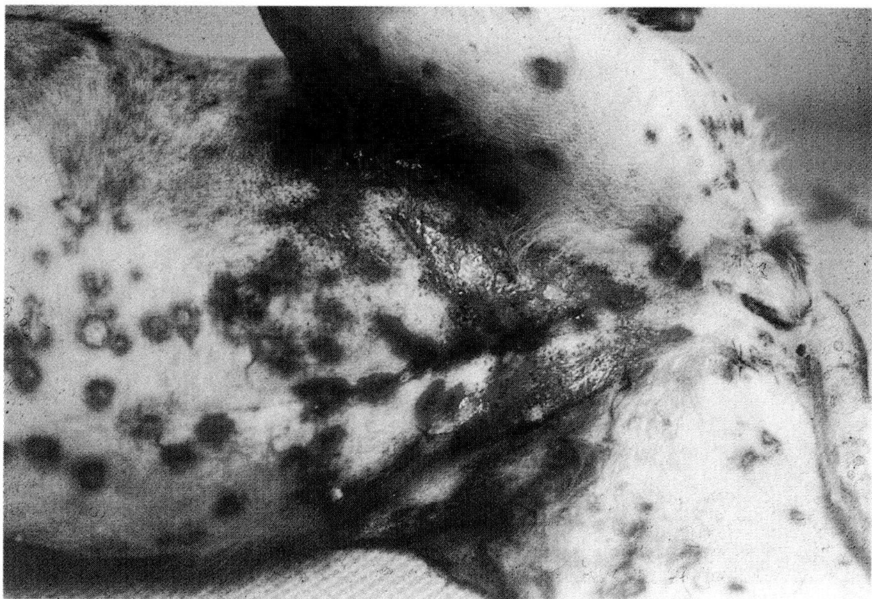

- Rocky Mountain spotted fever
- Staphylococcal hypersensitivity

Differential Diagnosis

Ear margin seborrhea, chemical and thermal burns, toxic epidermal necrolysis, erythema multiforme, and sepsis—biopsy representative lesions for histopathologic examination

Diagnostics

- Sepsis, disseminated intravascular coagulation, systemic lupus erythematosus, Rocky Mountain spotted fever, and rheumatoid arthritis—abnormalities may be noted
- Consider immunodiagnostics—ANA titer, Coombs test, and cold agglutinin tests
- Serologic tests may aid diagnosis of tick-related (i.e., rickettsial) disease
- ANA titer positive in patient with SLE, may also be positive in patients with other systemic illnesses
- Occult heartworm test positive in patient with dirofilariasis
- *Angiostrongylus* infestation diagnosed by fecal examination and cytologic examination of tracheal wash
- Radiographs help diagnose dirofilariasis and *Angiostronglyus* infection.
- Skin scrapings—possible demodicosis (with secondary sepsis)
- Biopsy of early lesion—submit to a dermatopathologist; findings depend on the underlying cause, but usually include neutrophilic (leukocytoclastic/non-leukocytoclastic), lymphocytic, eosinophilic, or granulomatous, mixed cells in and around the vessels; vascular necrosis and fibrin thrombi may be prominent; perivascular hemorrhage and edema may occur
- Vasculitis—perform representative cultures (blood, urine, skin, etc.) if CBC, chemistry screen, or urinalysis reveal systemic disease

Therapeutics

- Underlying disease—first priority in clinical management
- No systemic abnormalities—treat as outpatient with no alterations in food or water intake
- Systemic disease—inpatient care must be recommended
- Inform owner that the prognosis is guarded until a cause is found; prognosis is based on the cause.

Drugs

- First line of therapy while awaiting histopathology results, if no drug reaction is suspected—antibiotics
- Immune-mediated disease with concurrent vasculitis—prednisone (2–4 mg/kg q24h)
- No known underlying cause or prednisolone alone does not work—try dapsone (1 mg/kg q8h) or sulfasalazine (20–40 mg/kg q8h)

- Vasculitis—pentoxifylline; published doses vary; 400 mg q24–48h has been recommended
- Alkylating agents including chlorambucil and azathioprine have been added to regimens to decease the need for corticosteroids.

Contraindications/Possible Interactions

- Dapsone and sulfasalazine—not recommended with pre-existing renal disease, hepatic disease, or blood dyscrasias
- Sulfasalazine—not recommended with pre-existing or borderline keratoconjunctivitis sicca; use with caution in cats; may displace highly protein-bound drugs (e.g., methotrexate, warfarin, phenylbutazone, thiazide diuretics, salicylates, probenecid, and phenytoin); bioavailability decreased by antacids; may decrease bioavailability of folic acid or digoxin; blood levels may be decreased if concurrently administering ferrous sulfate or other iron salts
- Pentoxifylline—may increase prothrombin times; may decrease blood pressure

Comments

- Patients receiving prednisolone or dapsone—initially monitor every 2 weeks with a CBC, chemistry screen, and urinalysis if a specific underlying disease is found, then monitor appropriately
- If no underlying disease is found, vasculitis may be difficult to treat and the prognosis is guarded.
- Immunosuppressive therapies should always be reduced to the lowest possible therapeutic dose.

Abbreviation

ANA = antinuclear antibody

Suggested Reading

Greek JS. New therapeutics in dermatology. Vet Med 1996.

Mueller GH, Kirk RW, Scott DW, eds. Small animal dermatology. 4th ed. Philadelphia, Saunders, 1989.

Consulting Editor Karen Helton Rhodes

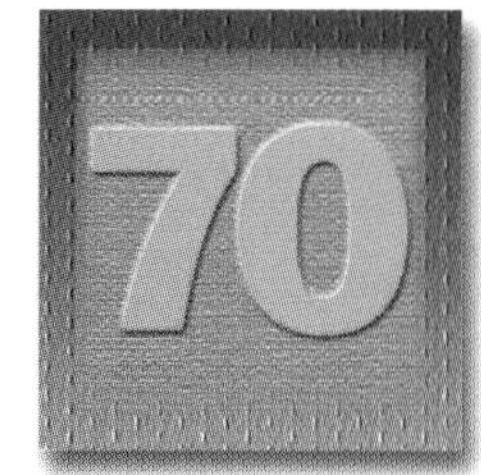

Uveodermatologic Syndrome—Vogt-Koyanagi Harada-Like Syndrome

W. Dunbar Gram

Definition/Overview

- Rare syndrome similar to Vogt-Koyanagi-Harada syndrome in humans
- Considered to be an autoimmune disorder resulting in concurrent granulomatous uveitis and depigmenting dermatitis and rare meningoencephalitis

Etiology/Pathophysiology

- Thought to be an autoimmune disease; antiretinal antibodies have been found in affected dogs.
- Exposure to sunlight—exacerbates symptoms

Signalment/History

- Reported in dogs, especially akitas, Samoyeds, and Siberian huskies
- No apparent age or sex predilections (Fig. 70-1)

Clinical Features

- Sudden-onset uveitis—may be painful and progress to blindness; concurrent or subsequent leukoderma of the nose, lips, and eyelids (Figs. 70-2, 70-3 and 70-4)
- Footpads, scrotum, anus, and the hard palate may also become depigmented.

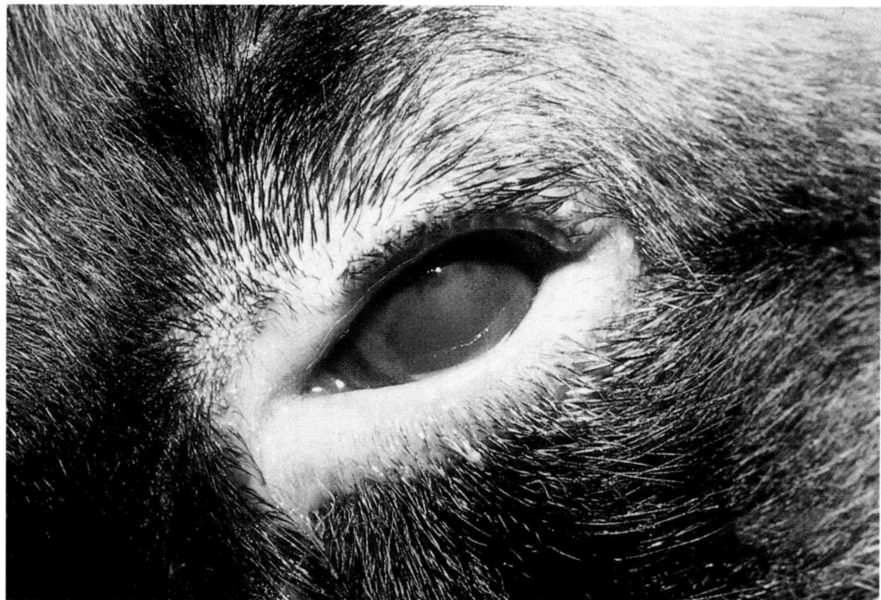

Figure 70-1 Uveodermatologic syndrome (VKH-like). Note the early evidence of uveitis, which is often the initial clinical feature recognized.

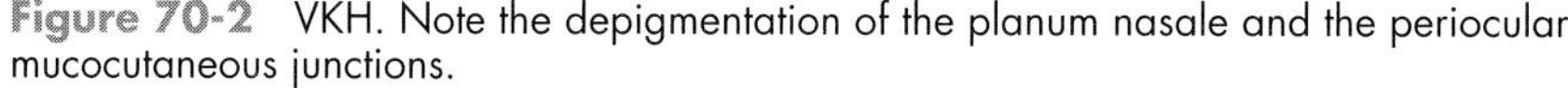

Figure 70-2 VKH. Note the depigmentation of the planum nasale and the periocular mucocutaneous junctions.

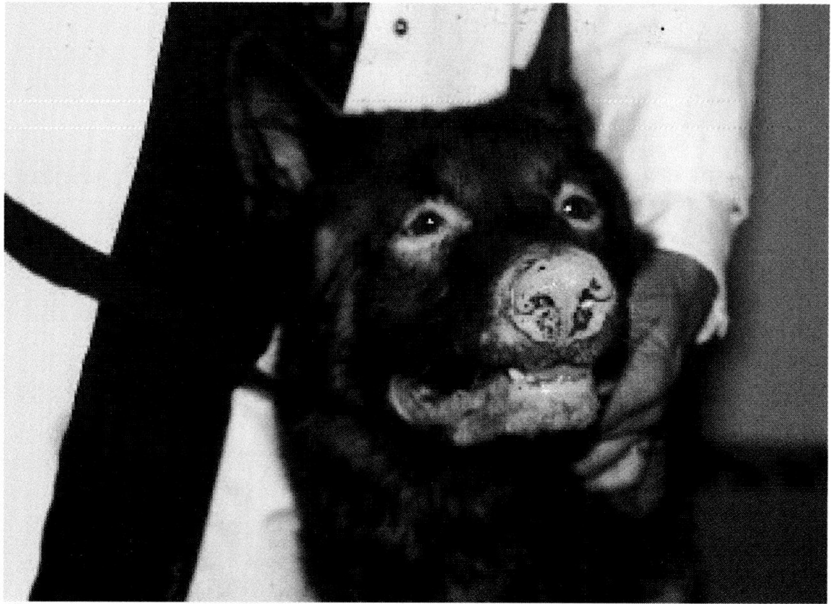

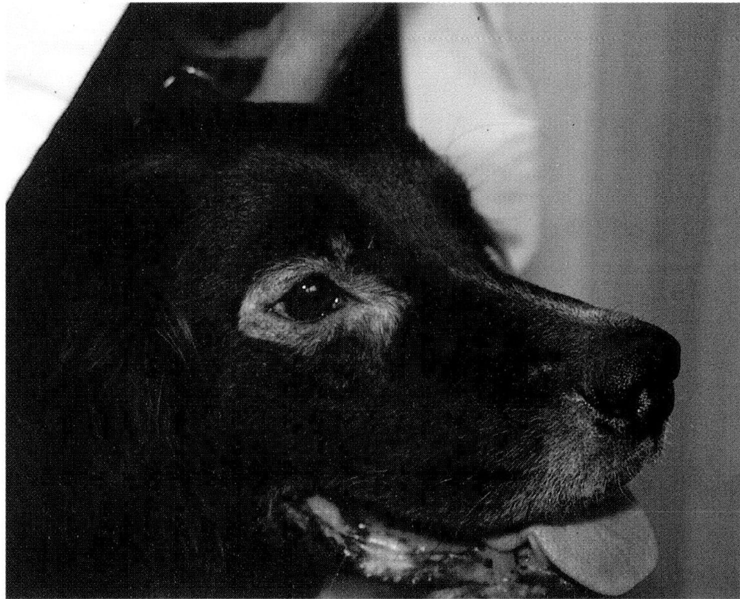

Figure 70-3 VKH. Depigmentation of the periocular region.

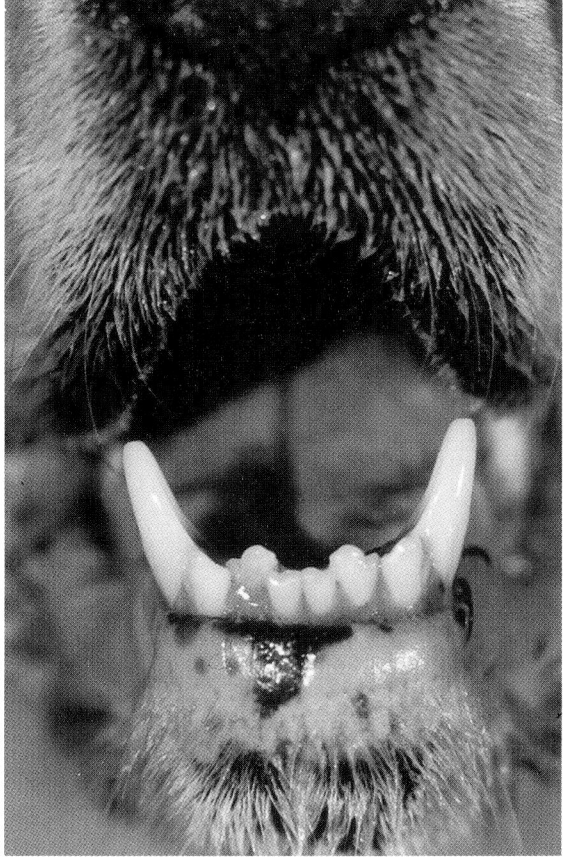

Figure 70-4 VKH. Note the depigmentation of the mucous membranes in this case.

- Ulcerations may develop.
- Meningoencephalitis—reported (rare)

Differential Diagnosis

- Immune-mediated skin diseases—pemphigus complex, systemic lupus erythematosus, and discoid lupus erythematosus, pemphigoid
- Neoplasia and numerous other inflammatory and infectious skin diseases that can cause depigmentation
- Skin biopsies, negative ANA titers, and a normal retinal examination—help differentiate these diseases

Diagnostics

- Biopsy and dermatopathology—best interpreted by a veterinarian experienced in detecting the sometimes subtle differences in pathologic patterns; early lesions have a lichenoid interface pattern with large histiocytes and pronounced pigmentary incontinence; hydropic degeneration of the epidermal basal cell rare
- Evaluate the retina.

Therapeutics

- Aggressive and rapid initiation of immunosuppressive therapy is recommended to prevent formation of posterior synechiae and secondary glaucoma, cataracts, or blindness.
- Retinal examinations—most important means of monitoring progress; improvement in dermatologic lesions may not reflect the retinal pathology.
- Enucleation—sometimes recommended because of pain

Drugs

- Corticosteroids—initial high doses of prednisone (1.1–2.2 mg/kg PO q12–24h) and azathioprine (1.5–2.5 mg/kg PO q24h) recommended; taper dosages and frequencies to every other day for chronic use; some patients may improve with the initial use of prednisone alone, but the potential sequelae of delayed aggressive therapy warrants the additional use of azathioprine.
- Topical or subconjunctival steroids and cycloplegics—may be indicated with anterior uveitis

Contraindications/Possible Interactions

Prednisone and azathioprine—anemia, leukopenia, thrombocytopenia, high serum alkaline phosphatase levels, vomiting, and pancreatitis; conduct biweekly serum chemistries and CBCs, including platelet counts, initially; decrease after the condition has stabilized and the dose and frequency have been tapered.

Comments

- Weekly or biweekly examinations including retinal evaluations—recommended initially for monitoring side effects associated with therapeutics; retinal examinations are important because improvement in dermatologic lesions may not indicate improvement in the retinal lesions.

- Azathioprine may be discontinued after a few months of therapy; prednisone may be necessary indefinitely.
- Iatrogenic hyperadrenocorticism—often a result of the steroid therapy

Suggested Reading

Scott DW, Miller WH, Griffen CE. Small animal dermatology. 5th ed. Philadelphia: Saunders, 1995.

Consulting Editor Karen Helton Rhodes

Epidermotrophic Lymphoma

K. Marcia Murphy

Definition/Overview

- A subset of cutaneous T cell lymphosarcoma
- An uncommon malignant neoplasia affecting many species, including dogs and cats

Etiology/Pathophysiology

- Mycosis fungoides and Sézary syndrome (mycosis fungoides with associated leukemia)—most common forms of cutaneous T cell lymphosarcoma
- Pagetoid reticulosis—rare; the lymphoid infiltrate is generally confined to the epidermis in the early stages of the disease.

Signalment/History

- More common in dogs than in cats
- Affects old dogs and cats; mean age 9–12 years
- No apparent breed or sex predilection

Historical Findings

- Chronic skin disease—months to years before diagnosis
- Erythema

- Depigmentation
- Scaling
- Alopecia
- Sometimes pruritus

Clinical Features

- Erythema
- Scaling
- Depigmentation (Fig. 71-1)
- Alopecia (Figs. 71-2, 71-3)
- Infiltrative plaques (Fig. 71-4)
- Ulceration
- Crusting (Fig. 71-5)
- Multiple nodules or mass formation
- Pruritus
- Lesions—throughout the skin; marked tendency for involvement of mucocutaneous junctions (lip, eyelids, nasal planum, anorectal junction, or vulva) or the oral cavity (gingiva, palate, or tongue)
- Usually three principal phases—patch, plaque, and tumor; progression to the tumor stage is very rapid in dogs (compared to humans); may also occur in tumor stage from the onset (tumor d'emblee form)

Figure 71-1 Note the areas of depigmentation of the footpads in this cocker spaniel with epidermotrophic lymphoma.

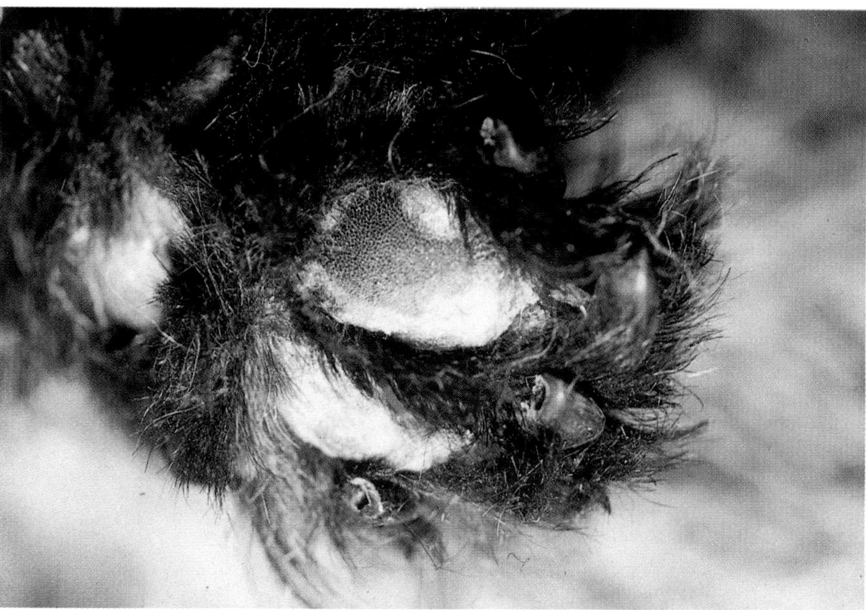

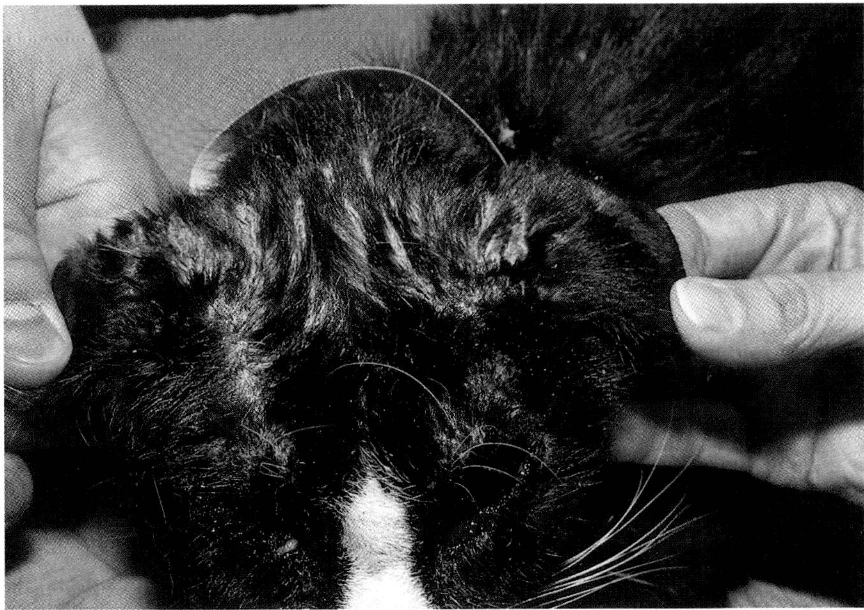

Figure 71-2 This cat had generalized diffuse scaling and alopecia associated with epidermotrophic lymphoma.

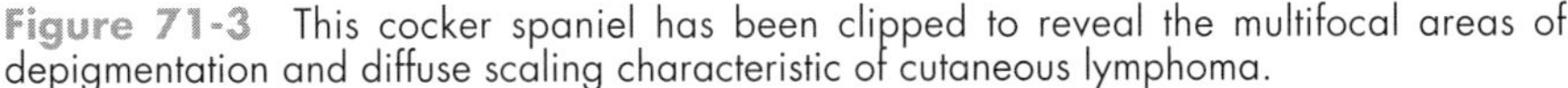

Figure 71-3 This cocker spaniel has been clipped to reveal the multifocal areas of depigmentation and diffuse scaling characteristic of cutaneous lymphoma.

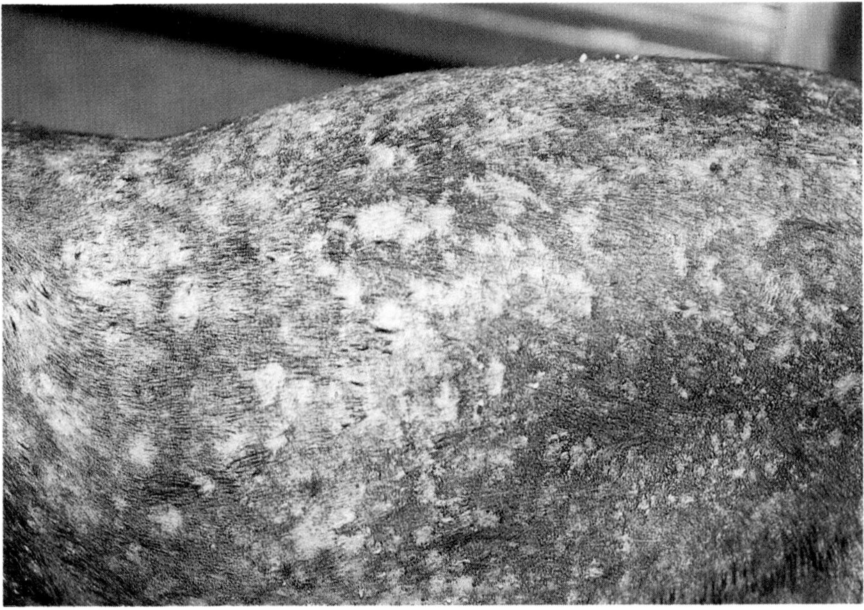

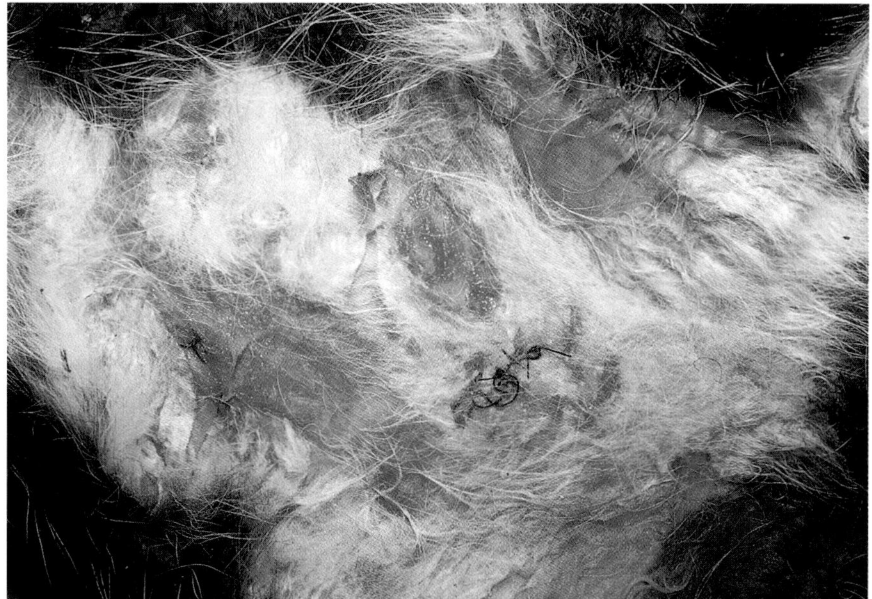

Figure 71-4 The ventral abdominal region of this cat with cutaneous lymphoma reveals erythematous plaques and ulcerations associated with advanced disease.

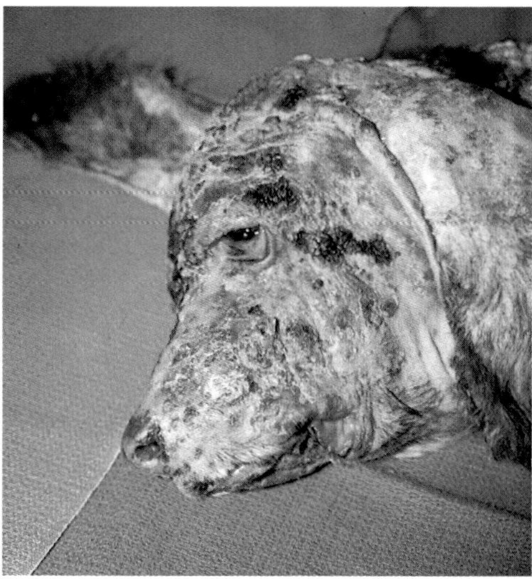

Figure 71-5 "End Stage" epidermotrophic lymphoma. Note the diffuse erythema, alopecia, crusting, and depigmentation (especially the planum nasale).

Differential Diagnosis

- Dermatophytosis, demodicosis—alopecia, erythema, scaling
- Allergies, scabies—generalized pruritus, erythema, scaling
- Cutaneous lupus erythematosus, erythema multiforme, other immune-mediated diseases—mucocutaneous depigmentation/ulceration
- Nonneoplastic chronic stomatitis—infiltrative and ulcerative oral mucosal disease
- Histiocytoma, cutaneous histiocytosis, mass cell tumor, or any other cutaneous neoplasia—nodule or mass formation

Diagnostics

- Laboratory abnormalities—vary, depending on the stage and form of cutaneous T cell lymphosarcoma (mycosis fungoides vs. Sezary syndrome)
- Generally not helpful in the early stages

Imaging

- Radiographs and ultrasound—not commonly used in the early stages; imaging is eventually necessary to confirm system disease and/or for tumor staging.

Diagnostic Procedures

- Skin scrapings and fungal culture—rule out demodicosis and dermatophytosis, if applicable.
- Skin biopsy—definitive diagnosis

Pathologic Findings

- Lymphoid infiltrate—into epidermis and epithelium of hair follicles and adnexal structures; distributed diffusely or as discrete Pautrier microaggregates within the epithelium
- Dermal infiltrate—polymorphous; also consists of malignant lymphocytes that obscure the dermoepidermal junction; in the patch and plaque stages, limited to the superficial dermis; in the tumor stage, extends to the deep dermis and subcutis
- Lymphocyte epitheliotropism—usually remains prominent throughout all stages

Therapeutics

- Inform the client that a cure is extremely unlikely.
- The goal is to maintain a good quality of life for as long as possible.
- Therapy is usually of little benefit; rarely, solitary nodules can be surgically excised resulting in long-term remissions.

Drugs

- Chemotherapy—several protocols used with limited to no success, including various combinations of prednisolone, chlorambucil, vincristine, cyclophosphamide, doxorubicin and methotrexate
- Topical chemotherapy—mechlorethamine (nitrogen mustard) has resulted in some success in managing early lesions; it has not been shown to alter the fatal course of the disease.
- α-Interferon, retinoids, extracorporeal photophoresis, and anti-T cell monoclonal antibodies—recently investigated in therapeutic trials with variable results

Contraindications/Possible Interactions

- Depends on the chemotherapeutic or treatment protocol
- Seek advice from a veterinary oncologist or dermatologist before initiating therapy if you are unfamiliar with cytotoxic drugs and/or to learn about the most recent treatment protocols.

Comment

- Prognosis grave
- Average survival time for dogs, from the onset of diagnosed skin lesions to death, is 5–10 months
- Death is usually the result of euthanasia.
- Rarely, dogs and cats may live for longer than 2 years after the diagnosis is made.

Suggested Reading

Moore PF, Olivry T. Cutaneous lymphomas in companion animals. Clin Dermatol 1994;12:499–505.

Scott DW, Miller WH, Griffin CE. Muller & Kirk's small animal dermatology. 5th ed. Philadelphia: Saunders, 1995.

Author K. Marcia Murphy

Consulting Editor Karen Helton Rhodes

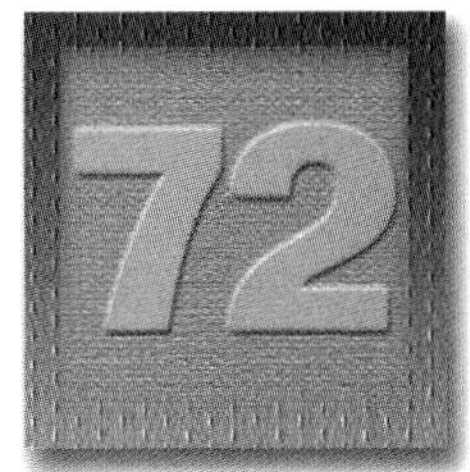

Hair Follicle Tumors

Joanne C. Graham

Definition/Overview

- Two main types—trichoepithelioma, which arises from keratinocytes in the outer root sheath of the hair follicle or from both the sheath and the hair matrix; pilomatricoma, which arises from the hair matrix
- Both types—generally benign; a few published reports of malignant pilomatricoma

Signalment/History

- Age—usually > 5 years
- No sex predisposition
- Trichoepithelioma—common in dogs; rare in cats; cocker spaniels and basset hounds may be predisposed; no breed predisposition in cats
- Pilomatricoma—uncommon in dogs and cats; Kerry blue terriers and poodles may be predisposed; no known breed predisposition in cats

Clinical Features

- Usually a solitary mass
- Trichoepithelioma—common on the back and head (cats)
- Pilomatricoma—common on the back, shoulders, flanks, and limbs
- Firm, round, elevated, well-circumscribed, hairless, or ulcerated dermoepithelial masses; cut surface gray (trichoepithelioma) or lobulated with white chalky areas (pilomatricoma) (Fig. 72-1)

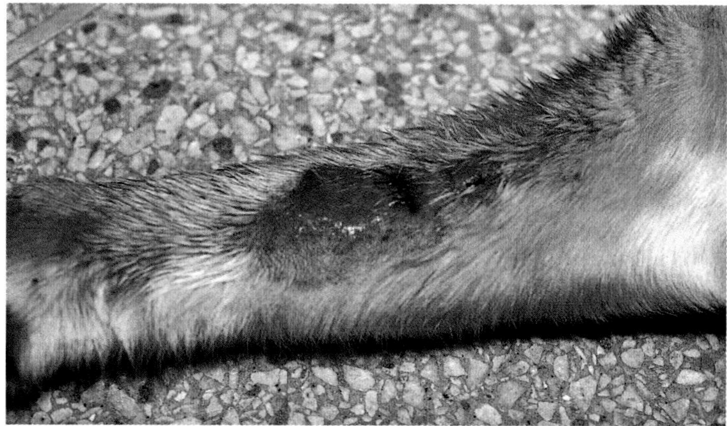

Figure 72-1 Solitary raised mass of the medial aspect of the forelimb diagnosed as a pilomatricoma.

Differential Diagnosis

Histopathologic examination—distinguish from basal cell tumor and squamous cell carcinoma

Diagnostics

Pathologic Findings

- Trichoepithelioma—varies in degree of differentiation and site of origin (root sheath or hair matrix); horn cysts, lack of desmosomes, and differentiation toward hair follicle–like structures and formation of hair common
- Pilomatricoma—characterized by a variable proliferation of basophilic cells resembling hair matrix cells and fully keratinized, faintly eosinophilic cells with a central unstained nucleus (shadow cells); calcification common

Therapeutics

- Complete excision—curative

Comments

- Monitor for local recurrence.
- Prognosis usually excellent

Suggested Reading

Muller GH, Kirk RW, Scott DW. Neoplastic diseases. In: Muller GH, Kirk RW, Scott DW, eds. Small animal dermatology. 4th ed. Philadelphia: Saunders, 1989:858–866.

Thomas RC, Fox LE. Tumors of the skin and subcutis. In: Morrison WB, ed. Cancer in dogs and cats: medical and surgical management. Philadelphia: Williams & Wilkins 1998:489–510.

Author Joanne C. Graham

Consulting Editor Karen Helton Rhodes

Cutaneous Hemangiosarcoma

Robyn Elmslie

Definition/Overview

- Malignant tumor arising from endothelial cells
- Primary tumor develops within dermal or subcutaneous tissues.
- Accounts for 14% of all hemangiosarcomas in dogs
- Prevalence (dogs)—0.3–2.0%

Signalment/History

- Dogs and rarely cats
- Pit bulls, boxers, and German shepherds—affected more commonly than other breeds
- Multicentric dermal hemangiosarcoma—whippet dogs and related breeds
- Median age, 9 years; range, 4.5–15 years
- Vascular stasis, radiotherapy, trauma, and sun exposure—predisposing factors in humans; may be risk factors in dogs

Clinical Features

- Usually solitary mass; may see multiple masses
- Dermal—firm, raised, dark nodules primarily on the limbs, prepuce, and ventral abdomen (Fig. 73-1)
- Subcutaneous—firm or soft, fluctuant masses with or without associated bruising; masses may appear to change size quickly because of intratumoral

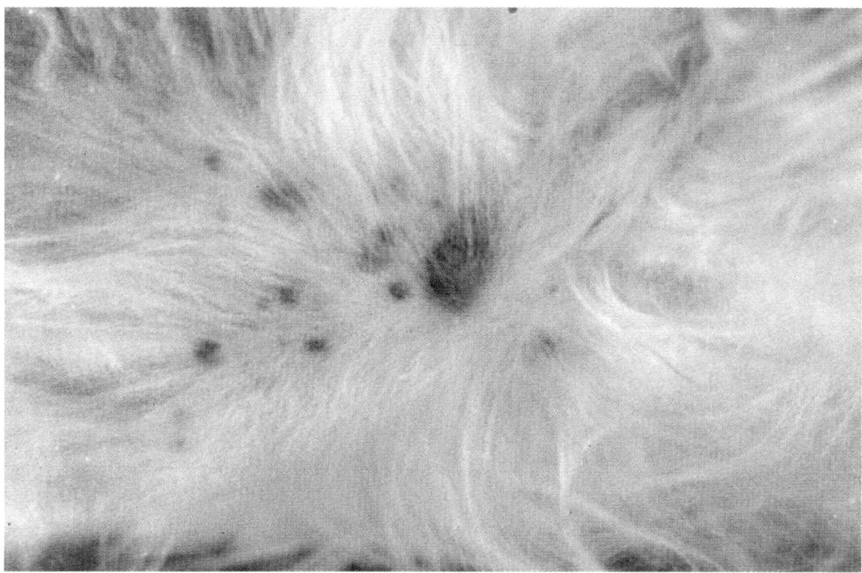

Figure 73-1 Cutaneous hemangiosarcoma in a dog. Note the raised dark nodules located on the ventral abdomen.

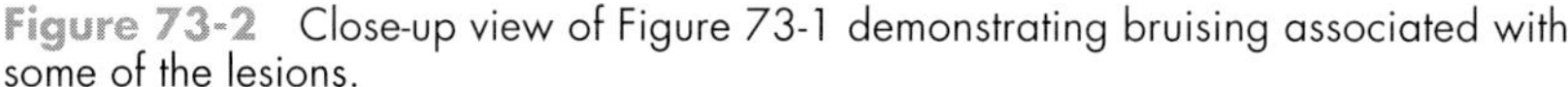

Figure 73-2 Close-up view of Figure 73-1 demonstrating bruising associated with some of the lesions.

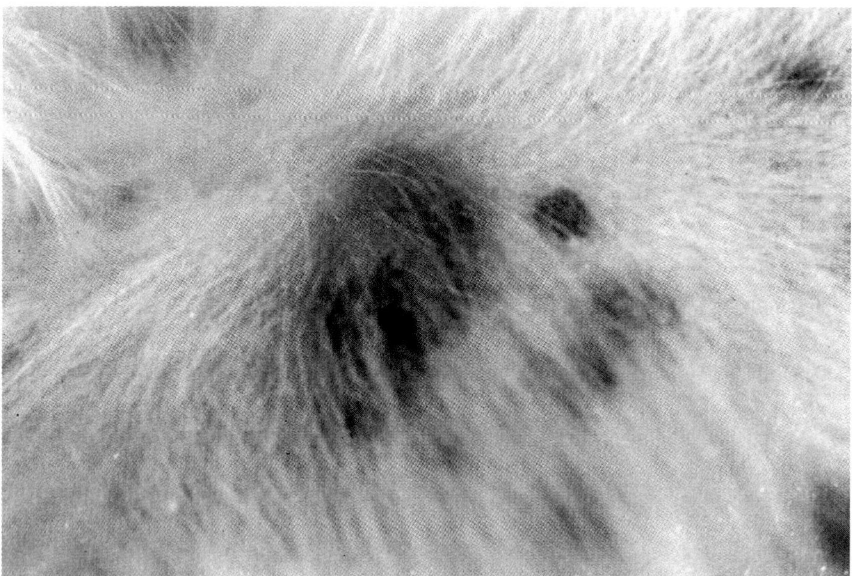

bleeding; typically larger than dermal; often found on the pelvic limbs, but may arise in any location (Fig. 73-2)

Differential Diagnosis

- Trauma—subcutaneous hematoma
- Other benign or malignant tumors

Diagnostics

- May see laboratory abnormalities compatible with DIC—prolonged bleeding times, thrombocytopenia, low fibrinogen, and high fibrin split products
- Thoracic radiographs—detect pulmonary metastasis
- CT or MRI—delineate extent of disease; often required to determine feasibility of surgery
- Skin biopsy—required to confirm diagnosis; differentiate between dermal and subcutaneous

Pathologic Findings

- Dermal—well circumscribed; confined to the dermis
- Subcutaneous—poorly circumscribed; very invasive

Therapeutics

- Aggressive surgical excision—treatment of choice; complete surgical excision of subcutaneous tumor difficult
- DIC and bleeding—important intraoperative and postoperative concerns
- Chemotherapy (subcutaneous tumor)—recommended after excision; may be administered to patients before surgery to cytoreduce tumor and increase the likelihood of successful surgical outcome; treatment with doxorubicin, cyclophosphamide, and vincristine shown to improve survival time in dogs
- Multicentric dermal—etretinate (0.75–1 mg/kg q24h) and vitamin E (400 IU PO q12h); author successfully induced partial remission in whippets with nonresectable disease

Comments

- Aspirin and other NSAIDs—avoid because of associated increased potential for bleeding
- Dermal—median survival, 780 days
- Subcutaneous—median survival, >6 months; depends on the degree of invasion
- Metastasis—may occur

Suggested Reading

Ward H, Fox LE, Calderwood-Mays MB, et al. Cutaneous hemangiosarcoma in 25 dogs: a retrospective study. J Vet Intern Med 1994:8:345–348.

Author Robyn Elmsie

Consulting Editor Karen Helton Rhodes

Histiocytoma

Joanne C. Graham

Definition/Overview

Benign skin tumor arising from Langerhans cells (e.g., histiocytes) of the skin

Signalment/History

- Common in dogs but extremely rare in cats
- More than 50% of patients are dogs <2 years old.
- Boxers, dachshunds, cocker spaniels, Great Danes, and Shetland sheepdogs—may be predisposed
- No breed predilection in cats
- No sex predilection in cats or dogs

Clinical Features

- Small, firm, dome- or button-shaped, dermoepithelial mass that may be ulcerated (Fig. 74-1)
- Fast growing, nonpainful, usually solitary
- Common sites—head, ear pinna, and limbs
- Occasionally multiple cutaneous nodules or plaques

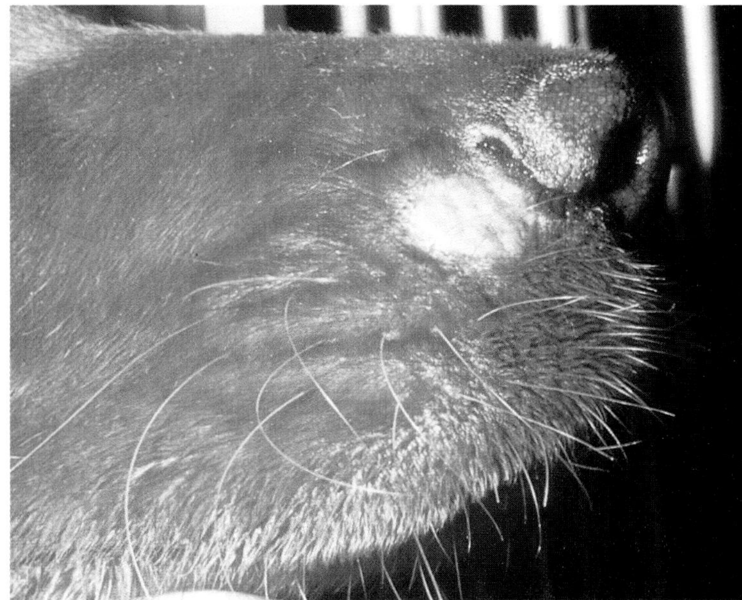

Figure 74-1 Histiocytoma. Note the raised alopecic nodule of the muzzle in this dog.

Differential Diagnosis

Histopathologic examination and immunohistochemical stains—distinguish from focal granulomatous inflammation, transmissible venereal tumor, lymphosarcoma, and mast cell tumor (latter stains positive with toluidine blue; histiocytoma does not)

Diagnostics

- Cytologic examination—fine-needle aspirate; reveals pleomorphic round cells, 12–24 μm in diameter; variable-sized and -shaped nuclei; variable amounts of pale blue cytoplasm that resemble monocytes
- Mitotic index usually high
- May see substantial lymphocyte, plasma cell, and neutrophil infiltration
- Histopathologic—characterized by uniform sheets of histiocytes that penetrate the dermis and subcutis; cells may be densely packed in deeper layers of the dermis
- Collagen fibers and skin adnexa—may be displaced
- Immunophenotyping—confirm cell origin

Therapeutics

- May spontaneously regress within 3 months
- Surgical excision or cryosurgery—generally curative
- Important to differentiate histiocytoma from malignant tumor if client elects the wait-and-see approach

Comments

- Surgical excision—recommended if mass has not spontaneously regressed within 3 months
- Prognosis—excellent with surgical removal
- Spontaneous regression possible within 3 months

Suggested Reading

Thomas RC, Fox LE. Tumors of the skin and subcutis. In: Morrison WB, ed. Cancer in dogs and cats: medical and surgical management. Baltimore: Williams & Wilkins 1998:489–510.

Author Joanne C. Graham

Consulting Editor Karen Helton Rhodes

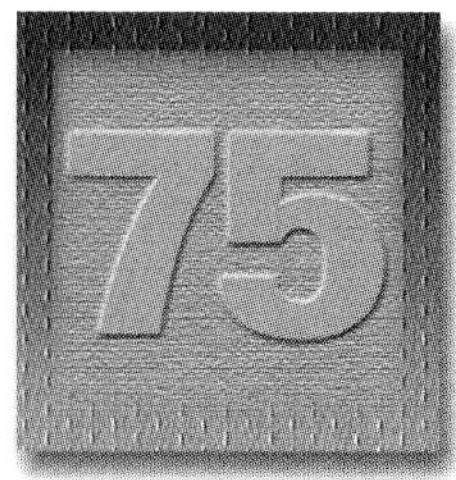

Mast Cell Tumors

Robyn E. Elmslie

Definition

Neoplasia arising from mast cells

Etiology/Pathophysiology

- Histamine and other vasoactive substances released from mast cell tumors—may cause erythema and edema; histamine may cause gastric and duodenal ulcers
- Heparin release—increases likelihood of bleeding
- Skin/Exocrine—skin and subcutaneous tissue most common tumor sites in dogs and cats
- Hemic/Lymphatic/Immune—spleen: common primary location in cats and uncommon primary location in dogs; common location for metastasis from the skin or subcutaneous sites
- Gastrointestinal—intestinal mast cell tumor uncommon in cats and rare in dogs; gastric and duodenal ulcers possible

Signalment/History

- Compose 20–25% of all skin and subcutaneous tumors in dogs
- Fourth most common skin tumor in cats (often benign in skin)
- Boxers and Boston terriers
- Siamese cats—predisposed to histiocytic cutaneous mast cell tumors

- Dogs—mean age, 8 years
- Cats—mean age, 10 years
- Reported in animals <1 year old and in cats as old as 18 years

Dogs

- Patient may have had skin or subcutaneous tumor for days to months at the time of examination.
- May have appeared to fluctuate in size
- Recent rapid growth after months of quiescence common
- Recent onset of erythema and edema most common with high-grade skin and subcutaneous tumors

Cats

- Anorexia—most common complaint with splenic tumor
- Vomiting—may occur secondary to both splenic and gastrointestinal tumors

Clinical Features

Dogs

- Extremely variable; may resemble any other type of skin or subcutaneous tumor (benign and malignant); may resemble an insect bite or allergic reaction
- Primarily a solitary skin or subcutaneous mass; but may be multifocal
- Approximately 50% located on the trunk and perineum; 40% on extremities; 10% on the head and neck region
- Regional lymphadenopathy—may develop when a high-grade tumor metastasizes to draining lymph nodes
- Hepatomegaly and splenomegaly—features of disseminated mast cell neoplasia

Cats

- Cutaneous—primarily found in the subcutaneous tissue or dermis; may be papular or nodular, solitary or multiple, and hairy or alopecic or have an ulcerated surface; slight predilection for the head and neck regions (Figs. 75-1, 75-2, 75-3, 75-4)
- Splenic—splenomegaly is only consistent finding
- Intestinal—firm, segmental thickenings of the small intestinal wall; measure 1–7 cm in diameter; metastases to the mesenteric lymph nodes, spleen, liver, and (rarely) lungs

Differential Diagnosis

- Any other skin or subcutaneous tumor, benign or malignant, including lipoma
- Insect bite or allergic reaction
- Splenic—most common cause of splenomegaly in cats; must differentiate from lymphoma
- Intestinal (cats)—may resemble any primary gastrointestinal disorder (e.g., inflammatory and neoplasia)

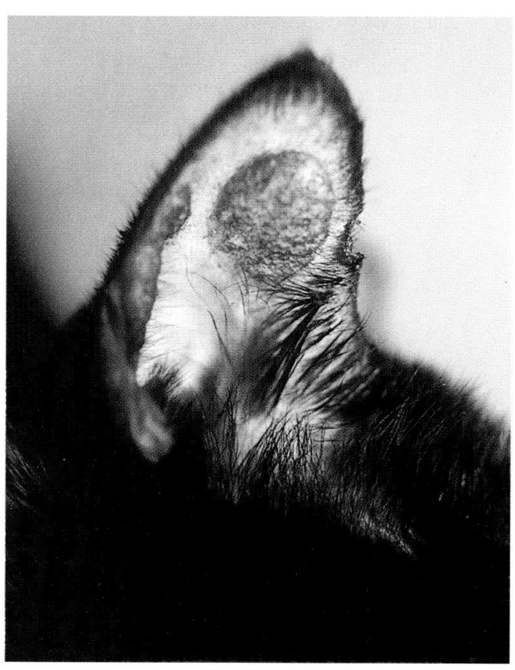

Figure 75-1 Multifocal mast cell tumors on the pinnae of a cat. These lesions were benign in behavior.

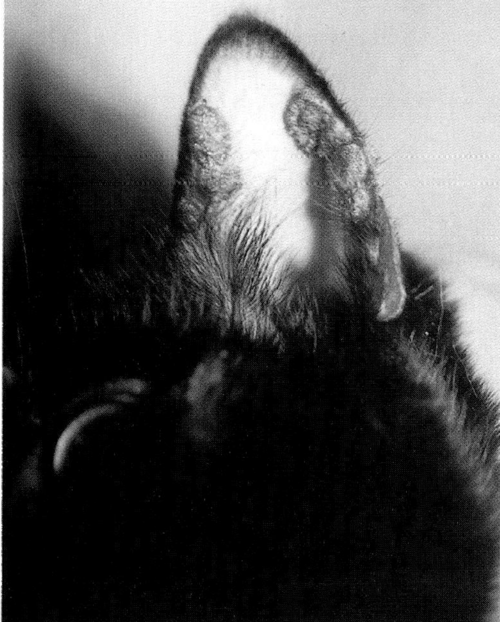

Figure 75-2 The other pinnae from the cat in Figure 75-1. Mast cell tumor (MCT).

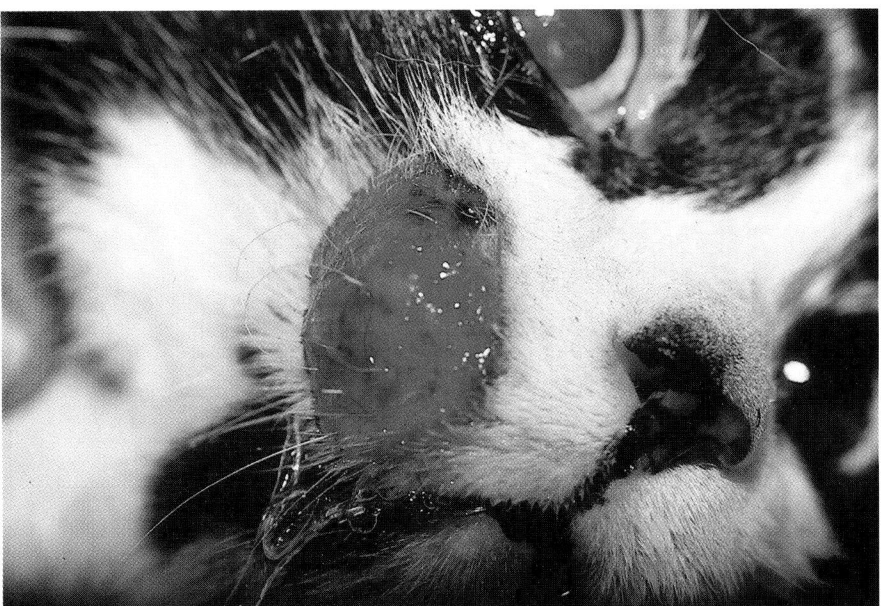

Figure 75-3 Ulcerative mast cell tumor on the face of a cat. Metastatic lesion from primary gastrointestinal MCT.

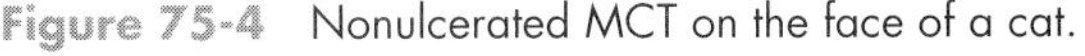

Figure 75-4 Nonulcerated MCT on the face of a cat.

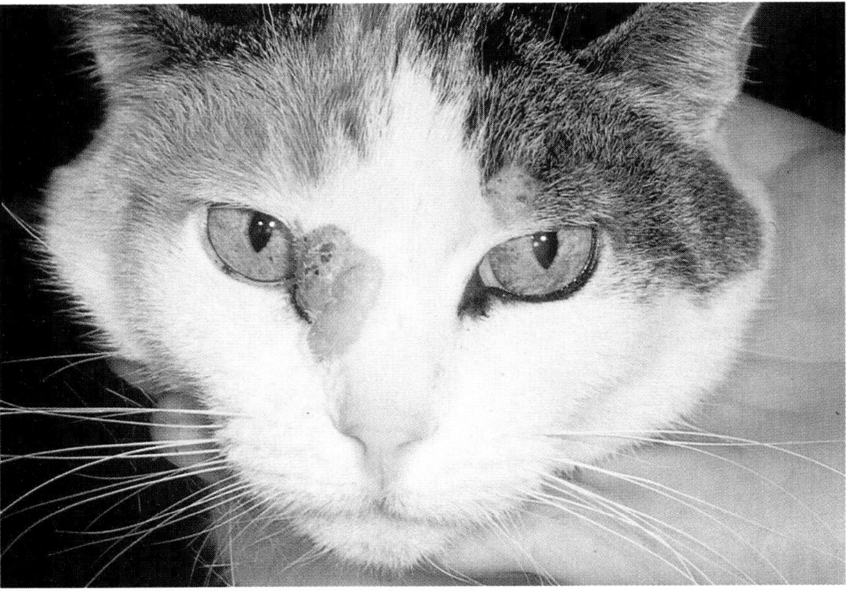

Diagnostics

- Anemia and mastocythemia—may find in cats with splenic tumor and dogs with systemic mastocytosis
- Abdominal radiography—may reveal splenomegaly in cats with splenic tumor and dogs with systemic mastocytosis
- Ultrasonography—helpful for evaluating visceral (liver, spleen) metastasis in dogs with high-grade tumors
- Cytologic examination of fine-needle aspirate—most important preliminary diagnostic test; reveals round cells with basophilic cytoplasmic granules that do not form sheets or clumps; if malignant mast cells are often agranular, occurrence of a large eosinophilic infiltrate may suggest mast cell tumor
- Tissue biopsy—necessary for definitive diagnosis and grading
- Staging—to determine the extent of disease and appropriate treatment
- Additional tests to achieve complete staging—cytologic examination or biopsy of local draining lymph node; cytologic examination of bone marrow aspirate; and thoracic radiography and abdominal ultrasonography with cytologic evaluation of hepatic and splenic aspirates
- Histopathologic examination (dogs)—grading of tumor to predict biologic behavior; graded I–III (III is the most aggressive type)
- Cats—grading system not beneficial; no correlation between histopathologic appearance of cutaneous tumor and prognosis

Therapeutics

Dogs

- Aggressive surgical excision—treatment of choice
- Histopathologic evaluation of the entire surgically excised tissue—essential to determine completeness of excision and predict the biologic behavior; if tumor cells extend close to the surgical margins, perform a second aggressive surgery as soon as possible.
- Lymph node involvement but no systemic involvement—aggressive excision of the affected lymph node(s) and the primary tumor required; follow-up chemotherapy useful to prevent further metastasis
- Primary tumor and/or affected lymph node cannot be excised—chemotherapy has minimal benefit.
- Systemic metastasis—excision of primary tumor and affected lymph nodes and follow-up chemotherapy have minimal effect on survival time.
- Radiotherapy—good treatment option for cutaneous tumor in a location that does not allow aggressive surgical excision; if possible, perform surgery before radiotherapy to reduce the tumor to a microscopic volume; tumors on an extremity respond better than do tumors located on the trunk.

Cats

- Surgery—treatment of choice for cutaneous tumors
- Splenectomy—treatment of choice for splenic tumor
- Splenectomy and chemotherapy—recommended when mastocythemia accompanies splenic tumor

Surgical Considerations

- Complete surgical excision with 2-cm margins in all planes—vital
- Excisional biopsy rather than incisional biopsy—necessary
- Biopsy of lymph nodes and other suspicious visceral organs—appropriate

Drugs

- Prednisone—has been mainstay; recent evidence suggests that, used alone, achieves only short-term remission
- Other drugs (e.g., vinblastine and cyclophosphamide)—add to lengthen the remission of prednisone-sensitive tumors
- Cutaneous tumor not controlled by surgery or radiotherapy—medical treatment appropriate; in author's experience, prednisone and chemotherapy not beneficial for aggressive tumors in cats
- Prednisone-resistant tumor—chemotherapy does not appear to be beneficial
- Intestinal tumor and systemic mastocytosis after splenectomy (cats)—prednisone and chemotherapy indicated
- Measurable tumor (dogs)—vincristine alone induced partial remission in 21% of patients

Combination Chemotherapy

- Author's preferred treatment
- Prednisone—1 mg/kg PO q24h; taper slowly after 4 months; discontinue after 7 months
- Vinblastine—2–3 mg/m^2 IV; administer on day 1 of each 21-day cycle; initiate at a dosage of 2 mg/m^2; increase by 10–30% with each subsequent cycle, depending on tolerance and response (e.g., check CBC 1 week after administration); perform CBC before each administration; continue for 6 months
- Cyclophosphamide—250–300 mg/m^2 PO divided over 4 days; administer on days 8, 9, 10, and 11 of each 21-day cycle; initiate at 250 mg/m^2 for two cycles; increase to 300 mg/m^2 for cycle 3 if well tolerated; continue for 6 months

Alternative Drugs

Histamine-blocking agents (e.g., cimetidine)—helpful, particularly for systemic mastocytosis or when massive histamine release is a concern

Comments

Client Education

- Warn client that a patient that has had more than one cutaneous tumor is predisposed to developing new mast cell tumors.
- Advise client that fine-needle aspiration and cytologic examination should be performed as soon as possible on any new mass.
- Inform client that appropriate surgical excision should be done as soon as possible.

Patient Monitoring

- Evaluate any new masses cytologically or histologically.
- Evaluate regional lymph nodes at regular intervals to detect metastasis of grade II or III tumor.

Possible Complications

- Bleeding
- Hemorrhagic gastroenteritis

Expected Course and Prognosis

Dogs

- Tumors in the inguinal region—tend to be more aggressive than similarly graded tumors in other locations; always consider to have the potential to metastasize
- Survival times 6 months after surgery (Bostock)—grade I, 77% alive; grade II, 45% alive; grade III, 13% alive
- Lymph node metastasis—survival may be prolonged if prednisone and chemotherapy are given after the primary tumor and affected lymph node(s) are aggressively excised
- Prednisone alone—effectively induced remission and prolonged survival time in 20% of patients with grade II or III tumors; only one of the five responding patients had documented lymph node metastasis when prednisone was initiated.

Cats

- Solitary cutaneous tumor—prognosis excellent; rate of recurrence low (16–36%) despite incomplete excision; <20% of patients develop metastasis
- Survival after splenectomy for splenic tumor—reports of >1 year
- Concurrent development of mastocythemia—prognosis poor; prednisone and chemotherapy may achieve short-term remission
- Intestinal tumor—prognosis poor; survival times rarely >4 months after surgery

Suggested Reading

Liska WD, MacEwen EG, Zaki FA, et al. Feline systemic mastocytosis: a review and results of splenectomy in seven cases. J Am Anim Hosp Assoc 1979;15:589–597.

McCaw DL, Miller MA, Ogilvie GK, et al. Response of canine mast cell tumors to treatment with oral prednisone. J Vet Intern Med 1994;8:406–408.

Molander-McCray H, Henry CJ, Potter K, et al. Cutaneous mast cell tumors in cats: 32 cases (1991–1994). J Am Anim Hosp Assoc 1998;34:281–284.

Patnaik AK, Ehler WN, MacEwen EG. Canine cutaneous mast cell tumors: morphologic grading and survival time in 83 dogs. Vet Pathol 1984;21:469–474.

Author Robyn Elmslie

Consulting Editor Karen Helton Rhodes

Melanocytic Tumors of the Skin and Digit

Joanne C. Graham

Definition/Overview

Benign or malignant neoplasm arising from melanocytes and melanoblasts (melanin-producing cells)

Etiology/Pathophysiology

- Locally invasive
- Malignant—may invade bone and metastasize to regional lymph nodes

Signalment/History

- Dogs—4–20% of all skin tumors
- Cats—0.8–7% of all skin tumors
- Dogs—Scottish terriers, Boston terriers, Airedale terriers, cocker spaniels, boxers, springer spaniels, Irish setters, Irish terriers, chow chows, Chihuahuas, and Doberman pinschers predisposed
- Dogs—9 years
- Cats—8–14 years
- Dogs—males may be predisposed
- Cats—none
- Slow or rapidly growing mass
- Lameness if digit is involved

Clinical Features

- Pigmented or nonpigmented (amelanotic) mass, usually solitary (Fig. 76-1)
- Develops anywhere but may be more common on face, trunk, feet, and scrotum in dogs and head and pinna in cats (Figs. 76-2, 76-3)
- Regional lymph nodes—may be large
- Advanced disease—may have dyspnea or harsh lung sounds because of pulmonary metastasis

Differential Diagnosis

- Histopathologic examination and special stains—may distinguish amelanotic melanoma from poorly differentiated mast cell tumors, lymphosarcoma, and carcinoma

Diagnostics

- Immunohistochemical stains—may help differentiate melanoma (especially amelanotic) from other tumors; melanoma stains positive with vimentin, S-100, neuron-specific enolase, and human melanosome-specific antigens
- Thoracic radiography—detect metastasis
- Area radiography—determine if underlying bone is involved, especially with melanoma of the digit
- Cytologic examination of fine-needle aspirate—reveals brown, rod-like intracellular granules (melanin) in cells of various sizes and shapes; pigment may be absent in the case of amelanotic melanoma; may see macrophages (melanophages) containing phagocytosed melanin

Figure 76-1 Solitary oral nonpigmented melanoma located at the mucocutaneous junction.

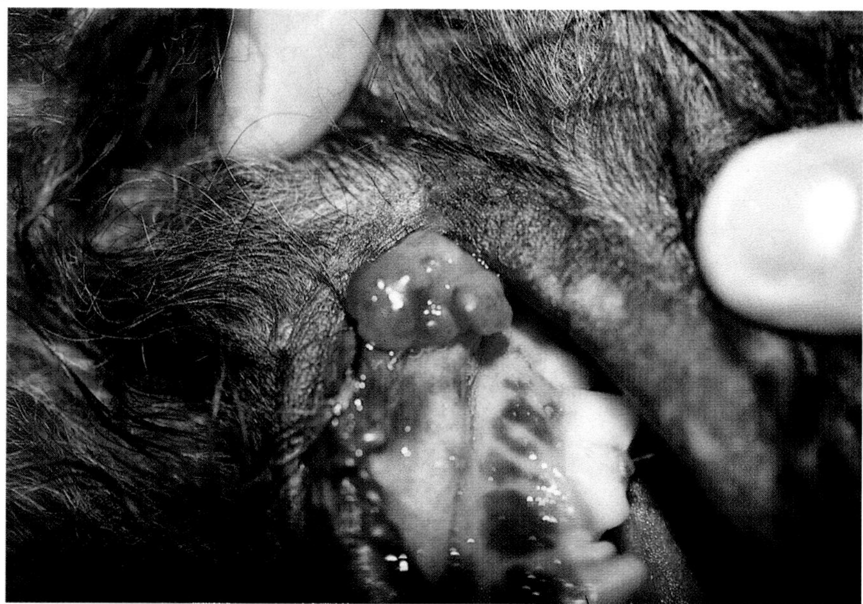

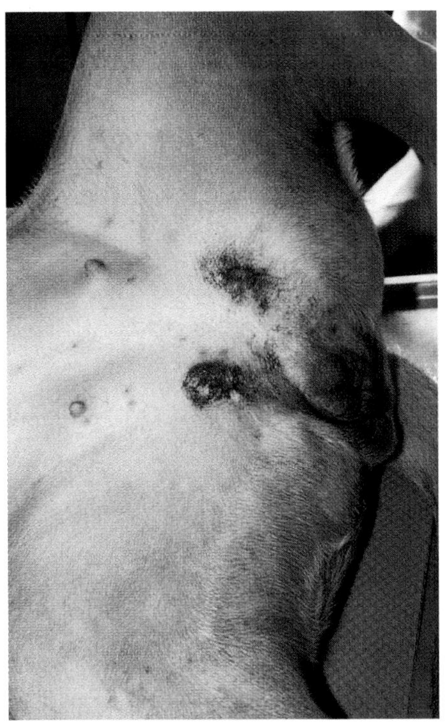

Figure 76-2 Melanoma of the inguinal region in a dog.

Figure 76-3 Close-up view of Figure 76-2.

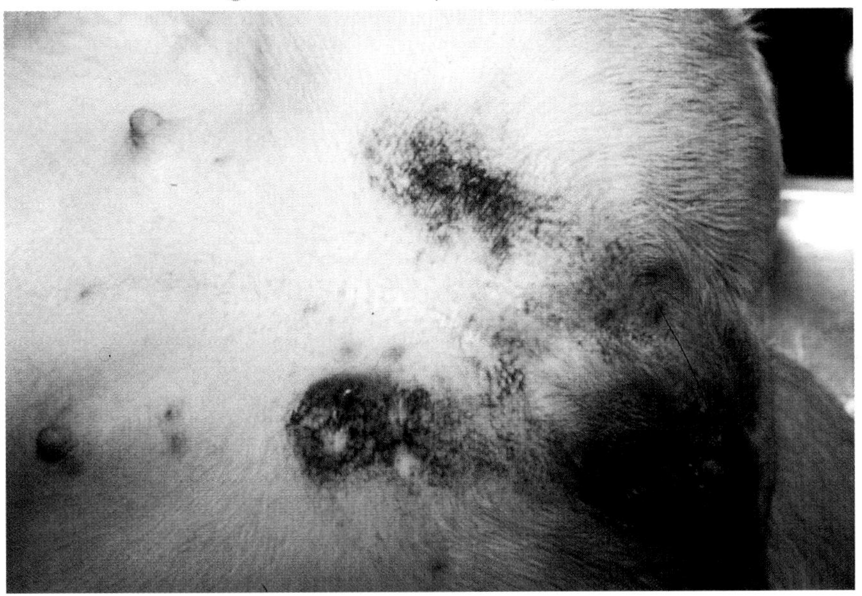

Gross Pathologic Findings

- Masses—vary in color and appearance; may be ulcerated
- Benign—generally slow-growing; brown to black; varies from macules and plaques to firm, dome-shaped nodules, 0.5–2 cm in diameter
- Malignant—generally rapidly growing; amelanotic to dark brown, gray, or black
- Melanomas of the digit (dog) and eyelid (cat) tend to be malignant.

Histopathologic Findings

- Often difficult to distinguish benign from malignant lesions because both may have cells that vary in shape (e.g., epithelioid, fusiform, dendritic, and mixed), degree of pigmentation, and cytoplasmic morphology
- Malignant—generally high mitotic index; nuclear and nucleolar pleomorphism; invasive into surrounding tissues; amelanotic may pose a diagnostic challenge; special stains may be particularly useful
- Benign and malignant—may note associated inflammation, predominantly lymphoplasmacytic

Therapeutics

Surgical Considerations

- Wide surgical excision—treatment of choice
- Amputation of digit—nail bed or digit affected

Drugs

- Adjunctive chemotherapy—recommended if surgical excision is incomplete or the mass is nonresectable
- Dacarbazine (DTIC), doxorubicin, and carboplatin—reported to induce partial and complete remission in a small number of animals; may be the drugs of choice

Contraindications

Doxorubicin—cardiotoxic; contraindicated with heart disease

Precautions

Veterinarians administering chemotherapeutics should follow published guidelines on the safe use of these drugs and should be familiar with potential side effects.

Alternative Drugs

Cimetidine—shown to be of some benefit in horses and humans with malignant melanoma; believed to act as a biologic response modifier by reversing suppressor T-cell–mediated immune suppression; has not been evaluated for this purpose in dogs and cats

Comments

Client Education

- Discuss the need for early surgical removal.
- Do not advise a wait-and-see approach.

- Warn client that malignant melanoma may metastasize early in the course of the disease; thus, prognosis is guarded.

Patient Monitoring

- Evaluate for evidence of recurrence and metastasis—1, 3, 6, 9, 12, 18, and 24 months after surgery; if the owner believes the mass is returning; if the patient is otherwise not normal
- Thoracic radiography—at the time of rechecks and periodically thereafter

Expected Course and Prognosis

- Dogs—25–50% of melanomas reported to be malignant; melanomas on the digit and scrotum have a greater likelihood of being malignant
- Survival with benign melanomas (dogs)—mean: skin, > 24 months; digit, 19.3 months; 2-year: skin, 94.3%; digit: 38%
- Survival with malignant melanoma (dogs)—skin: 8–13.5 months; digit: 16.9 months; 2-year: skin, 34.1%; digit: 22–36%
- Cats—35–50% of melanomas reported to be malignant
- Mean survival with melanoma of the skin or digit (cats)—not frequently reported; 4.5 months after surgery in one study of 57 cats

Abbreviation

DTIC = (dimethyltriazeno)imidazole carboxamide

Suggested Reading

Aronsohn MG, Carpenter JL. Distal extremity melanocytic nevi and malignant melanomas in dogs. J Am Anim Hosp Assoc 1990;26:605–612.

Bostock DE. Prognosis after surgical excision of canine melanomas. Ver Pathol 1979;16:32–40.

Miller WH, Scott DW, Anderson WI. Feline cutaneous melanocytic neoplasms: a retrospective analysis of 43 cases (1979–1991). Vet Dermatol 1993;4:19–26.

Pulley LT, Stannard AA. Tumors of the skin and soft tissues. In: Moulton JE, ed. Tumors in domestic animals. 3rd ed. Berkeley: University of California Press, 1990:75–82.

Thomas RC, Fox LE. Tumors of the skin and subcutis. In: Morrison WB, ed. Cancer in dogs and cats: medical and surgical management. Baltimore: Williams & Wilkins, 1998:489–510.

Author Joanne C. Graham

Consulting Editor Karen Helton Rhodes

Basal Cell Tumor

Robyn Elmslie

Definition/Overview

- Tumor that originates from the basal epithelium of the skin
- Includes benign (e.g., basal cell epithelioma and basaloid tumor) and malignant (e.g., basal cell carcinoma) tumors

Signalment/History

- Common—makes up 3–12% and 15–18% of all skin tumors in dogs and cats, respectively
- Age—dogs: 6–9 years; cats: 5–18 years (mean, 10.8 years)
- Cocker spaniels, poodles, and Siamese cats—more commonly affected than other breeds

Clinical Features

- Solitary, well-circumscribed, formed, hairless, intradermal raised mass, typically located on the head, neck, or shoulders (Fig. 77-1)
- Variable in size—0.2–10 cm in diameter
- Masses (cats)—often heavily pigmented, cystic, and occasionally ulcerated

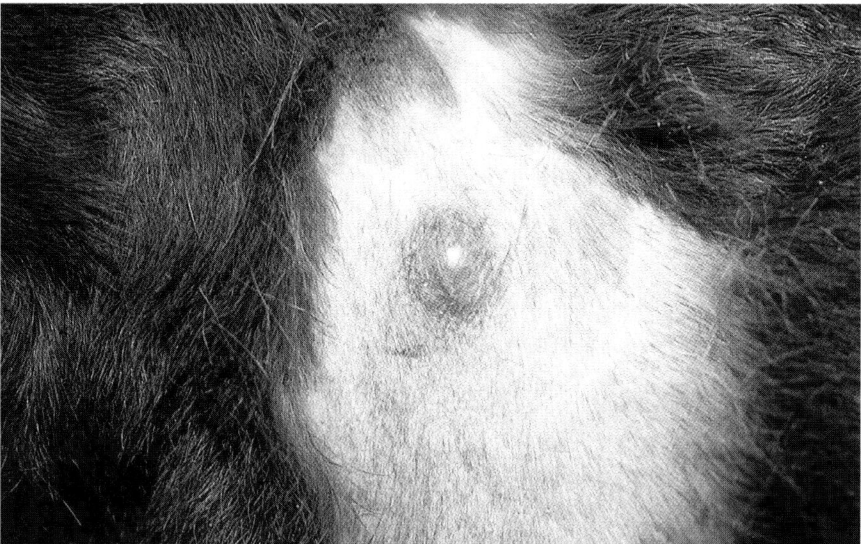

Figure 77-1 Small solitary firm dermal nodule located on the neck of a dog.

Differential Diagnosis

- Other skin tumors—mast cell tumor; melanoma; hemangioma; hemangiosarcoma
- Intradermal cysts

Diagnostics

- Histopathologic examination—definitive diagnosis
- Histologic cellular patterns—vary from solid to cystic to ribbon appearance
- Tumor cells—may contain melanin pigmentation; may have a fine eosinophilic stroma

Therapeutics

- Surgical excision—treatment of choice; generally curative

Comments

- Tumors—< 10% malignant
- Complete surgical excision—usually curative

Suggested Reading

Holzworth J. Diseases of the cat: medicine and surgery. Philadelphia: Saunders, 1987.

Thomas RC, Fox LE. Tumors of the skin and subcutis. In: Morrison WB, ed. Cancer in dogs and cats: medical and surgical management. Baltimore: Williams & Wilkins, 1998:489–510.

Author Robyn Elmslie

Consulting Editor Karen Helton Rhodes

Squamous Cell Carcinoma, Skin

Joanne C. Graham

Definition/Overview

- Malignant tumor of squamous epithelium
- Bowen disease (cats)—multicentric squamous cell carcinoma in situ

Etiology/Pathophysiology

Metastasis—to any site; more commonly to regional lymph nodes and lungs

Signalment/History

- Represents 9–25% of all skin tumors in cats and 4–18% in dogs
- More prevalent in sunny climates and high altitudes (high ultraviolet light exposure)

Breed Predilection

- Cats—none reported; patients often have light or unpigmented skin
- Dogs—Scottish terriers, Pekingese, boxers, poodles, Norwegian elkhounds, Dalmatians, beagles, whippets, and white English bull terriers may be predisposed; large breeds with black skin and haircoats may be predisposed to multiple squamous cell carcinoma involving the digits

Mean Age and Range

- Dogs—9 years
- Cats—9–12.4 years

Historical Findings

- Crusts, ulcer, or mass that may have been present for months and unresponsive to conservative treatment
- Bowen disease (cats)—skin becomes pigmented; ulcer forms in the center; followed by a painful scabby lesion that may expand peripherally
- Lips, nose, and pinna involvement—may start out as a shallow crusting lesion (Fig. 78-1) that progresses to a deep ulcer (Fig. 78-2)
- Facial skin involvement (cats)
- Nail bed involvement (dogs)

Clinical Features

- Proliferative or erosive skin lesions
- Most common sites—cats: nasal planum, eyelids, lips, and pinna; dogs: toes, scrotum, nose, legs, and anus
- Flank and abdomen involvement
- Bowen disease (cats)—may note 2 to > 30 lesions on the head, digits, neck, thorax, shoulders, and ventral abdomen; hair in the lesion epilates easily; crusts cling to the epilated hair shaft

Differential Diagnosis

- Often misdiagnosed as draining abscesses or infected wounds on the basis of gross appearance

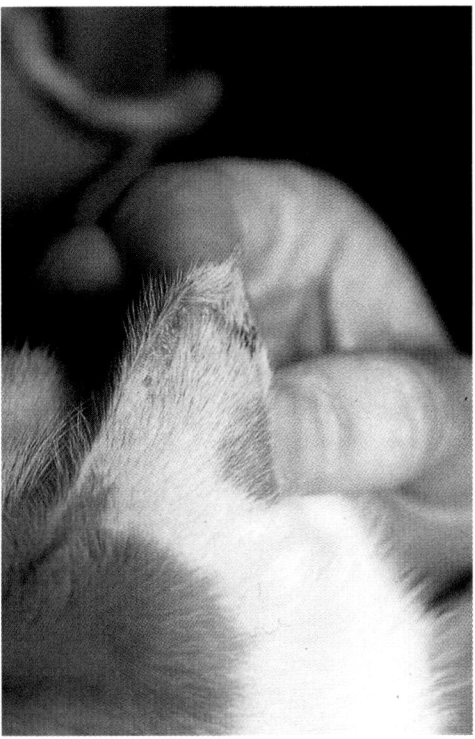

Figure 78-1 Early squamous cell carcinoma of the tip of the pinnae with minimal erythema and crusting.

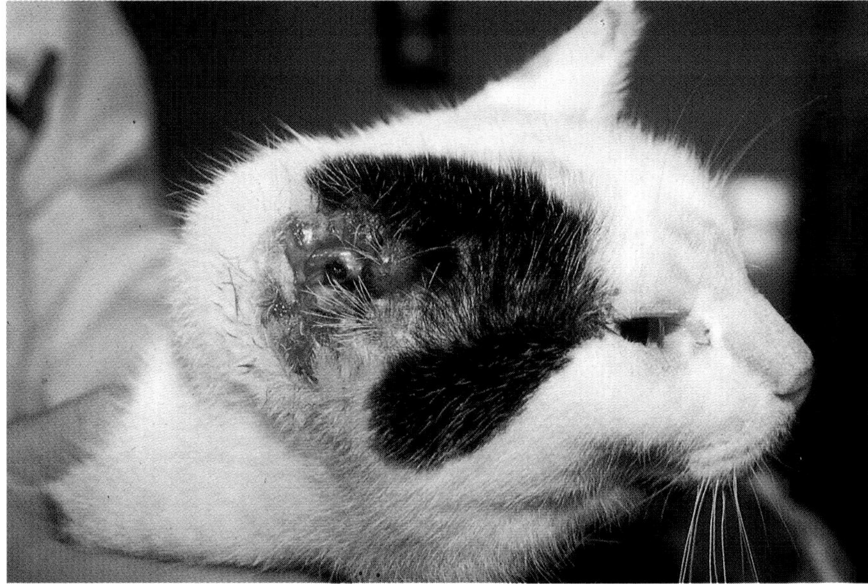

Figure 78-2 Advanced squamous cell carcinoma (SCC) that has eroded much of the pinnae.

- Digit involvement—sometimes confused with nail bed infection and osteomyelitis
- Biopsy and histopathology—distinguish from eosinophilic granuloma complex, immune-mediated disease, mast cell tumor, and cutaneous lymphosarcoma

Diagnostics

- Thoracic radiography—detects lung metastasis
- Abdominal radiography—evaluates and monitors sublumbar lymph nodes, if clinically relevant
- Radiography of extremities—with digital tumor; determines extent of underlying bone involvement
- Cytologic examination—fine-needle aspirate; evaluate large lymph nodes for metastasis
- Biopsy—needed to confirm diagnosis

Gross Pathology

- Ulcerative tumors—most common; may appear shallow and crusted and progress to deep craters
- Proliferative tumors—may have a cauliflower-like appearance; may ulcerate and bleed easily
- Bowen disease—painful ulcers that scab over and expand peripherally to reach more than 4 cm in diameter

Histopathology

- Cords or irregular masses of epidermal cells infiltrating into the dermis and subcutis

- Large numbers of horn (keratin) pearls in well-differentiated tumors
- Desmosomes and mitotic figures common
- Bowen disease—dysplastic, highly ordered keratinocytes proliferate, replacing normal epidermis, but do not penetrate the basement membrane into the surrounding dermis

Therapeutics

- Invasive tumors—inpatient; require aggressive surgical excision or radiotherapy
- Superficial tumors—surgery, cryosurgery, photodynamic therapy, or irradiation
- Topical synthetic retinoids—may be useful for early superficial lesions

Surgical Considerations

- Wide surgical excision—treatment of choice; skin flaps and body wall reconstruction sometimes required
- Digit involvement—amputation
- Pinna involvement—may require partial or total resection
- Invasive tumors of the nares—removal of the nasal planum recommended
- Radiotherapy—recommended for inoperable tumors or as adjunct to surgery

Drugs

- Adjunctive chemotherapy—recommended with incomplete surgical excision, nonresectable mass, and metastasis
- Cisplatin (dogs), carboplatin, and mitoxantrone—reported to induce partial and complete remission; generally of short duration; small number of patients
- Intralesional sustained-release chemotherapeutic gel implants (dogs)—contain either 5-fluorouracil or cisplatin; effective

Contraindications

- Cisplatin—do not use in cats, causes severe hydrothorax, pulmonary edema, and death; do not use in dogs with concurrent renal disease, potentially nephrotoxic
- 5-Fluorouracil—contraindicated in cats

Precautions

Chemotherapeutics—follow published guidelines and protocols for safe use; be familiar with potential side effects

Alternative Drugs

Topical synthetic retinoids—may be useful for early superficial lesions

Comments

Client Education

- Inform client about the benefit of early diagnosis and treatment.

- Discuss risk factors associated with the development of the tumor (ultraviolet light exposure).

Patient Monitoring

- Physical examination and radiography—1, 3, 6, 9, 12, 18, and 24 months after treatment or if the owner thinks the tumor is recurring
- Thoracic and abdominal radiography—at each recheck examination, if the lesion is on the caudal portion of the patient

Prevention/Avoidance

- Limit sun exposure, especially between the hours of 10:00 A.M. and 2:00 P.M.
- Yearly tattoos on nonpigmented areas may be helpful.
- Sunscreens—usually licked off by the patient; may help in some areas (e.g., pinna)

Expected Course and Prognosis

Prognosis—good with superficial lesions that receive appropriate treatment; guarded with invasive lesions and those involving the nail bed or digit

- Etretinate—0.75–1 mg/kg q24h; used successfully to prevent progression of precancerous lesions
- Vitamin E—400–600 IU PO q12h; may be beneficial to prevent or delay progression of precancerous lesions
- Bleomycin—10–20 IU/m^2 SC once per week; has been used systemically to treat advanced disease
- Chemotherapy—benefit not yet established

Suggested Reading

Himsel CA, Richardson RC, Craig JA. Cisplatin chemotherapy for metastatic squamous cell carcinoma in two dogs. J Am Vet Med Assoc 1986;189:1575–1578.

Marks S. Clinical evaluation of etretinate (Tegison) for the treatment of preneoplastic and early neoplastic cutaneous squamous cell carcinoma in dogs. Vet Can Soc Newslett 1990;14:4–5.

O'Brien MG, Berg J, Engler SJ. Treatment by digital amputation of subungual squamous cell carcinoma in dogs: 21 cases (1987–1988). J Am Vet Med Assoc 1992;201:759–761.

Peaston AE, Leach MW, Higgins RJ. Photodynamic therapy for nasal and aural squamous cell carcinoma in cats. J Am Vet Med Assoc 1993;202:1261–1265.

Thomas RC, Fox LE. Tumors of the skin and subcutis. In: Morrison WB, ed. Cancer in dogs and cats: medical and surgical management. Baltimore: Williams & Wilkins, 1998;489–510.

Author Joanne C. Graham

Consulting Editor Karen Helton Rhodes

Ceruminous Gland Adenocarcinoma, Ear

Joanne C. Graham

Definition/Overview

- Primary malignant tumor of the external auditory meatus arising from coiled tubular apocrine sweat glands (e.g., ceruminous glands)
- May be locally invasive but has a low rate of distant metastasis

Signalment/History

- Rare but the most common malignant tumor of the ear canal in dogs and cats
- Cocker spaniel may be predisposed.
- Mean age—dogs, 8–11 years; cats, 10.5–13 years
- No known sex predisposition
- Chronic inflammation may play a role in tumor development.

Clinical Features

- Similar to otitis externa
- Early appearance—pale pink, friable, ulcerative, bleeding nodular mass(es)
- Late appearance—large mass(es) filling the canal and invading through canal wall into surrounding structures
- Local lymphadenomegaly (Fig. 79-1)
- May see vestibular signs

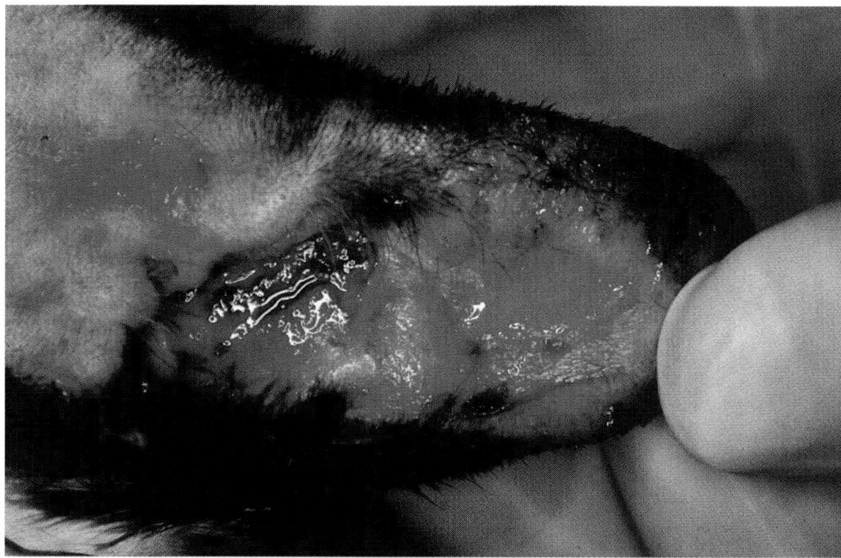

Figure 79-1 Ceruminous gland adenocarcinoma with involvement of the pinnae and metastasis to the submandibular lymph nodes. (Courtesy of Dr. Chris Hunt.)

Differential Diagnosis

- Nodular hyperplasia
- Pedunculated inflammatory polyps (cats)
- Squamous cell carcinoma
- Basal cell tumor
- Papilloma
- Sebaceous gland tumor
- Ceruminous gland adenoma

Diagnostics

- Skull radiography—determine involvement of tympanic bulla
- Thoracic radiography—evaluate for lung metastasis
- CT—useful before radiotherapy

Diagnostic Procedures

- Cytologic examination of aspirate from large lymph nodes
- Biopsy
- Histopathologic characteristics—apocrine type differentiation from ceruminous glands and local invasion into stroma
- Tumor cells—show moderate to marked nuclear atypia with frequent mitosis

Therapeutics

- Ear canal ablation and lateral bulla osteotomy—preferred over lateral ear resection
- Radiotherapy—large or incompletely excised masses

Comments

Patient Monitoring

Physical examination and thoracic radiography—at 1, 3, 6, 12, 16, and 24 months after treatment

Possible Complications

Permanent or transient Horner syndrome

Expected Course and Prognosis

- Median survival after lateral ear resection (cats)—10 months (1-year survival, 33.3%)
- Median survival after ear ablation and lateral bulla osteotomy (cats)—42 months (1-year survival, 75%)
- Median survival after radiotherapy (cats)—39.5 months (1-year survival, 56%)
- Poor prognosis associated with extensive tumor involvement and neurologic signs

Suggested Reading

Marino DJ, MacDonald JM, Matthisen DT, et al. Results of surgery in cats with ceruminous gland adenocarcinoma. J Am Anim Hosp Assoc 1994;30:54–58.

Morrison WB. Cancers of the head and neck. In: Morrison WB, ed. Cancer in dogs and cats: medical and surgical management. Philadelphia: Williams & Wilkins, 1998:511–519.

Author Joanne C. Graham

Consulting Editor Karen Helton Rhodes

Adenocarcinoma, Skin (Sweat Gland, Sebaceous)

Robyn Elmslie

Definition/Overview

Malignant growth originating from sebaceous and apocrine sweat glands within the skin

Signalment/History

- Sebaceous gland—rare in dogs and cats
- Apocrine sweat gland—rare in dogs and cats; occurs more frequently in cats than does sebaceous gland adenocarcinoma
- Both types—more common in old patients

Clinical Features

- Appear as solid, firm, raised lesions
- May be ulcerated and bleeding and accompanied by inflammation of the surrounding tissue
- Apocrine sweat gland—often poorly circumscribed; very invasive into underlying tissue (Fig. 80-1)
- Sebaceous gland—cats (rare) may have inflammation and swelling of multiple digits owing to metastasis of multicentric ungual adenocarcinoma from a distant cutaneous site (Fig. 80-2)

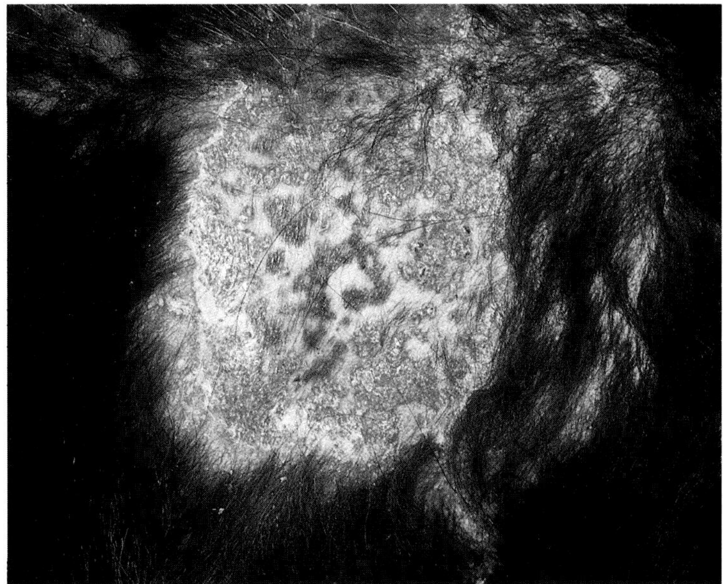

Figure 80-1 Poorly circumscribed canine apocrine gland adenocarcinoma on the lateral aspect of the trunk.

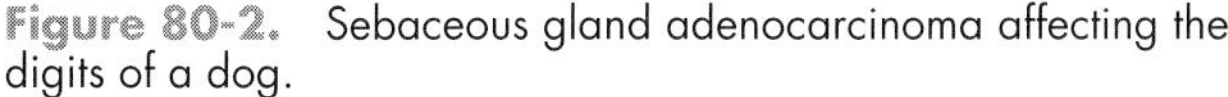

Figure 80-2. Sebaceous gland adenocarcinoma affecting the digits of a dog.

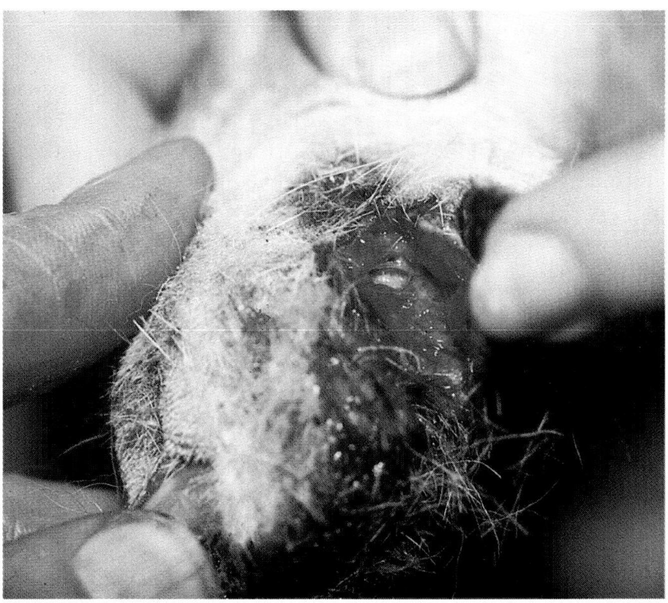

Differential Diagnosis

- Any other skin tumor
- Cellulitis

Diagnostics

- Thoracic radiographs and cytologic examination or biopsy of regional lymph nodes—required at the time of diagnosis; rule out metastatic disease
- Histopathologic examination—essential to confirm diagnosis
- Apocrine sweat gland—typically invasive into the underlying stroma and blood vessels; has poorly demarcated borders and a high mitotic index

Therapeutics

- Aggressive surgical excision required for both types
- Entire tissue specimen must be evaluated histologically to assess completeness of resection
- Radiotherapy—recommended for local control when complete surgical excision is not possible
- Apocrine sweat gland—chemotherapy after surgery recommended, particularly in cats; carboplatin most effective agent in author's experience

Comments

- Sebaceous gland—little known about the metastatic potential; prognosis good if complete surgical excision is achieved, particularly in dogs
- Apocrine sweat gland—associated with a very guarded prognosis; aggressive surgical resection required for local tumor control; postoperative chemotherapy recommended to delay or prevent development of metastasis

Suggested Reading

Carpenter JL, Andrews LK, Holzworth J. Tumors and tumor like lesions. In: Holzworth J, ed. Diseases of the cat: medicine and surgery. Philadelphia: Saunders, 1987:406–596.

Thomas RC, Fox LE. Tumors of the skin and subcutis. In: Morrison WB, ed. Cancer in dogs and cats: medical and surgical management. Baltimore: Williams & Wilkins, 1998:489–510.

Author Robyn Elmslie

Consulting Editor Karen Helton Rhodes

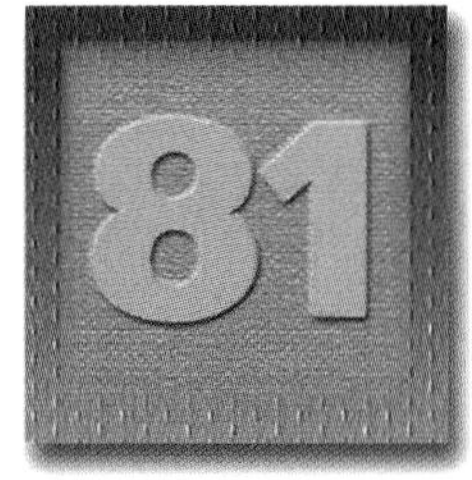

Feline Paraneoplastic Syndrome

Karen L. Campbell

Definition/Overview

- Rare—only seven reported cases
- Characterized by cutaneous lesions, which serve as markers of internal neoplasia

Etiology/Pathophysiology

- Most affected cats have had pancreatic adenocarcinomas with metastases to liver, lungs, pleura, and/or peritoneum; one report of bile duct carcinoma
- The link between internal malignancies and cutaneous lesions is unknown; may involve cytokines producing atrophy of the hair follicles
- Skin/Exocrine—alopecia
- Gastrointestinal—weight loss, anorexia
- Other systems—result of metastasis of the pancreatic or biliary tumor (e.g., liver, lungs, pleura, and/or peritoneal cavity)

Signalment/History

- All affected animals were mixed-breed or domestic shorthair cats.
- Mean age, 12.5 years; range of 9–16 years
- Six cases were male.
- Decrease in appetite followed by rapid weight loss and excessive shedding

- Pruritus—variable; sometimes with excessive grooming
- Hair loss—rapidly progressive
- Some affected cats may be reluctant to walk, owing to painful fissuring of the footpads.

Clinical Features

- Hairs epilate easily
- Severe alopecia—ventral neck, abdomen, and medial thighs (Fig. 81-1)
- The stratum corneum may "peel," leading to a glistening appearance to the skin (Fig. 81-2)
- Gray lentigines may develop in alopecic areas.
- Footpads may be fissured and/or scaly (Fig. 81-3).

Differential Diagnosis

- Hyperadrenocorticism—polyuria, polydipsia, and skin fragility
- Hyperthyroidism—polyphagia
- Hypothyroidism—spontaneous condition rare in cats; not associated with glistening skin
- Feline symmetrical alopecia—hair loss self-induced; not associated with easy epilation
- Demodicosis—mites are not associated with paraneoplastic alopecia
- Dermatophytosis—hair loss often associated with breakage, not spontaneous shedding; inappetence and weight loss rare

Figure 81-1 Twelve-year-old MC DSH with severe ventral alopecia in association with pancreatic adenocarcinoma.

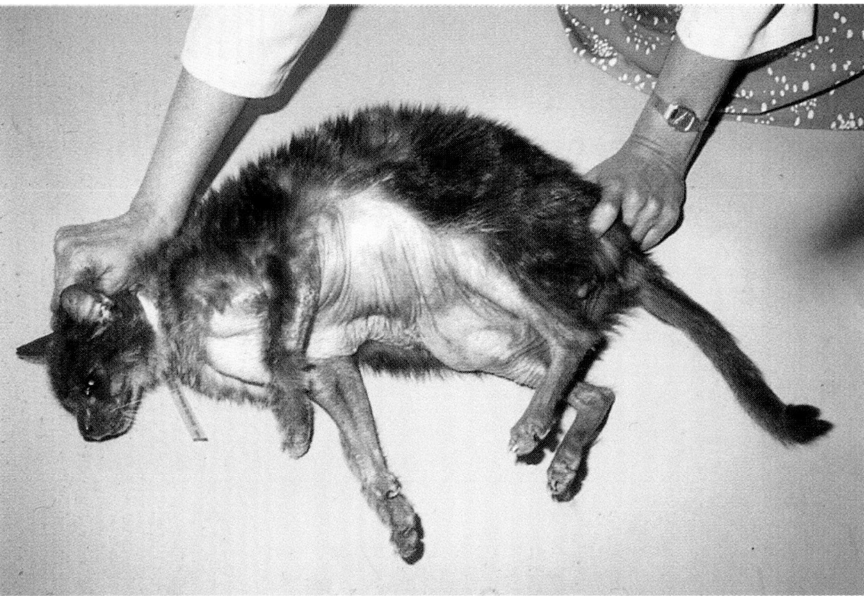

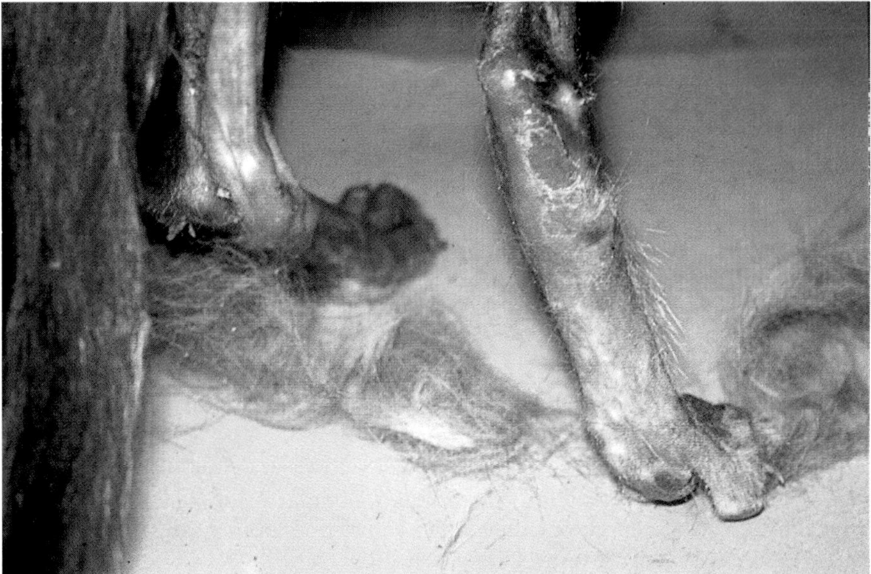

Figure 81-2 Rear limbs of cat in Figure 81-1; hairs epilate easily revealing the thin, glistening appearance of the skin.

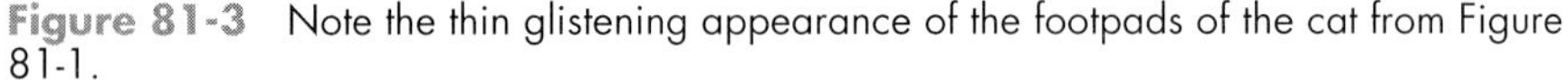

Figure 81-3 Note the thin glistening appearance of the footpads of the cat from Figure 81-1.

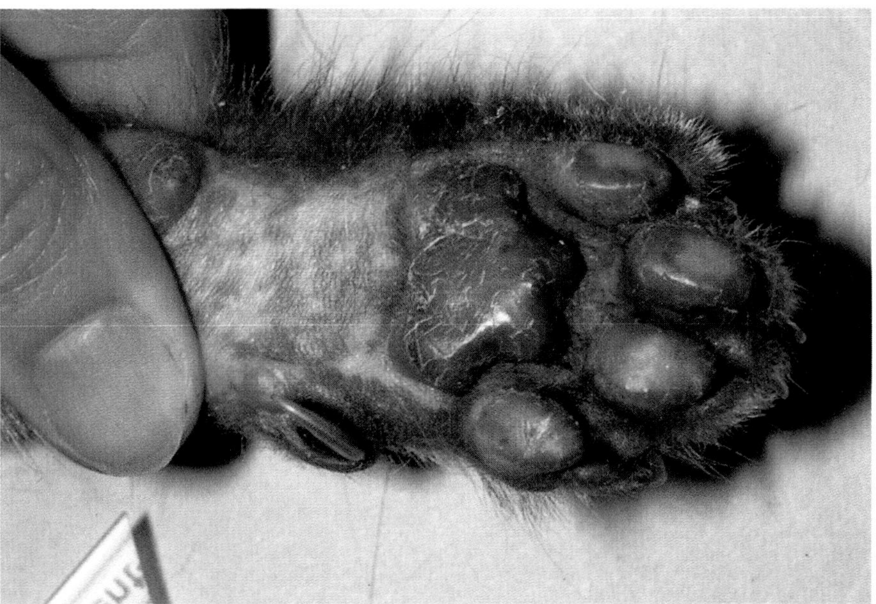

- Alopecia areata—rarely involves the entire ventral surface; inappetence and weight loss rare
- Telogen effluvium—not associated with miniaturization of hair follicles
- Skin fragility syndrome—fragile skin not associated with paraneoplastic alopecia
- Superficial necrolytic dermatitis—not associated with marked exfoliation and miniaturization of hair follicles

Diagnostics

- Endocrine (thyroid profiles and a dexamethasone suppression test)—rule out endocrine disease
- Skin scrapings—rule out demodicosis
- KOH examination of hairs and/or fungal culture—rule out dermatophytosis
- Ultrasonography—pancreatic mass and/or nodular lesions in the liver or peritoneal cavity; failure to demonstrate nodules does not exclude the diagnosis, because they may be too small for detection
- Thoracic radiographs—metastatic lesions in the lungs or pleural cavity
- Skin biopsies
- Laparoscopy or exploratory laparotomy—identify primary and metastatic tumors

Pathologic Findings

- Histopathologic examination of the skin—nonscarring alopecia; severe atrophy of hair follicles and adnexa; miniaturization of hair bulbs; mild acanthosis; variable absence of stratum corneum; variable mixed superficial perivascular infiltrates of neutrophils, eosinophils, and mononuclear cells
- Primary tumor—usually pancreatic adenocarcinoma, one case with a primary bile duct carcinoma
- Metastatic nodules—common in the liver, lungs, pleura, and peritoneum

Therapeutics

- Chemotherapy or other—no reported response; all cases have had metastatic disease at the time of diagnosis
- Affected animals rapidly deteriorate; euthanasia should be suggested as a humane intervention.
- Supportive care—only if owners refuse to consider euthanasia; feed highly palatable, nutrient-dense foods, and/or tube feed.

Comments

- Progressive deterioration
- Supportive care—ultrasonography and thoracic radiographs may demonstrate progression of metastatic disease
- Expect death to occur within 2–8 weeks after onset of skin lesions.

Suggested Reading

Brooks DG, Campbell KL, Dennis JS, et al. Pancreatic paraneoplastic alopecia in three cats. J Am Anim Hosp Assoc 1994;30:557–562.

Pascal-Tenorio A, Olivry T, Gross TL, et al. Paraneoplastic alopecia associated with internal malignancies in the cat. Vet Dermatol 1997;8:47–52.

Consulting Editor Karen Helton Rhodes

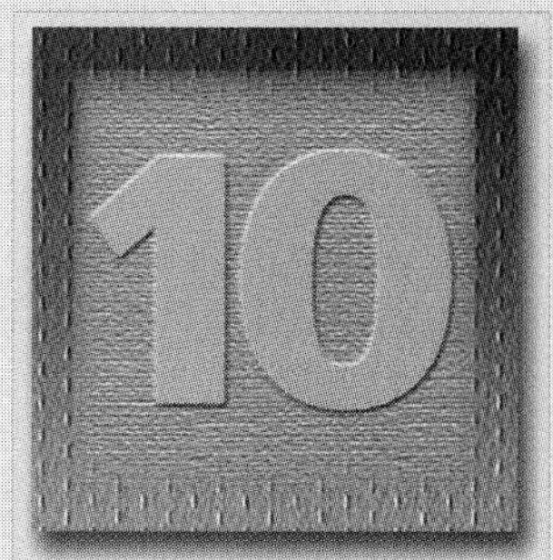

Exotic Pet Dermatology

GUINEA PIGS: ECTOPARASITE

Karen Rosenthal

Definition/Overview

The most common ectoparasite causing disease in guinea pigs is the sarcoptic mite, *Trixacarus caviae*. It is a burrowing mite and can be an unapparent infection or the cause of severe disease in pet guinea pigs (Fig. 82-1).

Etiology/Pathophysiology

The guinea pig sarcoptic mite can cause disease in solitary pet guinea pigs or in a group of guinea pigs. It spreads easily within a colony. When a clinical infection with *Trixacarus caviae* becomes apparent in a solitary older guinea pig, a primary disease process should be considered.

Clinical Features

Guinea pigs can be infected with *Trixacarus caviae* but show no signs of disease. In mild cases, a thinning hair coat and scaly skin is apparent. In more severe cases, alopecia and erythema caused by intense pruritus is seen. As the disease progresses, the skin becomes ulcerated and a mucopurulent discharge may be present. Some clinicians have reported that severe pruritus caused by mites can lead to seizure-like activity in guinea pigs.

Lab Findings

The complete blood count and plasma biochemistry findings are usually not affected by this disease. Occasionally, an eosinophilia may be observed in some

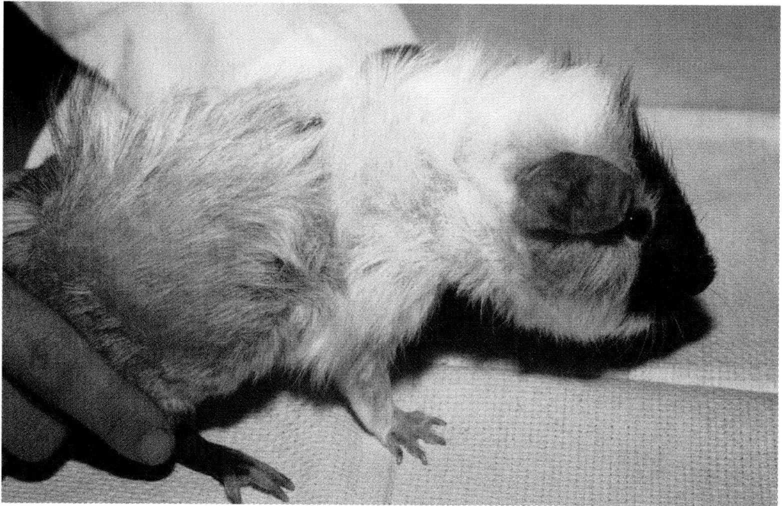

Figure 82-1 Infestation of *Trixacarus* in a guinea pig.

guinea pigs. If a severe secondary bacterial dermatitis is present, the white blood cell count may be elevated. If a primary disease is the cause of a secondary mite infestation, then there might be associated changes in the biochemistry panel.

Diagnostic Tests

Diagnose this disease by observing the mite, *Trixacarus caviae*, or its ova. This can be done by skin scrapes or the "scotch tape" method. Scotch tape is applied to the skin and the debris stuck to the tape is observed under the microscope. In some cases, the mites cannot be identified, and response to treatment is used to diagnose this disease.

Treatment

Various topical antiparasiticidal treatments have been recommended to treat this guinea pig mite. This should be viewed with caution as guinea pigs can be very susceptible to the negative side effects of these preparations. The safest method to treat this disease is with subcutaneous injections of ivermectin. Use a dose of 0.2 to 0.4 mg/kg once every 2 weeks for up to four treatments. Resistance to ivermectin has been reported and some clinicians have used dosages of up to 1 mg/kg. All guinea pigs in the house should be treated, even if clinical signs are not apparent. If a secondary bacterial dermatitis is present, treat with topical antibiotic preparations. If severe, systemic antibiotics may be necessary. The environment should also be cleaned. All materials that are disposable should be replaced. The cage and the housing areas should be treated with anti-parasiticidal applications. Care should be taken to cleanse these areas of all antiparasiticidal preparations before re-introducing the guinea pigs. If this is an older guinea pig that has an acute mite infestation, a primary disease should be investigated before successful treatment of *Trixacarus caviae* can be accomplished.

Prognosis

Excellent if there is no primary disease process

Hedgehog: Chorioptes Mites

Karen Rosenthal

Definition/Overview

African hedgehogs have recently entered the pet trade. A commonly reported problem in hedgehogs is quill loss (Fig. 83-1). Relatively few data about these animals are available to guide the clinician in regarding diagnostics and treatment.

Etiology/Pathophysiology

Chorioptes mites are the most common species of mange mite that appear to infect the African hedgehog.

Clinical Signs

Mite infestation can range from unapparent to mild or severe. In mild cases, the skin becomes flaky and a few quills are lost. As the disease progresses, pruritus is present and many quills fall out in patches around the body.

Lab Findings

It is unknown if there are any blood count or biochemistry changes associated with this disease.

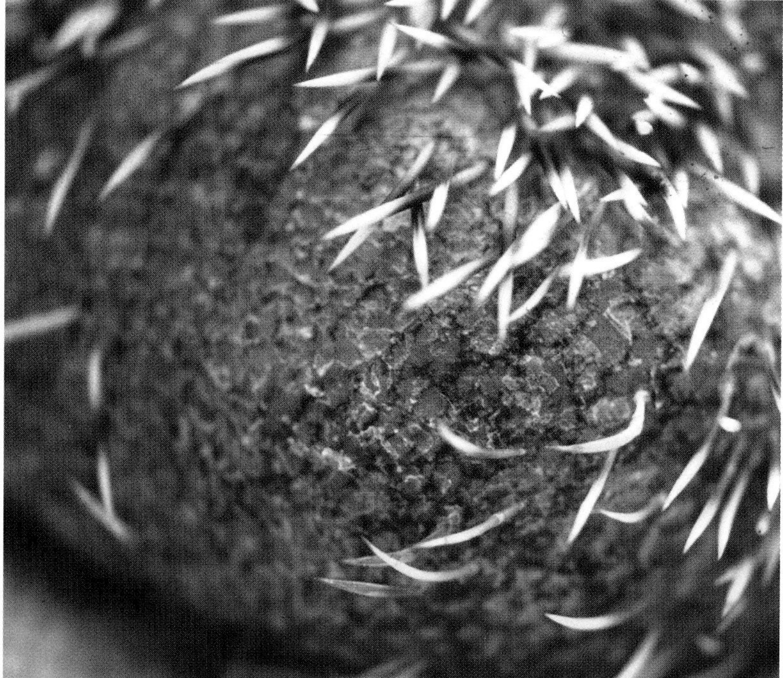

Figure 83-1 Note absence of quills along internal trunk

Diagnostic Tests

It is common to find the mites on either a skin scrape or microscopic examination of the quills. If the mites are not seen on examination, response to treatment is used as a diagnostic test.

Treatment

The treatment of choice appears to be ivermectin at 0.2 to 0.4 mg/kg SC given once and repeated one to two times at 2-week intervals. Environmental clean-up along with treatment of all other hedgehogs in the house is important to cure this problem.

Prognosis

The prognosis is good for this disease. If an older, solitary hedgehog acutely develops disease as a result of Chorioptes mites, a primary problem may be present.

Author Karen Rosenthal

Consulting Editor Karen Helton Rhodes

Rabbits: Urine Scald

Karen Rosenthal

Definition/Overview

When rabbit skin is exposed to urine for an extended length of time, inflammation of the skin with a secondary bacterial dermatitis can occur (Fig. 84-1).

Pathophysiology

Numerous systemic diseases will cause rabbits to sit for extended periods in a hunched position. In some cage settings, this will expose the perineal and ventral skin to the urine. Rabbits with cystitis and "bladder sludge syndrome" are also prone to urine scald.

Clinical Signs

Rabbits with urine scald emit a foul odor. The perineal and ventral skin can be erythematous and ulcerated. Palpation of this area can be painful and a mucopurulent discharge may be present.

Lab Findings

In some cases, the complete blood count and plasma biochemistry findings are not affected by this disease. But if a severe secondary bacterial dermatitis is present, an increase in the white blood cell count may be observed. Urine scald is always caused by a primary disease and these diseases may cause abnormalities in the biochemistry panel.

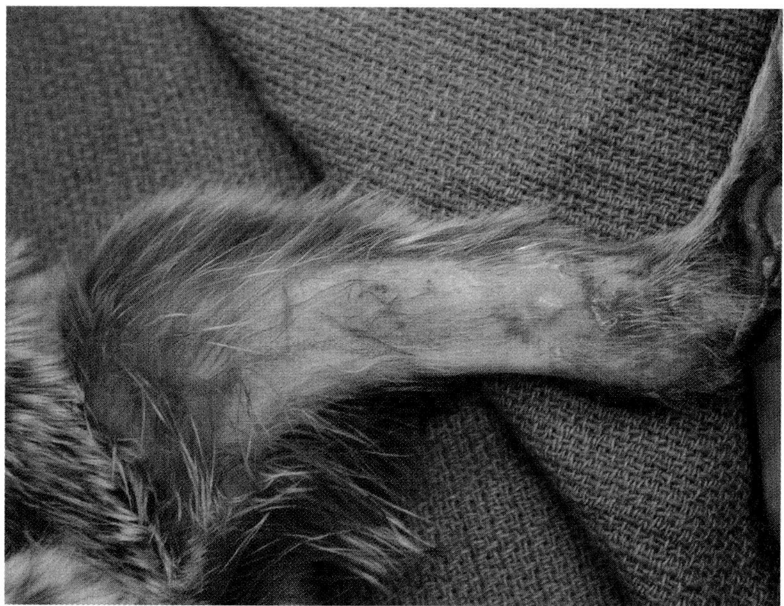

Figure 84-1 Erythema and alopecia of the medial aspect of the hindlimb secondary to urine scalding

Diagnostic Tests

Diagnosis is made by observing the lesions. A skin biopsy shows inflammation and, possibly, intralesional bacteria.

Treatment

Treatment has to include therapy for the primary disease; otherwise, urine scald cannot be cured. The severity of the skin lesion dictates how aggressive the therapy should be. In mild cases, drying agents and topical antibacterial preparations can be used. In more severe cases, systemic antibiotics should be added to the treatment regimen. Hydrotherapy, if inflammation is severe, aids in healing of urine scald. However, the owners must understand that if the primary problem is not addressed, urine scald cannot be cured.

Prognosis

Prognosis is excellent for a cure if the primary problem is resolved.

Author Karen Rosenthal

Consulting Editor Karen Helton Rhodes

MICE: ECTOPARASITES

Karen Rosenthal

Definition/Overview

Pet mice can develop infestations with mites. There are three species of mites that are commonly seen in mice: *Myobia musculi, Myocoptes musculinus, and Radfordia affinis*. More than one species at a time may be present and causing disease.

Etiology/Pathophysiology

Mite infestations are seen in young, recently purchased mice. They are also seen in mouse colonies. A mite infestation in an older, solitary mouse may signal a more serious, primary problem.

Clinical Signs

As with other ectoparasites, a mite infection may range from unapparent to mild or severe. A mild infection is characterized by slight pruritus, hair thinning, and white, flaky skin. A severe infection includes alopecia, severe pruritus, and ulcerated skin. A mucopurulent skin discharge may be present if a secondary bacterial dermatitis occurs.

Lab Findings

The complete blood count and plasma biochemistry findings are usually not affected by this disease. In severe disease, the white blood cell count may be elevated and an eosinophilia may be present.

Diagnostic Tests

Diagnose this disease by observing the mites, either *Myobia musculi, Myocoptes musculinus*, and *Radfordia affinis*, or their ova. This can be done by skin scrapes or the "scotch tape" method. Scotch tape is applied to the skin and the debris stuck to the tape is observed under the microscope. In some cases, the mites cannot be identified and response to treatment is used to diagnose this disease.

Treatment

Various topical antiparasiticidal treatments have been recommended to treat mouse mange. This should be viewed with caution as mice can be very susceptible to the negative side effects of these preparations. The safest method to treat this disease is with subcutaneous injections of ivermectin. Use a dose of 0.2 to 0.4 mg/kg once every 2 weeks for up to four treatments. Resistance to ivermectin has been reported and some clinicians have used dosages of up to 1 mg/kg. All mice in the house should be treated, even if clinical signs are not apparent. If a secondary bacterial dermatitis is present, treat with topical antibiotic preparations. If severe, systemic antibiotics may be necessary. If pruritus has caused a severe inflammation, some clinicians recommend using a short-acting steroid preparation until the inflammation resides. The environment should be cleaned. All materials that are disposable should be replaced. The cage and the housing areas should be treated with antiparasiticidal applications; however, be sure to cleanse these areas of all antiparasiticidal preparations before re-introducing the mice. If this is an older mouse that acutely has this disease, a primary disease should be investigated before successful treatment of mites can be accomplished.

Prognosis

The prognosis is usually good with this disease.

Author Karen Rosenthal

Consulting Editor Karen Helton Rhodes

Rabbits: Fur Mites

Karen Rosenthal

Definition/Overview

Cheyletiella parasitovorax is a common problem in pet rabbits. Other ectoparasites can be found on rabbits, but the fur mite is the most frequently found (Fig. 86-1). Disease can be unapparent to mild to severe. Secondary bacterial dermatitis can occur in severe infestations. Rabbit owners may know this disease as *walking dandruff*.

Pathophysiology

The rabbit fur mite can cause disease in a rabbitry and spread quickly from cage to cage. It is also common for a single rabbit to be affected by this mite. In the older, solitary rabbit that acutely develops disease caused by the fur mite, a primary problem causing immune suppression is likely present.

Clinical Signs

A rabbit with fur mite infestation may not present clinical signs of disease. When clinical signs are apparent, the owner usually reports seeing *dandruff*. In affected areas, the skin is white and scaly. Patches of alopecia are common. The rabbit may or may not be pruritic. The rabbit's fur will easily epilate.

Lab Findings

The complete blood count and plasma biochemistry findings are usually not affected by this disease. Possibly, an eosinophilia is observed with this disease.

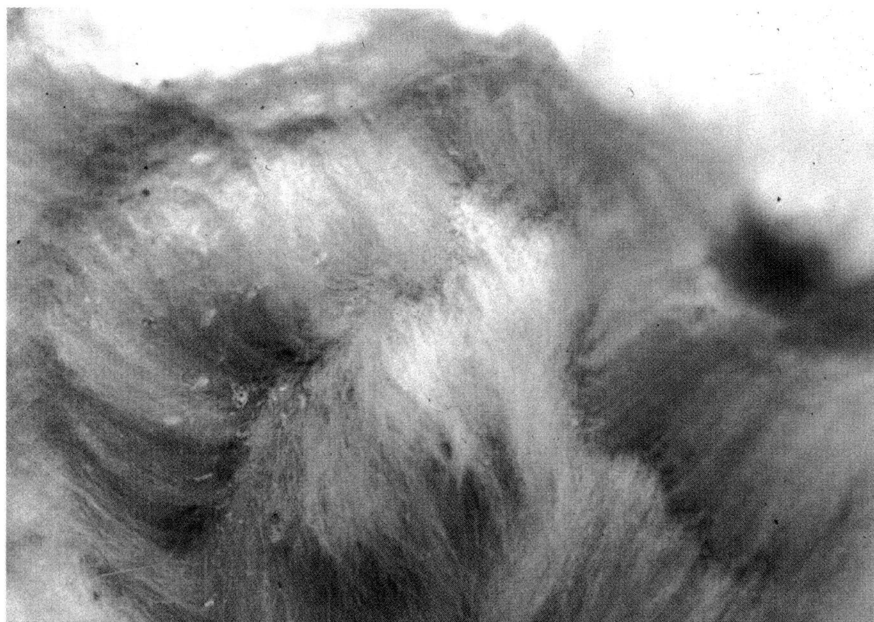

Figure 86-1 Note large flake "dandruff" associated with *Cheyletiella* infestation

Diagnostic Tests

Diagnose this disease by observing the mite, *Cheyletiella parasitovorax*, or its ova. This can be done by skin scrapes or the "scotch tape" method. Scotch tape is applied to the skin and the debris stuck to the tape is observed under the microscope. In some cases, the mites cannot be identified and response to treatment is used to diagnose this disease.

Treatment

Various topical antiparasiticidal treatments have been recommended to treat the fur mite. This should be viewed with caution as rabbits can be very susceptible to the negative side effects of these preparations. The safest method to treat this disease is with subcutaneous injections of ivermectin. Use a dose of 0.2 to 0.4 mg/kg once every 2 weeks for up to four treatments. Resistance to ivermectin has been reported and some clinicians have used dosages of up to 1 mg/kg. All rabbits in the house should be treated, even if clinical signs are unapparent. The environment should also be cleaned. If this is an older rabbit that acutely has this disease, a primary disease should be investigated before successful treatment of *Cheyletiella parasitovorax* can be accomplished.

Prognosis

The prognosis for this disease is excellent. If a primary disease is present, that must be addressed first before a fur mite infestation can be cured.

Guinea Pigs: Ovarian Cysts

Karen Rosenthal

Definition/Overview

Ovarian or follicular cysts are not uncommon in older female guinea pigs. The only clinical sign of this disease may be alopecia (Fig. 87-1).

Pathophysiology

It is assumed that ovarian cysts produce abnormal quantities of hormones causing an endocrine pattern of alopecia in guinea pigs.

Clinical Signs

The first sign of this disease is hair thinning along the flanks. Alopecia then typically becomes bilateral along the flanks. If the disease progresses further, alopecia continues along the entire dorsum.

Lab Findings

The complete blood count and plasma biochemistry findings are not affected by this disease.

Diagnostic Tests

In most cases, the ovarian cyst can be palpated on physical examination. One or both ovaries can be involved. A percutaneous aspirate of the cyst can be performed

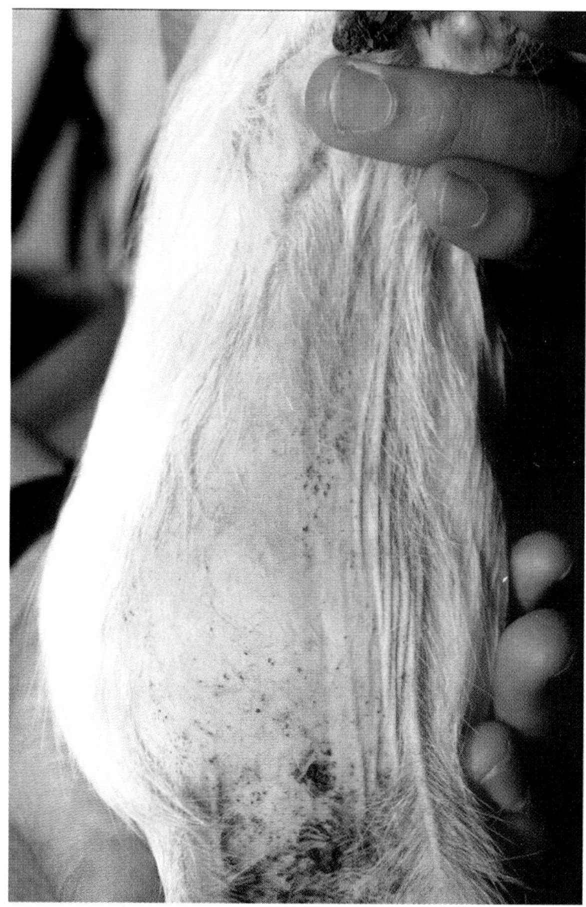

Figure 87-1 Ovarian cyst (advanced stage). Note confluent ventral alopecia

along with cytologic examination of the fluid. Radiographs and abdominal ultrasound will confirm the presence of these cysts. Response to treatment (hair regrowth) is also considered a diagnostic test for determining the presence of ovarian cysts. A skin biopsy will show histopathologic evidence of an endocrine alopecia.

Treatment

The ultimate treatment is abdominal surgery with removal of the ovarian cyst(s). Usually, these are benign cysts and removal is curative. Nonsurgical treatment includes percutaneous aspiration of as much of the cystic fluid as possible. Human chorionic gonadotropin has been given to guinea pigs to reduce the size of the cysts.

Prognosis

If the cysts are removed, the prognosis is excellent.

Author Karen Rosenthal

Consulting Editor Karen Helton Rhodes

Hamsters: Cushing's Disease

Karen Rosenthal

Definition/Overview

Cushing's disease occurs infrequently in pet hamsters. It may be more common than we recognize, but pet hamsters in the United States are not routinely brought to the veterinarian for treatment (Fig. 88-1).

Pathophysiology

Both adrenal glands appear enlarged with this disease and it is likely the result of pituitary abnormalities. High cortisol concentrations are present in these hamsters.

Clinical Signs

Bilateral, nonpruritic alopecia is seen with this disease in hamsters. Eventually, a hamster will lose all of its hair, except the whiskers. The skin may be flaky with hyperpigmentation. Other signs of this disease include profound polyuria and polydipsia. Polyphagia may also be present.

Lab Findings

High cortisol and alkaline phosphatase concentrations have been reported in hamsters with this disease.

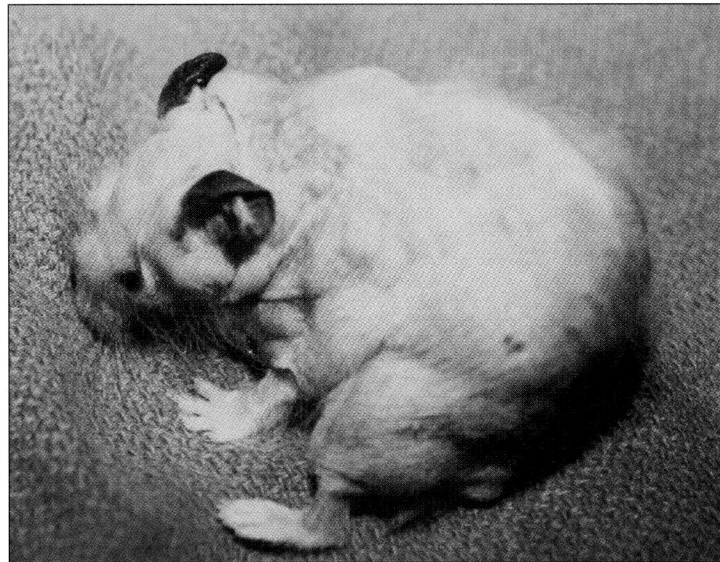

Figure 88-1 Advanced Cushing's disease; partial to complete alopecia

Diagnostic Tests

Because of their small size and the limitation of how much blood can be obtained, it is not always practical to perform such diagnostic tests as the ACTH stimulation test. An abdominal ultrasound should reveal bilateral adrenal gland enlargement.

Treatment

Mitotane therapy can be attempted but the pharmacokinetics of this drug for hamsters has not been determined.

Prognosis

The prognosis for hamsters with this disease is not known.

Author Karen Rosenthal

Consulting Editor Karen Helton Rhodes

FERRETS: ADRENAL GLAND DISEASE

Karen Rosenthal

Definition/Overview

Adrenal gland disease is common in pet ferrets older than 3 years. One or both adrenal glands are affected. The most common sign in both sexes is alopecia (Fig. 89-1).

Pathophysiology

Alopecia is caused by the overproduction of adrenal androgens from the diseased adrenal gland(s). One or more of these compounds are known to be elevated in ferrets with adrenal gland disease: estrogen, androstenedione, 17-OH-progesterone, and DHEAS.

Clinical Signs

The most common sign in ferrets with this disease is alopecia. Hair loss typically starts at the base of the tail or on the tail. Over a period of weeks or months, the alopecia progresses in a symmetrical fashion to include the rump, thigh area, ventrum, and finally along the dorsum to the shoulder blade area. In extreme cases, only guard hairs are left on the entire body. In females, an enlarged vulva is another common sign. In both males and females, pruritus may be present. Ferrets do not have to have alopecia to be pruritic.

Lab Findings

The complete blood count and plasma biochemistry findings are not affected by this disease. Typical tests for adrenal gland disease such as the ACTH stimulation test and the urine cortisol:creatinine ratio do not diagnose this disease.

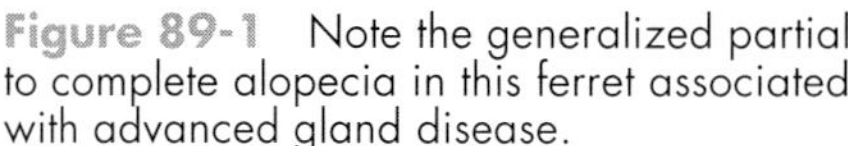

Figure 89-1 Note the generalized partial to complete alopecia in this ferret associated with advanced gland disease.

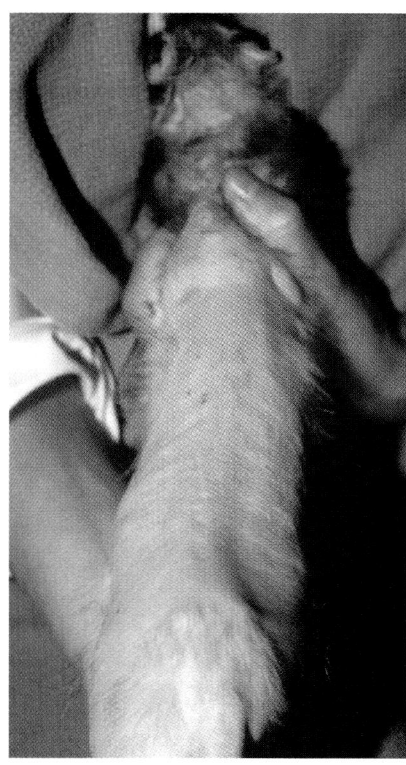

Diagnostic Tests

Abdominal ultrasound can detect an enlarged adrenal gland in some cases. Not all adrenal glands that are diseased are enlarged. Measurement of adrenal androgen concentrations is a more consistent method to diagnose this disease. In ferrets with adrenal gland disease, one or more adrenal androgens will be elevated above the normal range.

Treatment

Surgical removal of the diseased adrenal gland is currently the preferred treatment. If both adrenal glands are diseased, the clinician has the option of removing both glands or one whole gland and part of the other. If both glands are entirely removed, then glucocorticoid supplementation is required. In some ferrets, mineralcorticoid supplementation may also be needed. If one whole gland and part of the other is removed, then supplementation may not be necessary. However, in this instance, the signs of disease may not entirely dissipate if some of the diseased gland remains. Mitotane administration appears to cause signs to regress in some ferrets. Mitotane appears to work best in younger ferrets with this disease. Pruritus from adrenal gland disease appears to only respond to removal of the offending adrenal glands.

Prognosis

The prognosis with this disease is usually excellent. Once the diseased adrenal gland is removed, the clinical signs resolve. If the entire gland cannot be removed, depending on the amount of diseased gland remaining, signs may fully or partially resolve.

Rabbits: Dermatophytosis

Karen Rosenthal

Definition/Overview

Dermatophytosis (ringworm) is rare in rabbits. It is commonly included in the differential diagnosis of hair loss in rabbits but it should be considered an uncommon finding.

Pathophysiology

Trichophyton mentagrophytes is the more common dermatophyte in rabbits. *Microsporum* species is less common.

Clinical Signs

Signs include hair loss, scaly skin, and occasionally, pruritus. Hair loss can be in a ring pattern but patches of alopecia with easily epilating hair can also occur.

Lab Findings

The complete blood count and plasma biochemistry findings are not affected by this disease.

Diagnostic Tests

Diagnose dermatophytoses in rabbits by culture or by identifying organisms in skin scrapings treated with 10% potassium hydroxide.

Treatment

The safest treatment of this disease is by use of topical antifungal preparations. If the skin areas affected are small, this is the treatment of choice. If there is a more generalized infection, griseofulvin can be used, but as with all off-label use of drugs, the owners should be warned of potential negative side effects. The environment should also be cleaned.

Prognosis

The prognosis for this disease is good. Generalized cases, may be a secondary or primary disease process. If the primary disease process is not resolved, then the case carries a more guarded prognosis for a cure.

Author Karen Rosenthal

Consulting Editor Karen Helton Rhodes

Ferrets: Mast Cell Tumors

Karen Rosenthal

Definition/Overview

Cutaneous mast cell tumors are common causes of skin masses in ferrets. This is almost always a benign disease in ferrets. Rarely does cutaneous mast cell tumor disease lead to or result from mast cell metastasis (Fig. 91-1). Ferrets with cutaneous mast cell tumors have no other signs of disease.

Etiology/Pathophysiology

Cutaneous mast cell tumors have histopathologic characteristics common to mast cell tumors in other animals. The mast cells are well-differentiated, round to oval in shape, and are usually arranged in sheets. Because this is usually a benign disease, mitotic figures are rare.

Clinical Signs

Mast cell tumors appear as individual skin nodules. A ferret can have one or many nodules on different skin areas. The most common body area in which to find the nodules is the dorsum, especially near the shoulders. Nodules vary in size from a couple of millimeters to up to 3 centimeters. Although they can appear just as a nodule, typically, the mass is erythematous. Dried blood on and around the nodule is common. Mast cell tumors can either be flat or raised and both can appear at the same time on the same ferret. Occasionally, the area of the mast cell tumor will be pruritic. Infrequently, localized alopecia will accompany the mast cell tumor.

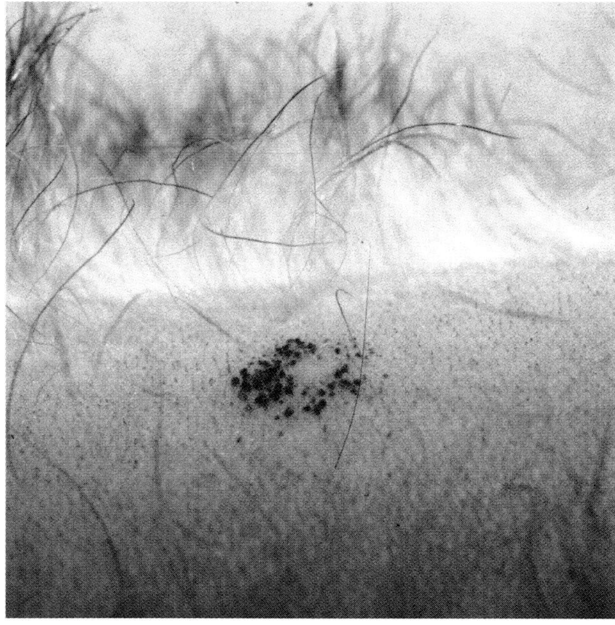

Figure 91-1 Mast cell tumor (MCT): Note the mildly erythematous base with dried blood adhered to the surface.

Lab Findings

The complete blood count and plasma biochemistry findings are not affected by cutaneous mast cell tumors.

Diagnostic Tests

The diagnostic test of choice is biopsy of the mast cell tumor. The ferret is tranquilized or anesthetized and the biopsy specimen is taken. An impression smear can also be used to diagnose this disease.

Treatment

Removal of the cutaneous tumors is the treatment of choice. These tumors do not require chemotherapy or radiation therapy. In some cases, these cutaneous tumors have been seen to dissipate without treatment.

Prognosis

The prognosis for cutaneous mast cell tumors in ferrets is excellent. Even without surgery, these cutaneous tumors do not appear to metastasize. Removal is still indicated though. If the nodules are pruritic, removal will improve the quality of life. Although it has not been shown that metastasis from cutaneous to systemic disease occurs, prevention by removal of the tumors is warranted for precautionary reasons.

Ferrets: Sarcoptic Mange

Karen Rosenthal

Definition/Overview

Sarcoptic mange is rarely seen in pet ferrets. *Sarcoptes scabiei*, which affects dogs and cats, is the cause of sarcoptic mange in ferrets. Two syndromes are seen with sarcoptes mites, either a generalized infestation or one that is localized to the feet only.

Etiology/Pathophysiology

Sarcoptic mange is rare in ferrets and therefore has not been extensively studied. In the generalized form, this is likely a secondary disease process and the existence of a primary disease should be investigated.

Clinical Signs

In the localized form, only the feet show signs of disease. The feet are swollen, erythematous, and the ferret may feel pain when walking. The pads may be cracked and bleeding. In the generalized form, there are patches of alopecia and the ferret is intensely pruritic. The skin may be erythematous and ulcerated because of the pruritus.

Lab Findings

Typically, the complete blood count and plasma biochemistry findings are not affected by this disease except for an eosinophilia. If secondary bacterial dermatitis is present, the white blood cell count may be slightly elevated.

Diagnostic Tests

This disease is diagnosed by a skin scrape revealing either the mite or ova. It can be difficult in chronic cases to demonstrate the mite on skin scrapes. A biopsy of the skin may show evidence of the mites and/or severe inflammation. In the localized form, it may be difficult to find areas on the foot to scrape for evidence of mites. It is not uncommon to use response to treatment as a diagnostic test for sarcoptic mites.

Treatment

Treat sarcoptic mites with ivermectin at 0.2 to 0.4 mg/kg SC once and repeat in 2 weeks. Other animals in the house may need to be treated, too. This includes other ferrets, dogs, and cats. Also, the environment the ferret lives in should be cleaned. If a primary problem is present, this must be addressed before successful treatment of sarcoptic mange can be attained.

Prognosis

The prognosis for a cure is excellent in the localized form. In the generalized form, unless the primary problem is resolved, the prognosis is more guarded.

Author Karen Rosenthal

Consulting Editor Karen Helton Rhodes

RABBITS: BARBERING

Karen Rosenthal

Definition/Overview

Rabbits will barber themselves for a variety of reasons. The most common reason is because of pregnancy or pseudopregnancy. Dominant rabbits will barber subordinate rabbits in a group. Infrequently, some rabbits appear to pull hair as a displacement reaction (Fig. 93-1).

Etiology/Pathophysiology

Barbering during gestation is used to build a nest. Barbering in a group is performed by the dominant rabbits on the subordinates.

Clinical Signs

Fur loss is the only sign of this disease. The skin is unaffected. In gestating rabbits, fur is typically pulled from the dewlap, forelegs, and abdomen. If a rabbit is being barbered by another rabbit, hair loss can occur anywhere on the body.

Lab Findings

The complete blood count and plasma biochemistry findings are not affected by this disease.

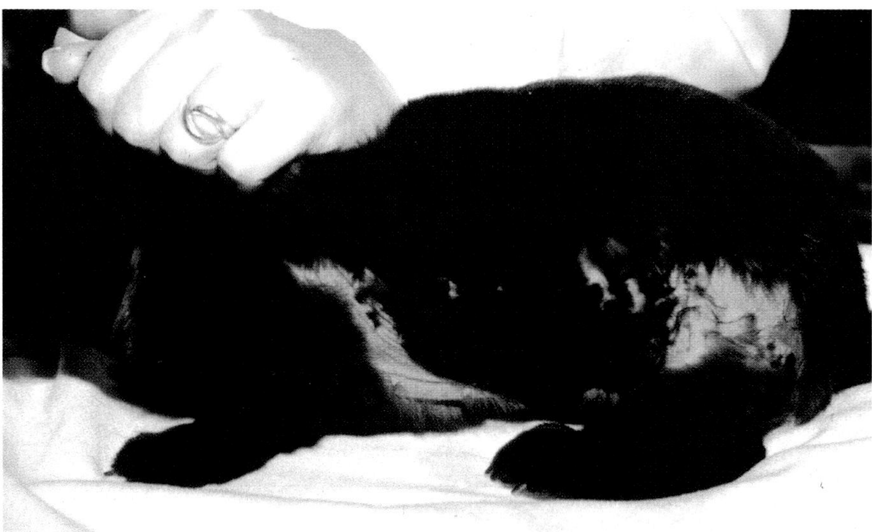

Figure 93-1 This rabbit demonstrates barbering by more dominant members of the group.

Diagnostic Tests

There are no specific tests for this disease. The removal of a rabbit from the group and cessation of signs is evidence for dominance barbering. In gestating rabbits, hair loss will stop once the rabbits are born. Skin biopsies have normal histologic characteristics. In some rabbits, this is a diagnosis of exclusion.

Treatment

There is no specific treatment for this disease. Separation of group members will stop dominance barbering.

Prognosis

The prognosis for this disease is excellent.

Author Karen Rosenthal

Consulting Editor Karen Helton Rhodes

Ferrets: Canine Distemper Virus

Karen Rosenthal

Definition/Overview

Canine distemper virus is fatal in ferrets. One manifestation of this disease is the dermatologic changes. In the scheme of things, the dermatologic signs are minor, but these changes are important for diagnostic purposes.

Etiology/Pathophysiology

Canine distemper virus causes respiratory, dermatologic, gastrointestinal, and neurologic disease in ferrets. Ferrets die from the viral infection or a severe, secondary bacterial pneumonia. Inclusion bodies can be found in all tissues post-mortem but are most common in the epithelium of the gastrointestinal tract, bladder, and skin.

Clinical Signs

The dermatologic clinical signs of canine distemper virus are mainly observed on the chin and footpads. The first signs of this disease are a mild upper respiratory infection including ocular and nasal discharges. In some cases, the dermatologic changes follow the upper respiratory signs or the skin changes can appear first. A chin rash including erythema and alopecia develops. The skin in this area then becomes swollen and crusty. As the disease progresses, hyperkeratosis of the footpads ensues. The footpads become hard, swollen, and crusted. In most cases, other clinical signs of disease accompany hyperkeratosis of the footpads, including neurologic signs and severe lower respiratory disease.

Lab Findings

The complete blood count may be elevated, reflecting the secondary bacterial pneumonia that accompanies canine distemper virus. Depending on the progression of the disease at the time of venipuncture, various biochemical abnormalities will be seen, including elevated hepatic enzymes.

Diagnostic Tests

The definitive diagnosis of canine distemper virus is usually made postmortem. Inclusion bodies are found in epithelial cells on histopathology. History of exposure to this virus in an unvaccinated ferret is common. Serum antibody tests and fluorescent antigen tests aid in the diagnosis. Biopsy of the affected areas of the skin is usually not practical as the ferret commonly succumbs to the disease before histopathology results are known. Very rarely, ferrets will develop atypical canine distemper virus infection. This usually is the result of improper vaccination procedures. In these ferrets, the only sign of disease may be the dermatologic changes.

In the early stages of canine distemper virus infection, the mild upper respiratory signs can mimic those of the much less serious disease, influenza virus infection. Dermatologic disease is not part of influenza viral infections. If a ferret has a mild upper respiratory infection accompanied by a chin rash, this is a signal that canine distemper viral infection is a more likely diagnosis than influenza viral infection.

Treatment

There is no treatment for canine distemper virus. Antibiotics can be used to treat the secondary bacterial infections.

Prognosis

The prognosis for this disease is very poor.

Author Karen Rosenthal

Consulting Editor Karen Helton Rhodes

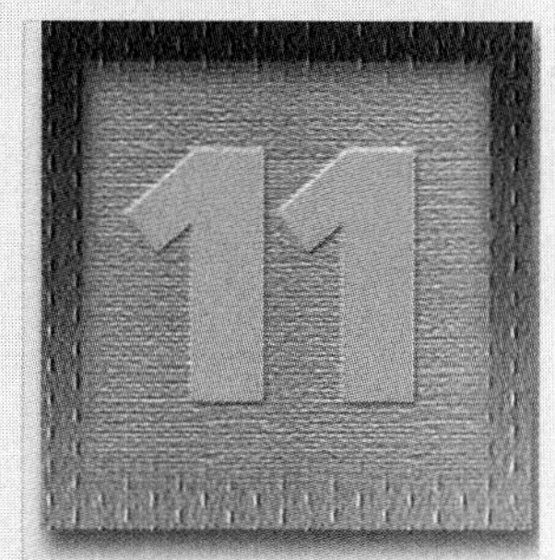

Selected Topics

Canine Familial Dermatomyositis

Linda Medleau and Keith A. Hnilica

Definition/Overview

An inherited inflammatory condition of dogs that involves the skin and muscle and, occasionally, the blood vessels

Etiology/Pathophysiology

- Exact pathogenesis unknown
- Although it is well accepted that there is a genetic predisposition, some researchers suspect an infectious agent (i.e., a virus) triggers the clinical signs; others believe an immune-mediated or autoimmune process may be involved.
- Skin/Exocrine—initially, variable dermatitis on the face, ears, and tail tip and over the bony prominences of the distal extremities develops
- Musculoskeletal—later, myositis, which can be subtle to severe, develops; usually, the temporal and masseter muscles are involved; in more severe cases, generalized muscle disease and involvement of the esophageal muscles may occur; generally, the more severe the dermatitis, the more severe the myositis
- Thought to be inherited as an autosomal dominant trait with variable expression in collies and Shetland sheepdogs

Signalment/History

Breed Predilection

- Collies, Shetland sheepdogs, and their crossbreeds

- Isolated reports—Australian cattle dogs, Welsh corgis, chow chows, German shepherds, and kuvaszes

Mean Age and Range

- Cutaneous lesions usually develop between 7 weeks and 6 months of age
- Mild disease—lesions may resolve in 3 months
- Moderate disease—lesions may persist for 6 months or more
- Severe disease—lesions usually persist throughout life
- Adult-onset disease—much less common

Risk Factors

- Trauma
- Sunlight
- Estrus
- Parturition
- Lactation

Clinical Features

- The clinical signs vary from subtle skin lesions and subclinical myositis to severe skin lesions and generalized muscle atrophy.
- Waxing and waning skin lesions—in dogs <6 months old; around the eyes, lips, face, inner ear pinnae, tail tip, and bony prominences of distal extremities; healing may lead to residual scarring
- Muscle atrophy of the masseter and/or temporal muscles may be evident.

Figure 95-1 Dermatomyositis in a collie. The dermatologic lesions consist of alopecia, crusting, and scarring. (Courtesy of Gail Kunkle, University of Florida College of Veterinary Medicine.)

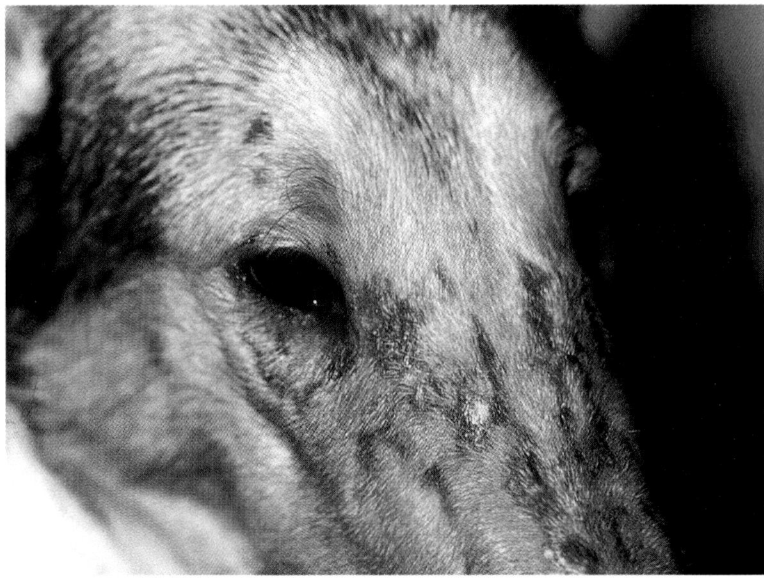

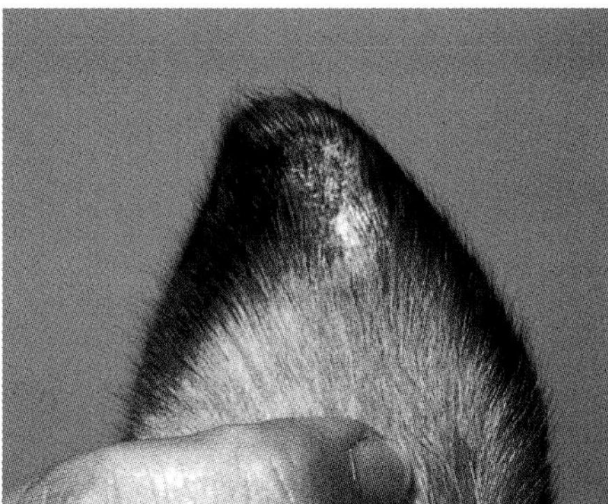

Figure 95-2 Skin lesions on the pinnae consisting of crusts and alopecia. Scarring may be a sequela of this disease. (Courtesy of Gail Kunkle, University of Florida College of Veterinary Medicine.)

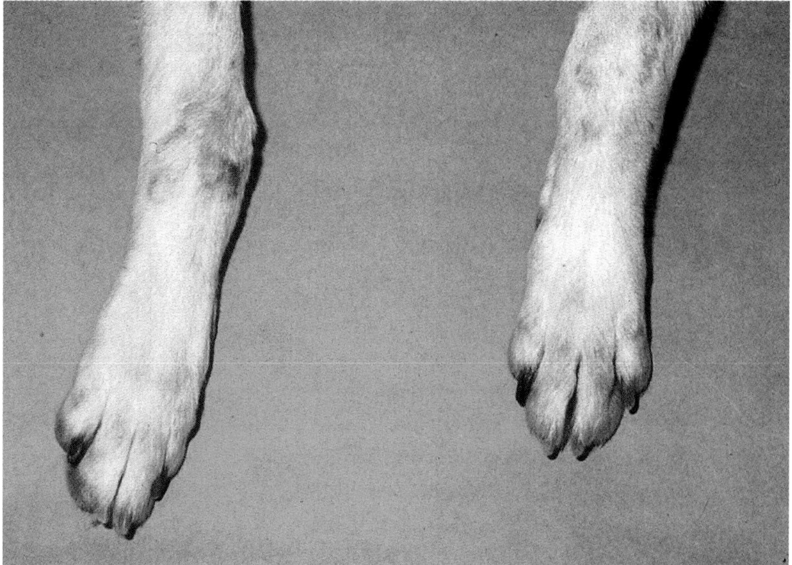

Figure 95-3 Crusting alopecic lesions on the distal extremities. (Courtesy of Gail Kunkle, University of Florida College of Veterinary Medicine.)

- Severely affected dogs may have difficulty eating, drinking, and swallowing; have stunted growth, be lame, have widespread muscle atrophy, and be infertile.
- Several litter mates may be affected, but the severity of the disease often varies significantly among the affected dogs.
- Skin lesions—characterized by papules and vesicles (rare); variable degrees of erythema; alopecia, scaling, crusting, ulceration, and scarring on the face, around the lips and eyes, in the inner ear pinnae, on the tail tip, and over bony prominences on the distal extremities (Figs. 95-1–95-4)
- Footpad and oral ulcers rare
- Myositis—vary from none to a bilateral symmetric decrease in the mass of the temporalis muscles to generalized symmetric muscle atrophy; lameness
- Aspiration pneumonia—with megaesophagus

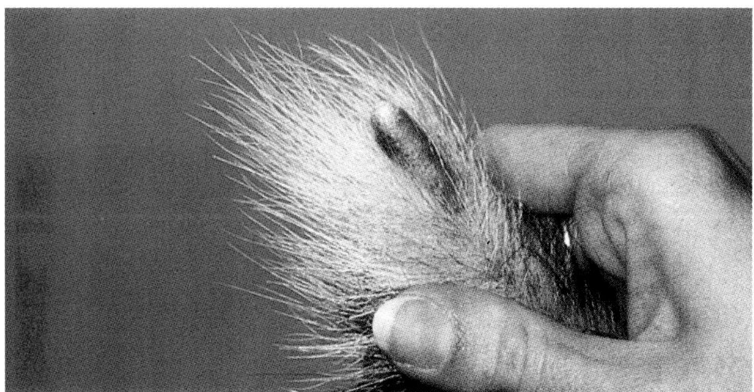

Figure 95-4 Tail tip lesions often consist of alopecia and crusting. (Courtesy of Gail Kunkle, University of Florida College of Veterinary Medicine.)

Differential Diagnosis

- Demodicosis
- Dermatophytosis
- Bacterial folliculitis
- Juvenile cellulitis
- Discoid lupus erythematosus
- Systemic lupus erythematosus
- Polymyositis

Diagnostics

- Nonregenerative anemia may occur with severe disease.
- Serum creatine kinase may be normal or slightly high.
- ANA titers and lupus erythematosus tests negative
- EMG—abnormalities in affected muscles; fibrillation potentials; bizarre high-frequency discharges; positive sharp waves
- Skin biopsy—choose papules, vesicles, or lesions that show alopecia and erythema; avoid infected and scarred lesions
- Muscle biopsy—difficult because pathologic changes may be mild, multifocal, or (in early states) absent; ideally, use EMG to select affected muscles; otherwise, use atrophied muscles; if muscles appear clinically normal, random biopsies may not be diagnostic

Skin Biopsy

- Scattered necrotic basal cells (colloid bodies) or vacuolated individual basal cells
- Occasionally, vesicles that contain small amounts of RBCs
- Superficial, mild, and diffuse dermal inflammatory infiltrates composed of lymphocytes and histiocytes with variable numbers of mast cells and neutrophils (especially perifollicularly)
- Usually, follicular basal cell degeneration and follicular atrophy
- Secondary epidermal ulceration and dermal scarring
- Combination of perifollicular inflammation, epidermal and follicular cell degeneration, and follicular atrophy strongly suggest the diagnosis.

Muscle Biopsy

- Variable multifocal accumulations of inflammatory cells, including lymphocytes, macrophages, plasma cells, neutrophils, and eosinophils
- Myofibril degeneration characterized by fragmentation, vacuolation, and increased eosinophilia of the myofibrils
- Myofiber atrophy and regeneration

Therapeutics

- Nonspecific symptomatic therapy includes hypoallergenic shampoo baths, treating secondary pyoderma and demodicosis, and avoiding trauma and intense sunlight.
- Avoid activities that may traumatize the skin.
- Keep indoors during the day to avoid exposure to intense sunlight.
- Because estrus exacerbates the disease, neutering intact females is recommended.

Drugs

- The therapeutic efficacy of medical treatment can be difficult to assess, because the disease tends to be cyclic and is often self-limiting.
- Vitamin E—100–400 IU PO q12–24h
- Prednisone—1–2 mg/kg PO q12h until remission; then alternate-day administration with the lowest dosage possible for long-term control
- Pentoxifylline (Trental)—400 mg PO with food q24h; human drug that increases microvascular blood flow and tissue oxygenation by lowering blood viscosity, inhibiting platelet aggregation, increasing RBC deformability, and reducing serum fibrinogen levels; sold as 400-mg tablets that should not be divided; beneficial in some dogs, but improvement may not be seen for 1–2 months

Contraindications

Pentoxifylline should not be used in dogs that are sensitive to methylxanthine derivatives (e.g., theophylline).

Precautions

- Pentoxifylline—can cause gastric irritation; animals with prolonged clotting times and those receiving anticoagulant therapy should be monitored carefully
- Glucocorticoids—discuss possible side effects with the owner

Comments

- Discuss the hereditary nature of the disease.
- Note that affected dogs should not be bred.
- Inform owner that the disease is not curable, although spontaneous resolution can occur.
- Discuss prognosis and possible complications, especially in severely affected dogs.
- Advise that medications may not help.

Client Education

- Prevention/avoidance
- Minimize trauma and exposure to sunlight.
- Spay intact females to prevent estrus, parturition, and lactation (all precipitating causes of active dermatomyositis).
- Do not breed affected animals.

Possible Complications

- Secondary pyoderma and demodicosis
- Mild to moderate disease—residual foci of alopecia, hypopigmentation, and hyperpigmentation in areas of previously active skin lesions; occur most frequently on the bridge of the nose and around the eyes
- Severe disease—extensive scarring; trouble chewing, drinking, and swallowing if the masticatory and esophageal muscles are involved; megaesophagus may develop, predisposing the dog to aspiration pneumonia
- Generalized myositis—growth may be stunted

Expected Course and Prognosis

- Long-term prognosis—varies, depending on the severity
- Minimal disease—prognosis good; tends to spontaneously resolve with no evidence of scarring
- Mild to moderate disease—tends to eventually spontaneously resolve; usually with residual scarring
- Severe disease—poor prognosis for long-term survival; dermatitis and myositis are severe and life-long

Associated Conditions

Idiopathic ulcerative dermatosis of Shetland sheepdogs and collies—poorly understood disease; described in adult collies and Shetland sheepdogs; characterized by well-demarcated serpiginous ulcers in the intertriginous areas of the groin and axillae; may occur alone or concurrently with dermatomyositis; may be a subgroup of dermatomyositis

Age-Related Factors

- Clinical signs are usually first seen in dogs <6 months old.
- Adult-onset—rare; more commonly seen in dogs that had subtle lesions as puppies; more noticeable lesions develop as a result of some precipitating event (i.e., trauma, estrus).

Pregnancy

- Do not breed affected dogs.
- Pregnancy exacerbates clinical symptoms.

Suggested Reading

Gross TL, Ihrke PJ, Walder E. Veterinary dermatopathology: a macroscopic and microscopic evaluation of canine and feline skin disease. St. Louis: Mosby, 1992.

Hargis AM, Mundell AC. Familial canine dermatomyositis. Comp Contin Educ 1992;14:855–864.

Hargis AM, Prieur DJ, Haupt KH, et al. Post-mortem findings in four litters of dogs with familial canine dermatomyositis. Am J Pathol 1986;123:480–496.

White SD, Shelton GD, Sisson A, et al. Dermatomyositis in an adult Pembroke Welsh corgi. J Am Anim Hosp Assoc 1992;28:398–401.

Authors Linda Medleau and Keith A. Hnilica

Consulting Editor Karen Helton Rhodes

Canine Keratinization Disorders

Linda Messinger

Definition/Overview

- Keratinization disorders are congenital or acquired abnormalities in the process of epidermopoiesis or cornification (skin renewal, maturation, and replacement), generally resulting clinically as excessive scaling or seborrhea.
- Greasiness and inflammation may sometimes be seen.
- Abnormalities may also be present in the apocrine or sebaceous glands.
- Keratinization disorders are classified as primary or secondary. Secondary keratinization disorders are caused by another disease process.

Etiology/Pathophysiology

- Keratinization disorders arise from an abnormality in epidermopoiesis or cornification resulting in excessive scale.
- Many primary keratinization disorders are congenital or familial defects in the process by which the epidermal cells of the skin are constantly being replaced by new cells.
- The defects tend to be genetic inborn errors of metabolism, primary cellular defects of the keratinocytes, abnormal humoral control of cell maturation and proliferation, abnormal cutaneous glandular function, or abnormal epidermal lipid production.
- Secondary keratinization disorders result from another disease process that causes changes in epidermopoiesis, cornification, or desquamation.
- Primary causes of secondary keratinization defects include endocrinopathies, allergies, infections, nutritional factors, neoplasia, immune-mediated dermatoses, and environmental factors.

- Also, overzealous or inappropriate topical therapies may result in signs of a secondary keratinization disorder.
- The exact mechanism by which other disease processes lead to keratinization disorders is not fully understood.

Signalment/History

Age

- Primary keratinization disorders usual appear during the first 2 years of life. Secondary keratinization disorders can occur at any age and depend on the underlying cause.

No Sex Predilection

Breed Predilections: Exist Depending on the Type of Primary Keratinization Disorder Present

- Acne: English bulldog, boxer, Doberman pinscher, Great Dane
- Disorder of cornification similar to CHILD syndrome: Rottweiler
- Ear margin dermatosis: Dachshund
- Epidermal dysplasia: West Highland white terrier
- Footpad hyperkeratosis: Irish terriers, dogue de Bordeaux
- Ichthyosis: West Highland White Terrier mostly, but also reported in the Doberman pinscher, Irish setter, collie, bull terrier, American Staffordshire terrier, Labrador retriever, Jack Russell terrier, Cavalier King Charles spaniel, English springer spaniel, Yorkshire terrier, Rottweiler, and mixed breeds
- Idiopathic seborrhea: Cocker spaniels, English springer spaniels, Basset hounds, West Highland White Terriers (Figs. 96-1, 96-2)
- Lichenoid-psoriasiform dermatosis: English springer spaniel
- Nasal digital hyperkeratosis: Cocker spaniel and English bulldog
- Schnauzer comedone syndrome: miniature schnauzer
- Sebaceous adenitis: Standard poodle, akita, vizsla, Samoyed
- Vitamin A–responsive dermatosis: Cocker spaniels, miniature schnauzers, Labrador retrievers (Fig. 96-3, 96-4)
- Zinc-responsive dermatosis: Alaskan malamutes, Siberian huskies

Historical Findings (Primary Keratinization Disorder)

Keratinization Disorders Are Often Secondary to a Pre-existing Underlying Disease. Thus, Obtaining a Thorough History Is of Prime Importance

- Excessive scale generally starts at an early age in primary keratinization disorders.
- Scaling, follicular casts, or comedones present before other signs such as pruritus, inflammation, alopecia, and pyoderma.
- Response to prior therapy for pyoderma reveals incomplete resolution of scale, comedones, or follicular casts (if treating the pyoderma results in complete resolution of signs, then a secondary keratinization disorder is more likely).

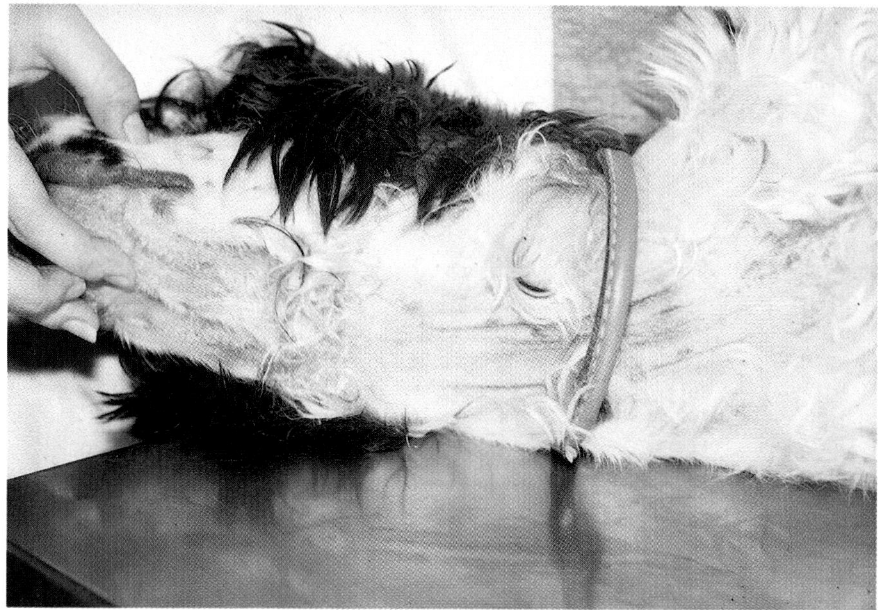

Figure 96-1 Cocker spaniel with primary keratinization disorder demonstrating erythema and partial alopecia with a thick greasy surface exudate of the ventral neck region.

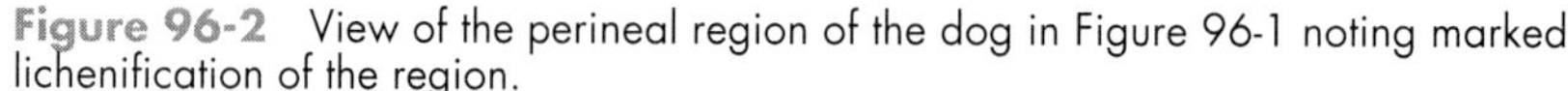

Figure 96-2 View of the perineal region of the dog in Figure 96-1 noting marked lichenification of the region.

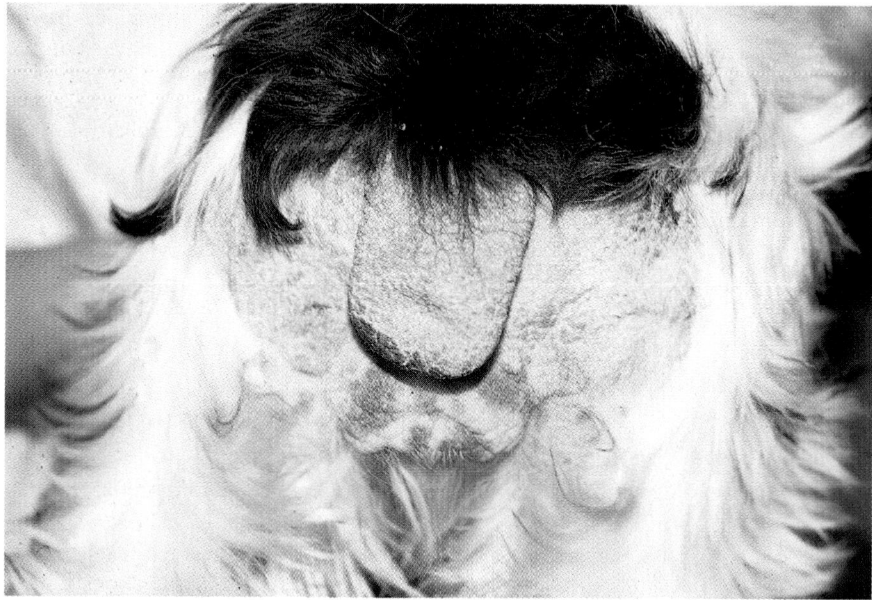

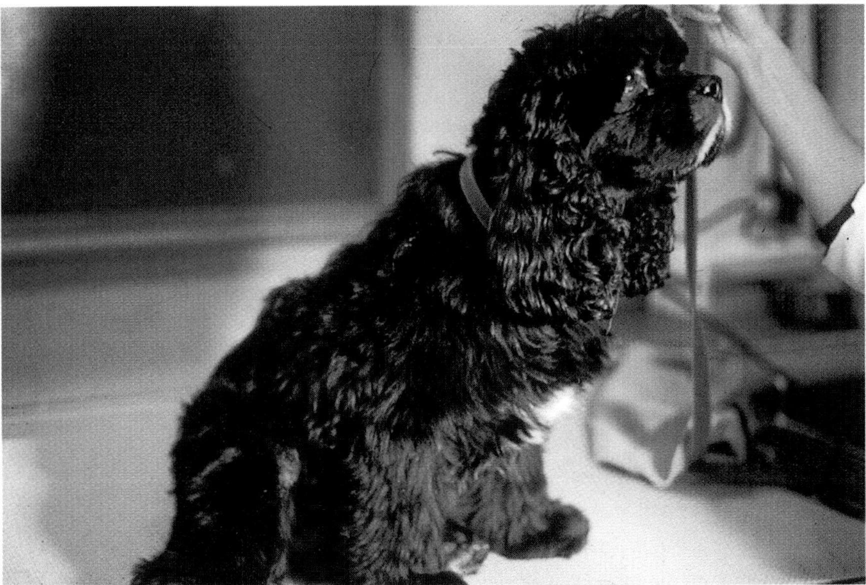

Figure 96-3 Vitamin A–responsive dermatosis. Cocker spaniel. Focal patches of hyperkeratosis over the trunk.

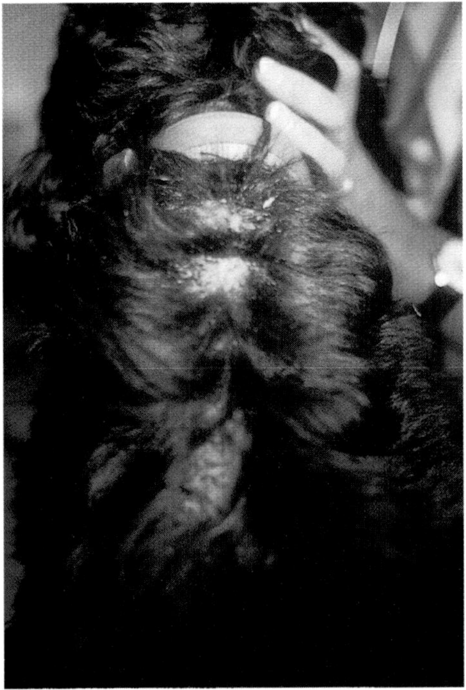

Figure 96-4 Close-up view of Figure 96-3.

- Remaining scale plus pruritus or inflammation after antibiotic therapy suggests a secondary keratinization disorder (secondary to ectoparasites or allergies), whereas resolution of pruritus or inflammation with remaining scale suggests a primary keratinization disorder or an endocrinopathy or environmental factors with a secondary keratinization disorder.
- Other historic aspects to help evaluate a primary versus a secondary keratinization disorder include seasonality, other members of the household having similar signs, and concurrent systemic signs.

Clinical Features

- Excess greasy, waxy, or dry scale
- Follicular casts
- Comedones
- Seborrheic odor (rancid)
- Ceruminous otitis externa
- Hyperkeratotic footpads
- Hyperkeratotic nasal planum
- Variable pruritus
- Secondary clinical signs include alopecia, crusts, pyoderma, inflammation, and excoriation.
- Secondary pyodermas or malasseziasis

Differential Diagnosis

- Differentiation between primary and secondary keratinization disorders is important.
- Causes of secondary keratinization disorders include endocrinopathies, allergies, infections, nutritional factors, neoplasia, immune-mediated dermatoses, environmental factors, and overzealous or inappropriate topical therapies. Historical findings are paramount (e.g., response to prior therapies, onset of pruritus, seasonality).

Diagnostics

- Laboratory work will reflect the underlying cause in secondary keratinization disorders and will be normal in primary keratinization disorders.
- Eosinophilia may suggest allergies or parasites.
- High serum alkaline phosphatase, a stress leukogram, low urine specific gravity, and abnormal cortisol values are suggestive of hyperadrenocorticism.
- Low thyroid levels would suggest hypothyroidism.
- Laboratory tests would generally be normal in primary keratinization disorders, except, for example, with advanced diagnostics such as cell proliferation kinetic studies (increased epidermal turnover time would be seen in primary idiopathic seborrhea).
- Skin biopsies (see histopathology) should be indicative of a keratinization disorder in primary keratinization disorders.
- With secondary keratinization disorders, diagnostic test results will be out of the normal range depending on the primary cause. For example, skin scrap-

ings will be positive for mites in acariases. Fungal cultures will be positive in dermatophytosis, and KOH preparations or Wood's lamp examination may be positive in dermatophytosis. Flea combing or response to flea control will be positive in the presence of fleas or flea allergy dermatitis. Skin cytologies will be positive for bacteria or yeast in pyoderma or malasseziasis, respectively. A strict food elimination diet trial can determine the presence of food allergy. Intradermal skin testing or in vitro allergy testing along with clinical signs and history can help explore the presence of atopy. Secondary keratinization disorders arising in environments with low humidity should respond to treatment with topical moisturizers. Histopathology will help determine if an immune-mediated or neoplastic process is present as the primary cause of a secondary keratinization disorder.

- Histopathologic findings will depend on the type of primary (or secondary) keratinization disorder present and include varying degrees of orthokeratotic and/or parakeratotic hyperkeratosis, follicular hyperkeratosis, follicular dilatation, follicular casts, dyskeratosis, epidermal hyperplasia, dystrophic hairs, pigmentary clumping, vacuolated keratinocytes, increased mitotic activity in basal keratinocytes, and other epidermal abnormalities.

Therapeutics

- In secondary keratinization disorders, treatment of underlying causes should resolve the keratinization disorder. In very chronic cases it may take 3 to 4 months to see complete resolution. Secondary pyoderma or malassezia infections need to be treated appropriately.
- In primary keratinization disorders, the specific keratinization disorder should be addressed to put the keratinization disorder in remission or to control it as best as possible.
- Topical therapies are generally used, aggressively at first, and then tapered to an "as-needed" basis.

Specific Recommended Therapy

Acne

- Mild cases: benign neglect
- Moderate to severe cases: benzoyl peroxide shampoos or gels or mupirocin ointment twice daily until controlled and then as needed. Warm water or epsom salt soaks may be needed.
- In recurrent or deeper infections: appropriate oral antibiotics for at least 3–8 weeks
- Short-term corticosteroids (prednisone, prednisolone) at 1.1 mg/kg q24h PO (dogs) and 1–2 mg/kg q24h PO (cats) are occasionally indicated to help reduce inflammation and scar tissue formation.
- Refractory cases: topical retinoids (tretinoin) q12h or systemic retinoids (isotretinoin) at 1–2 mg/kg q24h PO
- Dogs often outgrow their acne with the onset of sexual maturity.

Disorder of Cornification in the Rottweiler Similar to CHILD Syndrome of Humans

- Depends on severity of case and degree of systemic involvement
- Mild cases: benign neglect, topical antiseborrheics or keratolytic gels; advise against breeding

- Moderate to severe cases: no good therapies exist. Topical therapies with sulfur/salicylic acid or tar or benzoyl peroxide shampoos may be of temporary benefit.

Ear Margin Dermatosis

- Rarely curable
- Mild cases: topical therapy with antiseborrheic shampoo (sulfur/salicylic acid shampoos or benzoyl peroxide shampoos or benzoyl peroxide-sulfur shampoos) to help remove the accumulated scale and debris
- More advanced cases may require topical glucocorticoid creams or ointments or if severe inflammation is present, a short course of oral glucocorticoids (1 mg/kg q24h PO) is indicated. Other options include pentoxifylline (Trental), topical retinoids, EFAs, etc.
- Severe or extensive fissures may require pinnal surgery.

Epidermal Dysplasia of West Highland White Terriers

- Often refractory to medical therapy
- In cases with secondary malassezia dermatitis, significant improvement may be noted with a 3–4 week course of oral ketoconazole at 10 mg/kg q24h PO and 1–3 times per week baths with ketoconazole or miconazole shampoos or enilconazole rinses. The disease is kept controlled with topical baths or rinses and/or daily or alternate-day oral ketoconazole. A 50/50 white vinegar and water rinse 1 to 2 times weekly may prolong the interval between recurrences of the disease.
- Early cases may benefit from immunosuppressive doses of prednisone or prednisolone at 1.1–2.2 mg/kg q12h PO until in remission and then tapered to an every-other-day dosage for long-term management.

Footpad Hyperkeratosis

- Daily 50% propylene glycol soaks until improvement is noted (usually within 5 days), then taper to as needed
- Retinoids are postulated to help.

Ichthyosis

- Not curable; lifelong therapy is needed
- Topical therapies including warm water soaks and antiseborrheic shampoos, esp. sulfur salicylic shampoos, antiseborrheic gels (esp. KeraSolv), topical retinoids, and humectant or emollient sprays or rinse (esp. with lactic acid or propylene glycol), are used initially aggressively and frequently and then tapered to an "as-needed" basis.
- Good to excellent results are usually seen with systemic retinoids. Isotretinoin at 1–2 mg/kg q24h PO or soriatane at 1–2 mg/kg q24h PO may be used. Remission may take up to 3 months. Some dogs may be tapered to an alternate-day therapeutic regime.

Idiopathic Seborrhea

- Therapeutic goal is to identify best means of control with lifelong therapy
- Topical therapy with antiseborrheic shampoos based on type of seborrhea
- When presented with dry scale: moisturizing, hypoallergenic shampoos and rinses should be used. If dry scale is severe, sulfur/salicylic acid shampoos and moisturizing rinses should be used.

- When presented with greasy scale: degreasing, keratolytic, keratoplastic shampoos such as those with coal tar, benzoyl peroxide, or selenium sulfide are indicated. Occasionally, moisturizing rinses may be needed, esp. where low humidity is present.
- Oral supplementation with an omega-6/omega-3 fatty acid supplement may be beneficial.
- Oral retinoid therapy with soriatane (1 mg/kg q24h PO) has been beneficial. Response may take up to 2 months. Alternate-day therapy must be used for long-term management in some dogs.
- Ceruminous otitis is most refractory to therapies. Lifelong maintenance ear cleaning is generally needed.

Lichenoid-psoriasiform Dermatosis

- This condition waxes and wanes and may be refractory to medical therapy.
- Oral antibiotics (esp. erythromycin, trimethoprim-sulfadiazine or cephalexin) may help.
- Prednisone (2.2 mg/kg q24h PO) has allowed for improvement of some lesions.

Idiopathic Nasal Digital Hyperkeratosis

- Mild cases: daily hydration of area with water soaks or wet dressings followed by a petrolatum barrier seal or keratolytic agent such as KeraSolv. When in remission, therapy may be done "as needed."
- Moderate to severe cases: topical keratolytic gels or 0.01% tretinoin gel q12h until control is achieved, then as needed. Tretinoin may be irritating.
- If severe inflammation is present, corticosteroid or antibiotic ointments, creams, or gels may be indicated.
- If very profound hyperkeratotic projections are present (esp. of footpads) trimming dead tissue with scissors or nonaggressive debridement under general anesthesia may be undertaken.

Schnauzer Comedone Syndrome

- Mild cases: salicylic acid pads (Stridex) used daily or alternate day as a wipe over affected areas to help loosen or dissolve comedones
- Moderate to severe cases: regular benzoyl peroxide shampoos to flush hair follicles and control secondary pyodermas. Benzoyl peroxide gels may be used on focal adherent comedones. A Buff-Puff sponge can be used to help remove comedones.
- Systemic antibiotics are indicated with secondary pyodermas.
- Do not use corticosteroids as they may promote comedone formation.
- Isotretinoin at 1–2 mg/kg q24h PO is indicated in refractory cases.
- Some cases are aggravated when dogs are groomed or plucked very short.

Sebaceous Adenitis

- Keratolytic shampoos and emollient rinses may be beneficial in mild cases.
- Propylene glycol and water (50–75%) mixture sprayed on affected area once daily and tapered to as needed
- Weekly baby oil baths and soaks is an option, albeit labor-intensive.
- Essential fatty acid supplementation (omega-3/omega-6) q12h PO
- Evening primrose oil at 500 mg q12h PO

- Systemic retinoids (isotretinoin at 1–2 mg/kg q24h PO or etretinate at 1–2 mg/kg q24h PO) are used in cases refractory to topical therapies. If responsive, dose may be tapered to half the initial dose or to an alternate-day dosage.
- Cyclosporine at 5 mg/kg q12h PO may be used in refractory cases, esp. those that failed retinoid therapy.
- Azathioprine was used in a Vizsla with success. This dog was refractory to other therapies.
- Most cases are unresponsive to corticosteroids.
- Secondary pyodermas should be treated with appropriate antibiotic therapy and antibacterial and follicular flushing topical therapy.
- Spontaneous remission or seasonality has been noted in some dogs.

Vitamin A–Responsive Dermatosis

- Lifelong supplementation with vitamin A (retinol) at 625–800 IU/kg q24h PO or 10,000 IU/cocker spaniel q24h PO. Improvement is generally seen within 3–6 weeks and may take 10 weeks for complete clinical remission.
- Keratinolytic shampoos with benzoyl peroxide 1–2 times per week should be used as an adjunct therapy, esp. while awaiting improvement from vitamin A.

Zinc-Responsive Dermatosis

- Zinc sulfate at 10 mg/kg q24h PO or 5 mg/kg q12h PO or zinc gluconate at 5 mg/kg q24h PO or zinc methionine at 2 mg/kg q24h PO. Give with food.
- Correct dietary imbalances—e.g., diets high in calcium and phytates.
- Some cases require concurrent corticosteroid therapy—i.e., prednisone or prednisolone at 0.15 mg/kg q24h PO.
- Refractory cases may require intravenous sterile zinc sulfate at 10–15 mg/kg given once weekly for at least 4 weeks to resolve lesions, and then every 1–6 months to prevent relapses.

PRECAUTIONS

- Animals with hypersensitivities to a given medication should avoid that medication. Retinoids are teratogens and thus should be avoided in breeding animals (female and male) and pregnant animals. Do not use tar shampoos in cats.
- Topical retinoids may be irritating or cause xerosis.
- Systemic retinoids may cause lethargy, vomiting, diarrhea, polydipsia, hyperactivity, pruritus, erythematous mucocutaneous junctions, keratoconjunctivitis sicca, conjunctivitis, swollen tongue, arthralgia, and lameness. Laboratory abnormalities include hypertriglyceridemia, hypercholesterolemia, increased liver enzymes, and high platelet counts.
- Cyclosporine may cause vomiting, diarrhea, gingival hyperplasia, hirsutism, papillomatous skin lesions, nephrotoxicity, hepatotoxicity, and B-lymphocyte hyperplasia. Increased incidence of infection may also be seen.
- Zinc supplementation may cause vomiting.
- Azathioprine may cause anorexia, vomiting, bone marrow suppression, and increased risk of infection.
- Benzoyl peroxide products may cause cutaneous irritation or xerosis. They may bleach fabrics.
- Tar shampoos may cause cutaneous irritation, xerosis, photosensitization, and may stain light-colored coats. Tars are potentially carcinogenic. Tars are odiferous.

- Topical therapies may cause cutaneous irritation.
- Fatty acid supplementation may aggrevate pancreatitis. Rarely, vomiting and diarrhea may be noted.
- Corticosteroid side effects are legend and well known. They may mask signs of secondary pyodermas and interfere with the accurate diagnosis of primary disease.
- Antibiotics may cause vomiting and diarrhea and decreased appetite.
- Ketoconazole may cause anorexia, vomiting, and hepatotoxicity, as well as graying of the haircoat.

Comments

- Monitoring of potential side effects for the various therapies should be undertaken as indicated, generally every 2–3 weeks to start. Response to therapy should be evaluated and adjusted as needed. Patient monitoring should be done at regular intervals depending on the keratinization defect present and the therapies used.
- Animals with keratinization disorder with a genetic basis should not be bred.
- The use of cytotoxic immunosuppressive drugs, corticosteroids, retinoids, and therapeutic doses of vitamin A are contraindicated in pregnant animals or animals intended for breeding. Clients should be warned about the risk of accidental human ingestion of retinoids. Retinoids have strong teratogenic effects.

Suggested Reading

Griffin CE, Kwochka KW, MacDonald JM, eds. Current veterinary dermatology. St. Louis: Mosby Year Book, 1993.

Moriello K, Mason I. Handbook of small animal dermatology. Tarrytown, NY: Pergamon, 1995.

Scott DW, Miller WH, Griffin CE. Muller and Kirk's small animal dermatology. 5th ed. Philadelphia: Saunders, 1995.

Consulting Editor Karen Helton Rhodes

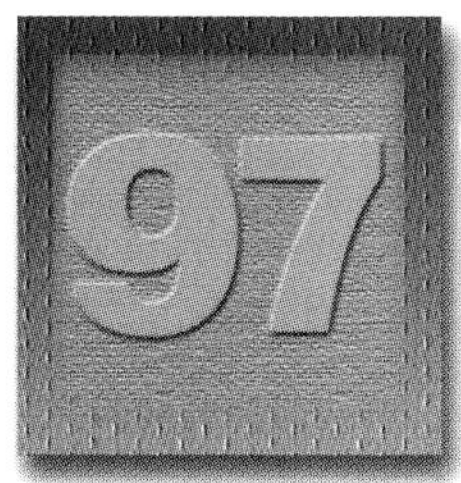

Sterile Nodular/ Granulomatous Dermatoses

Dawn E. Logas

Definition/Overview

Diseases whose primary lesions are nodules that are solid, elevated, and >1 cm in diameter

Etiology/Pathophysiology

- Nodules—usually result from an infiltration of inflammatory cells into the dermis and subcutis; may be secondary to endogenous or exogenous stimuli
- Inflammation is typically, but not always, granulomatous to pyogranulomatous.

Causes

- Amyloidosis
- Foreign body reaction
- Spherulocytosis
- Idiopathic sterile granuloma and pyogranuloma (Fig. 97-1)
- Canine eosinophilic granuloma
- Calcinosis cutis (Figs. 97-2, 97-3)
- Calcinosis circumscripta (Figs. 97-4, 97-5, 97-6)
- Malignant histiocytosis
- Cutaneous histiocytosis (Figs. 97-7, 97-8)
- Sterile panniculitis (Figs. 97-9, 97-10, 97-11)
- Nodular dermatofibrosis
- Cutaneous xanthoma (Fig. 97-12)

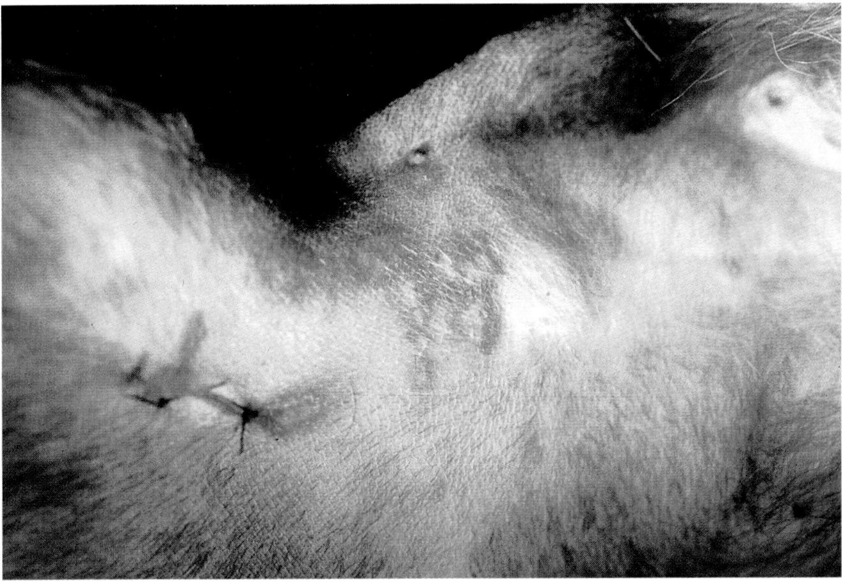

Figure 97-1 Sterile idiopathic periadnexal pyogranulomatous dermatitis of the axilla in a dog.

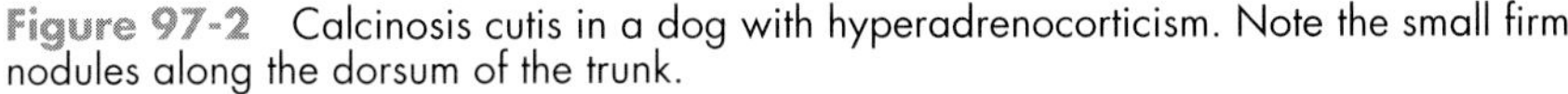

Figure 97-2 Calcinosis cutis in a dog with hyperadrenocorticism. Note the small firm nodules along the dorsum of the trunk.

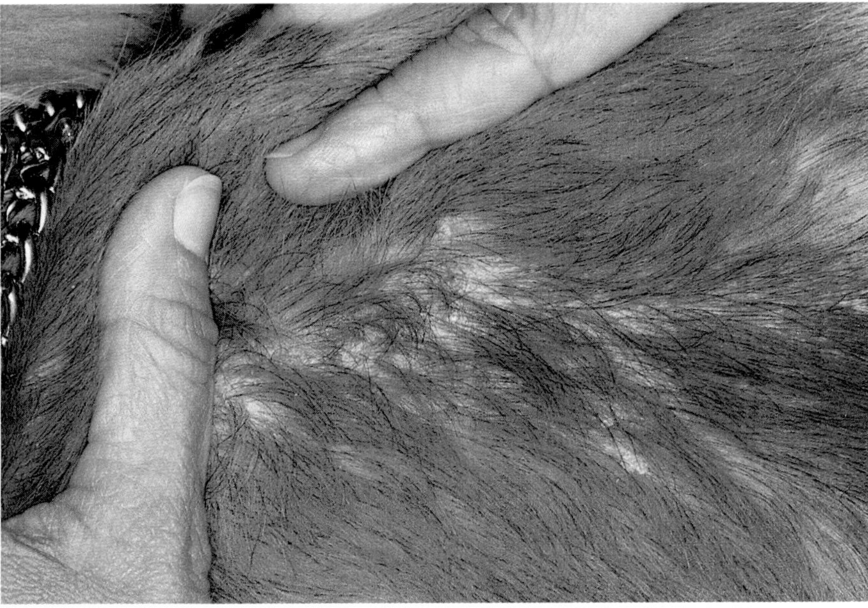

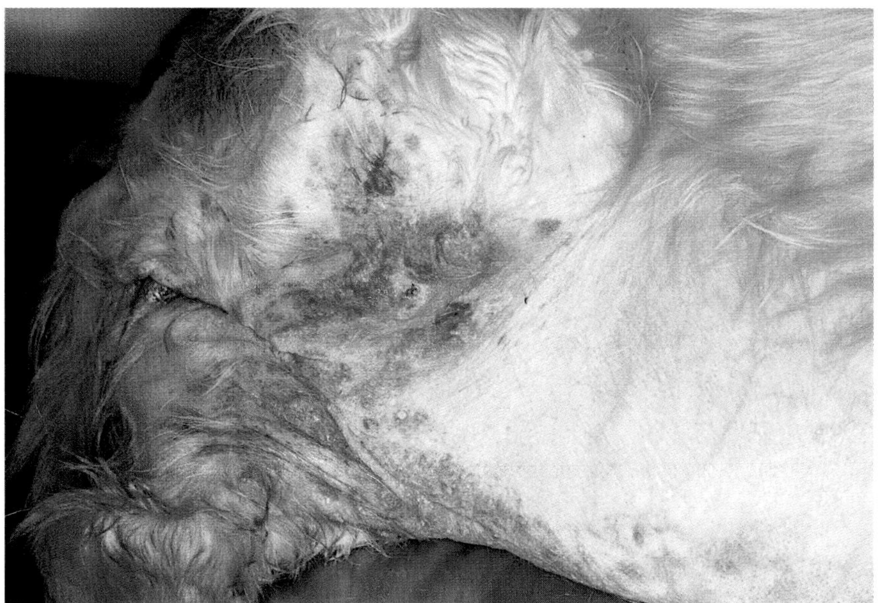

Figure 97-3 Inguinal region of the dog in Figure 97-2 demonstrating coalescing erythematous plaques with a yellow-pink discoloration.

Figure 97-4 Miniature pinscher with swollen digits caused by calcinosis circumscripta.

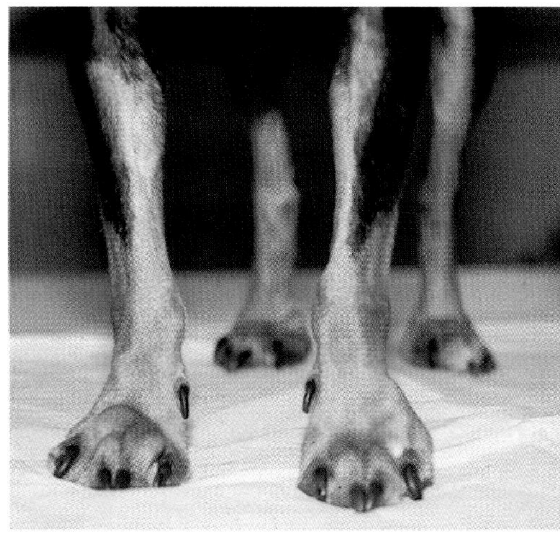

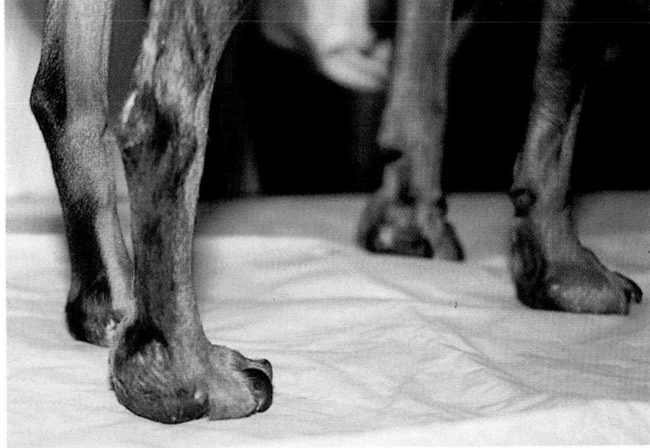

Figure 97-5 Rear view of the dog in Figure 97-4 revealing the extent of the swelling of the metatarsal pad.

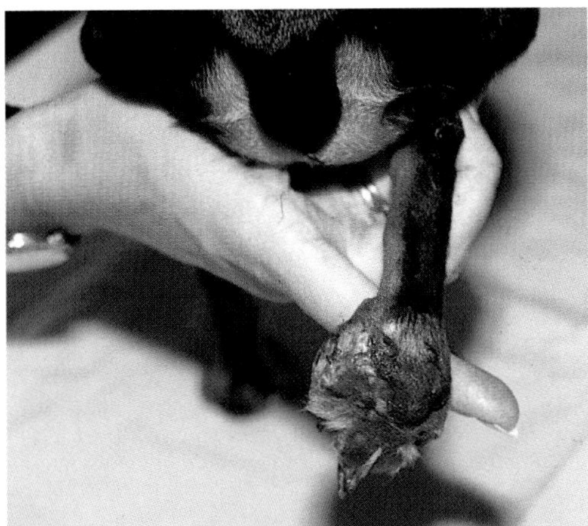

Figure 97-6 View of the footpad showing marked deformity caused by calcinosis circumscripta.

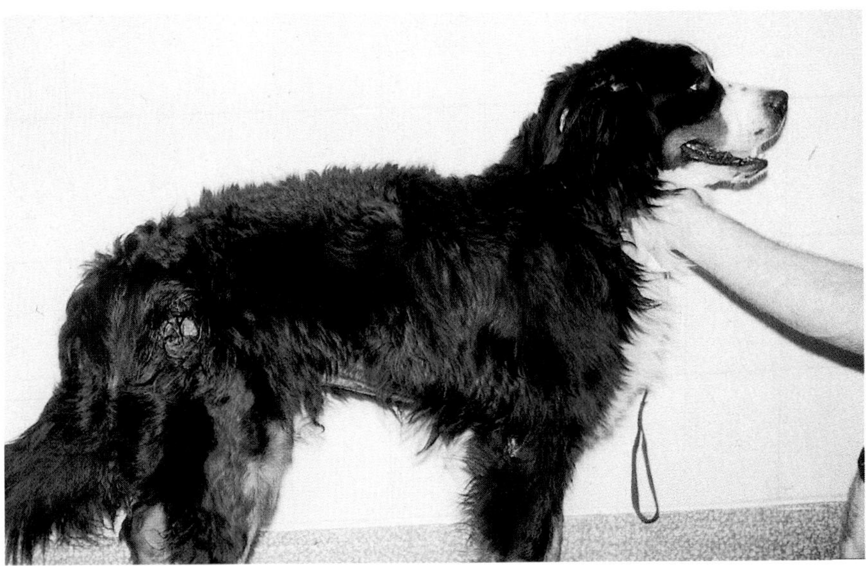

Figure 97-7 Bernese mountain dog with cutaneous histiocytosis.

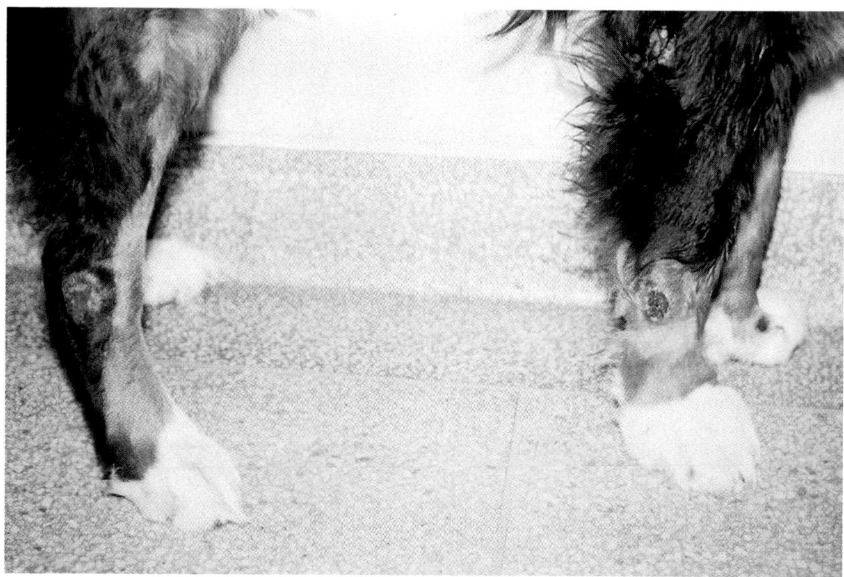

Figure 97-8 Cutaneous nodules caused by histiocytosis on the extremities.

Figure 97-9 Panniculitis in a 3.5-year-old Weimeraner. (Courtesy of Drs. Marcia Schwassmann and Dawn Logas.)

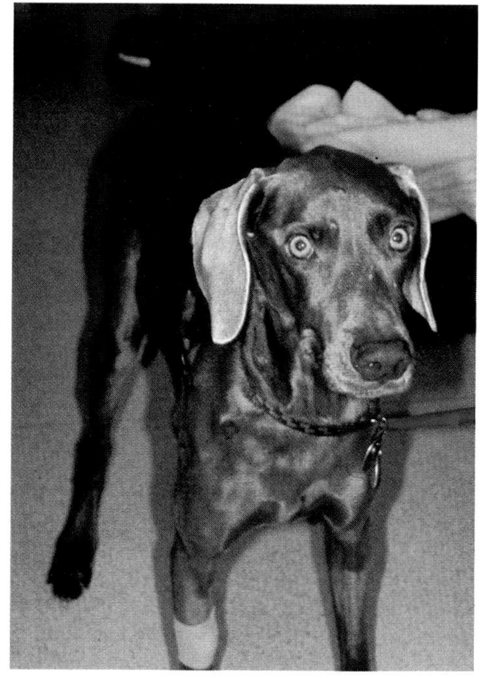

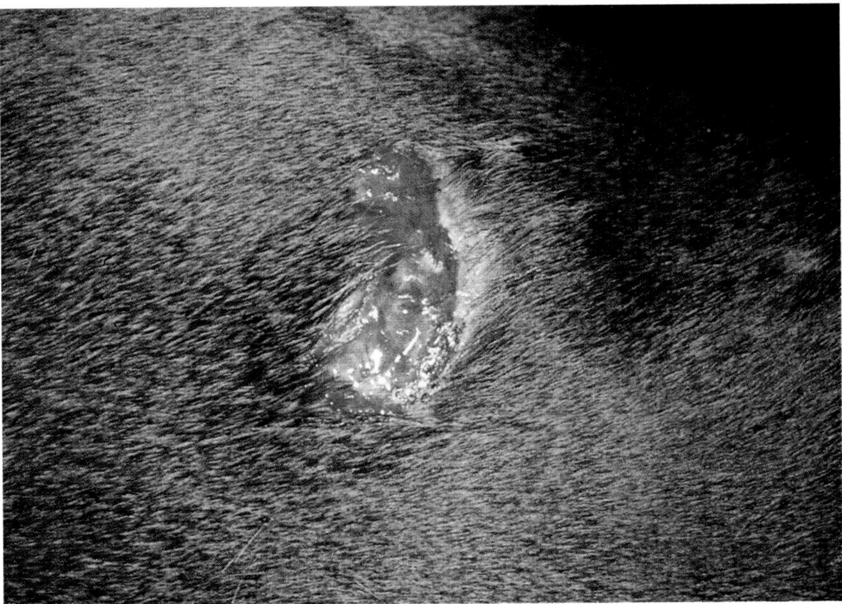

Figure 97-10 Ulcerative nodule of the trunk caused by sterile nodular panniculitis. (Courtesy of Drs. Marcia Schwassmann and Dawn Logas.)

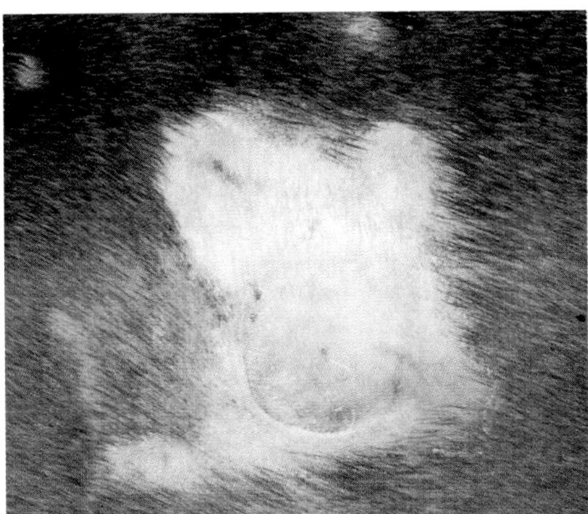

Figure 97-11 Scarred lesion from a healed wound secondary to panniculitis. (Courtesy of Drs. Marcia Schwassmann and Dawn Logas.)

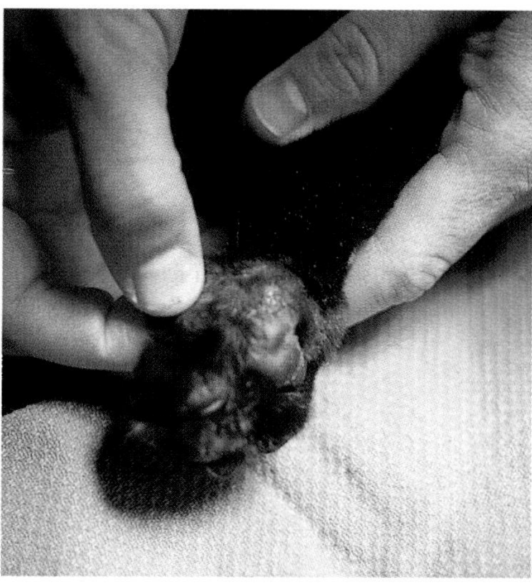

Figure 97-12 Firm yellow-pink nodule resulting from cutaneous xanthomatosis along the metacarpal pad of this cat.

Signalment/History

- Nodular dermatofibrosis—German shepherds, 3–5 years old
- Calcinosis circumscripta—German shepherds, <2 years old
- Malignant histiocytosis—Bernese mountain dogs
- May affect any age, breed, or sex, although Bernese mountain dogs are at higher risk for malignant histiocytosis and German shepherds are at higher risk for nodular dermatofibrosis

Risk Factors

- Foreign body reaction—induced by exposure to any irritating material (e.g., concrete dust or fiberglass)
- Hair foreign bodies—increased risk for large dogs that rest on very hard surfaces
- Calcinosis cutis—increased risk with exposure to high doses of exogenous glucocorticoids
- Panniculitis—increased risk with vitamin E–deficient diet

Differential Diagnosis

- Sterile nodular dermatoses—must be differentiated from deep bacterial and fungal infections and dermal neoplasias
- All of these diseases can be diagnosed by histopathology and deep tissue cultures.

Diagnostics

- Amyloidosis—possible changes in biochemistry and/or urinalysis if internal organs are affected
- Malignant histiocytosis—pancytopenia, serum ferritin levels—may be high with malignant histiocytosis but not with cutaneous histiocytosis

- Calcinosis cutis—changes characteristic of hyperglucocorticoidism (e.g., stress leukogram, high ALP, hyperglycemia, low urine specific gravity)
- Cutaneous xanthomas—may be glucosuria, hyperglycemia, and/or lipid profile abnormalities
- Radiology and ultrasonography—delineate involvement of internal organs in amyloidosis and histiocytosis
- Radiology—identify other areas of dystrophic calcification in dogs with calcinosis cutis
- Ultrasonography—identify cystadenocarcinomas in dogs with nodular dermatofibrosis
- Skin biopsies for histopathology and cultures (fungal, aerobic, and mycobacterial) are essential for nodular dermatoses.

Therapeutics

- Most of these disorders can be treated on an outpatient basis.
- A few of these disorders (e.g., malignant histiocytosis, amyloidosis, and nodular dermatofibrosis) are almost always fatal.
- Dogs with calcinosis cutis may need to be hospitalized for sepsis and intense topical therapy.

Drugs

- Amyloidosis—no known therapy, unless the lesion is solitary and can be surgically removed
- Spherulocytosis—only effective treatment is surgical removal
- Idiopathic sterile granuloma and pyogranuloma—prednisone (2.2–4.4 mg/kg divided PO q12h) is the first line of therapy; continue steroids for 7–14 days after complete remission; then taper dose; for cases that are refractory to glucocorticoids, azathioprine (2.2 mg/kg PO q48h) in combination with prednisone or sodium iodide may be tried.
- Foreign body reactions—best treated by removal of the offending substance if possible; for hair foreign bodies, the dog should be placed on softer bedding and topical therapy with keratolytic agents should be initiated; many dogs with hair foreign bodies also have secondary deep bacterial infections that need to be treated with both topical and systemic antibiotics
- Canine eosinophilic granuloma—prednisone (1.1–2.2 mg/kg PO q24h) produces a good response
- Malignant histiocytosis—no effective therapy; it is rapidly fatal
- Cutaneous histiocytosis—high-dose glucocorticoids and cytotoxic drugs result in remission; recurrences are common; L-asparginase has been helpful in some cases
- Calcinosis cutis—underlying disease must be controlled if possible; most cases require antibiotics to control secondary bacterial infections; hydrotherapy and frequent bathing in antibacterial shampoos minimize secondary problems; topical DMSO is useful (applied to no more than one-third of the body once daily until lesions resolve); if lesions are extensive, serum calcium levels should be monitored closely
- Calcinosis circumscripta—surgical excision is the therapy of choice in most cases
- Sterile panniculitis—single lesions can be removed surgically; prednisone (2.2 mg/kg PO q24h or divided PO q12h) is the treatment of choice; administered

until lesions regress; then tapered; some dogs remain in long-term remission, but others require prolonged alternate-day therapy; a few cases respond to oral vitamin E (400 IU q12h)

- Nodular dermatofibrosis—no therapy for most cases, because the cystadenocarcinomas are usually bilateral; for rare unilateral case of cystadenocarcinoma or a cystadenoma, removal of the single affected kidney may be helpful
- Cutaneous xanthoma—correction of the underlying diabetes mellitus or hyperlipoproteinemia is usually curative

Contraindications

Corticosteroids and other immunosuppressive drugs should be avoided, if possible, in any animal with a secondary infection.

Precautions

DMSO—handle with care; monitor serum calcium levels if used to treat calcinosis cutis.

Comments

Patient Monitoring

- Patients on long-term glucocorticoids should have a CBC, chemistry screen, urinalysis, and urine culture done every 6 months.
- Dogs being treated with DMSO for calcinosis cutis should have calcium levels checked every 7–14 days, starting at the beginning of therapy.

Possible Complications

Systemic amyloidosis, malignant histiocytosis, and nodular dermatofibrosis—invariably fatal

Associated Conditions

- Calcinosis cutis—hyperglucocorticoidism, chronic renal failure, and diabetes mellitus
- Calcinosis circumscripta—(occasionally) hypertrophic osteodystrophy and idiopathic polyarthritis
- Nodular dermatofibrosis—cystadenocarcinomas
- Cutaneous xanthoma—diabetes mellitus and hyperlipoproteinemia

Suggested Reading

Griffin CE, Kwochka KW, MacDonald JM, eds. Current veterinary dermatology. St Louis: Mosby, 1993.

Gross TL, Ihrke PJ, Walder EJ. Veterinary dermatopathology. St Louis: Mosby, 1992.

Scott DW, Miller BH, Griffin CE, eds. Muller & Kirk's small animal dermatology. 5th ed. Philadelphia: Saunders, 1995.

Author Dawn E. Logas

Consulting Editor Karen Helton Rhodes

Granulomatous Sebaceous Adenitis

Ellen C. Codner and Karen Helton Rhodes

Definition/Overview

An inflammatory disease process directed against the cutaneous adnexal structures (sebaceous glands)

Etiology/Pathophysiology

- May be genetically inherited, immune-mediated, or metabolic
- Initial defect—a keratinization disorder or an abnormality in lipid metabolism (accumulation of toxic intermediate metabolites)

Signalment/History

- Young adult to middle-aged dogs
- Two forms—one in long-coated and one in short-coated breeds
- Predisposed—standard poodles, akitas, Samoyeds, and vizslas (Fig. 98-1)

Clinical Features

Long-Coated Breeds

- Symmetrical, partial alopecia
- Dull brittle hair

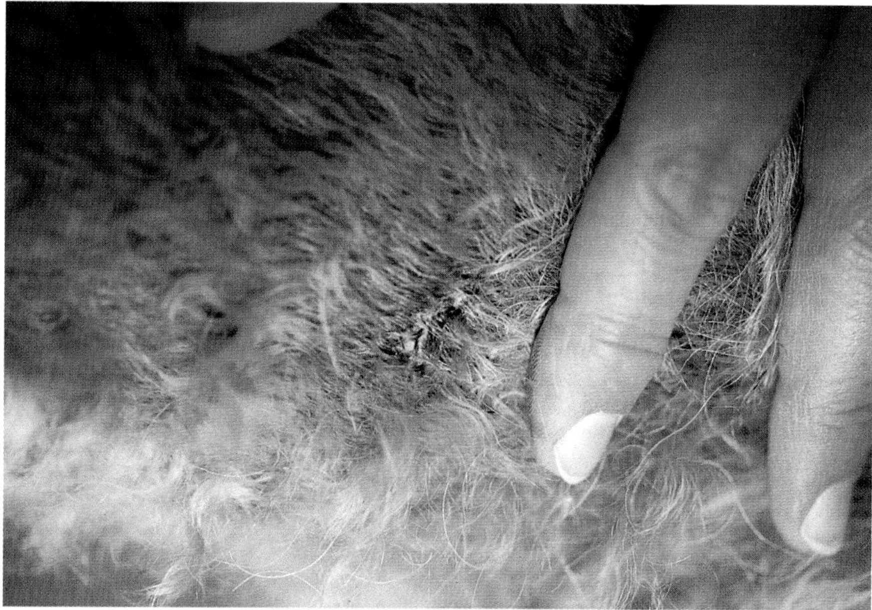

Figure 98-1 Loss of guard hairs (partial alopecia) with tightly adherent scale on the surface of the skin with follicular casts around hair shafts. Standard poodle.

- Tightly adherent silver-white scale
- Follicular casts around hair shaft
- Small tufts of matted hair
- Lesions—often first observed along dorsal midline and dorsum of the head
- Severe—secondary bacterial folliculitis, pruritus, and malodor
- Akitas—often relatively severely affected

Short-Coated Breeds

- Alopecia—moth-eaten, circular, or diffuse
- Mild scaling
- Affects the trunk, head, and ears
- Secondary bacterial folliculitis rare

Differential Diagnosis

- Primary seborrhea—keratinization disorder
- Bacterial folliculitis
- Demodicosis
- Dermatophytosis
- Endocrine skin disease

Diagnostics

- Skin scrapings—normal
- Dermatophyte culture—negative

- Endocrine function tests—normal
- Skin biopsies

Pathologic Findings

- Nodular granulomatous to pyogranulomatous inflammatory reaction at the level of the sebaceous glands
- Orthokeratotic hyperkeratosis and follicular cast formation; more prominent in long-coated breeds
- Advanced—complete loss of sebaceous glands; periadnexal fibrosis
- Destruction of entire hair follicle and adnexal unit rare

Therapeutics

- Clinical signs may wax and wane irrespective of treatment.
- Controlled studies have not been done to document efficacy of any therapy.
- Results extremely variable; response may depend on severity of disease at the time of diagnosis.
- Akita—breed most refractory to treatment

Drugs

- Propylene glycol and water—50–75% mixture; spray every 24 hr to affected areas
- Baby oil—soak affected areas for 1 hr; follow with multiple shampoos to remove oil and scales
- Derm Cap (1 extra-strength) and evening primrose oil (500 mg)—q12h PO; possible side effects include vomiting, diarrhea, and flatulence
- Isotretinoin (Accutane)—1 mg/kg q12h PO; reduce to 1 mg/kg q24h after 1 month and to 1 mg/kg q48h after 2 months; continue as needed for maintenance
- Cyclosporine (Sandimmune)—5 mg/kg q12h PO; side effects include vomiting, diarrhea, gingival hyperplasia, hirsutism, papillomatous skin lesions, increased incidence of infections, nephrotoxicity, and hepatotoxicity
- Bactericidal antibiotics and benzoyl peroxide shampoo—for secondary bacterial folliculitis

Comments

Urge owners to register affected dogs so that mode of inheritance can be determined.

Suggested Reading

Rosser EJ. Sebaceous adenitis. In: Griffin CE, Kwochka KW, MacDonald JM, eds. Current veterinary dermatology. St. Louis: Mosby, 1993:211–214.

Authors Ellen C. Codner and Karen Helton Rhodes

Consulting Editor Karen Helton Rhodes

CUTANEOUS ASTHENIA

Jon D. Plant and Karen Helton Rhodes

Definition/Overview

- Group of hereditary diseases characterized by abnormal skin hyperextensibility and fragility
- Also known as Ehlers-Danlos syndrome and dermatosparaxis

Etiology/Pathophysiology

- Abnormal collagen synthesis or fiber formation is responsible for the skin fragility in most syndromes; however, the biochemical defects have been elucidated in only a few dogs and cats.
- Varying modes of inheritance have been suspected.

Signalment/History

- Congenital syndrome—patients are usually presented quite young
- Dogs—beagles, dachshunds, boxers, St. Bernards, German shepherds, English springer spaniels, greyhounds, Manchester terriers, Welsh corgis, red kelpies, soft-coated Wheaten terriers, Irish setters, Keeshonds, English setters, and mongrels.
- Cats—domestic shorthairs, domestic longhairs, and Himalayans

Clinical Features

- Skin hyperextensibility (Figs. 99-1, 99-2)
- Easily torn skin
- Diminished skin elasticity
- Scars from previous trauma
- Widening of the bridge of the nose

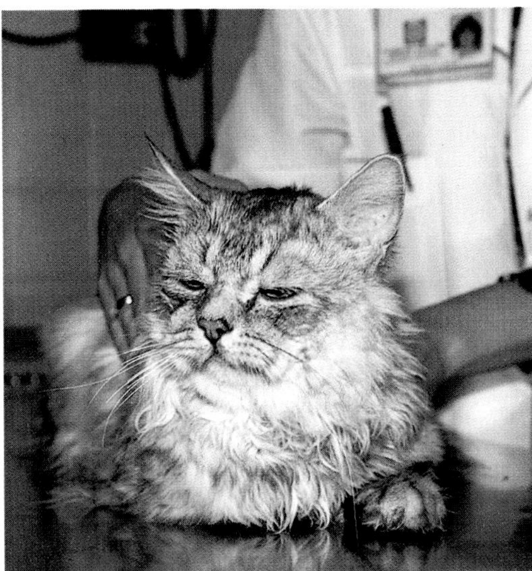

Figure 99-1 Cutaneous asthenia. This cat had a history of frequent and unexplained lacerations that was revealed during a routine examination for an upper respiratory infection.

Figure 99-2 Cutaneous asthenia. The cat from Figure 99-2 demonstrating the hyperextensibility of the skin.

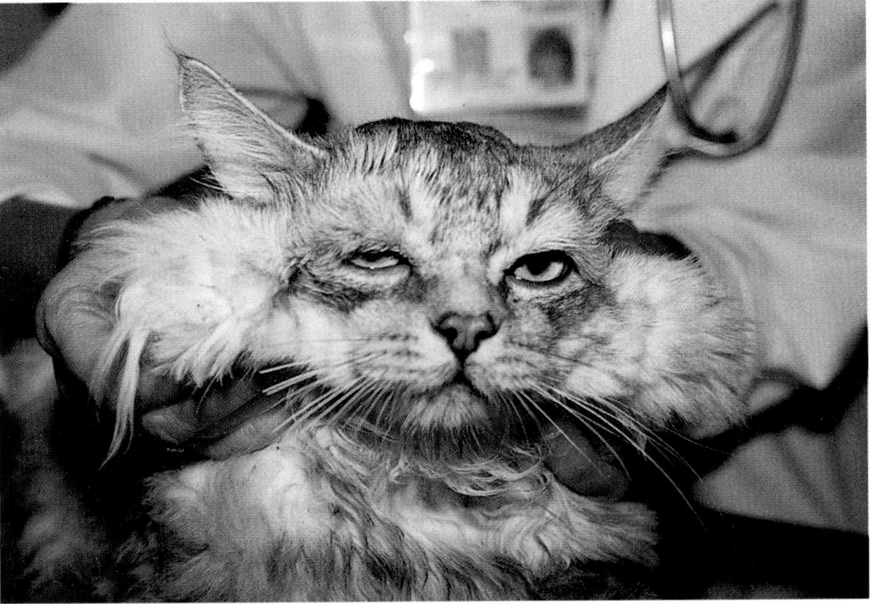

- Joint laxity
- Elbow hygromas
- Lens luxation
- Cataracts
- Even minor trauma to the skin can produce large skin tears.

Differential Diagnosis

Clinically characteristic syndrome

Diagnostics

- Skin extensibility index—identifies affected animals; calculated by dividing the maximal height of a dorsal lumbar skin fold by the body length (from the base of the tail to the occipital crest) and converting to a percentage; affected dogs >14.5% and affected cats >19% (Fig. 99-3)
- Histopathologic examination of the skin—either normal dermal architecture or collagen abnormalities (disoriented, fragmented, abnormal tinctorial properties or abnormal organization)
- Electron microscopy—ascertain collagen abnormalities more precisely

Therapeutics

- Because of poor prognosis, affected animals may be euthanatized.
- If the owner chooses to keep the animal—keep environment free of sharp corners and other animals; handle and restrain affected animal carefully to prevent large skin tears; keep resting areas well padded to prevent elbow hygromas.

Figure 99-3 Cutaneous asthenia. Note the exaggerated dorsal lumbar skin extensibility.

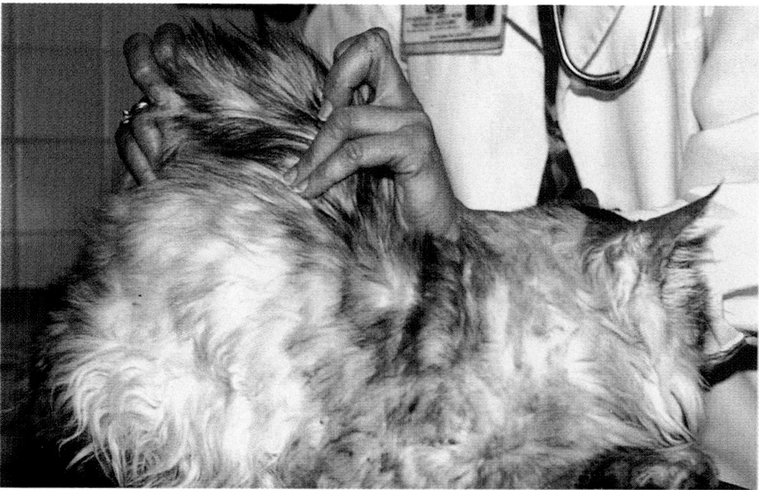

Comments

- Lacerations should be surgically repaired as they occur.
- Declawing may be necessary to prevent self-trauma

Suggested Reading

Scott DW, Miller WH, Griffin CE, eds. Congenital hereditary defects. In: Muller & Kirk's small animal dermatology. 5th ed. Philadelphia: Saunders, 1995:785–789.

Author Jon D. Plant

Consulting Editor Karen Helton Rhodes

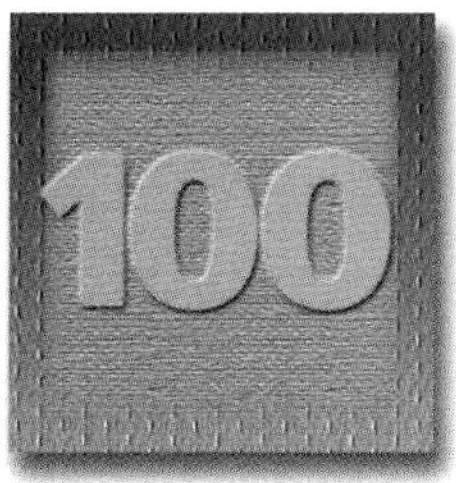

Feline Symmetrical Alopecia

David Duclos

Definition/Overview

- Alopecia in a symmetrical pattern with no gross changes in the skin
- Common clinical presentation in cats

Etiology/Pathophysiology

Manifestation of several underlying disorders

Signalment/History

No age, breed, or sex predilection

Clinical Features

- Total to partial hair loss; most often symmetrical but can occur in a patchy distribution (Fig. 100-1)
- Areas of the trunk most commonly affected are the ventrum, caudal dorsum, and lateral and caudal thighs. (Fig. 100-2)
- Sometimes patchy areas of hair loss (unsymmetrical) on the distal extremities or trunk (Fig. 100-3)

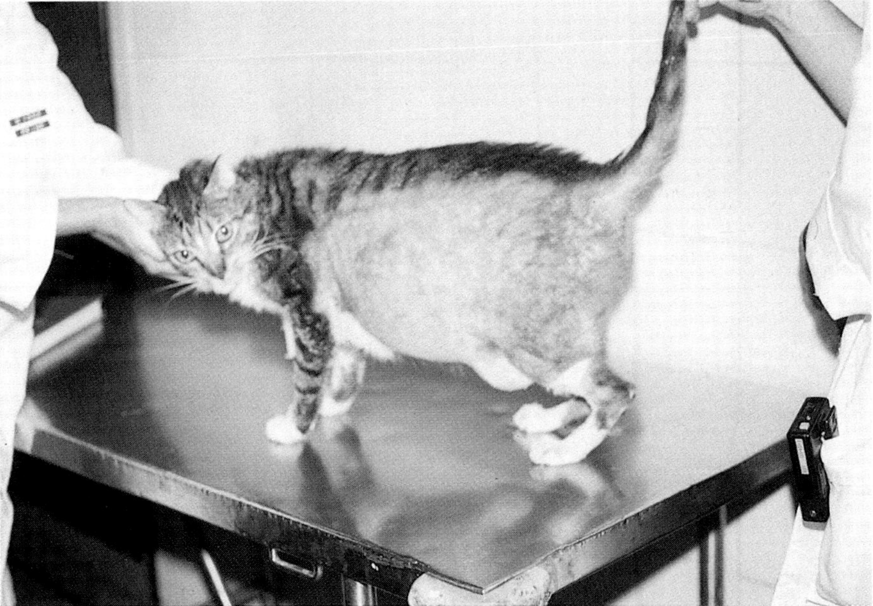

Figure 100-1 Feline symmetrical alopecia. Note the well-demarcated area of alopecia with no associated inflammation.

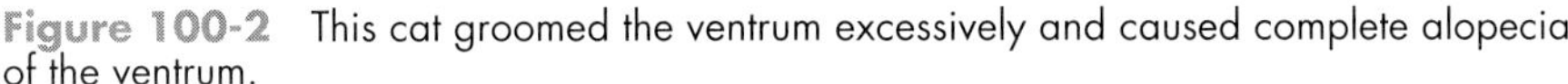

Figure 100-2 This cat groomed the ventrum excessively and caused complete alopecia of the ventrum.

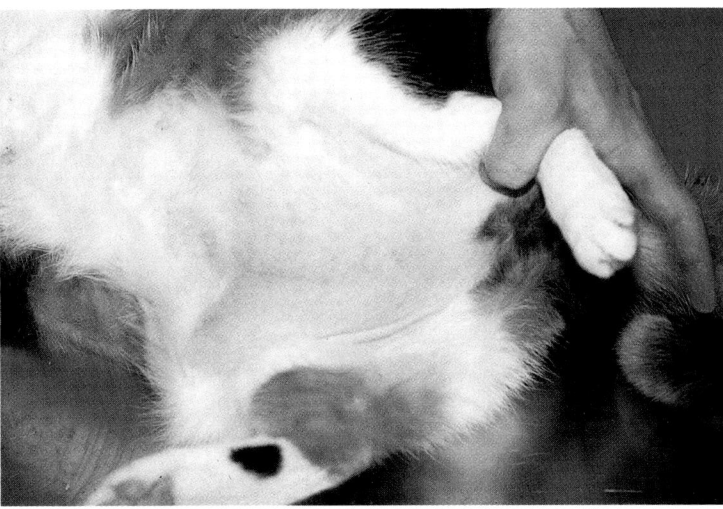

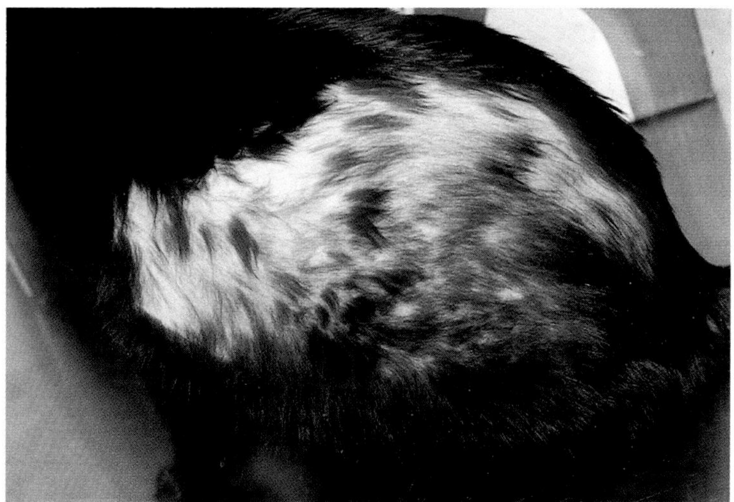

Figure 100-3 Patchy areas of alopecia with no inflammation resulting from psychogenic dermatoses.

Differential Diagnosis

- Hypersensitivity reactions—fleas, food, atopy
- Parasites—fleas, *Cheyletiella*
- Infections—dermatophytosis
- Neurologic/behavioral—psychogenic
- Stress/metabolic—telogen effluvium
- Neoplasia—pancreatic neoplasia (paraneoplastic alopecia)
- Hyperadrenocorticism
- Alopecia areata
- Hyperthyroid (early sign)

Diagnostics

CBC: Eosinophilia in some allergic cats
Serology: T_4-hyperthyroid

Diagnostic Procedures

- Flea combing—identify fleas, flea excrement, or both
- Microscopic examination of hair—self-induced hair loss results in broken ends, whereas endogenous hair loss results in tapered ends.
- Fecal examination—excess hair, mites, and ova (*Cheyletiella*), tapeworm, or fleas
- Food elimination diet trial—see Food Reactions (Dermatologic)
- Intradermal skin test—see Atopy
- Histopathologic examination—see below

Pathologic Findings

- Biopsies—help confirm underlying cause (e.g., allergic dermatitis, psychogenic, or rarely, systemic disease)

- Histopathologic findings—vary depending on the cause
- Feline psychogenic alopecia—hair follicles and skin normal
- High numbers of mast cells, eosinophils, lymphocytes, or macrophages suggest allergic dermatitis.
- Alopecia areata—lymphocytic inflammation that encircles the bulb portions of the hair follicles; rare

Therapeutics

- Effective management of the underlying causes is important.
- Inform the owner of the diagnostic plan and the time it could take to see a response (e.g., fleas, 4–6 weeks; diet, 3–12 weeks).

Drugs

- Antihistamines—e.g., chlorpheniramine, 0.5 mg/kg PO q8h
- Glucocorticoids—0.5 mg/kg PO, alternate-day therapy
- Amitriptyline—1–2 mg/kg PO daily
- Glucocorticoids—can cause alopecia, diabetes mellitus, polydipsia, polyuria, polyphagia, and weight gain; can suppress pruritus, making it difficult to determine the underlying cause
- Withdraw antipruritic medications (including glucocorticoids) as the diagnostic tests near completion (e.g., food hypersensitivity reactions)

Comments

- Frequent examinations are essential in confirming the differential diagnoses.
- Successful identification of the underlying cause offers the best prognosis, if the cause can be controlled (e.g., flea bites or food hypersensitivity).

Suggested Reading

O'Dair HA, Foster AP. Focal and generalized alopecia. Vet Clin North Am Small Anim Pract 1995;25:851–870.

Author David Duclos

Consulting Editor Karen Helton Rhodes

Hepatocutaneous Syndrome

Sheila M. Torres

Definition/Overview

- A rare canine disorder
- Usually a cutaneous marker for advanced hepatic disease or concurrent hepatic disease and diabetes mellitus
- Rarely associated with a glucagon-secreting pancreatic tumor
- Hepatocutaneous Syndrome—superficial necrolytic dermatitis

Etiology/Pathophysiology

- Lesions—pathogenesis unclear; result of keratinocyte degeneration and necrosis; hyperglucagonemia, hypoaminoacidemia, zinc and essential fatty acid deficiencies believed to play a direct or indirect role
- Skin/Exocrine—eroded, erythematous, and crusting lesions around the mouth and eyes and on the legs, feet, and genitalia
- Hepatobiliary—hepatic cirrhosis or vacuolar hepatopathy with parenchymal collapse and nodular hyperplasia
- Endocrine/Metabolic—glucagon-secreting pancreatic tumor

Causes & Risk Factors

- Specific cause unknown
- Keratinocyte degeneration and necrosis—probably result from cellular starvation or other nutritional imbalance
- Nutritional imbalance—probably hypoaminoacidemia or deficiencies in essential fatty acids and zinc; owing to metabolic abnormalities caused by high serum glucagon levels, liver dysfunction, or a combination
- No risk factors have been identified.

Signalment/History

- Dogs
- No breed predilection
- Often old dogs
- Males more likely affected

Clinical Features

- Skin lesions—usually precede clinical evidence of internal disease by weeks or months; usually the presenting complaint; consist of erythema, crusts, and erosions or ulcerations affecting the muzzle (Figs. 101-1, 101-2), mucocutaneous areas of the face, distal limbs, feet, and external genitalia (Figs. 101-3, 101-4, 101-5, 101-6, 101-7, 101-8)
- Footpads—usually hyperkeratotic and affected with fissures and ulcerations; pain associated with walking
- Secondary bacterial and/or fungal infections—often associated with footpad lesions

Differential Diagnosis

- Pemphigus foliaceus
- Systemic lupus erythematosus
- Zinc-responsive dermatosis
- Toxic epidermal necrolysis
- Drug eruption
- Distal extremity erythema and footpad hyperkeratosis—unique; strongly suggest the diagnosis

Figure 101-1 Superficial necrolytic dermatitis (SND). Note the ulcerations and crusting of the facial region.

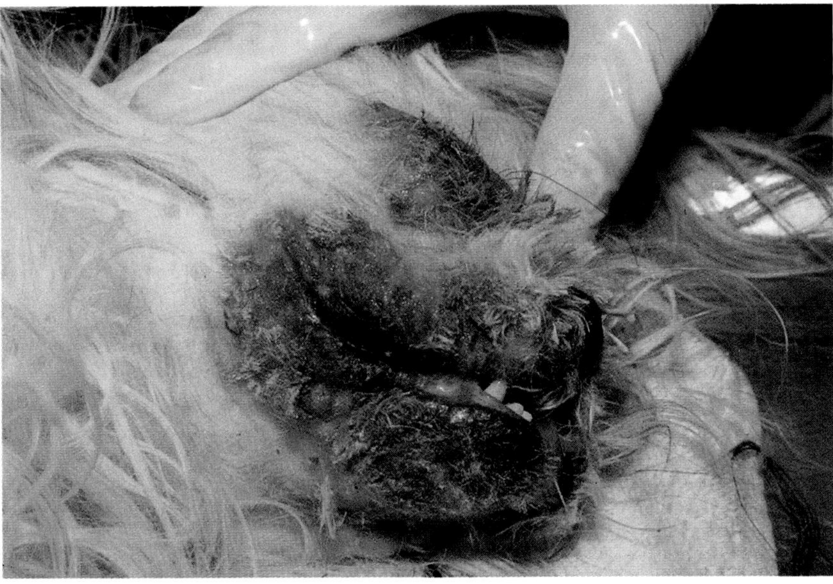

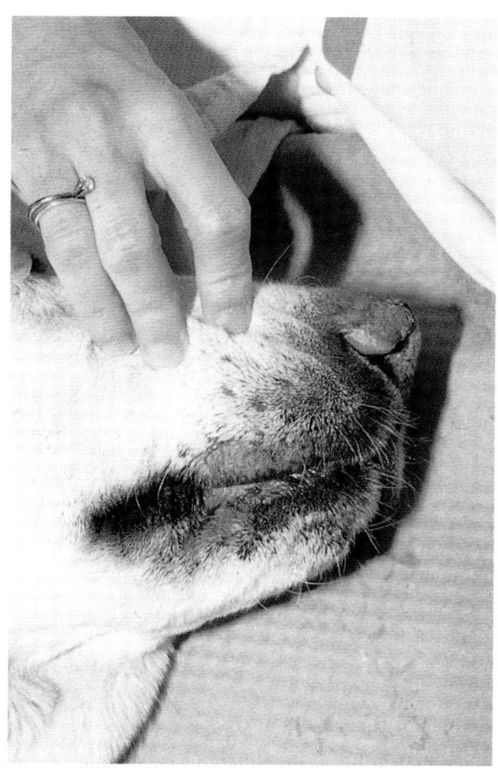

Figure 101-2 SND. Erythema, alopecia, and hyperkeratosis of the muzzle.

Figure 101-3 SND. Hyperkeratosis of the extremity.

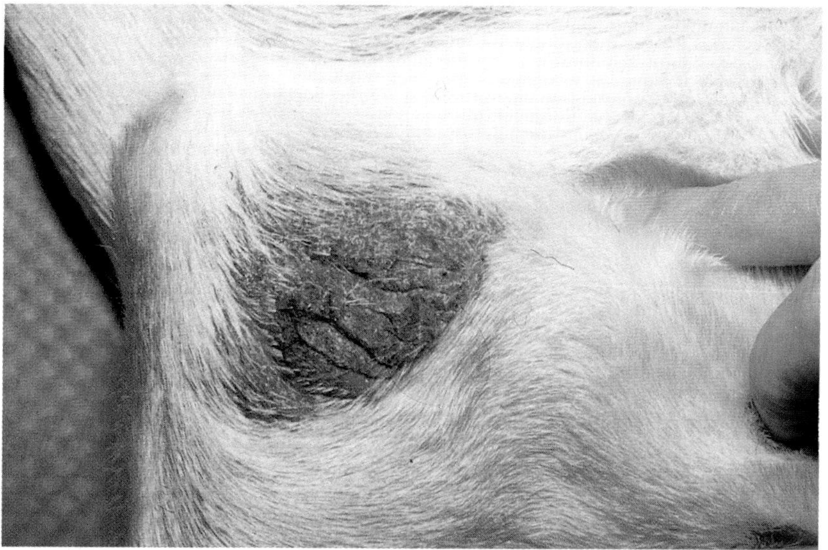

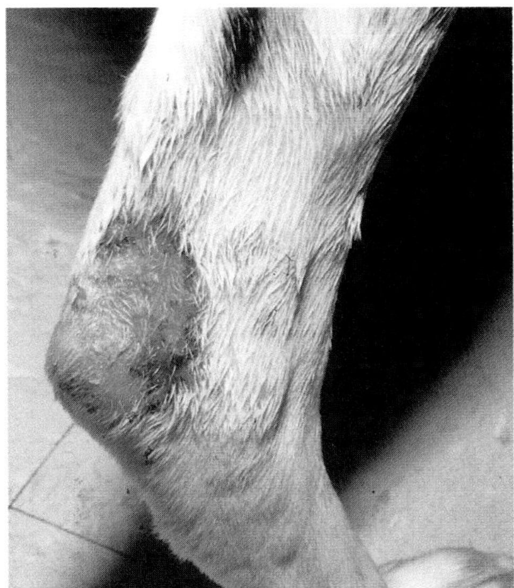

Figure 101-4 SND. Hyperkeratosis and crusting with erosion of the extremities.

Figure 101-5 SND. Hyperkeratosis, erythema, and crusting of the footpads.

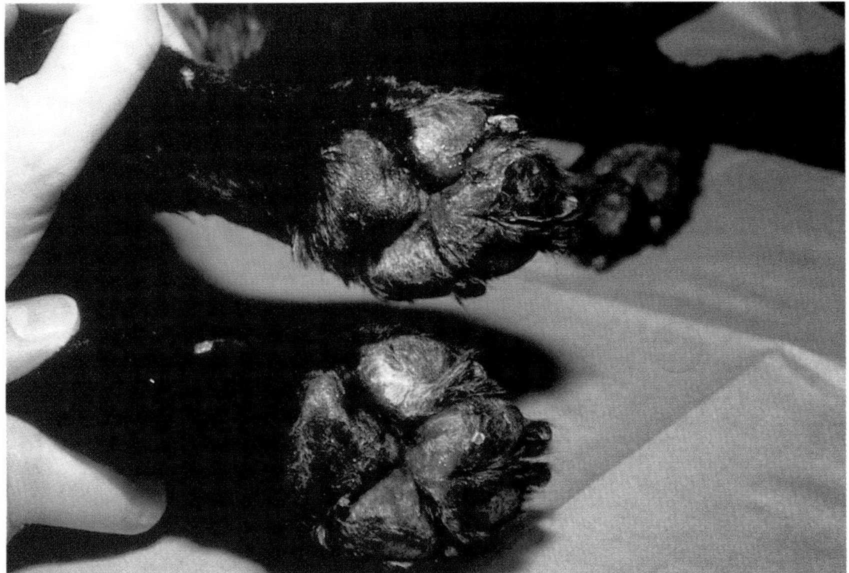

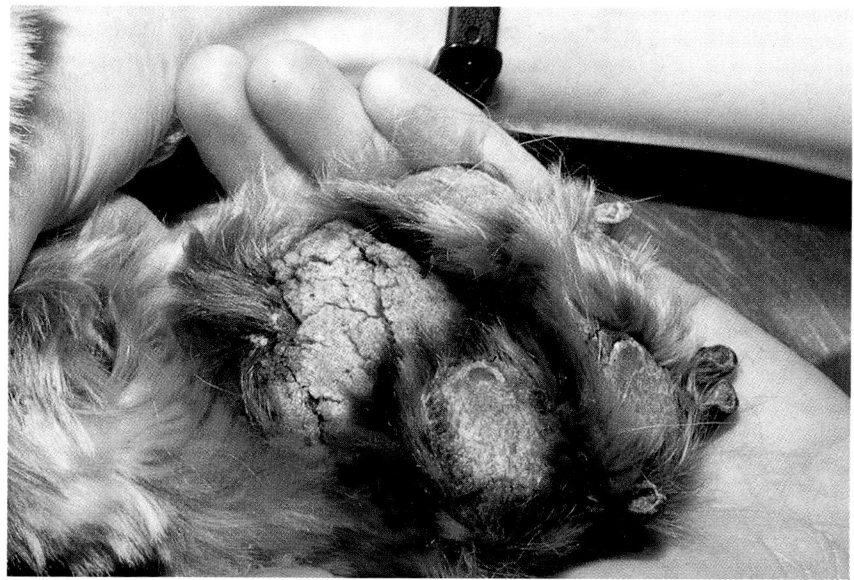

Figure 101-6 SND. Severe hyperkeratosis of the footpads.

Figure 101-7 SND. Severe ulceration of the extremities.

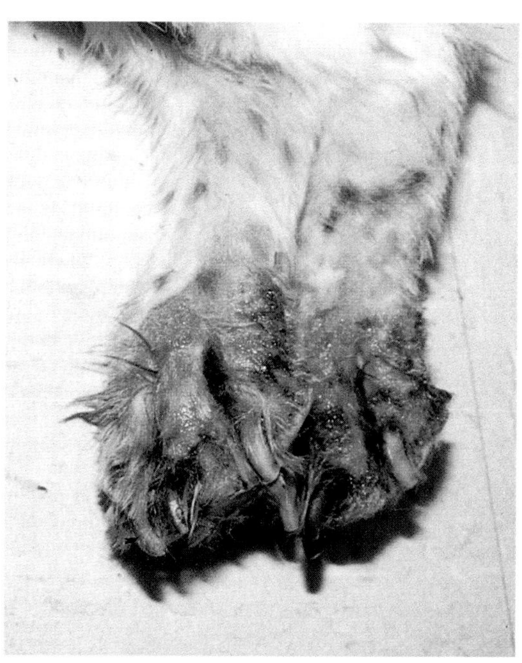

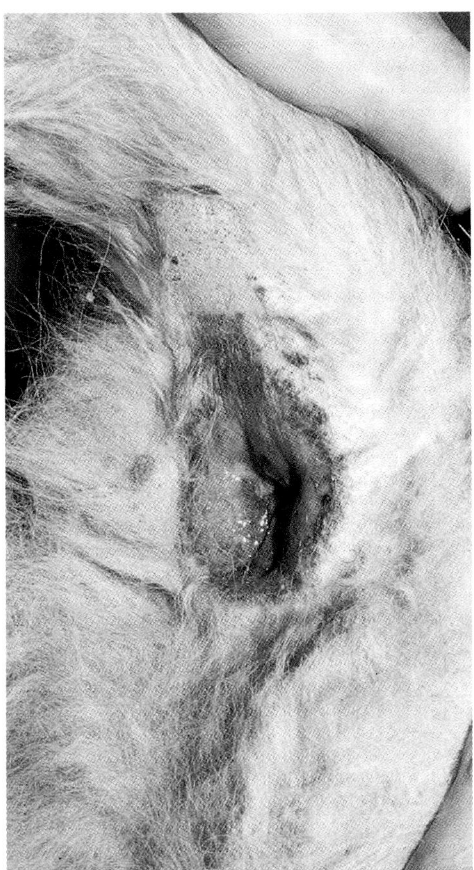

Figure 101-8 SND. Hyperkeratosis with erythema and crusting of the perianal region.

Diagnostics

- Anemia—may be noted; usually normocytic, normochromic, and nonregenerative
- RBC abnormalities—polychromasia; anisocytosis; poikilocytosis; and target cells
- ALP, ALT, and AST—high activity
- Total bilirubin and bile acid levels—high
- BSP retention
- Biochemistry abnormalities are not seen in dogs with glucagon-secreting tumors.
- Most patients develop borderline or frank hyperglycemia.
- Elevated plasma glucagon levels—consistently present with glucagon-secreting tumors; variably observed with chronic hepatic disorders
- Hypoaminoacidemia common
- High insulin levels may be noted.
- Abdominal radiography and ultrasonography—usually unremarkable with glucagon-secreting pancreatic tumors; abnormalities compatible with hepatic cirrhosis or vacuolar hepatopathy and nodular hyperplasia seen with advanced liver disease
- Skin biopsies—important diagnostic tool; sample early lesions because chronic lesions rarely show the unique epidermal edema

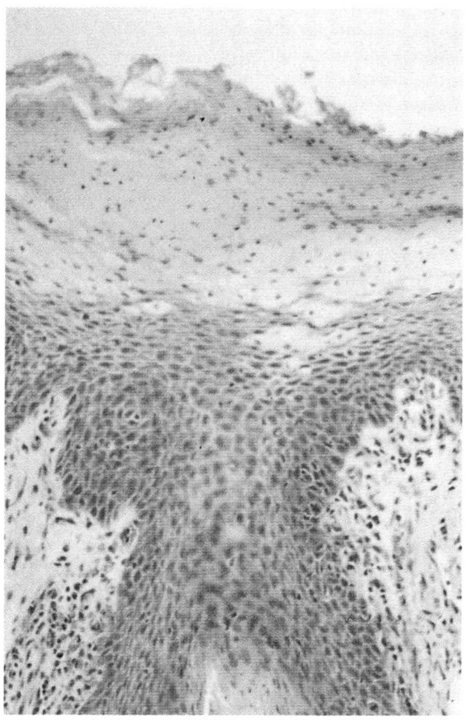

Figure 101-9 SND. Histopathology. Characteristic "red-white-blue" pattern noted in SND. Red=marked hyperkeratosis, white=spongiosis (edema), blue=epidermal hyperplasia.

Pathologic Findings

- Skin biopsies—diffuse parakeratotic hyperkeratosis with high-level intracellular and intercellular epidermal edema are unique; irregular epidermal hyperplasia and mild superficial perivascular dermatitis
- Chronic lesions—marked parakeratotic hyperkeratosis and epidermal hyperplasia; also noted with zinc deficiency (Fig. 101-9)

Therapeutics

- Usually as outpatients
- Patients with signs of liver failure may need to be hospitalized for supportive care.
- Surgical excision of glucagon-secreting tumors—can be curative if diagnosis is made before metastasis; unfortunately, this is rarely the case.
- Most cases are associated with chronic irreversible liver disease.
- Inform clients that this disorder indicates concurrent severe internal disease with a poor prognosis.
- Hydrotherapy and shampoos—help remove crusts; lessen pruritus and pain

Drugs

- Specific treatment—attempt to correct the underlying disease; not usually accomplished
- Nonspecific symptomatic therapy—antibiotics and antifungal drugs for secondary skin infections
- Glucocorticoids—improve skin lesions; may induce a diabetic crisis because patients are either prediabetic or overtly diabetic at diagnosis; may induce as-

cites if patient has chronic severe liver disease; prednisone or prednisolone: usual initial dosage of 0.5–1.0 mg/kg daily; maintain at lowest possible alternate-day dosage

- Zinc sulfate or gluconate—10 mg/kg daily; results unrewarding
- Essential fatty acids—not beneficial

Comments

Possible Complications

- Liver failure
- Secondary bacterial and/or fungal skin infections

Expected Course and Prognosis

Prognosis poor; survival time reported as 5 months after development of skin lesions

Associated Conditions

Diabetes mellitus—usually nonketoacidotic

Abbreviations

- ALP = alkaline phosphatase
- ALT = alanine aminotransferase
- AST = aspartate aminotransferase
- BSP = sulfobromophthalein

Suggested Reading

Scott DW, Miller WH, Griffin GE. Endocrine and metabolic diseases. In: Muller & Kirk's small animal dermatology. 5th ed. Philadelphia: Saunders, 1995:706–710.

Author Sheila M. Torres

Consulting Editor Karen Helton Rhodes

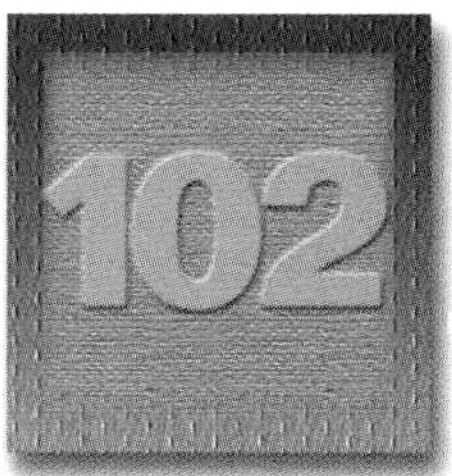

Lymphedema

Francis W. K. Smith, Jr.

Definition/Overview

- Abnormal accumulation of protein-rich lymph fluid into interstitial spaces, especially subcutaneous fat
- Chronic lymphedema causes tissue fibrosis.
- May be congenital or acquired

Etiology/Pathophysiology

- Hereditary/congenital malformation of the lymphatic system—aplasia, valvular incompetence, and lymph node fibrosis
- Excessive interstitial fluid production secondary to venous hypertension (associated with congestive heart failure and obstruction of venous drainage) or increased vascular permeability (associated with infection, trauma, heat, and irradiation)
- Secondary damage to lymphatic vessels or lymph nodes—associated with trauma, infection, and neoplasia

Signalment/History

- More common in dogs than cats
- Congenital in bulldogs and hereditary/congenital in a family of poodles; possible breed predilection in Labrador retrievers and Old English sheepdogs

- Primary/congenital—usually peripheral limb swelling at birth or develops in first several months
- Typically starts at distal extremity and slowly advances proximally

Clinical Features

- Most common in limbs, especially pelvic limbs; may be unilateral or bilateral
- Less common in ventral thorax, abdomen, ears, and tail
- Pitting, nonpainful; temperature of affected area is normal
- Pitting quality lost with chronicity as fibrosis occurs
- Lameness and pain uncommon unless cellulitis develops

Differential Diagnosis

- Edema caused by venous stasis (e.g., congestive heart failure and cirrhosis); look for varices, hyperpigmentation, and ulceration
- Arteriovenous fistulae—listen for machinery murmur; feel for pulsatile vessels; confirm with angiogram
- Edema caused by hypoproteinemia—protein-losing nephropathy or enteropathy, hepatic failure, serum loss from burns or hemorrhage; check serum protein concentration
- Trauma—review history; look for bruising and lacerations
- Neoplasia—if swelling firm, obtain aspirate for cytologic examination
- Cellulitis—look for fever, pain, and warm swelling

Diagnostics

Lymphography useful in documenting abnormalities within the lymphatic system; best results obtained with an injection of water-based contrast media directly into a lymphatic vessel.

Therapeutics

- No curative therapy—a number of surgical and medical treatments may be tried
- Rest and massage of the affected limbs—does not help
- Conservative care—long-term use of pressure wraps, coupled with skin care and use of antibiotics to treat cellulitis and lymphangitis; may be successful in some patients
- Surgical procedures—can be attempted when conservative care and medications fail; lymphangioplasty, bridging techniques, lymphaticovenous shunts, superficial and deep lymphatic anastomosis, and excisional procedures; none is consistently beneficial, and only excisional procedures reported in dogs
- In humans—microwave heating of affected areas appears beneficial and adds to the effect of benzopyrones (see Drugs)
- Diets severely restricted in long-chain triglycerides are being investigated in humans.

Drugs

- Benzopyrones reduce high-protein edema by stimulating macrophages to release proteases; beneficial effects recorded in experimental studies in dogs. Rutin, 50 mg/kg PO q8h, may benefit. A recent study in humans showed combined usage of oral and topical benzopyrones to be more effective than either alone.
- Diuretics, steroids, anticoagulants, and fibrinolytic agents have been used, but no confirmed benefit

Contraindications/Possible Interactions

Diuretics—initially reduce swelling but increase protein content of interstitial fluid, resulting in further tissue damage and fibrosis

Comments

- Puppies with severe lymphedema may die.
- Resolution seen in some puppies with pelvic limb involvement only

Suggested Reading

Fossum TW, King LA, Miller MW, et al. Lymphedema: clinical signs, diagnosis, and treatment. J Vet Intern Med 1992;6:312–319.

Fossum TW, Miller MW. Lymphedema: etiopathogenesis. J Vet Intern Med 1992;6:283–293.

Author Francis W. K. Smith, Jr.

Consulting Editor Karen Helton Rhodes

Canine Juvenile Cellulitis (Puppy Strangles)

Karen Helton Rhodes

Definition/Overview

- An uncommon granulomatous and pustular disorder of puppies
- Rarely seen in adult dogs
- The face, pinnae, and submandibular lymph nodes are the most common sites.
- Immunopathogenesis unknown

Etiology/Pathophysiology

- Cause and pathogenesis unknown
- An immune dysfunction with a heritable cause is suspected.

Signalment/History

- Dogs
- Age range—usually between 3 weeks and 4 months
- Predisposed breeds—golden retrievers, dachshunds, and Gordon setters

Clinical Features

- Acutely swollen face (eyelids, lips, and muzzle)
- Submandibular lymphadenopathy (Fig. 103-1)

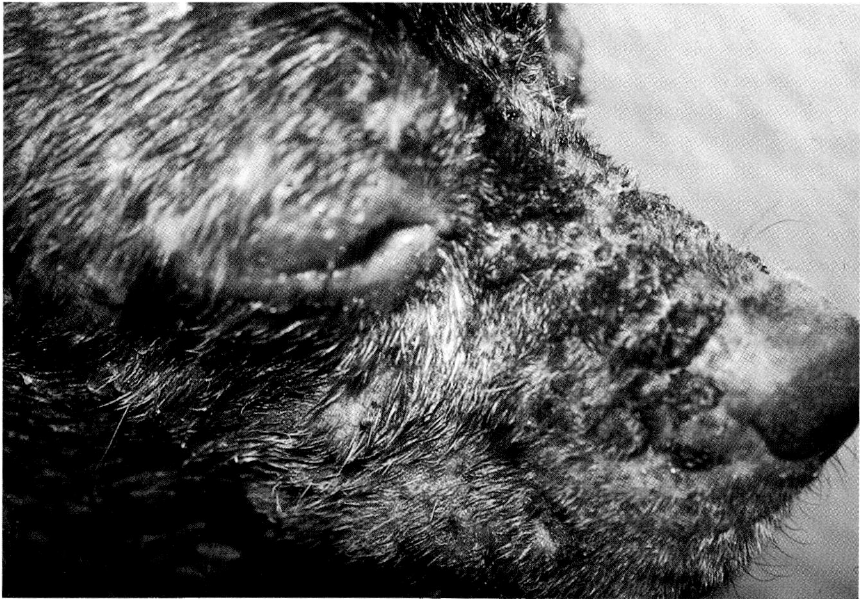

Figure 103-1 Canine juvenile cellulitis. This puppy had markedly swollen submandibular lymph nodes and a markedly exudative and crusting dermatitis.

- A marked pustular and exudative dermatitis, which frequently fistulates, develops within 24–48 hr.
- Purulent otitis externa
- Lesions often become crusted.
- Affected skin is usually painful.
- Lethargy—50% of cases
- Anorexia, pyrexia, and a sterile suppurative arthritis—25% of cases
- A sterile pyogranulomatous panniculitis (rare) over the trunk, preputial, or perianal area; lesions may appear as fluctuant subcutaneous nodules that fistulate.

Differential Diagnosis

- Staphylococcal dermatitis
- Demodicosis
- Drug eruption
- Deep fungal infection

Diagnostics

- Cytology—pyogranulomatous inflammation with no microorganisms; nondegenerate neutrophils
- Culture—sterile

Skin Biopsy

- Multiple discrete or confluent granulomas and pyogranulomas—clusters of large epithelioid macrophages and neutrophils

- Sebaceous glands and apocrine glands may be obliterated.
- Suppurative changes in the dermis—predominate in later stages
- Panniculitis

Therapeutics

- Early and aggressive therapy, because scarring may be severe
- Topical therapy—may be soothing and palliative; adjunct to corticosteroids
- Corticosteroids—high doses required; prednisone (2.2 mg/kg divided twice daily for at least 2 weeks)
- Do not taper too rapidly.
- Chemotherapeutics—rare resistant cases
- Adult dogs with panniculitis may require longer therapy.
- Antibiotics—if there is evidence of secondary bacterial infection; as an adjunct therapy with immunosuppressive doses of steroids

Comments

- Most cases do not recur.
- Scarring may be a problem, especially around the eyes.

Suggested Reading

Scott DW, Miller WH, Griffin CE, eds. Muller & Kirk's small animal dermatology. Philadelphia: Saunders, 1995:938–941.

Author Karen Helton Rhodes

Consulting Editor Karen Helton Rhodes

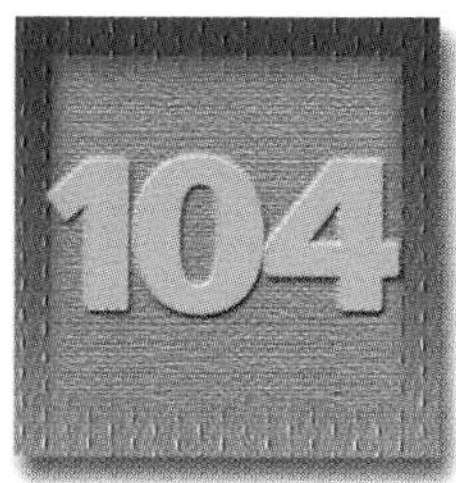

HISTIOCYTOSIS

Kenneth M. Rassnick

Definition/Overview

- Rare disorder resulting from proliferation of cells from the monocyte-macrophage lineage
- Many authors attempt to differentiate systemic from malignant disorders based on cytologic appearance of the histiocytes and tissue distribution.
- Organ systems affected include skin, hemic/lymphatic, nervous, ophthalmic, and respiratory.

Etiology/Pathophysiology

- Systemic—nonneoplastic disease
- Malignant—neoplastic disorder
- Both disorders—may represent variable manifestations of a common underlying defect; may represent stages in a range of histiocytic proliferative disorders, although intermediate stages have not been identified
- Familial disease of Bernese mountain dogs—polygenic mode of inheritance; heritability of 0.298; accounts for up to 25% of all tumors in this breed

Signalment/History

Systemic

- Young to middle-aged dogs (mean age at onset, 4 years)
- Usually male
- Usually Bernese mountain dogs (Fig. 104-1)

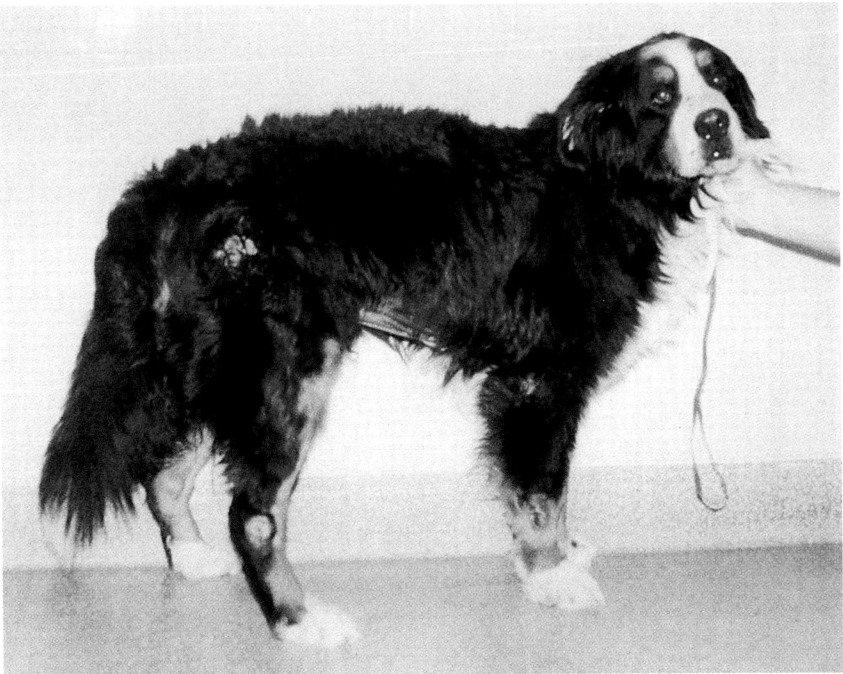

Figure 104-1 Bernese mountain dog with systemic histiocytosis.

Malignant

- Older male dogs (mean age at onset, 7 years)
- Most commonly reported in Bernese mountain dogs
- Has been documented in cats

Clinical Features

- Lethargy
- Anorexia
- Weight loss
- Respiratory stertor
- Coughing
- Dyspnea
- Dogs with systemic disorder may not have signs of systemic illness.
- Systemic histiocytosis
- Marked predilection for skin and lymph nodes
- Cutaneous masses—multiple; nodular; well-circumscribed; and often ulcerated, crusted, or alopecic; occur commonly on the muzzle, nasal planum, eyelids, flank, and scrotum (Figs. 104-2, 104-3)
- Moderate to severe peripheral lymphadenomegaly often present
- Ocular manifestations—conjunctivitis, chemosis, scleritis, episcleritis, episcleral nodules, corneal edema, anterior and posterior uveitis, retinal detachment, glaucoma, and exophthalmos
- Abnormal respiratory sounds and/or nasal mucosa infiltration
- Organomegaly occurs with systemic involvement.

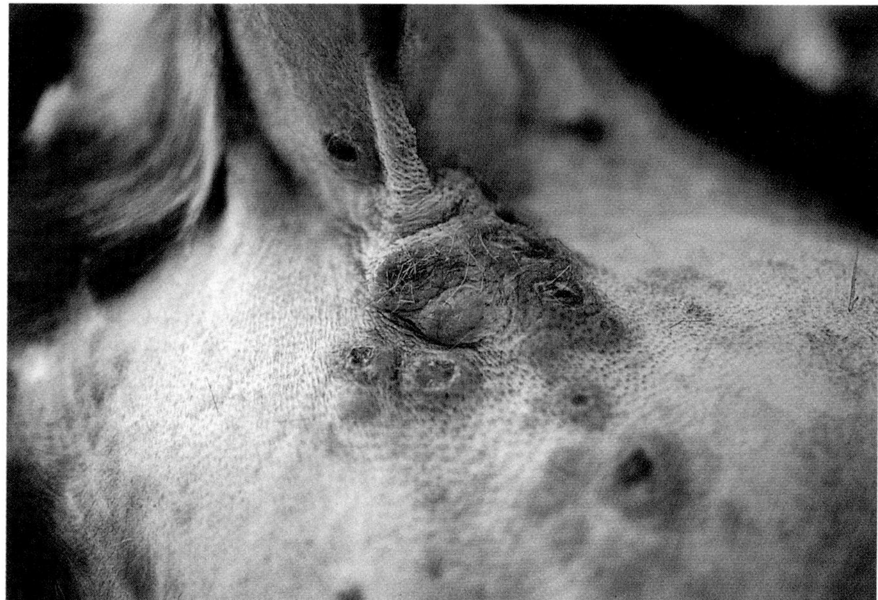

Figure 104-2 Advanced histiocytic lesion of the axillae and chest region.

Figure 104-3 Advanced lesions on the extremities.

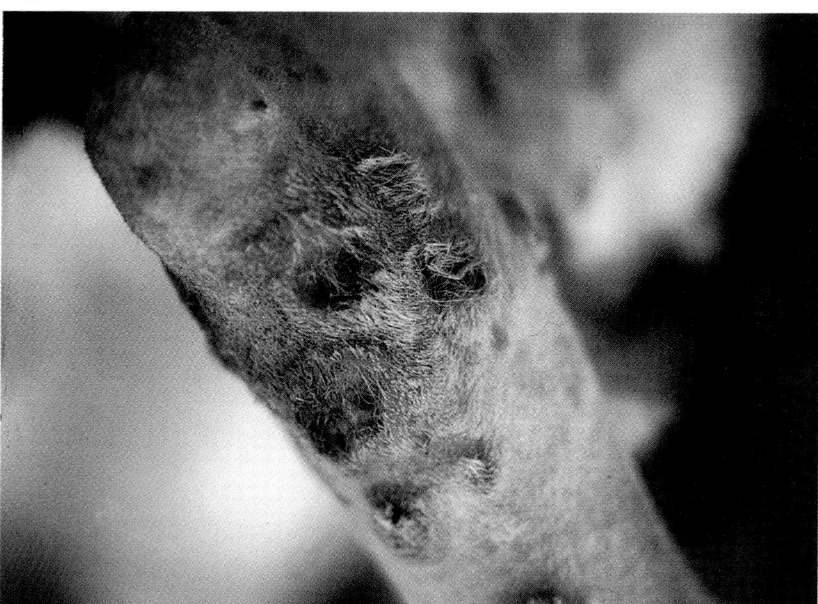

- Malignant histiocytosis
- Pallor, weakness, dyspnea with abnormal lung sounds, and neurologic signs (e.g., seizures, central disturbances, and posterior paresis) common
- Moderate to severe lymphadenomegaly and hepatosplenomegaly
- Occasionally, masses are palpated in the liver and/or spleen.
- Eyes and skin are rarely affected.

Differential Diagnosis

- Histiocytic lymphoma—differentiation and definitive diagnosis often require special staining for immunohistochemical markers
- Lymphomatoid granulomatosis—extensive pulmonary infiltrate of lymphocytes, plasma cells, histiocytes, and atypical lymphoreticular cells; affects young to middle-aged dogs, with respiratory disease as the chief complaint; lack of lymph node, organ, or bone marrow involvement
- Cutaneous histiocytosis—benign histiocytic proliferative disorder in young dogs of any breed; characterized by multiple dermal and subcutaneous nodules or plaques; no ocular involvement; fluctuating clinical course over months to years regardless of treatment
- Periadnexal multinodular granulomatous dermatitis—benign, well-demarcated cutaneous nodules, commonly on the muzzle and may affect the eye; histologically distinct granulomas and variable numbers of inflammatory cells; may be indistinguishable from cutaneous histiocytosis
- Cutaneous histiocytoma—common benign skin tumor of young dogs; solitary, alopecic, frequently ulcerated lesions; may regress without treatment
- Granulomatous diseases—dogs with infectious diseases (e.g., nocardiosis, actinomycosis, and mycotic diseases) may have nodular pulmonary opacities
- Malignant fibrous histiocytoma—locally aggressive soft tissue sarcoma composed of histiocytes and fibroblasts; no breed predilection; distant metastases rare
- Fibrous histiocytoma—lesion involving the eye(s), generally appearing as a raised limbal mass; involvement of the cornea, conjunctiva, nictitans, eyelid, and periocular areas possible
- Hemophagocytic syndrome (histiocytosis)—benign histiocytic proliferation secondary to infectious, neoplastic, or metabolic disease; can affect bone marrow, lymph nodes, liver, and spleen; causes cytopenia of at least two cell lines
- Anaplastic carcinoma or sarcoma—histopathologic findings in dogs with histiocytosis may indicate a poorly differentiated tumor; immunostaining for tissue-specific markers will differentiate

Diagnostics

- Mild to severe anemia (regenerative or nonregenerative) and thrombocytopenia common
- Biochemistry results reflect the degree of organ involvement.
- Serum ferritin—may be a tumor marker for malignant histiocytosis; one affected dog had very high serum ferritin concentration, suggesting secretion by neoplastic mononuclear phagocytes
- Thoracic radiographs—well-defined, nodular pulmonary opacities (single or multiple), pleural effusion, lung lobe consolidation, diffuse interstitial infiltrates, mediastinal masses, and sternal and bronchial lymphadenomegaly

- Abdominal radiographs—hepatomegaly, splenomegaly, abdominal effusion
- Biopsy of affected organs and/or lymph nodes
- Cytologic examination of bone marrow aspirate or biopsy may show histiocytic infiltration.
- Immunohistochemistry—diagnosis of histiocytosis may be difficult because results of cytologic/histologic examinations not always definitive; cytochemical staining may be useful in determining the histiocytic origin of the cells

Gross Findings

- Skin masses
- Lymphadenomegaly
- Ill-defined white foci in the spleen, lung, kidney, testes, liver, pancreas, skeletal muscles of the head
- Splenomegaly or hepatomegaly with possible mass lesions

Histopathologic Findings

Systemic

- Histiocytic infiltrates fail to demonstrate the bizarre cytologic characteristics of the mononuclear cells typical of malignant disorder.
- Histiocytes appear to target small blood vessels.
- Multinucleated giant cells rarely seen
- Immunohistochemistry—special stains for histiocytic markers such as lysozyme or α-1-antitrypsin may be required for a definitive diagnosis

Malignant

- Cytologic atypia is the hallmark characteristic in affected dogs.
- Histiocytes are large and pleomorphic with foamy cytoplasm.
- The mitotic index is generally high and abnormal mitotic figures may be present.
- Multinucleated giant cells often seen
- Classically, erythrophagocytosis by neoplastic histiocytes is evident.
- Occasionally, leukophagocytosis and thrombophagocytosis are evident.

Therapeutics

- Fluid therapy or blood transfusions may be required depending on clinical findings.

Drugs

- No definitive treatment
- Immunotherapy with a human leukemic T-cell line being investigated

Systemic

- Palliative responses to corticosteroids, lasting from 4 to 18 months, reported
- Anecdotal responses to bovine thymic extract reported

Malignant

Responses to corticosteroids, cyclophosphamide, vincristine, and doxorubicin-based protocols reported; optimal choice of drugs is unknown.

Comments

- Effectiveness of treatment is determined by repeated physical examinations, CBC and biochemistry profiles, and diagnostic imaging.
- Patients with systemic disorder have a fluctuating debilitating disease that can be characterized by multiple clinical episodes and asymptomatic periods.
- Prognosis for malignant disorder extremely poor; death usually occurs within a few months of diagnosis

Suggested Reading

Padgett GA, Madewell BR, Keller ET, et al. Inheritance of histiocytosis in Bernese mountain dogs. J Small Anim Pract 1995:36; 93–98.

Author Kenneth M. Rassnick

Consulting Editor Karen Helton Rhodes

Immunodeficiency Disorders, Primary

Paul W. Snyder

Definition/Overview

- Diminished ability to mount an effective immune response
- Caused by heritable defects in the immune system (secondary disease—diminished immune response acquired as a consequence of some other primary disease)

Etiology/Pathophysiology

- The identification of a specific defect in the immune response requires an adequate understanding of the cellular and genetic basis of the immune system.
- The types and causes are diverse; defects in the cell-mediated, humoral, complement, and phagocytic systems have all been described in the veterinary literature.
- Defects involving the humoral immune response—associated with a high susceptibility to bacterial infection
- Defects involving the cell-mediated immune response—associated with a high susceptibility to viral, fungal, and protozoal infections
- Defects in the phagocytic or complement system—associated with disseminated infection

Systems Affected

- Hemic/Lymph/Immune—defect in a specific cell population in lymphoid tissue
- Skin/Exocrine, Respiratory, Gastrointestinal—chronic or recurrent infections

- Musculoskeletal—failure to thrive
- Other organ systems—dissemination of infection

Genetics

Typically breed-specific with variable modes of inheritance

Signalment/History

Breed Predilections

- X-linked severe combined immunodeficiency—Bassett hounds
- IgA deficiency—beagles, German shepherds, and Chinese sharpeis
- IgM deficiency—Doberman pinschers
- Thymic hypoplasia—dwarfed Weimaraners
- Cyclic hematopoiesis—gray collies
- Chediak-Higashi syndrome—Persian cats
- Leukocyte adhesion deficiency—Irish setters
- Complement deficiency—Brittany spaniels
- Bactericidal defect—Doberman pinschers
- Transient hypogammaglobulinemia—Samoyeds

Mean Age and Range

Primary immunodeficiency diseases typically expressed in the first year of life

Predominant Sex

X-linked recessive severe combined immunodeficiency disease of Bassett hounds—males affected and females carriers for the defect

Clinical Features

- Depend on the level at which the immune response is defective; range from chronic respiratory and gastrointestinal signs and skin infections to life-threatening conditions
- High susceptibility to infection and failure to respond to appropriate, conventional antibiotic therapy
- Lethargy
- Anorexia
- Skin infection
- Failure to thrive
- Signs often appear when maternal antibody concentrations decline.
- Vaccine-induced disease by modified live virus preparation
- Hallmark—failure to thrive
- Clinical signs attributable to infections

Differential Diagnosis

- Patients must be rigorously evaluated for underlying disease process that may cause secondary (acquired) immunodeficient state (e.g., hyperadrenocorticism, FeLV, and FIV).

- Patients are typically young, with recurrent infection that fails to respond to conventional treatment.

Diagnostics

- CBC may indicate deficiencies in specifically affected cell lines or a chronic inflammatory process.
- Serum protein electrophoresis—demonstrates gross deficiency in immunoglobulin concentration
- Serum immunoglobulin quantitation—evaluate humoral immune system, identify selective immunoglobulin deficiency, support diagnosis of agammaglobulinemia
- The lymphocyte transformation test—evaluate the cell-mediated immune system and identify animals with T-lymphocyte deficiency.
- Bactericidal assays—evaluate neutrophil function
- Serum concentration of complement components—diagnose complement deficiency
- Enumeration of lymphocyte subsets by immunofluorescence with monoclonal antibodies—identify deficiency of specific cell lines
- Other more specific tests to evaluate immune function in veterinary species are available, but to get reliable results generally requires access to research laboratories that perform these tests.
- In some patients, bone marrow and lymph node biopsy aids in classifying the type of immune deficiency.

Pathologic Findings

- Lesions vary; depend on the specific defect; most the result of recurrent or opportunistic infection involving the skin, ear canal, and respiratory and gastrointestinal systems
- Lesions of septicemia common in animals with severe defects
- T-lymphocyte defects—hypoplastic or dysplastic lesions of the thymus and T-lymphocyte–dependent areas of secondary lymphoid tissues
- B-lymphocyte defects—hypoplastic or dysplastic lesions of the bone marrow or B-lymphocyte–dependent areas of secondary lymphoid tissues
- Lymphoid hypoplasia or hyperplasia may be seen, depending on the overall defect and the occurrence of infection.

Therapeutics

- Hospitalization may be necessary to control life-threatening infection.
- Outpatient management possible for some patients
- Dietary management may be required to ensure that the patient is maintained at an adequate level of nutrition.
- Potential sources of infectious agents such as raw meat must be avoided.

Drugs

- Antibiotics to control infections
- γ-Globulin or plasma preparations can be used in conjunction with antibiotics to control infection in patients with humoral defect.
- Symptomatic treatment for secondary disease states

CONTRAINDICATIONS

γ-Globulin or plasma preparations should not be administered to patients with selective IgA deficiency, because many affected patients have high concentrations of anti-IgA antibodies and may develop an anaphylactic reaction.

PRECAUTIONS

Modified live virus vaccines should not be administered to patients with suspected T-lymphocyte deficiencies, because it may induce disease in these patients.

CLIENT EDUCATION

- Inform client that the animal cannot be cured.
- Discuss why the patient has high susceptibility to infection.
- Discuss and advise as to the heritability of the disease.
- Discuss the possibility of other litter mates being affected.
- Avoid exposure to ill animals.

PATIENT MONITORING

- For clinical signs of secondary infection
- Routine physical examination to assess efficacy of antibiotic therapy in control of secondary infection

PREVENTION/AVOIDANCE

- Affected animals should not be bred.
- Pedigree analysis to determine the mode of inheritance and prevent propagating the defect

EXPECTED COURSE AND PROGNOSIS

- The severity of the defect determines the course of disease and prognosis.
- Patients with minor defects can be successfully managed.

ABBREVIATIONS

- FeLV = feline leukemia virus
- FIV = feline immunodeficiency virus

Suggested Reading

Guliford WG. Primary immunodeficiency diseases of dogs and cats. Compend Contin Educ Pract Vet 1987;9:641–648.

Lewis RM, Picut CA. Veterinary clinical immunology. Philadelphia: Lea & Febiger, 1989.

Author Paul W. Snyder

Consulting Editor Karen Helton Rhodes

SHAMPOO THERAPY

Anthony A. Yu

Shampoo treatment has gained increased usage as a therapeutic tool in veterinary dermatology and has thus sparked the emergence of several new medicated shampoos. A summary of some of the available products is included; however, it is not all-encompassing. When used correctly, veterinary shampoos can help control or prevent dermatopathies. Emphasis on client education when prescribing topical dermatologics is of utmost importance. These include the following:

- contact time — 5 to 15 minutes to allow for hydration of the epidermis and provide sufficient time for penetration and action of the shampoo
- frequency — discuss intervals of shampooing and any alterations with respect to improvement or deterioration.
- technique — treat severely affected areas first and rinse well.

The small amount of time spent by either a veterinarian or technician with the owner will promote client enthusiasm as he or she will feel essential to the pet's recovery/comfort.

Cleansing and Moisturizing Shampoos

Cleansing and moisturizing shampoos are mildly medicated and hypoallergenic products that clean without soap, using detergent soap substitutes and anionic/amphoteric surfactant systems. They mainly serve to rehydrate and cleanse the skin. They are particularly useful for xeroderma (dry, flaky skin) with little evidence of other disease.

- Allergroom (Allerderm) — contains NaCl, glycerin, lactic acid, and urea
  — rarely causes skin irritation
- HydraPearls (EVSCO) — contains Novasome technology in a pH balanced shampoo
- HyLyt EFA (DVM) — contains Na-lactate, coconut oil, lanolin, glycerin, protein, fatty acids
  — rarely causes skin irritation

Although veterinary products tend to provide excellent results, their costs may be prohibitive. The use of Johnson's Baby Shampoo, Palmolive, Ivory, or Mycodex shampoo for the removal of surface dirt may decrease costs and augment the efficacy of more expensive medicated shampoos.

Antiseborrheic Shampoos

Visible scale may result from abnormal cell migration, increased mitotic activity in the stratum basale, biochemical anomalies in keratin production, and aberrations in intercellular lipid production. Antiseborrheic shampoos are primarily directed at eliminating surface scale (keratolysis) and normalizing epidermal cell kinetics (keratoplasty). Conditions that are amenable to these shampoos include zinc responsive dermatosis, pemphigus foliaceus, ear margin dermatosis, and hypothyroidism.

Sulfur And Salicylic Acid

Properties of sulfur include:

- keratoplastic — cytostatic or related to the formation of cystine which is an important constituent of the stratum corneum, thus normalizing keratinization.
- keratolytic — primarily due to the formation of hydrogen sulfide and pentathionic acid from the combination of sulfur with cysteine.
- antifungal
- antibacterial
- antiparasitic
- antipruritic

Properties of salicylic acid include:

- keratoplastic
- keratolytic — decreases pH resulting in increased hydration of keratin and thus swelling of cells in the stratum corneum. As well, it solubilizes intercellular cement substance promoting the desquamation of attached surface cells.
- antipruritic
- bacteriostatic

A synergistic keratolytic effect is observed when sulfur and salicylic acid are incorporated in equal proportions. Examples of these shampoos include:

- SebaMoist (EVSCO) — contains 2% sulfur, 2% salicylic acid
  — incorporates Novasome rehydrating technology
- Sebolux (Allerderm) — 2% sulfur, 2.3% Na-salicylate
  — mild antibacterial effects
  — lathers extremely well

- SeboRx (DVM) — 2% sulfur, 3% salicylic acid, 0.5% Triclosan
  — mild to moderate antibacterial effects
  — more pleasing than the SebaLyt

Tar Shampoos

Tar shampoos are a product of distillation of bituminous coal or woods such as pine and juniper. Crude coal tar is a composition of thousands of elements. Work has been done recently to define the active ingredients to eliminate the odor and staining properties. As a result, this process has led to the development of fractionated tar shampoos with the same activity and fewer unwanted attributes, promoting better owner compliance. Owners should still be forewarned to discontinue treatment if drying or irritation should occur. I tend to save the tars for severe cases of greasy, scaly skin disorders such as that seen on the Bassett hound with *Malassezia*, the cocker spaniel with a primary keratinization disorder, and the West Highland white terriers with epidermal dysplasia.

Properties of tars include:

- antimitotic — occurs by suppression of epidermal growth and DNA synthesis of the stratum basale
- keratolytic
- antipruritic
- degreasing
- anti-inflammatory — vasoconstrictive action

Several tar shampoos exist that have undergone different production techniques. Because of this, one is advised to read the labels CAREFULLY. Tar solutions contain only 20% equivalent of crude tar extract. I RARELY use the 3–4% tar shampoos for any length of time because of their potential irritating and photosensitizing effects. Thus, when dispensing the higher concentration tars, I would only use 8-oz bottles so that I am assured that the owner will return for a recheck. The tar shampoos that I use include the following:

Milder Tar Shampoos

- EVSCO-Tar — contains 5% coal tar solution (equivalent to 1% coal tar)
  — incorporates Novasomes as a rehydrating vehicle
- NuSal-T (DVM) — contains 2% coal tar, 3% salicylic acid, 1% menthol
  — cooling and degreasing
- T-Lux (Allerderm) — 4% solubilized coal tar (equivalent to 2% coal tar), 2% sulfur, 2.3% Na-salicylate
  — has less odor and clear gold in color

Stronger Tar Shampoos

- AllersebT (Allerderm) — 4% coal tar, 2% sulfur, 2% salicylic acid
  — strongest tar shampoo with odor and color
- LyTar (DVM) — 3% refined juniper tar, 2% sulfur, 2% salicylic acid
  — stronger tar shampoo with odor and color

Selenium Sulfide

Antiseborrheic with limited usage owing to its staining, drying, and irritating properties—especially to mucous membranes and the scrotum. I have used this product with success in some of the really greasy *Malassezia* cases.

Properties of selenium sulfide include:

- keratoplastic — depresses epidermal cell turnover rate and interferes with
- keratolytic — hydrogen bond formation in the keratin.
- degreasing
- Selsun Blue (Ross) — 1% selenium sulfide
  — do NOT use in cats
  — contact irritant, discolors, dries excessively

Benzoyl Peroxide

Benzoyl peroxide is included with antiseborrheic agents but also has superior antimicrobial activity. It is often formulated at 2.5% to 3% in veterinary products owing to its irritating effects at higher concentrations. Also, the excellent drying activity of benzoyl peroxide shampoos often necessitates the use of emollients or alternating treatments with a milder product. Cases in which benzoyl peroxides are of value include greasy pets with secondary bacterial dermatoses, dogs with demodicosis, cases of chin acne, and schnauzer comedo syndrome. Owners should be warned of the potential for bleaching fabrics and hair coats.

Properties of benzoyl peroxide:

- keratlytic
- antibacterial
- follicular flushing
- degreasing

This, along with tar-based shampoos, should be dispensed by prescription ONLY, and should be purchased from reputable suppliers as the bottle design is important in keeping the ingredients intact. The following are benzoyl peroxides that I would recommend:

- Benzoyl-Plus (EVSCO) — contains 2.5% benzoyl peroxide with Novasomes
- Pyoben (Allerderm) — 3% benzoyl peroxide
  — seems to lather better than others
- SulfOxyDex (DVM) — 2.5% benzoyl peroxide, 2% sulfur
  — sulfur offers additional descaling activity

Antimicrobials

Benzoyl Peroxide

- The most active antibacterial agent with residual effects of 48 hours
- See above for products

Chlorhexidine

Chlorhexidine is a synthetic biguanide with broad-spectrum activity against bacteria, fungi, and yeasts. It is characterized by a rapid kill and 36-hour residual activity. Available products include:

- ChlorhexiDerm (DVM) — contains 2 or 4% chlorhexidine gluconate
- Hexadene (Allerderm) — contains 2% chlorhexidine gluconate

- SebaHex (EVSCO)
  - contains 2% sulfur, 2% salicylic acid, 2% chlorhexidine gluconate
  - good for scaly skin with a secondary bacterial dermatitis
- Universal Medicated (Vet Solutions)
  - contains 2% sulfur, 2% salicylic acid, and supposedly 2% chlorhexidine (recent formulations have not been stable)

Iodine

Iodine preparations have decreased in popularity as a result of their unwanted properties and the development of more efficient products. Iodine has good activity against bacteria, viruses, fungi, and spore formers, especially when combined with pyrrolidone nitrogen. Residual activity lasts 6–8 hours and may cause irritation and staining.

- Iodine Shampoo (EVSCO)
  - 2% povidone iodine
  - also has Novasome technology

Imidazoles

Imidazoles act by interfering with ergosterol synthesis of fungal and yeast organisms, thereby increasing cellular permeability, suppressing metabolic function, and inhibiting growth. There has also been evidence that ketoconazole exerts an antiproliferative effect on keratinocytes in culture. These shampoos are of value when trying to address dermatophyte or *Malassezia* infections.

- Dermazole (Allerderm)
  - a 2% miconazole, 0.5% chlorhexidine formulation
  - it is available in 6- and 16-oz sizes @ $20 and $44
- Miconazole Shampoo (EVSCO)
  - contains 2% miconazole nitrate, chlorhexidine
  - it is available in a 12-oz size @ $20
- Nizoral (Janssen)
  - a human preparation contains 2% ketoconazole
  - only available in 4-oz bottles @ $28 each
- Malaseb (DVM)
  - chlorhexidine and miconazole
- Ketochlor (DVM)
  - ketoconazole and chlorhexidine

Ethyl Lactate

Ethyl lactate has excellent antibacterial activity in a nondrying, degreasing shampoo formulated at a 10% concentration, called Etiderm (Allerderm). My use for this product has been limited to the Xoloitzcuintle breed (the Mexican Hairless), although many colleagues have used it with favorable results. I find the shampoo extremely watery with a distinct odor, and it doesn't seem to lather as well as other shampoos. There have also been reported cases in which the shampoo seems to be irritating.

Topical Antipruritics

Topical antipruritic therapy is gaining increasing interest—in particular when trying to control itch prior to an intradermal allergy test. Ideal withdrawal times for anti-inflammatory medication before testing are as follows:

- corticosteroid injections: 8–12 weeks
- corticosteroid tablets: 4–6 weeks
- topical corticosteroids: 2 weeks
- oral antihistamines: 2 weeks

Thus, a 2-week interval remains in which other means of abating pruritus must be implemented. Oatmeal-based shampoos act by ADsorbing surface allergens and pruritic mediators to the ultra-fine colloidal oatmeal particles, which are then gently rinsed away. Several products are available.

- Dermal-Soothe (EVSCO) — 2% oatmeal-based shampoo and conditioner
  — also contains 1% pramoxine HCl, a local anesthetic
- Episoothe (Allerderm) — 2% oatmeal-based shampoo and conditioner
- Relief (DVM) — 2% oatmeal-based shampoo, 20% oatmeal-based conditioner
  — also contains 1% pramoxine HCl, a local anesthetic

The luxury of these formulations is that they do not have to be withdrawn prior to the IDAT. A powdered oatmeal formulation to be added to a cool bath is also available as EPISOOTHE and AVEENO.

Other Anti-Inflammatory Shampoos

Shampoos containing 2% diphenhydramine or 1% hydrocortisone, omega-6 fatty acids and 2% colloidal oatmeal (Histacalm and CortiCalm by Allerderm) and 0.01% fluocinolone acetonide with 8% colloidal oatmeal (FS Shampoo by Meridian Veterinary Products) are also available. Only anecdotal reports concerning the shampoos are available. The shampoos have not proven to be as effective as I had hoped. Owing to their potential interference with intradermal allergy testing, I have used the pramoxine HCl base products with greater frequency. With any of the above shampoos, contact time is crucial—i.e., 2–10 minutes.

Final Comments

When selecting a shampoo, base your decision on the active ingredients within a product, and then consider the company's quality control measures (development, stability trials, adherence to FDA requirements). With the advent of alternative medicine, many fly-by-night companies are producing shampoos whose formulations are not consistent with what is in the bottle, nor have they undergone any rigid testing before they reach the market.

Author Anthony A. Yu

Consulting Editor Karen Helton Rhodes

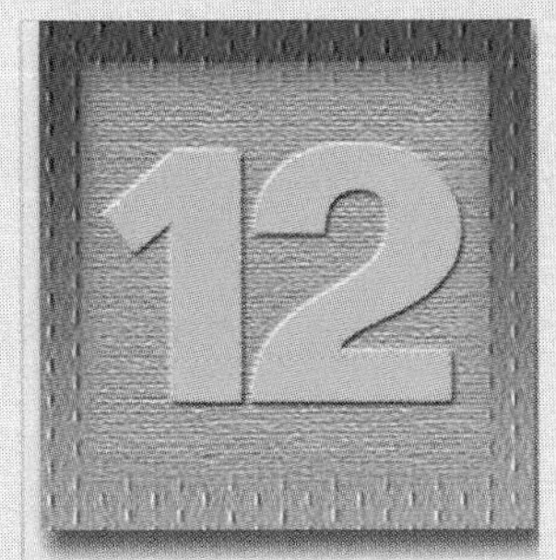

Laboratory Tests/Interpretation

ACTH Response Test

Ellen N. Behrend and Robert Kemppainen

Definition/Overview

- ACTH gel or synthetic ACTH is used.
- Dogs—if ACTH gel (Acthar, Rhone-Poulenc Rorer Pharmaceuticals) is used, collect a pre-ACTH blood sample and then give 2.2 U/kg IM; one post-ACTH sample is collected 2 hr later
- Cats—use the same dose of ACTH, but take blood samples before and 1 and 2 hr after injection
- If using synthetic ACTH (Cosyntropin, Organon Inc.), give the drug intravenously; use 5 μg/kg for dogs, with a maximum of 250 μg/dog, or 0.125 mg (125 μg)/cat; in both species, draw blood samples before and 1 hr after injection.
- Baseline, resting, or pre-ACTH cortisol concentration in dogs is 10–160 nmol/L (0.4–6.0 μg/dL) and in cats, 10–110 nmol/L (0.4–4.0 μg/dL).
- Normal dogs and cats have a post-ACTH plasma cortisol concentration of 220–560 nmol/L (8–20 μg/dL) and 220–330 nmol/L (8–12 μg/dL), respectively; normal values vary slightly between laboratories.

Etiology/Pathophysiology

- The dose of ACTH maximally stimulates cortisol secretion.
- The test can be used to screen for hyperadrenocorticism (Cushing's syndrome), hypoadrenocorticism (Addison's disease), and adrenal reserve in dogs or cats receiving exogenous glucocorticoids or mitotane (Lysodren) or cats receiving progestins.

- An above-normal response is consistent with a diagnosis of Cushing's syndrome but could also be a nonspecific finding in dogs with nonadrenal illness; a below-normal response is consistent with hypoadrenocorticism, previous glucocorticoid administration, Lysodren therapy in dogs or cats, or progestin treatment in cats.
- Cushing's syndrome can be caused by either an ACTH-secreting pituitary tumor (i.e., pituitary-dependent hyperadrenocorticism, PDH) or a cortisol-secreting AT; with PDH, constant overstimulation of the adrenal cortex by excess ACTH leads to bilateral adrenal hyperplasia and increased secretory ability; the adrenal tumor mass can similarly increase the ability to release cortisol; thus, ACTH usually elicits an above-normal cortisol response.
- An increased response to ACTH in dogs may also be a result of nonadrenal illness and associated nonspecific activation of the hypothalamic-pituitary-adrenal axis and adrenal cortical hyperplasia; the effect of nonadrenal illness on ACTH response in cats is unknown.
- A false-negative response is seen in ~15% of patients with canine or feline Cushing's syndrome; in PDH, this may be attributable to early hyperadrenocorticism in which adrenal cortical hyperplasia is minimal; in AT, the tumor tissue may not have receptors for ACTH and so does not respond to an injection of ACTH.
- A below-normal response can be seen with destruction or atrophy of the adrenal cortex; destruction can be caused by spontaneous primary Addison's disease or mitotane therapy; during long-term glucocorticoid therapy, a patient's ACTH secretion may be suppressed by negative feedback by the exogenous steroids on the pituitary; lack of ACTH in turn leads to atrophy of the adrenocortical zonae reticularis and fasciculata; thus, when therapy is discontinued, the adrenals secrete subnormal amounts of glucocorticoids; long-term glucocorticoid therapy results in adrenal atrophy and severely reduced or no response to ACTH; short-term glucocorticoid therapy can reduce the ACTH response moderately.
- Progestin therapy in cats also suppresses ACTH release; similarly, secondary Addison's disease, loss of ability to secrete ACTH, causes adrenal atrophy and a subnormal ACTH response.
- Because of the ability to detect hyper- and hypoadrenocorticism, this test is preferred if an animal has a definitive or questionable history of receiving exogenous glucocorticoids and signs compatible with Cushing's syndrome; the response to ACTH will differentiate spontaneous hyperadrenocorticism (an above-normal response in association with the clinical signs) from iatrogenic Cushing's syndrome (a below-normal response in association with the clinical signs).

Results

Above-Normal Response

- Cushing's syndrome—dogs and cats
- Nonadrenal illness—dogs, cats unknown

Below-Normal Response

- Primary or secondary hypoadrenocorticism—dogs and cats
- Glucocorticoid therapy—dogs and cats
- Mitotane therapy—dogs and cats
- Progestin therapy—cats

Differential Diagnosis

FINDINGS

Above-Normal Response

- Historical findings of hyperadrenocorticism include polyuria/polydipsia, alopecia or failure to regrow hair, abdominal enlargement, polyphagia, obesity, panting, lethargy, muscle weakness, anestrus, and heat intolerance.
- Physical examination findings of hyperadrenocorticism include thin skin, abdominal enlargement, bilaterally symmetrical alopecia, abdominal enlargement, hepatomegaly, pyoderma, seborrhea, cutaneous hyperpigmentation, muscle wasting of extremities, calcinosis cutis, bruising, and testicular atrophy.
- Findings vary depending on which nonadrenal illness is present.

Below-Normal Response

- Findings of glucocorticoid or mineralocorticoid deficiency are the same regardless of the cause. (See Hypoadrenocorticism.)
- A history of glucocorticoid, mitotane, or progestin administration helps to define the cause.

Laboratory Findings

DRUGS THAT MAY ALTER LABORATORY RESULTS

- Prednisone, prednisolone, and hydrocortisone cross-react in many cortisol radioimmunoassays and cause an artifactually high measured cortisol concentration.
- A subnormal cortisol concentration may be obscured, and a patient with subnormal or normal plasma cortisol concentrations may appear to have an above-normal ACTH response.

DISORDERS THAT MAY ALTER LABORATORY RESULTS

- Delayed separation of plasma from blood cells may falsely lower measured cortisol concentration.
- Use plasma, preferably collected with EDTA as the anticoagulant; cortisol is stable stored at $\leq$ 25°C for 5 days; storage at higher temperatures or use of serum may lead to decay of cortisol and a spurious decrease in apparent cortisol concentration.

VALID IF RUN IN HUMAN LABORATORY?

Yes, if assay is validated for dogs and cats

CBC/Biochemistry/Urinalysis

FINDINGS

Above-Normal Response

- CBC with hyperadrenocorticism—a mature leukocytosis, neutrophilia, lymphopenia, eosinopenia, or mild polycythemia

- Biochemistry—increased ALP, (elevation may be extreme), alanine aminotransferase (ALT), cholesterol, fasting blood glucose, and lipase can be seen with hyperadrenocorticism; may see lipemia and decreased BUN
- Urinalysis—dilute urine (e.g., specific gravity < 1.015) and bacteriuria with or without pyuria have been associated with Cushing's syndrome

Below-Normal Response

CBC, biochemistry, and urinalysis will be the same regardless of the underlying cause of hormone deficiency; hyperkalemia and hyponatremia are seen with loss of mineralocorticoids but not if only glucocorticoids were lacking.

Other Laboratory Tests

Findings

Above-Normal Response

- Other tests used to screen for Cushing's syndrome include urinary cortisol:creatinine ratio (UCCR) and a low-dose dexamethasone suppression test (LDDST).
- If an ACTH stimulation test indicates Cushing's syndrome but the diagnosis is questionable (e.g., nonadrenal illness or results borderline), the diagnosis is best confirmed with the LDDST, which is more sensitive than the ACTH response; if the LDDST is normal, consider another diagnosis.
- If the ACTH response is normal but suspicion of Cushing's syndrome remains high, an LDDST can be performed; a positive LDDST but normal ACTH response may represent a false-negative ACTH response with a true-positive LDDST result.
- If the ACTH response is above normal and a diagnosis of Cushing's syndrome is likely on the basis of historical and clinical findings, perform a high-dose dexamethasone suppression test or measure endogenous ACTH concentrations to differentiate between PDH and AT.

Below-Normal Response

- Measuring endogenous ACTH concentration and/or serum aldosterone concentrations pre- and post-ACTH injection can differentiate spontaneous primary and secondary Addison's disease.
- Measuring serum aldosterone concentrations can assess mineralocorticoid secretory ability after mitotane therapy.

Diagnostics

Imaging

Above-Normal Response

- Abdominal radiography and ultrasonography can be used to differentiate PDH from AT.
- Computed tomography (CT) and magnetic resonance imaging (MRI) can reveal a pituitary tumor.

Below-Normal Response

CT and MRI can reveal a pituitary abnormality (e.g., space-occupying lesion destroying the pituitary) in spontaneous secondary Addison's disease.

DIAGNOSTIC PROCEDURES

Above-Normal Response

- With hyperadrenocorticism, urinary protein: creatinine ratio and systemic blood pressure may be mildly elevated, but neither are specific.
- A skin biopsy can confirm the diagnosis of calcinosis cutis, a pathognomonic finding for hyperadrenocorticism; other skin changes may suggest an endocrinopathy but are not specific.
- A liver biopsy can show changes consistent with steroid hepatopathy, a sensitive but nonspecific marker of Cushing's syndrome.

Below-Normal Response

N/A

Treatment

Above-Normal Response

- Lack of suppression does not need to be treated.
- If the test result indicates nonadrenal illness, direct therapy toward resolution of that disease.
- If Cushing's syndrome is believed present, direct therapy toward managing hyperadrenocorticism; unless a complication of Cushing's syndrome requires hospitalization (e.g., pulmonary thromboembolism), treat as outpatients.

Below-Normal Response

- An acute addisonian crisis is a medical emergency requiring hospitalization and intensive fluid therapy (see Hypoadrenocorticism).
- Patients with chronic hypoadrenocorticism can be hospitalized or not, depending on the severity of clinical signs.
- Feeding must be altered if vomiting is present.
- Limit activity and avoid stress until the patient is stable and glucocorticoid replacement therapy has begun.

Medications

ABOVE-NORMAL RESPONSE

None needed while completing all tests for the diagnosis

BELOW-NORMAL RESPONSE

- Acute addisonian crisis requires glucocorticoids and fluid therapy.
- See Hypoadrenocorticism.
- Chronic glucocorticoid deficiency—may give physiologic doses of prednisone (0.2 mg/kg/day) as needed, depending on the severity of the deficiency
- If cortisol lack is a result of long-term steroid administration, taper the steroid dose slowly, if possible, to physiologic doses of prednisone, and then discontinue as adrenal function recovers; if the patient is receiving a synthetic glucocorticoid other than prednisone, taper medication slowly and then replace with prednisone; if a cat is receiving progestins, stop this medication and give physiologic doses of prednisone.
- A repeat test can indicate when the adrenal reserve has returned to normal.

Precautions

Above-Normal Response

N/A

Below-Normal Response

Any medication that can lower blood pressure (e.g., calcium-channel blockers, phenothiazine tranquilizers, α_2-agonists); if administered, observe the patient for weakness or syncope and monitor mucous membrane color and heart rate; pale or cyanotic mucous membranes or tachycardia are consistent with severe hypotension.

Comments

Patient Monitoring

Above-Normal Response

- If hyperadrenocorticism, follow-up depends on the type of therapy chosen (see Hyperadrenocorticism)
- If nonadrenal illness is present and considered a possible cause of the abnormal response, treat the illness; once the animal is stable, repeat the ACTH response test after 4–8 weeks.

Below-Normal Response

- If spontaneous Addison's disease, monitoring depends on the type of therapy chosen (see Hypoadrenocorticism)
- If subnormal response is caused by glucocorticoid, mitotane, or progestin administration, use sequential ACTH response tests to assess recovery of glucocorticoid secretory ability; test every 7–14 days at first; subsequent frequency depends on how quickly the secretory ability is returning
- Rate of recovery after glucocorticoid or progestin administration depends on the form, route, and length of administration.
- After mitotane therapy, if only glucocorticoids are deficient, secretory ability usually returns within 2 months but can take up to 18; if mineralocorticoids are deficient as well, loss of both hormones is likely to be permanent.

Possible Complications

Above-Normal Response

Untreated hyperadrenocorticism can lead to development of all classic signs if not already present (e.g., polyuria, polydipsia, panting, polyphagia) as well as such life-threatening complications as pulmonary thromboembolism or diabetes mellitus.

Below-Normal Response

Untreated glucocorticoid deficiency can be fatal; if mineralocorticoids are deficient as well, clinical deterioration and death may occur rapidly.

Age-Related Factors

Above-Normal Response

- Nonadrenal illness can occur in an animal of any age.
- Hyperadrenocorticism is typically a disease of middle-aged to old cats and dogs but has been reported in dogs 1 year old.

Below-Normal Response

- Spontaneous hypoadrenocorticism is seen in dogs < 1–12 years, with a median of 4 years, and mainly in middle-aged cats, but the reported range is 1–9 years.
- Glucocorticoids can suppress the adrenal cortex in dogs or cats of any age.
- Similarly, progestin therapy can cause adrenal atrophy in cats of any age.
- Mitotane suppression of the adrenal cortex can be seen any time during the course of therapy; since this drug is used to treat dogs with Cushing's syndrome, it is mainly administered to middle-aged and older dogs.

Suggested Reading

Feldman EC, Nelson RW. Hyperadrenocorticism (Cushing's syndrome). In: Canine and feline endocrinology and reproduction. 2nd ed. Philadelphia: Saunders, 1996:187–265.

Guptill L, Scott-Moncrieff JC, Widmer W. Diagnosis of canine hyperadrenocorticism. Vet Clin North Am Small Anim Pract 1997;27:215–235.

Kaplan AJ, Peterson ME, Kemppainen RJ. Effects of disease on the results of diagnostic tests for use in detecting hyperadrenocorticism in dogs. J Am Vet Med Assoc 1995;207:445–451.

Kintzer PP, Peterson ME. Primary and secondary canine hypoadrenocorticism. Vet Clin North Am Small Anim Pract 1997;27:349–358.

Van Liew CH, Greco DS, Salman MD. Comparison of results on adrenocorticotropic hormone stimulation and low-dose dexamethasone suppression tests with necropsy findings in dogs: 81 cases (1985–1995). J Am Vet Med Assoc 1997;211:322–325.

Authors Ellen N. Behrend and Robert Kemppainen

Consulting Editor Karen Helton Rhodes

Low-Dose Dexamethasone Suppression Test

Ellen N. Behrend and Robert Kemppainen

Definition/Overview

- To perform an LDDST, administer dexamethasone (0.01–0.015 mg/kg IV for dogs and 0.1 mg/kg for cats).
- Can use dexamethasone or dexamethasone sodium phosphate as long as calculations are based on the concentration of the active ingredient
- Draw blood before and 4 and 8 hr after injection.
- At baseline (i.e., pre-dexamethasone), normal plasma cortisol concentrations in dogs are 10–160 nmol/L (~0.4–6.0 μg/dL) and in cats, 10–110 nmol/L (~0.4–4.0 μg/dL).
- A normal animal has a cortisol concentration below ~30 nmol/L (1.0 μg/dL) at both 4 and 8 hr post-dexamethasone. (**Note:** normal values vary slightly between laboratories.)
- Dexamethasone should be diluted in sterile saline if necessary for cats and small dogs, so that the patient is dosed accurately.
- If part or all of the dexamethasone is given out of the vein, the test should be stopped and attempted again after at least 48 hr.

Etiology/Pathophysiology

- Used to screen for hyperadrenocorticism (Cushing's syndrome); lack of suppression in response to a low dose of dexamethasone is consistent with a diagnosis of hyperadrenocorticism but can be a nonspecific finding in dogs with nonadrenal illness.

- Cushing's syndrome can be caused either by an ACTH-secreting pituitary tumor (i.e., pituitary-dependent hyperadrenocorticism, PDH) or by a cortisol-secreting AT.
- Normally, dexamethasone feeds back onto the pituitary and turns off ACTH secretion; when systemic ACTH concentration falls, the secretory stimulus to the adrenal cortex diminishes, and cortisol release decreases; thus, 4 and 8 hr after dexamethasone, plasma cortisol concentration is low (<30 nmol/L).
- With PDH, the pituitary tumor is relatively resistant to feedback, and secretion of ACTH and, in turn, cortisol continues.
- Because of the continued autonomous secretion of cortisol from an AT, endogenous ACTH is already suppressed, administration of an exogenous glucocorticoid has no further effect on the pituitary, and autonomous cortisol secretion continues despite dexamethasone administration.
- A diagnosis of either PDH or AT is supported by a 4- and/or 8-hr post-dexamethasone plasma cortisol concentration > 30 nmol/L; in addition, if the 4-hr post-dexamethasone concentration is < 30 nmol/L but the 8-hr sample is > 30 nmol/L or if one or both are less than 50% of baseline, PDH is likely; however, if both post-dexamethasone concentrations are > 30 nmol/L and neither of these values is less than 50% of baseline, either PDH or AT is possible.
- A lack of suppression in dogs during an LDDST can also be an effect of nonadrenal illness and associated nonspecific activation of the hypothalamic-pituitary-adrenal axis; the effect of nonadrenal illness on the LDDST in cats is unknown.
- A false-negative test result is seen in ~5% of patients with Cushing's syndrome; this may be owing to early PDH in which the tumor still responds to glucocorticoid feedback.

Differential Diagnosis

- Historical findings of hyperadrenocorticism include polyuria/polydipsia, bilaterally symmetrical alopecia or failure to regrow hair, abdominal enlargement, polyphagia, obesity, panting, lethargy, muscle weakness, anestrus, and heat intolerance.
- Physical examination findings of hyperadrenocorticism include thin skin, abdominal enlargement, bilaterally symmetrical alopecia, hepatomegaly, pyoderma, seborrhea, cutaneous hyperpigmentation, muscle wasting of extremities, calcinosis cutis, bruising, and testicular atrophy.
- Historical and physical examination findings vary, depending on the nonadrenal illness present.

Laboratory Findings

Drugs That May Alter Laboratory Results

- Phenobarbital administration may cause lack of suppression.
- Prednisone, prednisolone, and hydrocortisone cross-react in many cortisol radioimmunoassays and cause an artifactual increase in measured cortisol concentration; suppression in response to dexamethasone may be obscured.
- Prolonged glucocorticoid therapy may affect the pituitary-adrenal axis by continuously activating normal negative feedback mechanisms.
- The LDDST is unreliable in these patients because it may not cause adequate suppression, leading to a false-positive test result.

Disorders That May Alter Laboratory Results

- Delayed separation of plasma from blood cells may falsely lower measured cortisol concentration.
- Use plasma collected with EDTA as an anticoagulant because cortisol will be stable if stored at ≤25°C for 5 days; storage at higher temperatures or use of serum may lead to decay of cortisol and a spurious decrease in apparent cortisol concentration.

Valid If Run in Human Laboratory?

Yes, if assay is validated for dogs and cats

CBC/Biochemistry/Urinalysis

- CBC—with hyperadrenocorticism, a mature leukocytosis, neutrophilia, lymphopenia, eosinopenia, or mild polycythemia
- Biochemistry—increased alkaline phosphatase (ALP; elevation may be extreme), alanine aminotransferase (ALT), cholesterol, fasting blood glucose, and lipase can be seen with hyperadrenocorticism; lipemia and decreased BUN may also be noted
- Urinalysis—dilute urine (e.g., specific gravity < 1.015) and bacteriuria with or without pyuria have been associated with Cushing's syndrome

Other Laboratory Tests

- Other tests used to screen for Cushing's syndrome include a urinary cortisol:creatinine ratio (UCCR), an ACTH response test, and a combined high-dose dexamethasone suppression/ACTH response.
- An elevated UCCR is a highly sensitive but nonspecific finding for Cushing's syndrome; a normal ratio signifies the patient has <10% chance of having hyperadrenocorticism.
- An ACTH response and the combined high-dose dexamethasone suppression/ACTH response are both less sensitive but more specific for Cushing's syndrome than the LDDST; if a patient does not suppress in response to dexamethasone but has a normal ACTH response or combination test, consider whether a nonadrenal illness is causing a false-positive LDDST result.
- If the results of the LDDST are abnormal but borderline (e.g., 4- and 8-hr postdexamethasone cortisol concentrations are slightly above 30 nmol/L), retest the patient or, ideally, perform an ACTH response test to confirm the diagnosis of Cushing's syndrome.
- If nonadrenal illness is present and possible cause of abnormal LDDST results, treat the illness; when the patient is stable, perform an ACTH response test after 4–8 weeks.
- If there is no suppression on the LDDST, no nonadrenal illness known to be present, and the diagnosis of hyperadrenocorticism is likely on the basis of historical and clinical findings but the test did not determine if the cause was PDH, a high-dose dexamethasone suppression test can be performed or endogenous ACTH concentration measured for differentiation.

Diagnostics

Imaging

- Abdominal radiography and ultrasonography can be used to differentiate PDH from AT.
- CT and magnetic resonance imaging (MRI) can reveal a pituitary tumor.

Diagnostic Procedures

- With hyperadrenocorticism, urinary protein:creatinine ratio and systemic blood pressure may be mildly elevated, but neither is specific.
- A skin biopsy can confirm the diagnosis of calcinosis cutis, a pathognomonic finding for hyperadrenocorticism; other skin biopsy changes may suggest an endocrinopathy but are not specific.
- A liver biopsy can show changes consistent with steroid hepatopathy, a sensitive but nonspecific marker of Cushing's syndrome.

Treatment

- Lack of suppression per se does not need to be treated.
- If the test result is an effect of nonadrenal illness, direct therapy toward resolution of that disease.
- If Cushing's syndrome is believed to be present, direct therapy toward managing hyperadrenocorticism; unless a complication of Cushing's syndrome requires hospitalization (e.g., pulmonary thromboembolism), patients can be treated as outpatients.

Follow-Up

Patient Monitoring

- If hyperadrenocorticism is present, follow-up depends on the type of therapy chosen (see Hyperadrenocorticism).
- If nonadrenal illness is present and believed possibly to be the cause of abnormal LDDST results, treat the illness; when the patient is stable, perform an ACTH response test after 4–8 weeks.

Possible Complications

Untreated hyperadrenocorticism can lead to development of all classic signs not already present (e.g., polyuria, polydipsia, panting, polyphagia), as well as such life-threatening complications as pulmonary thromboembolism or diabetes mellitus.

Age-Related Factors

- Nonadrenal illness can occur in an animal of any age.
- Hyperadrenocorticism is typically a disease of middle-aged to old cats and dogs, although it has been reported in dogs 1 year old.

Suggested Reading

Feldman EC, Nelson RW, Feldman MS. Use of low- and high-dose dexamethasone tests for distinguishing pituitary-dependent from adrenal tumor hyperadrenocorticism in dogs. J Am Vet Med Assoc 1996;209:772–775.

Feldman EC, Nelson RW. Hyperadrenocorticism (Cushing's syndrome). In: Feldman EC, Nelson RW, eds. Canine and feline endocrinology and reproduction. 2nd ed. Philadelphia: Saunders, 1996.

Guptill L, Scott-Moncrieff JC, Widmer W. Diagnosis of canine hyperadrenocorticism. Vet Clin North Am Small Anim Pract 1997;27:215–235.

Kaplan AJ, Peterson ME, Kemppainen RJ. Effects of disease on the results of diagnostic tests for use in detecting hyperadrenocorticism in dogs. J Am Vet Med Assoc 1995;207:445–451.

Van Liew CH, Greco DS, Salman MD. Comparison of results on adrenocorticotropic hormone stimulation and low-dose dexamethasone suppression tests with necropsy findings in dogs: 81 cases (1985–1995). J Am Vet Med Assoc 1997;211:322–325.

Authors Ellen N. Behrend and Robert Kemppainen

Consulting Editor Karen Helton Rhodes

High-Dose Dexamethasone Suppression Test and Plasma ACTH Levels

Peter P. Kintzer

Definition/Overview

Tests used to differentiate PDH from hyperadrenocorticism owing to cortisol-secreting AT; not used to diagnose HAC

Etiology/Pathophysiology

- A high dose of dexamethasone (0.1 or 1.0 mg/kg administered IV or IM, depending on the laboratory used) will, through negative feedback, shut off ACTH production in most (75–80%) animals with PDH, with a subsequent decrease in serum cortisol concentration.
- Cortisol secretion by ATs is autonomous; cortisol levels are not suppressed following administration of high doses of dexamethasone.
- Plasma ACTH levels are high normal to increased in PDH and undetectable-to-low in AT, although in rare cases overlap can be seen unless multiple samples are evaluated.

Differential Diagnosis

- PDH
- Cortisol-secreting AT

Laboratory Findings

- High-dose dexamethasone suppression test—suppression of serum cortisol levels below 1.5 μg/dL at 8 hr excludes an adrenal tumor; failure to suppress means an approximately 50/50 chance of the patient having an adrenal tumor versus nonsuppressible PDH; use of an absolute cutoff value of 8 hr is recommended; use of percentage suppression does not appear to be as accurate.
- ACTH levels—normal-to-elevated levels are consistent with PDH; undetectable-to-low levels are consistent with AT

Imaging

- Recommended to back up results; necessary if test is inconclusive
- Use of ultrasound, CT, or MRI preferred

Drugs of Choice

- Lysodren, ketoconazole, or *l*-deprenyl for PDH
- Surgery, Lysodren, or ketoconazole for AT (see section on HAC)

Abbreviations

- AT = adrenocortical tumor
- HAC = hyperadrenocorticism
- PDH = pituitary-dependent hyperadrenocorticism

Suggested Reading

Guptill L, Scott-Moncrieff JC, Widmer WR. Diagnosis of canine hyperadrenocorticism. Vet Clin North Am Small Anim Pract 1997;27:215–236.

Kintzer PP, Peterson ME. Diagnosis and management of canine cortisol-secreting adrenal tumors. Vet Clin North Am Small Anim Pract 1997.

Peterson ME. Hyperadrenocorticism. In: Kirk RW, ed. Current veterinary therapy IX. Philadelphia: Saunders, 1986.

Author Peter P. Kintzer

Consulting Editor Karen Helton Rhodes

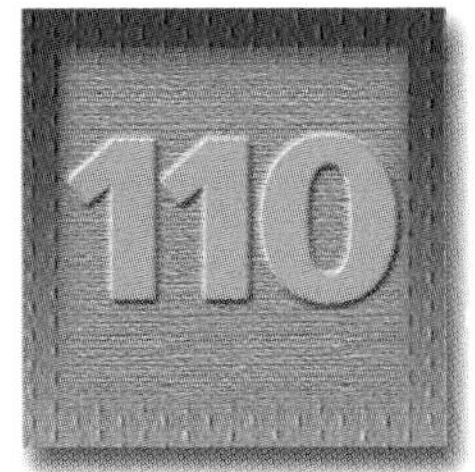

Urine Cortisol: Creatinine Ratio

Ellen N. Behrend and Robert Kemppainen

Definition/Overview

- To measure a urine cortisol: creatinine ratio (UCCR), a single midstream free-catch urine sample is used; cortisol and creatinine are both measured and the concentrations converted into the same units; the UCCR is simply the ratio of the two values.
- A normal UCCR is less than approximately $10–30 \times 10^{-6}$ depending on the laboratory; this value has no units and is typically reported without the scientific notation, e.g., 10×10^{-6} would be reported as 10.

Eitiology/Pathophysiology

- A UCCR is used to screen for spontaneous hyperadrenocorticism (Cushing's syndrome).
- Urine cortisol excretion increases as a reflection of augmented adrenal secretion of the hormone; this can be caused by either excess stimulation by a pituitary adrenocorticotropin (ACTH)-secreting tumor (i.e., pituitary-dependent hyperadrenocorticism, PDH) or by an autonomously functioning adrenal tumor (AT).
- Since creatinine excretion is relatively constant while kidney function is stable, dividing the urine cortisol concentration by the creatinine concentration negates the effect of urine volume in interpreting urine cortisol concentration.
- The finding of an elevated UCCR is a sensitive marker of hyperadrenocorticism, being present in 90–100% of affected animals.

- An elevated UCCR can also be a result of nonadrenal illness and nonspecific activation of the hypothalamic-pituitary-adrenal axis in dogs and cats.
- The chance of a false-positive is great since only about 25–30% of dogs with an elevated UCCR actually have Cushing's syndrome while the other 70–75% have nonadrenal illness.

Differential Diagnosis

- Historical findings of hyperadrenocorticism include polyuria/polydipsia, alopecia or failure to regrow hair, abdominal enlargement, polyphagia, obesity, panting, lethargy, muscle weakness, anestrus, and heat intolerance.
- Physical examination findings of hyperadrenocorticism include thin skin, abdominal enlargement, bilaterally symmetrical alopecia, hepatomegaly, pyoderma, seborrhea, cutaneous hyperpigmentation, muscle wasting of extremities, calcinosis cutis, bruising, and testicular atrophy.
- Historical and physical examination findings vary depending on which nonadrenal illness is present.

Laboratory Findings

Drugs That May Alter Laboratory Results

Prednisone, prednisolone, and hydrocortisone will cross-react on a radioimmunoassay and cause an artifactual increase in measured cortisol concentration; the ratio will be elevated as well.

Disorders That May Alter Laboratory Results

An elevated UCCR may be seen in dogs with nonadrenal illness; this is a highly sensitive but nonspecific test for Cushing's syndrome; the specificity is approximately 25–30%.

Valid If Run in Human Laboratory?

Yes, if assay validated for dogs and cats

CBC/Biochemistry/Urinalysis

- CBC: With hyperadrenocorticism, a mature leukocytosis, neutrophilia, lymphopenia, eosinopenia, or mild polycythemia
- Biochemistry: Increased alkaline phosphatase (ALP, elevation may be extreme), alanine aminotransferase (ALT), cholesterol, fasting blood glucose, and lipase can be seen with hyperadrenocorticism. Lipemia and decreased BUN may also be noted.
- Urinalysis: Dilute urine (e.g., urine specific gravity < 1.015) and bacteriuria with or without pyuria have been associated with Cushing's syndrome.

Other Laboratory Tests

- An elevated UCCR is consistent with but *not* diagnostic for hyperadrenocorticism.

- An ACTH response test, a low-dose dexamethasone suppression test (LDDST), or a combined high-dose dexamethasone suppression/ACTH response test must be done to confirm the diagnosis.
- If nonadrenal illness is present, the ACTH response test may be preferred as it is more specific, and normal findings would suggest an elevated UCCR is a result of nonadrenal illness.

Diagnostics

Imaging

- Abdominal radiography and ultrasonography can be used to differentiate PDH from AT.
- CT and MRI can reveal a pituitary tumor.

Diagnostic Procedures

- With hyperadrenocorticism, a urine protein:creatinine ratio and systemic blood pressure may be mildly elevated, but neither are specific findings.
- A skin biopsy can confirm the diagnosis of calcinosis cutis, a pathognomonic finding for hyperadrenocorticism; other skin biopsy changes may be suggestive of an endocrinopathy but are not specific.
- A liver biopsy can show changes consistent with steroid hepatopathy, a sensitive but nonspecific marker of Cushing's syndrome.

Treatment

- Lack of suppression itself does not need to be treated.
- If the test result is owing to nonadrenal illness, therapy should be directed toward resolution of that disease.
- If Cushing's syndrome is believed to be present, therapy is directed toward management of hyperadrenocorticism; unless a complication of Cushing's syndrome is present that requires hospitalization (e.g., pulmonary thromboembolism), patients can be treated as outpatients.

Comments

Patient Monitoring

- If hyperadrenocorticism is present, follow-up is done depending on the type of therapy chosen (see Hyperadrenocorticism).
- If nonadrenal illness is present and believed possibly to be the cause of the abnormal UCCR results, the illness should be treated; once the animal is stable, the UCCR should be repeated or an ACTH response test should be performed after 4–8 weeks.

Possible Complications

Untreated hyperadrenocorticism can lead to development of all classic signs if not already present (e.g., polyuria, polydipsia, panting, polyphagia) as well as life-threatening complications such as pulmonary thromboembolism or diabetes mellitus.

AGE-RELATED FACTORS

- Nonadrenal illness can occur in an animal of any age.
- Hyperadrenocorticism is typically a disease of middle-aged to older cats and dogs, although it has been reported in dogs 1 year old.

Suggested Reading

Galac S, Kooistra HS, Teske E, Rijnberk A. Urinary corticoid/creatinine ratios in the differentiation between pituitary-dependent hyperadrenocorticism and hyperadrenocorticism due to adrenocortical tumour in the dog. Vet Q 1997;19:17–20.

Henry CJ, Clark TP, Young DW, Spano JS. Urine cortisol: creatinine ratio in healthy and sick cats. J Vet Intern Med 1996;10:123–126.

Jensen AL, Iversen L, Koch J, Hoier R, Petersen TK. Evaluation of the urinary cortisol: creatinine ratio in the diagnosis of hyperadrenocorticism in dogs. J Small Anim Pract 1997;38:99–102.

Kaplan AJ, Peterson ME, Kemppainen RJ. Effects of disease on the results of diagnostic tests for use in detecting hyperadrenocorticism in dogs. J Am Vet Med Assoc 1995;207:445–451.

Smiley LE, Peterson ME. Evaluation of a urine cortisol: creatinine ratio as a screening test for hyperadrenocorticism in dogs. J Vet Intern Med 1993;7:163–168.

Authors Ellen N. Behrend and Robert Kemppainen

Consulting Editor Karen Helton Rhodes

Thyroid Hormones

Deborah S. Greco

Definition/Overview

Serum concentrations of T_4, T_3, free thyroxine, or endogenous canine TSH outside the normal range

Etiology/Pathophysiology

- The thyroid gland regulates basal metabolism; two molecules, *tyrosine* and *iodine,* are important for thyroid hormone synthesis.
- The tyrosyl ring can accommodate two iodide molecules; if one iodide attaches, it is called *monoiodotyrosine* (MIT); if two iodide molecules attach to the tyrosyl ring, it is called *diiodotyrosine* (DIT).
- Two DIT molecules form T_4; one MIT coupled with one DIT molecule forms T_3.
- T_4 is the major storage form of thyroid hormone; T_3 is the active form of the hormone; most T_3 is formed outside the thyroid gland by deiodination of T_4.
- Another type of T_3 is formed when an iodide molecule is removed from the inner phenolic ring of T_4; this compound is called *reverse* T_3 and increases in nonthyroidal illness.
- Thyrotropin, or TSH, is the most important regulator of thyroid activity.
- TSH secretion is regulated by thyroid hormones via negative feedback inhibition of the synthesis of TRH at the level of the hypothalamus and by inhibition of the activity of TSH at the level of the pituitary.
- With thyroid gland failure, the pituitary gland senses decreases in serum free thyroxine (FT_4) and TT_4, resulting in increased serum endogenous TSH concentration.

- The use of endogenous TSH alone is not recommended as a method of assessing thyroid function.
- FT_4 concentrations are measured by equilibrium dialysis (gold standard) or analogue immunoassays.

Systems Affected

- Ophthalmic
- Nervous
- Endocrine/Metabolism
- Gastrointestinal
- Hepatobiliary
- Cardiovascular
- Renal
- Reproductive

Risk Factors

Greyhounds have approximately half the normal TT_4 and FT_4 concentrations of other dogs.

Laboratory Findings

Sample Handling

- Collect blood samples for TT_4, cTSH, and TT_3 and spin and freeze serum for submission; it should be mailed and arrive at laboratory cool; ice is not necessary.
- Plasma and serum samples for FT_4 by dialysis should arrive at laboratory frozen; may require the use of dry ice

Drugs That May Alter Laboratory Results

- Anesthetics
- Phenobarbital
- Primidone
- Diazepam
- Trimethoprim-sulfas
- Quinidine
- Phenylbutazone
- Salicylates
- Glucocorticoids

Disorders That May Alter Laboratory Results

- Any nonthyroidal illness
- Hyperadrenocorticism
- Renal failure
- Diabetes mellitus

- Liver disease
- Pregnancy

Valid If Run in Human Laboratory?

- Serum concentrations of thyroid hormone (TT_4) are much lower in dogs than in humans; therefore, TT_4 assays must be run in a veterinary diagnostic endocrine laboratory.
- Endogenous TSH is species-specific; therefore, TSH assays do not cross-react with canine or feline TSH.

CBC/Biochemistry/Urinalysis

- Normocytic, normochromic anemia resulting from erythropoietin deficiency, decreased bone marrow activity, and decreased serum iron and iron-binding capacity are observed in about 25–30% of hypothyroid dogs; clinicopathologic features of hyperthyroidism include erythrocytosis and excitement leukogram (neutrophilia, lymphocytosis).
- Hypercholesterolemia is seen in approximately 75% of hypothyroid dogs because of altered lipid metabolism, decreased fecal excretion of cholesterol, and decreased conversion of lipids to bile acids.
- Hyponatremia, a common finding in humans with hypothyroidism, is observed as a mild decrease in serum sodium in about 30% of hypothyroid dogs.
- Increased serum CPK, possibly as a result of hypothyroid myopathy
- Hyperthyroid cats may exhibit increased BUN.
- Serum activities of liver enzymes (ALT, AST) increase in most hyperthyroid cats.

Other Laboratory Tests

- The antithyroglobulin autoantibody test (ATAA)—the presence of antithyroglobulin antibodies theoretically presages the onset of hypothyroidism in dogs with autoimmune thyroiditis
- TSH stimulation test—was considered the gold standard for diagnosis of hypothyroidism in dogs; does not differentiate between early hypothyroid dogs and those with "euthyroid-sick" syndrome, nor does it identify dogs with secondary or tertiary hypothyroidism; exogenous bovine TSH is no longer commercially available
- TRH stimulation test
- FT_4 by dialysis (along with TT_4)
- Dynamic endocrine testing (see T_3 suppression test)

Diagnostics

Imaging

Thyroid scan with technetium-99m

Comments

Associated Conditions

- "Euthyroid-sick" syndrome is characterized by decreased serum TT_4 and increased reverse T_3.
- Concurrent illnesses such as diabetes mellitus, CRF, hepatic insufficiency, and infections can cause euthyroid-sick syndrome, resulting in decreased serum TT_4 concentrations.

Age-Related Factors

- Puppies exhibit serum TT_4 concentrations 2–5 times those of adult dogs.
- There is an age-related decline in serum TT_4 concentrations and response to TSH stimulation in dogs.

Pregnancy

May affect serum total T_4 concentrations because of changes in protein binding

Suggested Reading

Moncrieff JC, Nelson RW, Bruner JM, et al. Comparison of serum concentrations of thyroid-stimulating hormone in healthy dogs, hypothyroid dogs, and euthyroid dogs with concurrent disease. J Am Vet Med Assoc 1998;212:387–391.

Peterson ME, Melian C, Nichols R. Measurement of serum total thyroxine, triiodothyronine, free thyroxine and thyrotropin concentrations for diagnosis of hypothyroidism in dogs. J Am Vet Med Assoc 1997;211:1396–1402.

Author Deborah S. Greco

Consulting Editor Karen Helton Rhodes

Antinuclear Antibody (ANA) Titer/Lupus Erythematosus (LE) Cell Test

Albert H. Ahn and Francis W. K. Smith, Jr.

Definition/Overview

Indicated in animals suspected of having SLE

Positive ANA Test

- Indicates development of autoantibodies directed against a wide variety of normal cellular components, which may be associated with several immune-mediated diseases, most notably SLE
- In dogs, primarily IgG directed against individual histones
- A more sensitive test for SLE than the LE cell test, but a positive result may be seen in animals with other diseases

Positive LE Cell Test

- Indicates neutrophils are phagocytizing nuclear material that has been depolymerized and opsonized by ANA
- Typically, these neutrophils contain a large pink-purple cytoplasmic inclusion (LE body) that causes peripheral displacement of the nucleus; the LE body is void of any nuclear chromatin material
- Neutrophils containing LE bodies are referred to as LE cells; their presence establishes a positive test result
- Can be performed in the clinic
- Less sensitive than the ANA test but more specific for SLE; does not require species-specific reagents

Etiology/Pathophysiology

- In animals with SLE, autoantibody formation to cell tissue–nonspecific autoantigens is responsible for multisystemic lesions, which are generally characterized by a type III hypersensitivity reaction.
- In animals with SLE, autoantibody formation to cell tissue–specific autoantigens (involving antigens found on platelets and erythrocytes) results in fairly well-defined or specific lesions, typical of a type II hypersensitivity response.
- LE cells develop in vitro when fresh clotted blood from a patient with ANAs is incubated.

Systems Affected

- Musculoskeletal—symmetric nonerosive polyarthritis with shifting leg lameness; painful and swollen joints (especially the carpi, tarsi, metatarsi, stifle, and elbows); up to 75% of patients have symmetric polyarthritis during the course of disease
- Renal/Urologic—glomerulonephritis (with deposition of immune complexes) in up to 50% of patients; urinalysis reveals proteinuria
- Skin/Exocrine—dermatologic disease (bullous dermatitis) in up to 50% of patients
- Hemic/Lymph/Immune—peripheral lymphadenopathy in up to 30% of patients; hemolytic anemia in 25% of dogs with SLE; thrombocytopenia in 20% of dogs with SLE
- Nervous—depression and seizures may be seen in dogs

Signalment

Species

- Dogs and cats
- Healthy animals frequently have low positive ANA titer.

Breed Predilection

Shetland sheepdogs, poodles, Irish setters, Old English sheepdogs, German shepherds, beagles, collies

Mean Age and Range

- Middle-aged dogs (mean, 5.8 years)
- Reported in 2–12-year-old dogs

Signs

General Comments

- Severity of clinical signs does not parallel the magnitude of the titer.
- Vary with cause of positive test results

Historical Findings

- Lethargy
- Shifting leg lameness
- Dermatologic lesions
- Signs may modulate and change over time.

Physical Examination Findings

- Fever
- Lymphadenomegaly
- Swollen and painful joints
- Dermatologic lesions (e.g., scaling, ulceration, alopecia, and erythema), symmetric or focal
- Lesions involving the mouth and other mucocutaneous junctions commonly observed

Skin Disorders

- SLE—ANA titer (1:80−>1:160) most consistently high
- Pemphigus erythematosus (seldom pemphigus vulgaris)
- Discoid lupus
- Generalized demodicosis
- Flea bite hypersensitivity
- Plasma cell pododermatitis

Hematologic Disorders

- Immune-mediated hemolytic anemia
- Immune-mediated thrombocytopenia

Cardiopulmonary Disorders

- Bacterial endocarditis
- Heartworm disease

Drugs

- Griseofulvin
- Hydralazine
- Procainamide
- Sulfonamides
- Tetracyclines

Other Disorders

- Cholangiohepatitis
- FeLV
- FIP
- Rheumatoid arthritis
- Lymphocytic thyroiditis

- Various neoplasms
- Ulcerative autoimmune stomatitis—ANA titer 1:80–1:160

Differential Diagnosis

- Polyarthritis/myositis, proteinuria, bullous dermatitis/vasculitis, hemolytic anemia, and thrombocytopenia—consider SLE; positive ANA test and/or an LE cell test in conjunction with appropriate clinical signs establishes diagnosis; ANA titer is preferred by most veterinary labs; however, no single test is diagnostic
- Fever, murmur, shifting leg lameness—consider bacterial endocarditis
- Chronic cough, dyspnea, ascites—consider heartworm disease
- Exposure to causative drugs—consider drug-induced positive test result
- Icteric cat—consider cholangiohepatitis and FIP
- Dermatologic condition with low-moderate ANA titer—consider pemphigus erythematosus and pemphigus vulgaris
- Evidence of mass or tumor—consider neoplasia

Laboratory Findings

Drugs That May Alter Laboratory Results

- Cytotoxic drugs and chronic or high-dose corticosteroids lower ANA concentration.
- LE test more sensitive than ANA test to effects of corticosteroids

Disorders That May Alter Laboratory Results

LE cell test—low levels of complement or excessive amounts of heparin can cause false-negative test results

Valid If Run in Human Laboratory?

- ANA requires species-specific reagent.
- LE test valid

CBC/Biochemistry/Urinalysis

- Regenerative anemia and thrombocytopenia—consider SLE
- Eosinophilia—consider heartworm disease
- Leukocytosis—consider heartworm disease
- Proteinuria—consider glomerulonephritis secondary to SLE, endocarditis, and heartworm disease

Other Laboratory Tests

Serologic tests for FeLV and heartworm disease

Diagnostics

IMAGING

- Radiographs of affected joints—nonerosive arthritis characteristic of SLE
- Thoracic radiographs—rule out neoplasia and heartworm disease
- Echocardiography—rule out bacterial endocarditis in dogs with heart murmur
- Abdominal ultrasound—rule out neoplastic disease and cholangiohepatitis, if indicated

DIAGNOSTIC PROCEDURES

- Arthrocentesis of affected joints for fluid analysis—generally with SLE, fluid is characterized by a high neutrophil count and bacterial culture is negative
- Patients with skin lesions—biopsy for immunofluorescent and histopathologic testing
- Urine protein:creatinine ratio and possibly renal biopsy—might be indicated in dogs with marked proteinuria

ABBREVIATIONS

- FeLV = feline leukemia virus
- FIP = feline infectious peritonitis
- SLE = systemic lupus erythematosus

Suggested Reading

Lewis RM, Picut CA. Veterinary clinical immunology: classroom to clinic. Philadelphia: Lea & Febiger, 1989.

Meyer DJ, Harvey JW. Veterinary laboratory medicine: interpretation and diagnosis. 2nd ed. Philadelphia: Saunders, 1998.

Willard MD, Tvedten H, Turnwald GH. Small animal clinical diagnosis by laboratory methods. Philadelphia: Saunders, 1989.

Authors Albert H. Ahn and Francis W. K. Smith, Jr.

Consulting Editor Karen Helton Rhodes

Coombs' Test

Albert Ahn

Definition/Overview

- Positive results indicate the presence of RBCs that have been coated with antierythrocyte autoantibody as a result of primary AIHA or secondary IMHA.
- Test indicated in patients with anemia, especially regenerative anemia

Etiology/Pathophysiology

- Intravascular or extravascular hemolysis resulting in anemia can occur as a sequela to certain bacterial and parasitic infections, chemical and plant exposures, immune-mediated diseases, erythrocyte defects, fragmentation processes, and electrolyte abnormalities.
- Immune-mediated disease—antierythrocyte autoantibody production; RBCs bearing these immunoglobulins on their surface are phagocytized and cleared by the liver, spleen, lymph nodes, and macrophages
- Affected animals may be severely anemic.
- Animals with intravascular hemolysis exhibit the classic signs of icterus, dark red (wine-colored) urine, and pallor; occasionally, they develop thromboembolic disorders and even DIC.

Systems Affected

If Accompanied by Anemia

- Hemic/Lymph/Immune—hemolysis can result in marked reduction of PCV

- Hepatobiliary—hemolysis can lead to hyperbilirubinemia with development of icterus
- Respiratory—response to hypoxia in severely anemic patients includes compensatory mechanisms that lead to tachypnea
- Cardiovascular—response to hypoxia results in a compensatory increase in heart rate
- Renal/Urologic—reduced perfusion and hypoxia can cause tubular necrosis

Signalment

Primary AIHA

- Dogs and rarely cats
- Any age
- Predilection for females
- Cocker spaniels, poodles, Old English sheepdogs, Irish setters, English springer spaniels, and collies

Signs

Historical Findings

- No signs, associated with the positive test result
- Signs, if any, relate to associated anemia and its cause (e.g., weakness, exercise intolerance, lethargy, syncope, tachypnea, and dyspnea).

Physical Examination Findings

Findings associated with IMHA

- Hepatomegaly
- Splenomegaly
- Icterus
- Pale mucous membranes
- Tachypnea
- Tachycardia

Secondary IMHA

- Infectious agents—viruses or modified live virus vaccines, *Hemobartonella, Babesia, Leptospira, Dirofilaria, Ehrlichia,* feline leukemia virus
- Microangiopathic processes
- Drugs—cephalosporins, heparin, quinidine, methimazole, propylthiouracil, sulfa compounds
- Neoplasia—especially lymphoma, malignant histiocytosis, and hemangiosarcoma

Differential Diagnosis

- Secondary problems must be ruled out.
- Some dogs with AIHA have nonregenerative anemia with or without a positive test.
- Between 25–30% of dogs with AIHA have a negative test.

Positive Test (Dogs)

- In animal with signs of hemolytic anemia, confirms an immune-mediated cause
- Rare in normal dogs

Other Causes of Hemolysis

- Dogs—onion and zinc ingestion, splenic torsion, and pyruvate kinase deficiency
- Cats—oxidant toxicity (e.g., acetaminophen, propylene glycol, and methylene blue) and anemia secondary to retrovirus infection

Laboratory Findings

Drugs That May Affect Laboratory Results

- Cephalosporins rarely reported to cause positive test
- Antibodies to transfused RBCs (alloantibodies) may be present in dogs.
- Previous treatment with steroids not likely to interfere if hemolysis is ongoing

Disorders That May Alter Laboratory Results

None

Valid If Run in Human Laboratory?

Species-specific reagent must be used.

CBC/Biochemistry/Urinalysis

In Patients with Concurrent Anemia

- CBC—anisocytosis, polychromasia, presence of spherocytes and nucleated RBCs, neutrophilic leukocytosis with left shift, hemoglobinemia, and elevation of MCV
- Biochemistry—high concentration of ALT and hyperbilirubinemia
- Urinalysis—bilirubinuria and hemoglobinuria

Other Laboratory Tests

- Serologic tests for appropriate infectious agents
- Coagulation profile to diagnose DIC
- Platelet count to diagnose Evan's syndrome or early DIC
- Reticulocyte count to determine if anemia is regenerative

Radiography

- Splenomegaly
- Hepatomegaly

ULTRASONOGRAPHY

- Hepatomegaly—with hyperechoic or hypoechoic parenchymal changes
- Splenomegaly
- Hyperdynamic cardiac changes consistent with anemic state

Diagnostic Procedures

Bone marrow aspiration typically reveals erythroid hyperplasia, although some animals with nonregenerative anemia may have low numbers of erythroid precursors.

Suggested Reading

Duncan JR, Prasse KW, Mahaffey EA. Veterinary laboratory medicine: clinical pathology. 3rd ed. Ames, IA: Iowa State University Press, 1994.

Lewis RM, Picut CA. Veterinary clinical immunology. Philadelphia: Lea & Febiger, 1989.

Meyer DJ, Coles EH, Rich LJ. Veterinary laboratory medicine: interpretation and diagnosis. Philadelphia: Saunders, 1992.

Author Albert H. Ahn

Consulting Editor Karen Helton Rhodes

APPENDIX I

CLIENT EDUCATION HANDOUT

STAPHYLOCCAL BLEPHARITIS: ANOTHER MANIFESTATION OF ALLERGIC DERMATITIS

Karen Helton Rhodes, DVM, Dip. ACVD
Ilene Katz, Dermatology Technician

Many canine patients with allergy are extremely pruritic in the periocular region. In some of these cases we may only see erythema or conjunctivitis, which readily respond to antiinflammatory ophthalmics. A small subset of these dogs will present with marked erythema, swelling/induration, and a papular eruption along the lid margins. These cases may have a primary staphylococcal blepharitis OR the infection and hypersensitivity may be secondary to allergic dermatitis. Some of these cases are so severe they may mimic autoimmune disorders. A biopsy of the periocular tissue will confirm the diagnosis.

THERAPY:

1. Eyelid scrubs: 1 drop of baby shampoo mixed in a cup of warm water; gently "scrub" the periocular and lid region with a wash cloth; often recommended as a twice-weekly protocol
2. Ophthalmic ointment: erythromycin ophthalmic (ocular & periocular) tid for 7–10 days
3. Cephalexin @ 10 mg/# PO tid for 21 days
4. After the initial 10 days of antibacterial ophthalmic ointment, I often recommend an antiinflammatory ointment (such as neomycin/polymyxin/dexamethasone) as a preventative to be used twice weekly during the allergy season; this step may be avoided if the case appears to be primary staphylococcal blepharitis rather than secondary to allergic dermatitis

ANTIHISTAMINE THERAPY

Karen Helton Rhodes, DVM, DVM, Dip. ACVD

—Antihistamines are effective in approximately 50% of allergic patients.
—To determine which antihistamine is effective for your pet, it is advisable to trial the selected drug for a minimum of 7–10 days before assuming that it is ineffective in controlling your pet's itchiness.
—Be sure to use the antihistamines one at a time.
—"Over-the-counter" medications may be used first before the prescription medications.
—Sometimes it is beneficial to grade the response to each drug on a scale of 0–5 so that at the end of the trials you will be able to easily determine which was most effective for your pet.
—It is not necessary to use each antihistamine if you find one that is effective for your pet.

"Over-the-counter" antihistamines:

1. Diphenhydramine (BENADRYL) 25-mg capsules: use________caps 3 times daily for 7–10 days & then as needed
2. Chlorpheniramine (CHLORTRIMETON) 4-mg tabs: use_______tabs 3 times daily for 7–10 days & then as needed
   8-mg tabs: use_______ tabs 3 times daily for 7–10 days & then as needed
3. Clemastine (TAVIST-1) 1.34-mg tabs: use______tabs twice daily for 7–10 days & then as needed

PRESCRIPTION ANTIHISTAMINES: * to be provided by Dr. Karen Helton Rhodes

1. Misoprostol (CYTOTEC)
2. Hydroxyzine (ATARAX)
3. Trimeprazine-prednisone (TEMARIL-P)—The combination allows for a lower dose of cortisone
4. Doxepin (SINEQUAN)
5. Cyproheptadine (PERIACTIN)
6. Amitriptyline (ELAVIL)

NOTES:

PHONE COMMUNICATION INFORMATION FOR DERMATOLOGY PATIENTS

Karen Helton Rhodes, DVM, Dip. ACVD
DERMATOLOGY CONSULTATIONS

1. The dermatology service is available for clinic visits @ the animal emergency & referral center.
2. Your veterinarian has a complete report of each dermatology examination in your file. We fax a detailed referral letter the same day as the examination. Your referring veterinarian may be able to assist if you have an immediate question and are unable to contact the dermatology service.
3. Dermatology is a specialty service and is not available at all times for your calls. A phone mail system has been installed for any questions that you may have. Please be advised that these calls will be monitored and returned as frequently as possible. A busy clinic schedule may necessitate your leaving a daytime and an evening telephone number. Every attempt will be made to return your call within 24 hours.
4. Please remember, phone call reports on the clinical progress of your pet are no substitute for a follow-up examination. Re-check examinations are generally suggested approximately 3–4 weeks after the initial visit.

"PHONE MAIL" NUMBER FOR DERMATOLOGY: 973-226-3282

DERMATOLOGY CONSULTATIONS
@
ANIMAL EMERGENCY AND REFERRAL CENTER
WEST CALDWELL, NJ
973-226-3282

KAREN HELTON RHODES, DVM
DIP, AMERICAN COLLEGE OF VETERINARY DERMATOLOGY

ILENE KATZ
DERMATOLOGY TECHNICIAN

CANINE ALLERGIC DERMATITIS

Karen Helton Rhodes, DVM, Dip. ACVD
Ilene Katz, Dermatology Technician

Canine allergy is a common and frustrating problem in veterinary practice. A wide variety of breeds suffer from allergic dermatitis and otitis. The usual, yet not exclusive, age of onset is between 2 and 6 years of age. Pure-breed dogs will often exhibit clinical signs at an earlier age.

HOW DOES AN ALLERGIC REACTION OCCUR?

—The body is constantly exposed to environmental allergens (molds, pollens, dust mites, fleas). Both healthy and allergic dogs will produce antibodies (IgE, IgG, IgM) to combat these foreign proteins.
—The allergic dog is thought to produce significantly higher levels of IgE (considered the most important antibody in producing allergic signs/symptoms) than the clinically normal dog.
—There is no specific level of IgE that will produce pruritus (itching)—each dog has its own "threshold" (an allergic dog is often thought to have a lower threshold or "tolerance" which makes it more susceptible).
—Classic clinical signs of allergy:
- biting, chewing, scratching
- feet, face, axillae, inguinal regions are predominant
- chronic ear infections/ inflammation
- chronic irritation from pruritus may lead to lichenification (thickened & pigmented skin)
- flea allergy: often near the tail and rump region

—You cannot clinically tell the difference between food allergy and inhalant/percutaneous allergy (note: there is no valid serum test for food allergy from any lab—you must do a food elimination diet trial).
—"Pathway" of allergic reaction:
- allergen exposure—body produces IgE specific for that allergen
- IgE binds to the mast cells in the skin and "coats" them
- Re-exposure to the allergen
- Allergen binds to the allergen-specific IgE
- Allergen: IgE: Mast cell binding causes the mast cell to degranulate (rupture)
- Mast cells contain pruritic (itchy) compounds—histamines, leukotrienes, prostaglandins, etc.

TYPES OF ALLERGY TESTING

1. "*in vitro*" (serum/plasma). . . . . . . RAST (radioallergosorbant test): uses radioactive tag
. . . . ELISA (enzyme-linked immunosorbant assay): uses an enzyme tag
2. "*in vivo*" (intradermal skin testing)

—The pet is tranquilized and an area is shaved on the side of the chest.
—Anywhere from 50–80 allergens are then injected intradermally (into the skin).

—The reactions are then measured against a positive and negative control.

—Intradermal Skin Testing (IDST) is considered the "gold standard" of allergy testing.

PREPARATION FOR THE PROCEDURE (IDST)

—Certain medications may interfere with the test results and should be withdrawn prior to the test date (see the chart below for guidelines).

Medication	Approximate Withdrawal Time Prior to Testing
Steroids (oral, otic, ophthalmic, topical)	3–4 weeks
Steroids (injectable DepoMedrol)	6–8 weeks
Antihistamines	10–14 days
Ketoconazole	2 weeks
Phenobarbital	>3 weeks
Acepromazine	>1 week

CANINE ALLERGY: INTRADERMAL SKIN TESTING PREPARATION

Karen Helton Rhodes, DVM, Dip. ACVD

Canine allergy is a common and frustrating problem in veterinary practice. A wide variety of breeds suffer from allergic dermatitis and otitis. The usual, yet not exclusive, age of onset is between 2 and 6 years of age. Pure bred dogs will often exhibit clinical signs at an earlier age.

Many antipruritic medications are either ineffective or inappropriate for the individual patient. Intradermal skin testing (IDST) is a readily available option for the client. This procedure (IDST) is still considered by veterinary dermatologists to be the "gold standard" for evaluating allergic dermatitis in the dog and cat. Serum testing still has many drawbacks in the veterinary patient that have not yet been overcome. The decision to pursue allergy testing should be carefully considered by the client and the veterinarian since the hyposensitization process requires a year-long commitment. The vaccine protocol requires frequent subcutaneous injections, with an average response noted within 6–12 months after initiation.

Preparation for the procedure is quite simple. Certain medications can interfere with the test results and should be withdrawn prior to the test date (see the chart below for guidelines). The procedure generally requires that the pet stay at the hospital for most of the day. Clients may elect to "drop off" their pet for the day and return at a later time (after work, etc.). We will try to accommodate the owner and make the procedure as convenient as possible. I will examine the pet and discuss all of the details of the procedure and the hyposensitization process with the owners.

Please feel free to call with any questions you may have regarding the procedure.

Medication	Withdrawal Time Prior to Testing
Steroids (oral, otic, ophthalmic, topical)	3–4 weeks
Steroids (Injectable Depo-Medrol)	6–8 weeks
Antihistamines	10 DAYS to 2 weeks
Ketoconazole	2 weeks
Phenobarbital	>3 weeks
Acepromazine	>1 week

GENERAL INFORMATION
ALLERGY VACCINE: HYPOSENSITIZATION

Karen Helton Rhodes, DVM, Dip. ACVD
Ilene Katz, Dermatology Technician
DERMATOLOGY CONSULTATIONS

TECHNIQUE FOR INJECTIONS: SUBCUTANEOUS (UNDER THE SKIN)

1. Keep the vaccine refrigerated.
2. Syringes and needles are disposable and should only be used once. Please bring the used syringes and needles to us or your referring veterinarian for safe disposal as medical waste.
3. Insert the needle underneath the skin over the neck, shoulder, or back area. Once in position, push the plunger and release the contents under the skin. Pull the needle out of the skin and discard. Vary your injection sites to avoid pain.

HOW ALLERGEN EXTRACTS WORK:

1. Hyposensitization (allergy vaccine) is an attempt to induce immunologic tolerance to allergens that currently cause allergic symptoms.
2. The rate at which an animal may respond to allergy vaccine is varied and the animal may take up to 6 months or even a year to build up enough "protective" antibodies to eliminate the allergic symptoms.
3. Hyposensitization is not a "cure" for allergies. Maintenance injections must be continued for the life of the pet. The interval between injections will vary with each animal but is generally given on a monthly basis once a good clinical response is achieved. DO NOT STOP THE VACCINE UNLESS YOU AND YOUR VETERINARIAN DECIDE THAT HYPOSENSITIZATION IS NOT ACCEPTABLE FOR YOUR PET.
4. Try to adhere to the suggested schedule of injections.

ADVERSE REACTIONS:

1. Reactions to allergy vaccine are rare.
2. There may be mild itchiness or irritation at the injection site for a few minutes after the injection.
3. Always give the injection when you will be able to watch your pet for at least 1 hour afterward.
4. During the early stages of hyposensitization, an increase in itchiness is common 1 or 2 days after the injection. If this is a problem for your pet, you may need to use topical therapy or antihistamines to help control the clinical signs.
5. The most severe reaction is anaphylactic shock. Your pet is being given very small amounts of allergens slowly to help prevent this occurrence. If anaphylaxis occurs, it will manifest within 30 minutes to 1 hour after the injection is given. This severe reaction will appear as vomiting, diarrhea, generalized hives, swollen face, and/or difficulty breathing and weakness. Take your pet to a veterinarian immediately.

INTERACTIONS WITH OTHER MEDICATIONS AND VACCINES:

1. Allergy vaccines will not interfere with other routine vaccines (distemper, parvo, rabies, etc.).
2. Large doses of prednisone or other corticosteroids may decrease or retard the effectiveness of the vaccine and should therefore be avoided if at all possible. Low doses are certainly acceptable.

BACTERIAL INFECTIONS:

1. Superficial pyoderma (bacterial folliculitis) is an infection of the skin and hair follicles recognized by the appearance of a rash, pimples, pustules, scabs, and "hot spots."
2. In certain short-coated breeds, these infections can appear merely as patches of circular hair loss.
3. *Staphylococcus intermedius* (Staph infection) is the frequent cause of this condition and is often seen in association with allergies.
4. Staphylococcal bacteria are part of the normal flora of the skin and are thus not considered contagious to you or other pets in the household.
5. Shampoo therapy and, often, oral antibiotics are needed to control superficial pyoderma in allergic patients.
6. Bacterial infections can contribute to your pet's itchiness.

FLEA CONTROL:

1. Flea control is vitally important for the allergic pet.
2. You do not have to see fleas in order for them to be a contributing factor in your pet's itchiness.
3. A flea-allergic pet does not generally have a severe flea infestation but rather a massive reaction to the saliva of the flea.

YEAST INFECTIONS:

1. *Malassezia pachydermatis* (yeast) overgrowth is a common cutaneous opportunist in allergic patients.
2. The organism may colonize the skin and/or the ear canal.
3. Allergic patients produce excess amounts of wax in the ear canal, which is a good microenvironment for yeast and bacterial overgrowth.
4. Yeast organisms may cause excessive pruritus and inflamed skin.
5. These organisms are not contagious to you or other pets in the household.

REMEMBER:

1. Hyposensitization is only a component or an integral part in controlling your pet's allergic symptoms.
2. Shampoo therapy should be part of your routine protocol.
3. Antihistamines or other medications may be necessary.
4. Hyposensitization is effective for approximately 75% of all tested patients. Vaccine therapy should be continued for at least 1 year before results can be evaluated.
5. Please contact your veterinarian or the dermatology service @ 973-226-3282 if you have any questions or problems with your pet. A re-check appointment is generally recommended 6 months (@ no charge) into the vaccine protocol.

ALLERGY VACCINE SCHEDULE

Karen Helton Rhodes, DVM, Dip. ACVD
DERMATOLOGY CONSULTATIONS

ALLERGY VACCINE SCHEDULE:

DAY	VIAL 1	VIAL 2	VIAL 3
1	0.1cc		
2			
3	0.2cc		
4			
5	0.4cc		
6			
7	0.6cc		
8			
9	0.8cc		
10			
11		0.1cc	
12			
13		0.2cc	
14			
15		0.4cc	
16			
17		0.6cc	
18			
19		0.8cc	
20			
21			0.1cc
22			
23			0.2cc
24			
25			0.4cc
26			
27			0.6cc
28			
29			0.8cc
30			
31			1.0cc

** CONTINUE WITH VIAL # 3 AS THE MAINTENANCE VIAL AND SLOWLY INCREASE THE INTERVAL BETWEEN INJECTIONS

34.. 1.0cc
40.. 1.0cc
47.. 1.0cc

Continue with weekly injections until you start to see an improvement in clinical symptoms (itching)

* AFTER an improvement is noted, the interval can be varied from weekly to monthly (as needed to control the symptoms); at the 6-month re-check visit we can discuss altering the maintenance volume (0.6cc to 1.0cc)

KEEP ALL VACCINES REFRIGERATED—DO NOT FREEZE
(Extreme heat and extreme cold are to be avoided)

ALL VACCINES ARE TO BE GIVEN SUBCUTANEOUSLY—"UNDER THE SKIN"

SCHEDULE A RE-CHECK APPOINTMENT (NO CHARGE) WITHIN 6 MONTHS OF STARTING THE VACCINE SERIES

RE-ORDER INFORMATION:
Call 973-226-3282 to re-order the vaccine (vial #3) approximately 2 weeks prior to finishing vial #3. Vials 1 & 2 from the starter set can be discarded. Only vial #3 will be used as the maintenance vial.

CONTACTS: KAREN HELTON RHODES, DVM, DIP. ACVD
ILENE KATZ, DERMATOLOGY TECHNICIAN

HOUSE DUST MITE: CONTROLLING EXPOSURE

Karen Helton Rhodes, DVM, Dip. ACVD
DERMATOLOGY CONSULTATIONS

House dust mites are microscopic and ubiquitous. They feed on human and animal dander, skin scales, and hair. They are frequently found in beds, mattresses, carpets, sofas, and pet bedding. Mites can flourish in the home environment because the temperature and humidity are optimum (50–70% relative humidity).

Hypersensitivity to house dust mites is a common problem for both animals and humans.

It is difficult and even impossible to eliminate mites from the environment of an allergic patient. An effective environmental control regimen can help to decrease the numbers of mites and therefore minimize the patient's discomfort. Also, hyposensitization therapy (allergy vaccines) can be effective in controlling or reducing the clinical symptoms associated with mite allergy.

The following steps may help control mite populations (special attention should be given to the sleeping areas of the allergic pet):

1. Avoid the use of carpeting. Bare floors, such as hardwood, vinyl, or tile are best; if carpet must be used, low pile is preferable.
2. Remove upholstered furniture, books, records, piles of newspapers and magazines, stuffed animals, wall hangings, and other "dust collectors" from the room.
3. Use only synthetic material in the pet's bedding. Feathers, wool, or horsehair stuffing should be avoided. Remember, cedar shavings are often a source of allergic dermatitis in the dog.
4. Wash all bedding frequently in hot water.
5. If your pet sleeps on the bed, encase mattresses and box springs in airtight plastic and seal zippers on these casings with tape. Use washable blankets and mattress pads. The most dust-free type of bed is a waterbed.
6. Plants can also be "dust collectors" and should be removed.
7. Change the furnace and air conditioning filters frequently. Electrostatic filters may be more effective in filtering out dust, mites, and inhalant particles. No specific research has been performed on these filters and their performance in controlling clinical signs of allergy in the dog.
8. Use air conditioning to control the temperature during warm months. Central air conditioning is preferred, but window units are also helpful. Try to maintain the humidity levels between 30 and 50%. Dehumidifiers may prove beneficial.
9. Vacuum floors, wet mop, and dust with a damp cloth daily. The room should be properly aired after vacuuming.
10. Groom animal frequently, preferably outside of the house environment.

MOLD ALLERGIES: CONTROLLING EXPOSURE

Karen Helton Rhodes, DVM, Dip. ACVD
DERMATOLOGY CONSULTATIONS

Most fungi and molds grow best in warm and humid climates yet they may be found in all types of regions from the tropics to the arctic and desert regions. Because of their ubiquitous nature, molds may be a source of environmental inhalant allergens in the home. Fungi generally depend on other organic substances for nutrients and energy. Molds are often found in refrigerators, shower stalls, basements, houseplant mulch, filters used with evaporate coolers, and humidifiers.

The following are most often found in the home:

1. *Alternaria:* windows, doorways, basements, evaporative coolers and humidifiers
2. *Aspergillus:* houseplants, kitchen mold
3. *Cladosporium* & *hormodendrum:* bathrooms, shower stalls, condensate on tile, behind baseboards, wood paneling, and wood floors
4. *Penicillium:* kitchen mold
5. *Rhizopus:* kitchen mold

Mold allergies can contribute to year-round clinical symptoms, with flare-ups during the winter months or during humid seasons. Spray wherever possible with fungicidal products to help eliminate spores. Change filters on cooling systems, furnaces, and humidifiers frequently. Use dehumidifiers to reduce the population of mold spores. Avoid houseplants, as the mulch tends to encourage mold growth.

CONTACT DERMATITIS

Karen Helton Rhodes, DVM, Dip. ACVD
DERMATOLOGY CONSULTATIONS

Contact hypersensitivity is the result of sensitization to an environmental allergen with subsequent reaction upon contact. It is classically a delayed (type IV) hypersensitivity, which may be the result of sensitization to any number of substances. Sensitization often results from introduction of new materials into the animals' environment; however, cases of hypersensitivity after previously uneventful contact with a substance for periods of time (months to years) are also reported. Fabrics and chemicals are probably the most common offending agents. Leafy plants used for ground cover have also been incriminated. Very thorough investigation is often necessary to determine the material responsible for the hypersensitivity. Patch testing, as is used in humans, has been used in dogs but the results have been equivocal. Isolation from suspect substances with subsequent challenge is the best method to detect an offending agent.

PLAN:

1. T-SHIRTS TO AVOID ANY POTENTIAL CONTACTANT AND HELP PREVENT SELF-TRAUMA
2. ORAL MEDICATIONS:____
3. TOPICAL MEDICATIONS:_____________________________________

SHAMPOO THERAPY: INSTRUCTIONS

Karen Helton Rhodes, DVM, Dip. ACVD
DERMATOLOGY CONSULTATIONS

A specific shampoo therapy has been selected for your pet. This shampoo is medicated and the instructions must be followed closely if your pet is to receive the full benefit of the treatment. Most shampoos and topical rinses are to be used as an adjunct to other forms of therapy (oral medication, hyposensitization, etc.). Often, shampoo therapy is recommended as a maintenance protocol to guard against relapse of the dermatologic condition and to prolong the health of the skin.

Steps to follow:

1. The air temperature in the bathing area should be warm; the water temperature should be lukewarm, unless otherwise specified. Wet the coat thoroughly.
2. Pay particular attention to the affected areas of your pet's skin. Apply sufficient shampoo to these affected areas and rub in well. Then proceed to lather the rest of your pet's haircoat. Some shampoos will lather better than others will, although the active ingredients may be equally effective.
3. Allow the shampoo to remain on the coat for **15–20 minutes.** Contact time with the shampoo is very important. For best results, use a timer. If bathing in the backyard, you may allow the dog to run free while soapy for the required 15–20 minutes.
4. Rinsing is as important as shampooing. Unrinsed shampoo may cause irritation to the skin.
5. Apply a medicated conditioner or rinse to the skin and coat, if indicated. Lightly rinse the coat after application.
6. Towel dry. You may use a blow dryer, but be sure that the temperature is warm, not hot.
7. Repeat the shampoo therapy every_____days for _____ weeks.
   and then. . . . ___________________

MEDICATED SHAMPOO	MEDICATED RINSE	TOPICAL OINTMENT/ SPRAY/ETC.
___________	___________	____________________

additional Tx:

CANINE OTITIS EXTERNA

Karen Helton Rhodes, DVM, Dip. ACVD
Ilene Katz, Dermatology Technician
DERMATOLOGY CONSULTATIONS

Otitis externa is a common clinical problem among dogs and is often a frustrating disease to cure or even control.

PRIMARY AND PREDISPOSING CAUSES OF OTITIS EXTERNA:

1. Parasites
2. Allergy
3. Contact irritant
4. Keratinization disorders (epidermal maturation problems)
5. Autoimmune disorders
6. Foreign body
7. Metabolic diseases
8. Conformational abnormalities (alter the microenvironment)
9. Microanatomy variability among species (e.g., cockers, labs, spaniels have been found to have more apocrine glands and hair follicles than mongrel dogs)
10. Excessive moisture (medications, swimming, etc. can macerate the tissue)
11. Obstructive ear disease can trap moisture and debris
12. Overzealous cleaning

SECONDARY INVADERS:

1. Yeast (*malassezia pachydermatis*)
2. Gram-positive bacteria (e.g., *staphylococcus*)
3. Gram-negative bacteria (e.g., *pseudomonas, proteus,* etc.)

COMPLICATIONS THAT CONTRIBUTE TO CHRONICITY OF LESIONS:

1. Chronic inflammation causes the epithelial lining of the ear canal to be thrown into proliferative folds, which hinder cleansing.
2. Chronic inflammation stimulates epidermal thickening, enlarged ceruminous glands, and fibrosis (scar), which may lead to a stenotic (narrowed) canal.
3. Scar tissue and calcification may result from chronic inflammation: may cause excessive discomfort and trap infection

THERAPY:

1. Routine cleansing with______number of times per week______
*Remember to wait 15 minutes after cleansing before medication is applied (the cleanser may dilute the medication)
2. Topical medication(s)
_______ # OF DROPS______ # TIMES PER DAY_________ FOR ______WEEKS
_______ # OF DROPS______ # TIMES PER DAY_________ FOR ______WEEKS
3. ORAL MEDICATION________________ RE-CHECK IN_____DAYS/WEEKS

MALASSEZIA DERMATITIS (YEAST):

Karen Helton Rhodes, DVM, Dip. ACVD
Ilene Katz, Dermatology Technician

Malassezia pachydermatis is a saprophytic yeast that is commonly found on both normal and abnormal skin. It is often difficult to ascertain if the yeast organisms are a primary contributor (yeast hypersensitivity) to the clinical lesions present or if they function as merely secondary invaders (underlying etiology; allergic dermatitis, etc.) of compromised skin. Clinical lesions most commonly associated with malassezia dermatitis include: erythema, scaling dermatitis (yellow-gray), greasy surface, crusting, and malodorous. The animal is extremely pruritic (itchy) and uncomfortable. Many of these cases have been poorly responsive to common therapeutics used to control pruritus. Approximately 50% of affected animals have an underlying cause, which must be explored.

Specific and accurate diagnosis of malassezia dermatitis is often difficult and may rely heavily on clinical evaluation of the cutaneous lesions. Treatment involves a combination of oral (ketoconazole or itraconazole) and topical (ketoconazole shampoo, selenium sulfide, or "malaseb" shampoo) anti-fungal medications. Many of these cases require chronic maintenance shampoo therapy to maintain the yeast population at an acceptable and nonclinical level.

Notes:

CANINE BACTERIAL INFECTIONS

Karen Helton Rhodes, DVM, Dip. ACVD
Ilene Katz, Dermatology Technician

Bacterial infections (pyoderma) of the skin and hair follicles are very common problems in the dog. These lesions often represent an infection of "overcolonization" of the skin by *staphylococcus intermedius.* Pyoderma often manifests in a characteristic sequence of lesions: follicular papule, pustule, crust from a ruptured pustule, epidermal collarette (central clearing with peripheral ring of scale), and a final hyperpigmented macule. In certain breeds, these infections can appear as merely patchy and circular areas of hair loss. The causative organism ("staph") is considered normal "resident" flora. There are several reasons that the "staph" are given the opportunity to cause disease and those reasons must be identified in order to prevent recurrences. Common causes include: allergies, parasite infestation, hormonal imbalances, keratinization disorders, immunodeficiencies, etc.

SUPERFICIAL PYODERMA (FOLLICULITIS):

Superficial folliculitis (pyoderma) may be a primary condition or secondary to other underlying diseases such as allergic dermatitis, endocrine abnormalities, immunosuppression, etc. Most cases of superficial pyoderma are associated with minimal pruritus (itching), although some dogs may experience marked pruritus owing to a presumed hypersensitivity to the staphylococcal bacteria. When pruritus is a feature, it is often necessary to evaluate the response of the patient to antibiotic therapy to determine if an underlying problem may be contributing to the clinical picture. Antibiotics must be used for a minimum of 3 weeks and given in conjunction with topical shampoo therapy. Steroids must be avoided during this evaluation period.

RECURRENT SUPERFICIAL PYODERMA:

Recurrent superficial pyoderma is a common and frustrating problem in the dog. If a specific underlying etiology cannot be determined (allergy, hypothyroidism, hyperadrenocorticism, diabetes mellitus, neoplasia, etc.) then efforts must be made to control the cutaneous bacterial population and/or stimulate the patient's immune status. Various methods may be trialed to manipulate the patient's response to it's normal flora: intermittent antibiotic therapy, subminimal inhibitory concentrations of antibiotics, aggressive shampoo and other topical therapy, immunomodulators, etc. An important aspect of managing these chronic cases is the establishment of an effective and acceptable therapeutic maintenance protocol.

DEEP PYODERMA:

Folliculitis and furunculosis, deep pyoderma, is a common and frustrating problem in the canine patient. Most of these cases involve a staphylococcal infection of the hair follicles which has become severe and caused a rupture of the follicular epithelium. This allows the hair shaft, keratin, and damaged collagen access to the dermis and thus initiates a "foreign body" reaction. The massive amount of inflammation accumulated as a result of this reaction accounts for the clinical signs of erythema and swelling with exudation. The tendency for this type of inflammation to be granulomatous causes a therapeutic problem in that treatment must be specific and continued for an extended period of time.

A complete metabolic diagnostic work-up is recommended to eliminate the possibility of underlying disease acting as a contributory factor. A cutaneous biopsy and surgically obtained culture are sometimes helpful in characterizing this disease.

Systemic antibiotic therapy is often necessary for a minimum of 6–8 weeks. Shampoo therapy with a benzoyl peroxide or chlorhexidine product should be used in conjunction with oral therapy. Often, the hair must be shaved to prevent the formation of a sealing crust and to allow the topical agents to contact the diseased skin. Hydrotherapy (soaks and/or whirlpool) with an antiseptic is beneficial in the early stages of therapy to allow for removal of crusts, decreasing the surface bacterial counts, promoting epithelialization, and to decrease discomfort.

PODODERMATITIS:

Pododermatitis is a form of deep pyoderma that affects the interdigital areas of the paws. Often in cases of deep pyoderma, this will be the last area to respond to therapy. A complete diagnostic work-up is necessary to rule out causes other than bacterial (i.e., demodicosis, *malassezia,* etc.). Oral antibiotics for an extended period (6–8 weeks) in association with topical therapy are necessary. Successful therapy requires a commitment from the owner because of the extensive protocol involved:

Step 1. Shampoo the feet with a benzoyl peroxide or chlorhexidine product. Allow the feet to soak in the shampoo for at least 15–20 minutes. Initial protocol—daily, and then the interval can be lengthened.
Step 2. Dry the feet and apply an astringent liberally to the area (i.e., domboros. Let air dry—this step may be needed on a once-daily or tid regimen.
Step 3. Apply a topical ointment or gel (mupirocin ointment or benzoyl peroxide gel). Use a tid regiment in the initial stages, and then the frequency may be tapered.
Note** Step 2 may be eliminated when the area becomes less moist and exudative.

Remember that a maintenance protocol should be instituted that includes both shampoo and topical therapy. The frequency of application required to control the clinical lesions will vary with the patient.

Notes:

CANINE DEMODICOSIS

Karen Helton Rhodes, DVM, Dip. ACVD
Ilene Katz, Dermatology Technician

Canine demodicosis is an inflammatory parasitic disease characterized by the presence of greater than normal numbers of *demodex canis* mites in the hair follicles and on the skin. The reason for this proliferation is poorly understood but a genetic defect in the T-cell portion of the immune system is suspected.

There are two forms of demodicosis: 1) localized and 2) generalized. The localized form is characterized by small focal regional lesions. The lesions associated with localized demodicosis are typically focal mild erythema with partial alopecia and variable amounts of scale. The most frequently affected sites of lesions in this form are the periocular and perioral regions, with the forelegs and the trunk as the second most common site. Most of the localized demodicosis cases are benign and regress spontaneously; however, approximately 10% of cases will progress to the generalized form. The generalized form may be divided into juvenile (dogs less than 1 year of age), adult onset, and pododemodicosis. Generalized demodicosis can be quite severe and the lesions include erythema, alopecia, crust, scale, and exudation. Pruritus is variably present. Some dogs may have pododemodicosis only, without involvement of other sites. Secondary pyoderma is a consistent feature in generalized demodicosis.

LOCALIZED DEMODICOSIS THERAPY

Treatment of localized demodicosis is not always necessary as the majority of cases will spontaneously cure. Treatment will not prevent progression to the generalized form. The general health status of the patient should be evaluated—i.e., intestinal parasitism, diet, etc.—to ensure that underlying abnormalities do not contribute to the animal's predisposition to demodicosis. Topical therapy for localized cases include Goodwinol ointment or benzoyl peroxide gel.

GENERALIZED DEMODICOSIS THERAPY

Therapy for generalized demodicosis requires dedication and time and may be expensive for the owner. In many cases, only control of the disease may be established rather than a complete cure. The following steps are recommended for the treatment of generalized demodicosis:

1. Shave the dog (long-haired pets) if the skin is markedly crusted and exudative.
2. Gently remove all heavy crusts from the skin.
3. Protect the eyes with opthalmic ointment.
4. Shampoo the dog with a benzoyl peroxide shampoo and/or soak in a whirlpool bath with an antiseptic solution.
5. Towel dry.
6. Repeat on a weekly or twice-weekly basis.
7. Systemic antibiotics should be given for an extended period of time.

TX OPTION A

8. Apply Amitraz (mitaban) solution at a concentration of 5 ml/gallon water (12.5%, 250 ppm) on a weekly basis—do not rinse off—let air dry (may require 6–8 weeks of therapy) Remember** Amitraz should be applied in a well-ventilated area. Gloves should be worn to prevent the possibility of contact hypersensitivity. Side effects of amitraz commonly noted include sedation for 12–24 hours, pruritus, and polydipsia/polyuria.
9. Re-check every 3–4 weeks to evaluate mite status.

TX OPTION B

8. Administer oral ivermectin daily for a minimum of 60–90 days.
9. Re-check every 3–4 weeks to evaluate mite status.

TX OPTION C

8. Administer oral milbemycin daily for a minimum of 60–90 days.
9. Re-check every 3–4 weeks to evaluate mite status.

PODODEMODICOSIS THERAPY

The following steps should be taken when treating dogs with pododemodicosis:

1. Shave the feet.
2. Shampoo the feet with a benzoyl peroxide shampoo every other day.
3. Soak the feet in an antiseptic solution for 15 minutes.
4. Towel dry.
5. Liberally apply an astringent to the feet and let air dry (domeboro solution).

TREATMENT OPTION A

6. Alternate days with the application of mupirocin ointment (or oxydex gel) and mitaban solution @ a concentration of 0.3 ml mitaban/30 ml mineral oil.
   Remember*** the mitaban solution should be stored in a dark bottle and made fresh on a weekly basis.
7. Re-check every 3–4 weeks to evaluate mite status.

TREATMENT OPTION B

6. Oral ivermectin daily for a minimum of 60–90 days.
7. Daily application of mupirocin ointment or benzoyl peroxide gel.
8. Re-check every 3–4 weeks for evaluation of mite status.

TREATMENT OPTION C

6. Oral milbemycin daily for a minimum of 60–90 days.
7. Daily application of mupirocin ointment or benzoyl peroxide gel.
8. Re-check every 3–4 weeks for evaluation of mite status.

Notes:

DERMATOPHYTOSIS (RINGWORM)

Karen Helton Rhodes, DVM, Dip. ACVD
Ilene Katz, Dermatology Technician

Dermatophytosis (*M. canis, M. gypseum, T. mentagrophytes*) implies a cutaneous infection with a number of keratinophilic species of fungi. Transmission is by direct contact or contact with infected hairs and scale in the environment. Infected hairs in the environment may remain contagious for months to years. Zoonosis is a frequent problem and is most often associated with the Persian breed and other long-haired cats which can be asymptomatic carriers.

Treatment should be aimed at eliminating the infection from the host and cleaning the environment. Optimally, affected animals should be separated from other pets in the household. Every confirmed case of dermatophytosis should be treated topically. Total body clipping may be beneficial to decrease environmental contamination by infected hairs and to allow for topical applications. The efficacy of topical antiseptic baths and rinses vary, but each is effective in removing scale, crust, exudate, and loose infected hairs. Systemic therapy is often needed to hasten recovery. Medications most often used include: griseofulvin (serious side effects may be associated with the use of this medication in the cat—leukopenia), ketoconazole, and itraconazole. Fungal vaccines have shown little efficacy in controlling dermatophytosis. Animals receiving this vaccine may demonstrate suppressed clinical signs but will culture positive, posing a zoonotic threat.

Environmental decontamination is an important feature in these cases. Re-exposure and re-contamination are a constant problem. All contaminated equipment, toys, feed containers, transport cages, scratching posts, grooming supplies, bedding, etc. must be removed from the environment. Any item that cannot be washed in a bathtub or washing machine should be destroyed. Salvaged items must be washed in hot water using an antifungal soap (Nolvasan scrub), rinsed, and then soaked in a 1:30 dilution of 0.5% sodium hypochlorite (Chlorox) for 10 minutes. This should be repeated a minimum of 3 times. All surfaces in the environment should be vacuumed, scrubbed, rinsed, and wiped down with a 1:30 dilution of chlorox. Vacuum bags should be burned or saturated with chlorox. Furnace and air conditioner filters will need to be changed and discarded once a week. Daily spraying of filters with a Nolvasan (2% chlorhexidine) solution at a 1:4 dilution will help decrease the number of fungal spores that are recirculated. Books, lamps, bric-a-brac, bed linens, and furniture must also be vacuumed and wiped once a week with an antifungal liquid (Chlorox, Nolvasan). Rugs that cannot be destroyed or removed should be washed with an antifungal disinfectant. Steam cleaning fails to maintain water temperatures of above 43°C at the carpet level and may not be a reliable method to kill fungal spores unless an antifungal disinfectant (Nolvasan) is added to the water. This massive clean-up is mandatory if the owner wishes to effectively remove fungi from the premises.

Notes:

CYCLIC FLANK ALOPECIA

Karen Helton Rhodes, DVM, Dip. ACVD
DERMATOLOGY CONSULTATIONS

Cyclic flank alopecia is a poorly understood follicular dysplasia. Symmetric trunkal alopecia or marked thinning of the haircoat is a prominent feature. The areas of alopecia may be characterized by a large "spot" on the lateral flank region or may appear more serpiginous or "snake-like" along the trunkal region. The alopecia may be seasonal or remain constant. The skin tends to be hyperpigmented and, because of follicular keratosis (plugged hair follicles), prone to secondary infections.

THERAPY:

1. There is no current effective therapy for hair regrowth.
2. Melatonin is often trialed as a stimulus for hair regrowth.
3. Secondary bacterial infections can be minimized by antibiotics and antibacterial shampoos.

PLAN:

1. ORAL MEDICATIONS:____
2. TOPICAL MEDICATIONS:______________________________________

GRANULOMATOUS SEBACEOUS ADENITIS

Karen Helton Rhodes, DVM, Dip. ACVD
Ilene Katz, Dermatology Technician

—Alopecic and scaling disorder of the skin owing to a granulomatous destruction of the sebaceous glands
—Breeds affected include: standard poodle, akita, samoyed, vizsla, as well as other pure and mixed breeds
—Suspect an autosomal recessive mode of inheritance
—Cause/pathogenesis: unknown—theories include:
1. Sebaceous gland destruction is a developmental and inherited defect.
2. Sebaceous gland destruction is an immune-mediated disease directed against a component of the sebaceous gland.
3. The initial defect is a keratinization defect that leads to obstruction of the sebaceous ducts, with resultant inflammation and destruction.
4. The sebaceous adenitis and the keratinization defects are the result of a defector abnormality in lipid metabolism (toxic intermediate metabolite, etc.).

—Clinical presentation: bilaterally symmetric heavy adherent scale on the dorsum of the body to include the head and the extremities (silver-white scale that encases tufts of matted hair)—lesions are usually not malodorous and are not greasy.
—Secondary bacterial infections are common, especially in the akita breed.

DIAGNOSTIC TESTS CURRENTLY AVAILABLE:

1. Cutaneous biopsy

Treatment: not curable—only controllable (in some cases)

TOPICAL THERAPY:

1. Keratolytic shampoos____
2. Keratolytic rinses and sprays__________________________________
3. Emollient rinses, soaks, and sprays____________________________

ORAL THERAPEUTICS AVAILABLE:

1. Essential fatty acids—variable success
2. Retinoids—lifetime therapy if beneficial
   expensive
   variable success rate
3. Corticosteroids—decrease associated pruritus (itching) if present
4. Cyclosporne—variable success
   potential toxicity
5. Other experimental medication trials

DERMATOHISTOPATHOLOGY: OBTAINING A DIAGNOSTIC BIOPSY

Karen Helton Rhodes, DVM, Dip. ACVD

The skin biopsy is one of the most important diagnostic tools available. Three factors are key in obtaining a diagnostic biopsy: site selection, tissue handling, and a good dermatopathologist. There are a number of recognized dermatopathologists available through a variety of commercial and private laboratories. Your area board-certified dermatologist(s) may be helpful in providing names and locations of laboratories. The art of site selection and tissue handling are the responsibility of the submitting veterinarian.

THE DECISION TO BIOPSY

There are a number of cutaneous disorders for which the biopsy is the only helpful diagnostic tool. The biopsy is equally important for what appears to be a "classic case" that continues to fail conventional therapy. The following "rules" apply to the question of

When to Biopsy:

1. Persistent lesions
2. Any neoplastic or suspected neoplastic disorder
3. Any scaling dermatoses
4. Vesicular dermatosis
5. Undiagnosed alopecias
6. Any unusual dermatoses

SITE SELECTION

It is often difficult to decide which area to biopsy. We have been taught to sample the periphery of the lesion so that both normal and abnormal areas will be available for inspection. This is a problem in many cases and may facilitate a poor section when only a small portion of the pathology is present in the tissue. It is more productive to choose representative lesions and submit multiple pieces of skin for evaluation. Most laboratories will allow the clinician to submit up to 4 or 5 sections of skin for the same fee, as multiple sections will aid the pathologist in making a diagnosis. Remember, if the lesion is present on the planum nasale, then submit a section of the planum nasale and not the surrounding skin. Although the area bleeds profusely when cut, it heals nicely with minimal scarring and you will increase the likelihood of an accurate diagnosis. The following "rules" apply to the question of

Where to Biopsy:

1. Choose several representative lesions as they may represent various stages of the same disorder or multiple problems.
2. Include lesions characterized by scale, crust, erythema, erosion, ulceration, etc.
3. It is not always necessary to biopsy the edge of a lesion, although a sample taken from the center of an ulcer is rarely diagnostic.
4. Pustules and vesicles should not be biopsied with a punch, as the twisting motion of the punch will rupture or remove the roof of the lesion and disrupt the architecture of the sample; these lesions should be excised "in total."
5. Ulcers or deep draining lesions are best taken by excision, rather than a punch, because the twisting motion may separate the pathologic tissue from the more normal tissue—leaving important clues behind (i.e. vasculitis, panniculitis, etc.).

6. Don't be afraid to biopsy a footpad or the planum nasale—wedge samples are easier to close than circular punched samples.
7. Crusted lesions are good sites for biopsy. Remember, if the crust falls off the lesion during sampling, be sure to include it in the formalin jar and make a notation for the technician to "please cut in the crust."
8. Heavily scaled areas are often good diagnostic sites.

BIOPSY TECHNIQUE

One of the most important points to remember is that cutaneous biopsy sites should not be scrubbed and cleaned as this will remove important clues regarding the diagnosis. It is often difficult for veterinarians to feel comfortable cutting through crust and scale without scrubbing the area. Most cutaneous biopsies can be taken with local anesthesia via lidocaine injection into the subcutaneous region. Some fractious animals may require sedation such as with a ketamine/valium cocktail. Excisional biopsies or ellipses are often the best choice. When punch biopsies are chosen, remember to use a 6-mm and avoid the 2- and 4-mm punches as the sections are too small for good sample size. The following "rules" apply to the question of

How to Biopsy:

1. Never scrub or cleanse the area prior to excision—the surface crust may contain the pathologic changes necessary to make a diagnosis.
2. Use a surgical blade to obtain a wedge-shaped or elliptical biopsy when sectioning the nose, footpad, vesicles, bullae, deep lesions (vasculitis, panniculitis, etc.).
3. When using a punch biopsy, choose the 6-mm size.
4. When using a punch biopsy, rotate in one direction only and do not re-use the tool as the blade is easily dulled and may cause the tissue to tear during the procedure.
5. When using lidocaine, place the anesthesia in the subcutaneous compartment and not intradermally.
6. Try not to handle the tissue with forceps (crushing artifact) but rather use a small-gauge needle to manipulate the tissue.
7. Place the sample immediately in the formalin.
8. Small or thin specimens may be placed on a small piece of a tongue depressor with the haired portion on the outside to prevent curling and then floated upside down in the formalin.
9. Avoid freezing.

Remember to provide your pathologist with a thorough history and clinical description of the lesions. I routinely include a copy of the referral letter with the biopsy request. That letter outlines the history, clinical signs, differential diagnoses considered, and a plan. You and your pathologist should become a diagnostic team. It is unrealistic to expect that the pathologist can consistently provide answers if we do not supply the appropriate tissue or information.

APPENDIX II

5-MINUTE CONSULT DRUG FORMULARY

Drug Name (Trade or Other Names)	Pharmacology and Indications	Adverse Effects and Precautions	Dosing Information and Comments	Formulations	Dosage
Acetaminophen (Tylenol, and many generic brands)	Analgesic agent. Exact mechanism of action is not known. Not a prostaglandin synthesis inhibitor.	Well tolerated in dogs at doses listed. High doses have caused liver toxicity. Do not administer to cats.	Many OTC formulations available. Acetaminophen with codeine may have greater analgesic efficacy in some animals.	120, 160, 325, 500 mg tablets.	Dogs: 15 mg/kg, q8h PO. Cats: not recommended.
ACTH	See Corticotropin.				
Amoxicillin trihydrate (Amoxi-Tabs, Amoxi-drops, Amoxil, and others)	β-lactam antibiotic. Inhibits bacterial cell wall synthesis. Generally, broad-spectrum activity, but resistance is common.	Use cautiously in animals allergic to penicillin-like drugs.	Dose requirements vary depending on susceptibility of bacteria.	50, 100, 200, 400 mg tablets. 50 mg/mL oral suspension.	6–20 mg/kg q8–12h PO.
Amphotericin B (Fungizone)	Antifungal drug. Fungicidal for systemic fungi, by damaging fungal membranes.	Produces a dose-related nephrotoxicosis. Also produces fever, phlebitis, and tremors.	Administer IV via slow infusion diluted in fluids, and monitor renal function closely. When preparing IV solution, do not mix with electrolyte solutions (use D_5W, for example); administer NaCl fluid loading before therapy. (One study administered this drug subcutaneously: Aust Vet J 73:124, 1996)	50 mg injectable vial.	0.5 mg/kg IV (slow infusion) q48h, to a cumulative dose of 4–8 mg/kg.
Ampicillin + Sulbactam (Unasyn)	Ampicillin plus a β-lactamase inhibitor (sulbactam). Sulbactam has similar activity as clavulanate.	Same as ampicillin.	Same as amoxicillin + clavulanate.	2:1 combination for injection. 1.5 and 3 g vials.	10–20 mg/kg IV, IM q8h.
Ampicillin trihydrate (Polyflex)	β-lactam antibiotic. Inhibits bacterial cell wall synthesis.	Use cautiously in animals allergic to penicillin-like drugs.	Absorption is slow and may not be sufficient for acute serious infection.	10, 25 mg vials for injection.	Dogs: 10–50 mg/kg q12–24h IM, SC. Cats: 10–20 mg/kg q12–24h IM, SC.

Aspirin (many generic and brand names [Bufferin, Ascriptin])	Nonsteroidal anti-inflammatory drug. Anti-inflammatory action is generally considered to be caused by inhibition of prostaglandins. Used as analgesic, anti-inflammatory, and anti-platelet drug.	Narrow therapeutic index. High doses frequently cause vomiting. Other gastrointestinal effects can include ulceration and bleeding. Cats susceptible to salicylate intoxication because of slow clearance. Use cautiously in patients with coagulopathies because of platelet inhibition.	Analgesic and anti-inflammatory doses have primarily been derived from empiricism. Antiplatelet doses are lower because of prolonged effect of aspirin on platelets. When administering aspirin, buffered forms, or administration with food may decrease stomach irritation. Enteric-coated formulations are not recommended for dogs and cats.	81, 325 mg tablets.	Mild analgesia: (dog) 10 mg/kg q12h. Anti-inflammatory: Dogs: 20–25 mg/kg q12h; Cats: 10–20 mg/kg q48h. Antiplatelet: Dogs: 5–10 mg/kg q24–48h; Cats: 80 mg q48h
Azathioprine (Imuran)	Thiopurine immunosuppressive drug. Acts to inhibit T-cell lymphocyte function. This drug is metabolized to 6-mercaptopurine, which may account for immunosuppressive effects. Used to treat various immune-mediated disease.	Bone marrow suppression is most serious concern. Cats particularly are susceptible. There has been some associaton with development of pancreatitis when administered with corticosteroids.	Usually used in combination with other immunosuppressive drugs (such as corticosteroids) to treat immune-mediated disease. Some evidence suggests that it is contraindicated in cats because of bone-marrow effects. Doses of 2.2 mg/kg to cats have produced toxicity.	50 mg tablets; 10 mg/mL for injection.	Dogs: 2 mg/kg q24h PO initially, then 0.5–1 mg/kg q48h. Cats (use cautiously): 1 mg/kg q48h PO.
Azithromycin (Zithromax)	Azalide antibiotic. Similar mechanism of action as macrolides (erythromycin), which is to inhibit bacteria protein synthesis via inhibition of ribosome. Spectrum is primarily Gram-positive.	Has not been in common use in veterinary medicine to establish adverse effects. Vomiting is likely with high doses. Diarrhea may occur in some patients.	Azithromycin may be better tolerated than erythromycin. Primary difference from other antibiotics is the high intracellular concentrations achieved.	250 mg capsules, 250 and 600 mg tablets, 100 or 200 mg/5 mL oral suspension, and 500 mg vials for injection.	Dogs: 10 mg/kg, PO, once every 5 days, or 3.3 mg/kg, once daily for 3 days. Cats: 5 mg/kg PO every other day.
Bactrim (sulfamethoxazole + trimethoprim)	See Trimethoprim-sulfonamide combinations.				

Drug Name (Trade or Other Names)	Pharmacology and Indications	Adverse Effects and Precautions	Dosing Information and Comments	Formulations	Dosage
Betamethasone (Celestone)	Potent, long-acting corticosteroid. Anti-inflammatory and immunosuppressive effects are approximately 30 times more than cortisol. Anti-inflammatory effects are complex, but primarily via inhibition of inflammatory cells and suppression of expression of inflammatory mediators. Use is for treatment of inflammatory and immune-mediated disease.	Side effects from corticosteroids are many, and include polyphagia, polydipsia/polyuria, and HPA-axis suppression. Adverse effects include gastrointestinal ulceration, hepatopathy, diabetes, hyperlipidemia, decreased thyroid hormone, decreased protein synthesis and wound healing, and immunosuppression.	Dosing schedules are based on desired effect. Anti-inflammatory effects are seen at doses of 0.1–0.2 mg/kg, immunosuppressive effects at 0.2–0.5 mg/kg.	600 μg (0.6 mg) tablets; 3 mg/mL sodium phosphate injection.	0.1–0.2 mg/kg q12–24h PO.
Cefaclor (Ceclor)	Cephalosporin antibiotic. Action is similar to other β-lactam antibiotics, which is to inhibit synthesis of bacterial cell wall leading to cell death. Cephalosporins are divided into 1st, 2nd, or 3rd generation, depending on spectrum of activity. Consult package insert or specific reference for spectrum of activity of individual cephalosporin. Cefaclor is a 2nd-generation cephalosporin.	All cephalosporins are generally safe; however, sensitivity can occur in individuals (allergy). Rare bleeding disorders have been known to occur with some cephalosporins.	Used primarily when resistance has been demonstrated to 1st-generation cephalosporins.	250, 500 capsule; 25 mg/mL oral suspension.	4–20 mg/kg q8h PO.

Cefadroxil (Cefa-Tabs, Cefa-Drops)	See Cefaclor. Cefadroxil is a 1st-generation cephalosporin.	See Cefaclor. Cefadroxil has been known to cause vomiting after oral administration in dogs.	Spectrum of cefadroxil is similar to other 1st-generation cephalosporins. For susceptibility test, use cephalothin as test drug.	50 mg/mL oral suspension; 50, 100, 200, 1000 mg tablet.	Dogs: 22 mg/kg q12h, up to 30 mg/kg q12h PO. Cats: 22 mg/kg q24h PO.
Cefazolin sodum (Ancef, Kefzol, and generic)	See Cefaclor. Cefazolin is a 1st-generation cephalosporin.	See Cefaclor. For cefazolin, use cephalothin to test susceptibility.	Commonly used 1st-generation cephalosporin as injectable drug for prophylaxis for surgery as well as acute therapy for serious infections.	50 and 100 mg/50 mL for injection.	20–35 mg/kg q8h IV, IM. For perisurgical use: 22 mg/kg every 2 hr during surgery.
Cefixime (Suprax)	See Cefaclor. Cefixime is a 3rd-generation cephalosporin.	See Cefaclor.	Although not approved for veterinary use, pharmacokinetic studies in dogs have provided recommended doses.	20 mg/mL oral suspension; 200 and 400 mg tablets.	10 mg/kg q12h PO; for cystitis: 5 mg/kg q12–24h PO.
Cefotaxime (Claforan)	See Cefaclor. Cefotaxime is a 3rd-generation cephalosporin. Cefotaxime is used when resistance is encountered to other antibiotics, or when infection is in central nervous system.	See Cefaclor.	3rd-generation cephalosporin used when resistance encountered to 1st- and 2nd-generation cephalosporins.	500 mg; 1, 2, and 10 g vials for injection.	Dogs: 50 mg/kg, IV, IM, SC, q12h. Cats: 20–80 mg/kg q6h IV, IM.
Cefotetan (Cefotan)	See Cefaclor. Cefotetan is a 2nd-generation cephalosporin.	See Cefaclor.	2nd-generation cephalosporin similar to cefoxitin, but may have longer half-life in dogs.	1, 2, and 10 g vials for injection.	30 mg/kg q8h IV, SC.
Cefoxitin sodium (Mefoxin)	See Cefaclor. Cefoxitin is a 2nd-generation cephalosporin. May have increased activity against anaerobic bacteria.	See Cefaclor.	2nd-generation cephalosporin, which is often used when activity against anaerobic bacteria is desired.	1, 2, and 10 g vials for injection.	30 mg/kg q6–8h IV.

Drug Name (Trade or Other Names)	Pharmacology and Indications	Adverse Effects and Precautions	Dosing Information and Comments	Formulations	Dosage
Ceftiofur (Naxcel [ceftiofur sodium]; Excenel [ceftiofur HCL]).	See Cefaclor. Ceftiofur is a unique cephalosporin that does not fit into a distinct class; however, its spectrum resembles many of the 3rd-generation cephalosporins.	See Cefaclor. Ceftiofur is primarily used only for urinary tract infections.	Available as powder for reconstitution prior to injection. After reconstitution stable for 7 days when refrigerated or 12 hr at room temperature, or frozen for 8 weeks. Excenel is not approved for use in dogs.	50 mg/mL injection.	2.2–4.4 mg/kg SC q24h (for urinary tract infections).
Cephalexin (Keflex and generic forms)	See Cefaclor. Cephalexin is a 1st-generation cephalosporin.	See Cefaclor. For cephalexin, use cephalothin to test susceptibility.	Although not approved for veterinary use, trials in dogs with pyoderma show similar efficacy.	250, 500 mg capsules; 250, 500 mg tablets; 100 mg/mL or 125, 250 mg/5 mL oral suspension.	10–30 mg/kg q6–12h PO; for pyoderma, 22–35 mg/kg q12h PO.
Chlortetracycline (generic)	Tetracycline antibacterial drug. Inhibits bacterial protein synthesis by interfering with peptide elongation by ribosome. Bacteriostatic agent with broad spectrum of activity.	Avoid use in young animals; may bind to bone and developing teeth. High doses have caused renal injury.	Broad-spectrum antibiotic. Used for routine infections and intracellular pathogens.	Powdered feed additive.	25 mg/kg q6–8h PO.
Cimetidine (Tagamet [OTC and prescription])	Histamine-2 antagonist (H-2 blocker). Blocks histamine stimulation of gastric parietal cell to decrease gastric acid secretion. Used to treat ulcers and gastritis.	Adverse effects usually seen only with decreased renal clearance. In people, CNS signs may occur with high doses. Drug interactions: May increase concentrations of other drugs used concurrently (e.g., theophylline), because of inhibition of hepatic enzymes.	Precise doses needed to treat ulcers have not been established. Doses are derived from gastric secretory studies.	100, 150, 200, 300 mg tablets and 60 mg/mL injection.	10 mg/kg q6–8h IV, IM, PO (in renal failure, administer 2.5–5 mg/kg q12h IV, PO).

Clavamox	See Amoxicillin/ Clavulanic acid.				
Clavulanic acid	See Amoxicillin/ Clavulanic acid.				
Colony-stimulating factor (Amgen)	Stimulates granulocyte development in bone marrow. Used primarily to regenerate blood cells to recover from cancer chemotherapy or other therapy.		Doses based on limited experimental information performed in dogs. (JAVMA 200: 1957, 1992)		2.5 μg/kg q12h SC.
Corticotropin (ACTH) (Acthar)	Used for diagnostic purposes to evaluate adrenal gland function. Stimulates normal synthesis of cortisol from adrenal gland.	Adverse effects unlikely when used as single injection for diagnostic purposes.	Doses established by measuring normal adrenal response in animals. See also Cosyntropin.	Gel 80 U/mL.	Response test: Collect pre-ACTH sample and inject 2.2 IU/kg IM. Collect post-ACTH sample at 2 hr in dogs and at 1 and 2 hr in cats.
Cosyntropin (Cortrosyn)	Cosyntropin is a synthetic form of corticotropin (ACTH) used for diagnostic purposes only. In humans, it is preferred over corticotropin because it is less allergenic.	Same as for corticotropin.	Same as for corticotropin. Use for diagnostic purposes only; not intended for treatment of hypoadrenocorticism.	250 μg per vial.	Response test: collect pre-ACTH sample and inject 5 μg/kg IV (dog) or 0.125 mg IV (cat), and collect post sample at 30, 60 min.
Cyclophosphamide (Cytoxan, Neosar)	Cytotoxic agent. Bifunctional alkylating agent. Disrupts base-pairing and inhibits DNA and RNA synthesis. Cytotoxic for tumor cells and other rapidly dividing cells. Used primarily as adjunct for cancer chemotherapy and as immunosuppressive therapy.	Bone marrow suppression is most common adverse effect. Can produce severe neutropenia (that usually is reversible). Vomiting and diarrhea may occur in some patients. Dogs are susceptible to bladder toxicity (sterile hemorrhagic cystitis). May cause hair loss when used in some chemotherapeutic protocols.	Cyclophosphamide is usually administered with other drugs (other cancer drugs in cancer protocols or corticosteroids) when used for immunosuppressive therapy. Consult specific anticancer protocols for specific regimens.	25 mg/mL injection; 25, 50 mg tablet.	Anticancer: 50 mg/m^2 once daily 4 days/week PO, or 150–300 mg/m^2 IV, and repeat in 21 days. Immunosuppressive therapy: 50 mg/m^2 (approx. 2.2 mg/kg) q48h PO, or 2.2 mg/kg once daily for 4 days/week. Cats: 6.25–12.5 mg/cat once daily 4 days/week.

Drug Name (Trade or Other Names)	Pharmacology and Indications	Adverse Effects and Precautions	Dosing Information and Comments	Formulations	Dosage
Deprenyl (L-deprenyl)					
Dexamethasone (Dexamethasone solution and dexamethasone sodium phosphate) (Azium solution in polyethylene glycol. Sodium phosphate forms include: Dexaject SP, Dexavet, and Dexasone. Tablets include Decadron and generic)	Corticosteroid. Dexamethasone has approximately 30 × potency of cortisol. Multiple anti-inflammatory effects (see Betamethasone).	Multiple side effects. (See Betamethasone.)	Doses based on severity of underlying disease (see Betamethasone). Dexamethasone is used for testing hyperadrenocorticism. Low-dose dexamethasone suppression test: dogs 0.01 mg/kg IV, cats 0.1 mg/kg IV, and collect sample at 0, 4, and 8 hours. For high-dose dexamethasone suppression test: dogs 0.1 mg/kg, cats 1.0 mg/kg.	Azium solution, 2 mg/mL. Sodium phosphate forms are 3.33 mg/mL. 0.25, 0.5, 0.75, 1, 1.5, 2, 4, 6 mg tablets.	Anti-inflammatory: 0.07–0.15 mg/kg q12–24h IV, IM, PO. For shock, spinal injury: 2.2–4.4 mg/kg IV (of sodium phosphate form). Dexamethasone suppression test: dogs 0.01 mg/kg IV, cats 0.1 mg/kg IV, and collect sample at 0, 4, and 8 hours.
Diethylstilbestrol (DES) (DES, generic [no longer manufactured in US, but available from compounding pharmacist])	Synthetic estrogen compound. Used for estrogen replacement in animals. DES is most commonly used to treat estrogen-responsive incontinence in dogs. Also has been used to induce abortion in dogs.	Side effects may occur that are caused by excess estrogen. Estrogen therapy may increase risk of pyometra and estrogen-sensitive tumors.	Doses listed are for treating urinary incontinence, and vary depending on response. Titrate dose to individual patients. Although used to induce abortion, it was not efficacious in one study that administered 75 μg/kg.	1, 5 mg tablet; 50 mg/mL injection.	Dogs: 0. 1–1.0 mg/dog q24h PO. Cats: 0.05–0.1 mg/cat q24h PO.
Dihydrotachysterol (Vitamin D) (Hytakerol, DHT)	Vitamin D analogue. Used as treatment of hypocalcemia, especially hypoparathyroidism associated with thyroidectomy. Vitamin D promotes absorption and utilization of calcium.	Overdose may cause hypercalcemia. Avoid use in pregnant animals because it may cause fetal abnormalities. Use cautiously with high doses of calcium-containing preparations.	Available as oral solution, tablets, and capsules. Doses for individual patients should be adjusted by monitoring serum calcium concentrations.	0. 125 mg tablet; 0.5 mg/mL oral liquid.	0.01 mg/kg/day PO; for acute treatment, administer 0.02 mg/kg initially, then 0.01–0.02 mg/kg q24–48h PO thereafter.

Enrofloxacin (Baytril)	Fluoroquinolone antibacterial drug. Acts via inhibition of DNA gyrase in bacteria to inhibit DNA and RNA synthesis. Bactericidal. Broad spectrum of activity.	Adverse effects include: seizures in epileptic animals, arthropathy in dogs 4–28 weeks of age, vomiting in dogs and cats at high doses. Drug interactions: May increase concentrations of theophylline if used concurrently. Coadministration with di- and trivalent cations (e.g., sucralfate) may decrease absorption.	Low dose of 5 mg/kg/day is used for sensitive organisms with MIC of 0.12 µg/mL or less, or urinary tract infection; dose of 5–10 mg/kg/day is used for organisms with MIC of 0.12–0.5 µg/mL; dose of 10–20 mg/kg/day is used for organisms with MIC of 0.5–1.0 µg/mL. Solution is not approved for IV use, but has been administered via this route safely if given slowly.	68, 22.7, and 5.7 mg tablet. Taste Tabs are 22.7 and 68 mg. 22.7 mg/mL injection.	5–20 mg/kg/day (see dosing information guidelines).
Epinephrine (Adrenaline and generic forms)	Adrenergic agonist. Nonselectively stimulates α- and β_2-adrenergic receptors. Used primarily for emergency situations to treat cardiopulmonary arrest and anaphylactic shock.	Overdose will cause excessive vasoconstriction and hypertension. High doses can cause ventricular arrhythmias. When high doses are used for cardiopulmonary arrest, an electrical defibrillator should be available.	Doses are based on experimental studies, primarily in dogs. Clinical studies are not available. IV doses are ordinarily used, but endotracheal administration is acceptable when intravenous access is not available. Intraosseous route also has been used and doses are equivalent to IV. When endotracheal route is used, the dose is higher and duration of effect may be longer than IV administration. There appears to be no advantage to intracardiac injection compared with IV administration.	1 mg/mL (1:1000) injection solution.	Cardiac arrest: 10–20 µg/kg, IV; *or* 200 µg/kg endotracheal (may be diluted in saline before administration). Anaphylactic shock: 2.5–5 µg/kg IV; *or* 50 µg/kg endotracheal (may be diluted in saline).

Drug Name (Trade or Other Names)	Pharmacology and Indications	Adverse Effects and Precautions	Dosing Information and Comments	Formulations	Dosage
Famotidine (Pepsid)	H-2 receptor antagonist. (See Cimetidine for details.)	See Cimetidine.	See Cimetidine. Clinical studies for famotidine have not been performed; therefore, optimal dose for ulcer prevention and healing are not known.	10 mg tablet; 10 mg/mL injection.	0.5 mg/kg q12–24h IM, SC, PO.
Fluconazole (Diflucan)	Azole antifungal drug. Similar mechanism as other azole antifungal agents. Inhibits ergosterol synthesis in fungal cell membrane. Fungistatic. Efficacious against dermatophytes, and variety of systemic fungi.	Adverse effects have not been reported from fluconazole administration. Compared with ketoconazole, has less effect on endocrine function. However, increased liver enzyme plasma concentrations and hepatopathy are possible. Compared with other oral azole antifungals, fluconazole is absorbed more predictably and completely, even on an empty stomach.	Doses for fluconazole are primarily based on studies performed in cats for treatment of cryptococcosis. Efficacy for other infections has not been reported. The primary difference between fluconazole and other azoles is that fluconazole attains higher concentrations in the CNS.	50, 100, 150, or 200 mg tablets; 10 or 40 mg/mL oral suspension; 2 mg/mL IV injection.	Dogs: 10–12 mg/kg/day PO. Cats: 50 mg/cat q12h PO, or 50 mg/cat per day PO.
Flucytosine (Ancobon)	Antifungal drug. Used in combination with other antifungal drugs for treatment of cryptococcosis. Action is to penetrate fungal cells and is converted to fluorouracil, which acts as antimetabolite.	Adverse effects have not been reported in animals.	Flucytosine is used primarily to treat cryptococcosis in animals. Efficacy is based on flucytosine's ability to attain high concentrations in CSF. Flucytosine may be synergistic with amphotericin B.	250 mg capsule; 75 mg/mL oral suspension.	25–50 mg/kg q6–8h PO (up to a maxiumum dose of 100 mg/kg q12h PO).

Gentamicin (Gentocin)	Aminoglycoside antibiotic. Action is to inhibit bacteria protein synthesis via binding to 30S ribosome. Bactericidal. Broad spectrum of activity except streptococci and anaerobic bacteria.	Nephrotoxicity is the most dose-limiting toxicity. Ensure that patients have adequate fluid and electrolyte balance during therapy. Ototoxicity, vestibulotoxicity also are possible. Drug interactions: When used with anesthetic agents, neuromuscular blockade is possible. Do not mix in vial or syringe with other antibiotics.	Dosing regimens are based on sensitivity of organisms. Some studies have suggested that once-daily therapy (combining multiple doses into a single daily dose) is as efficacious as multiple treatments. Activity against some bacteria (e.g., *Pseudomonas*) is enhanced when combined with a β-lactam antibiotic. Nephrotoxicity is increased with persistently high trough concentrations.	50 and 100 mg/mL solution for injection.	Dogs: 2–4 mg/kg q6–8h, or 6–10 mg/kg q24h IV, IM, SC. Cats: 3 mg/kg q8h, or 9 mg/kg q24h IV, IM, SC.
Hydrocortisone (Cortef, and generic)	Glucocorticoid anti-inflammatory drug. Hydrocortisone has weaker anti-inflammatory effects and greater mineralocorticoid effects, compared with prednisolone or dexamethasone (see dexamethasone for other details). Also used for replacement therapy.	Adverse effects are attributed to excessive glucocorticoid effects (see Betamethasone).	Dose requirements are related to severity of disease.	5, 10, 20 mg tablet.	Replacement therapy: 1–2 mg/kg q12h PO. Anti-inflammatory: 2.55 mg/kg q12h PO.
Hydrocortisone sodium succinate (Solu-Cortef)	Same as hydrocortisone, except that this is a rapid-acting injectable product.	Same as hydrocortisone.	Same as hydrocortisone. Prepare vials according to manufacturer.	Various size vials for injection.	Shock: 50–150 mg/kg IV. Anti-inflammatory: 5 mg/kg q12h IV.
Iodide					

Drug Name (Trade or Other Names)	Pharmacology and Indications	Adverse Effects and Precautions	Dosing Information and Comments	Formulations	Dosage
Isotretinoin (Accutane)	Keratinization stabilizing drug. Isotretinoin reduces sebaceous gland size and inhibits sebaceous gland activity, and decreases sebum secretion. In people, it is primarily used to treat acne. In animals, has been used to treat sebaceous adenitis.	Absolutely contraindicated in pregnant animals. Adverse effects not reported for animals, although experimental studies have demonstrated that it can cause focal calcification (such as in myocardium and vessels).	Use in veterinary medicine is confined to limited clinical experience and extrapolation from human reports.	10, 20, 40 mg capsules.	1–3 mg/kg/day (up to a maximum recommended dose of 3–4 mg/kg/day PO.
Itraconazole (Sporanox)	Azole (triazole) antifungal drug. Active against dermatophytes and systemic fungi, such as *Blastomyces*, *Histoplasma* and *Coccidioides*.	Itraconazole is better tolerated than ketoconazole. However, vomiting and hepatotoxicosis are possible, especially at high doses. In one study, hepatotoxicosis was more likely at high doses. 10–15% of dogs will develop high liver enzyme levels. High doses in cats caused vomiting and anorexia.	Doses are based on studies in animals in which itraconazole has been used to treat blastomycosis in dogs. In cats, lower doses have been effective for dermatophytes (see dosing section). Other uses or doses are based on empiricism or extrapolation from human literature.	100 mg capsules and 10 mg/mL oral liquid.	Dogs: 2.5 mg/kg q12h, or 5 mg/kg q24h PO. Cats: 5 mg/kg q12h PO. For dermatophyte infection in cats: 1.5–3.0 mg/kg (up to 5 mg/kg) q24h PO for 15 days.
Levamisole (Levasole, Tramisol, Ergamisol)	Antiparasitic drug of the imidazothiazole class. Mechanism of action due to neuromuscular toxicity to parasites. Levamisole has been used for endoparasites in dogs and as microfilaricide. In people, levamisole is used as immunostimulant to aid in treatment of colorectal carcinoma and malignant melanoma.	May produce cholinergic toxicity. May cause vomiting in some dogs.	In heartworm-positive dogs, it may sterilize female adult heartworms. Levamisole has also been used as an immunostimulant; however, clinical reports of its efficacy are not available.	0.184 g bolus; 11.7 g per 13 g packet; 50 mg tablet (Ergamisol).	Dogs (hookworms): 5–8 mg/kg once PO (up to 10 mg/kg PO for 2 days). Microfilaricide: 10 mg/kg q24h PO for 6–10 days. Immunostimulant: 0.5–2 mg/kg 3 times/week PO. Cats: 4.4 mg/kg once PO; (for lungworms: 20–40 mg/kg q48h for 5 treatments PO).

Lufenuron (Program)	Antiparasitic. Used for controlling fleas in animals. Inhibits development in hatching fleas. Antifungal	Adverse effects have not been reported. Appears to be relatively safe during pregnancy and in young animals.	Lufenuron may control flea development with administration once every 30 days in animals.	45, 90, 135, 204.9, 409.8 mg tablets; 135 and 270 mg suspension per unit pack.	Dogs: 10 mg/kg PO q30 days. Cats: 30 mg/kg PO q30 days. Cat injection: 10 mg/kg SC every 6 mos.
6-Mercaptopurine (Purinethol)	Anticancer agent. Antimetabolite agent that inhibits synthesis of purines in cancer cells.	Many side effects are possible that are common to anticancer therapy (many of which are unavoidable), including bone marrow suppression and anemia.	Used for various forms of cancer, including leukemia and lymphoma. Consult specific anticancer protocol for specific regimen.	50 mg tablets.	50 mg/m^2 q24h PO.
Methylprednisolone (Medrol)	Glucocorticoid anti-inflammatory drug. (See Betamethasone). Compared with prednisolone, methylprednisolone is 1.25 × more potent.	Same as for other glucocorticoids (see Betamethasone). Manufacturer suggests that methylprednisolone causes less PU/PD than prednisolone.	Use of methylprednisolone is similar to other corticosteroids. Dose adjustment should be made to account for difference in potency. (See dose section.)	1, 2, 4, 8, 18, 32 mg tablets.	0.22–0.44 mg/kg, q12–24h PO. Compared with prednisolone, methylprednisolone is 1.25 × more potent.
Methylprednisolone acetate (Depo-Medrol)	Depot form of methylprednisolone. Slowly absorbed from IM injection site, producing glucocorticoid effects for 3–4 weeks in some animals. Used for intralesional therapy, intra-articular therapy, and for inflammatory conditions.	Many adverse effects possible from use of corticosteroids (see Betamethasone).	Use of methylprednisolone acetate should be evaluated carefully because one injection will cause glucocorticoid effects that persist for several days to weeks.	20 or 40 mg/mL suspension for injection.	Dogs: 1 mg/kg (or 20–40 mg/dog) IM q1–3 weeks. Cats: 10–20 mg/cat IM q1–3 weeks.
Methylprednisolone sodium succinate (Solu-Medrol)	Same as methylprednisolone, except that this is a water-soluble formulation intended for acute therapy when high IV doses are needed for rapid effect. Used for treatment of shock and CNS trauma.	Adverse effects are not expected from single administration; however, with repeated use, other side effects are possible (see Betamethasone).	Results of clinical studies in animals have not been reported. Use in animals (and doses) is based on experience in people, or anecdotal experience in animals.	1 and 2 g and 125 and 500 mg vials for injection.	For emergency use: 30 mg/kg IV and repeat at 15 mg/kg in 2–6 hr, IV.

Drug Name (Trade or Other Names)	Pharmacology and Indications	Adverse Effects and Precautions	Dosing Information and Comments	Formulations	Dosage
Methyltestosterone (Android, generic)	Anabolic androgenic agent. Used for anabolic actions or testosterone hormone replacement therapy (androgenic deficiency). Testosterone has been used to stimulate erythropoiesis.	Adverse effects caused by excessive androgenic action of testosterone. Prostatic hyperplasia is possible in male dogs. Masculinization can occur in female dogs. Hepatopathy is more common with oral methylated testosterone formulations.	See also Testosterone cypionate, Testosterone propionate. Use of testosterone androgens has not been evaluated in clinical studies in veterinary medicine. Use is based primarily on experimental evidence or experiences in people.	10, 25 mg tablets.	Dogs: 5–25 mg/dog q24–48h PO. Cats: 2.5–5 mg/cat q24–48h PO.
Milbemycin oxime (Interceptor, Interceptor Flavor Tabs, and Safe Heart)	Antiparasitic drug. Action is similar to ivermectin. Acts as GABA agonist in nervous system of parasite. Used as heartworm preventative, miticide, and microfilaricide. Used to control infections of hookworm, roundworms, and whipworms. At high doses, it has been used to treat *Demodex* infections in dogs.	In susceptible dogs (collie breeds), milbemycin may cross the blood–brain barrier and produce CNS toxicosis (depression, lethargy, coma). At doses used for heartworm prevention, this effect is less likely.	Doses vary, depending on parasite treated. Consult dose column. Treatment of *Demodex* requires high dose administered daily (JAVMA 207:1581, 1995). See also Sentinel tablets, which contain milbemycin oxime and lufenuron.	2.3, 5.75, 11.5, 23 mg tablet.	Dogs: microfil aricide: 0.5 mg/kg: *Demodex*: 2 mg/kg q24h PO for 60–120 days; heartworm prevention and control of endoparasites: 0.5 mg/kg q30 days PO. Cats: for heartworm and endoparasite control, 2.0 mg/kg q30 days PO.
Minocycline (Minocin)	Tetracycline antibiotic. Similar to doxycycline in pharmacokinetics.	See other tetracycline (Doxycycline). Adverse effects have not been reported for minocycline. Oral absorption is not affected by calcium products as with other tetracyclines.	Minocycline has received little attention for clinical use in North America. Clinical use has not been reported, but properties are similar to doxycycline.	50, 100 mg tablets; 10 mg/mL oral suspension.	5–12.5 mg/kg q12h PO.

Misoprostol (Cytotec)	Prostaglandin E_2 analogue. Prostaglandins provide a cytoprotective role in the gastrointestinal mucosa. Misoprostol is used to prevent gastritis and ulcers associated with NSAID (aspirin-drugs) therapy.	Adverse effects are caused by effects of prostaglandins. Most common side effect is gastrointestinal discomfort, vomiting, and diarrhea. Do not administer to pregnant animals; may cause abortion.	Doses and recommendations are based on clinical trials in which misoprostol was administered to prevent gastrointestinal mucosal injury caused by aspirin.	0.1 mg (100 μg), 0.2 mg (200 μg) tablets.	Dogs: 2–5 μg/kg q6–8h PO. Cats: dose not established.
Mitotane (o,p′-DDD) (Lysodren, op-DDD)	Adrenocortical cytotoxic agent. Causes suppression of adrenal cortex. Used to treat adrenal tumors and pituitary-dependent hyperadrenocorticism (PDH).	Adverse effects, especially during induction period, include lethargy, anorexia, ataxia, depression, vomiting. Corticosteroid supplementation (e.g., hydrocortisone or prednisolone) may be administered to minimize side effects.	Dose and frequency often are based on patient response. Adverse effects are common during initial therapy. Administration with food increases oral absorption. Maintenance dose should be adjusted on the basis of periodic cortisol measurements and ACTH stimulation tests. (See also Vet Record 122:486, 1988.) Cats usually have not responded to mitotane treatment.	500 mg tablet.	Dogs: For PDH: 50 mg/kg/day (in divided doses) PO for 5–10 days, then 50–70 mg/kg/week PO; for adrenal tumor: 50–75 mg/kg/day for 10 days, then 75–100 mg/kg/week PO.
Ormetoprim	Trimethoprim-like drug used in combination with sulfadimethoxine. (See Primor.)				
Oxacillin (Prostaphlin, and generic)	β-lactam antibiotic. Inhibits bacterial cell wall synthesis. Spectrum is limited to Gram-positive bacteria, especially staphylococci.	Use cautiously in animals allergic to penicillin-like drugs.	Doses based on empiricism or extrapolation from human studies. No clinical efficacy studies available for dogs or cats. Administer if possible on empty stomach.	250, 500 mg capsules; 50 mg/mL oral solution.	22–40 mg/kg q8h PO.

Drug Name (Trade or Other Names)	Pharmacology and Indications	Adverse Effects and Precautions	Dosing Information and Comments	Formulations	Dosage
Penicillin G potassium; Penicillin G sodium (many brands)	β-lactam antibiotic. Action is similar to other penicillins (see Amoxicillin). Spectrum of penicillin G is limited to Gram-positive bacteria and anaerobes.	Same as for other penicillins (see Amoxicillin).	See other penicillins (Amoxicillin).	5–20 million U vials.	20,000–40,000 U/kg q6–8h IV, IM.
Penicillin V (Pen-Vee)	Oral penicillin. Otherwise same as other penicillins. Not highly absorbed, and narrow spectrum in comparison with other penicillin derivatives.	Same as other penicillins (see Amoxicillin).	Same as other penicillins (amoxicillin). Penicillin V should be administered on an empty stomach for maximum absorption (250 mg = 400,000 units).	250, 500 mg tablets.	10 mg/kg q8h PO.
Pentoxifylline (Trental)	Methylxanthine. Pentoxifylline is used primarily as a rheological agent in people (increases blood flow through narrow vessels). It may have anti-inflammatory action via inhibition of cytokine synthesis. Used in dogs for some dermatoses (dermatomyositis) and vasculitis.	May cause similar signs as other methylxanthines Nausea, vomiting have been reported in people. When broken tablet is administered to cats, the taste is unpleasant.	Results of clinical studies in animals have not been reported. Use in animals (and doses) is based on experience in people, or anecdotal experience in animals.	400 mg tablets.	Dogs: dermatologic use: 10 mg/kg q12h PO. For other uses: 10 mg/kg q8–12h PO, or 400 mg/dog for most animals. Cats: 1/4 of a 400 mg tablet (100 mg) q8–12h PO.
Prednisone (Deltasone and generic; Meticorten for injection)	Same as prednisolone, except that, after administration, prednisone is converted to prednisolone.	Same as prednisolone.	Same as prednisolone. There are no known contraindications in which prednisolone is preferred over prednisone.	1, 2.5, 5, 10, 20, 25, 50 mg tablets. 1 mg/mL syrup (Liquid-Pred in 5% alcohol) and 1 mg/mL oral solution (in 5% alcohol); 10, 40 mg/mL prednisone suspension for injection.	Same as prednisolone.

Primor (Ormetoprim + Sulfadimethoxine) (Primor)	Antibacterial drug. Ormetoprim inhibits bacterial dihydrofolate reductase, sulfonamide competes with PABA for synthesis of nucleic acids. Bactericidal/bacteriostatic. Broad antibacterial spectrum and active against some coccidia.	Several adverse effects have been reported from sulfonamides. No adverse effects reported from ormetoprim.	Doses listed are based on manufacturer's recommendations. Controlled trials have demonstrated efficacy for treatment of pyoderma on once-daily schedule.	Combination tablet (ormetoprim + sulfadimethoxine).	27 mg/kg on first day, followed by 13.5 mg/kg q24h PO.
Progesterone, repositol	See Medroxyprogesterone acetate (Depo-Provera).				
Promethazine (Phenergan)	Phenothiazine with strong antihistamine effects. Used for treatment of allergy and as antiemetic (motion sickness).	Adverse effects include sedation and antimuscarinic (atropine-like) effects. Both phenothiazine effects and anticholinergic) effects are possible in some patients.	Results of clinical studies in animals have not been reported. Use in animals (and doses) is based on experience in people, or anecdotal experience in animals.	6.25 and 25 mg/5 mL syrup; 12.5, 25, 50 mg tablets; 25, 50 mg/mL injection.	0.2–0.4 mg/kg q6–8h IV, IM PO (up to a maximum dose of 1 mg/kg).
Septra (sulfmethoxazole + trimethoprim) See Trimethoprim/ sulfonamides (Tribrissen)					
Terfenadine	Seldene: No longer available.				

Drug Name (Trade or Other Names)	Pharmacology and Indications	Adverse Effects and Precautions	Dosing Information and Comments	Formulations	Dosage
Testosterone cypionate ester (Andro-Cyp, Andronate, Depo-Testosterone, and other forms)	Testosterone ester. Similar effects as methyltestosterone. Testosterone esters are administered IM to avoid first-pass effects. Esters in oil are absorbed more slowly from IM injection. Esters are then hydrolyzed to free testosterone.	See Testosterone, Methyltestosterone.	See Methyltestosterone.	100, 200 mg/mL injection.	1–2 mg/kg q2–4 weeks IM (see also Methyltestosterone).
Testosterone propionate ester (Testex, [Malogen in Canada])	Testosterone ester for injection. Similar effects as methyltestosterone. Testosterone esters are administered IM to avoid first-pass effects. Esters in oil are absorbed more slowly from IM injection. Esters are then hydrolyzed to free testosterone.	See Testosterone, Methyltestosterone.	See Methyltestosterone.	100 mg/mL injection.	0.5–1 mg/kg 2–3 times/week IM.
Tetracycline (Panmycin)	Tetracycline antibiotic. Mechanism of action of tetracyclines is to bind to 30S ribosomal subunit and inhibit protein synthesis. Usually bacteriostatic. Broad spectrum of activity including bacteria, some protozoa, *Rickettsia*, *Ehrlichia*.	Tetracyclines in general may cause renal tubular necrosis at high doses. Tetracyclines can affect bone and teeth formation in young animals. Tetracyclines have been implicated in drug fever in cats. Hepatotoxicity may occur at high doses in susceptible individuals. Drug interactions: Tetracyclines bind to calcium-containing compounds, which decreases oral absorption.	Pharmacokinetic and experimental studies have been conducted in small animals, but no clinical studies. Do not use outdated solutions.	250, 500 mg capsule; 100 mg/mL suspension.	15–20 mg/kg q8h PO; or 4.4–11 mg/kg q8h, IV, IM.

Thyroid hormone	See Levothyroxine and Liothyronine.				
Thyrotropin, Thyroid-stimulating hormone (TSH) (Thytropar)	Thyroid-stimulating hormone is used for diagnostic testing. Stimulates normal secretion of thyroid hormone.	Adverse reactions rare. In people, allergic reactions have occurred.	To prepare solution, add 2 mL NaCL to 10-U vial. Reconstituted solutions retain potency for 2 weeks at 2–8°C. Consult testing laboratory for specific guidelines for thyroid testing.	10-U vial.	Dogs: Collect baseline sample, followed by 0.1 U/kg UIV (maximum dose is 5 U); collect post-TSH sample at 6 hr.
Ticarcillin (Ticar, Ticillin)	β-lactam antibiotic. Action similar to ampicillin/amoxicillin. Spectrum similar to carbenicillin. Ticarcillin is primarily used for Gram-negative infections, especially those caused by *Pseudomonas*.	Adverse effects are uncommon. However, allergic reactions are possible. High doses can produce seizures and decreased platelet function. Drug interactions: Do not combine in same syringe or in vial with aminoglycosides.	Ticarcillin is synergistic with, and often combined with aminoglycosides (e.g., amikacin, gentamicin). 1% lidocaine may be used for reconstitution to decrease pain from IM injection.	6 g/50 mL vial; vials containing 1, 3, 6, 20, and 30 g.	33–50 mg/kg q4–6h IV, IM.
Ticarcillin + Clavulanate (Timentin)	Same as ticarcillin, except clavulanic acid has been added to inhibit bacterial β-lactamase and increase spectrum. Clavulanate does not increase activity against *Pseudomonas*, however.	Same as ticarcillin.	Same as ticarcillin.	3 g per vial for injection.	Dose according to rate for ticarcillin.
Tobramycin (Nebcin)	Aminoglycoside antibacterial drug. Similar mechanism of action and spectrum as amikacin, gentamicin.	Adverse effects similar to amikacin, gentamicin.	Dosing requirements vary depending on bacterial susceptibility.	40 mg/mL injection.	2–4 mg/kg q8h IV, IM, SC.

Drug Name (Trade or Other Names)	Pharmacology and Indications	Adverse Effects and Precautions	Dosing Information and Comments	Formulations	Dosage
Triamcinolone (Vetalog, Trimtabs, Aristocort, generic)	Glucocorticoid anti-inflammatory drug. See Betamethasone for details. Triamcinolone has potency that is approximately equal to methylprednisolone (about 5× cortisol and 1.25× prednisolone), although some dermatologists suggest that potency is higher.	Adverse effects are similar to other corticosteroids (see β-methasone).	Note that cats may require higher doses than dogs (sometimes 2×).	Veterinary (Vetalog) 0.5 and 1.5 mg tablets. Human form: 1, 2, 4, 8, 16 mg tablets; 10 mg/mL injection.	Anti-inflammatory: 0.5–1 mg/kg q12–24h PO, then taper dose to 0.5–1 mg/kg q48h PO. (However, manufacturer recommends doses of 0.11 to 0.22 mg/kg/day.)
TSH (thyroid-stimulating hormone)	See Thyrotropin.				
Vancomycin (Vancocin, Vancoled)	Antibacterial drug. Mechanism of action is to inhibit cell wall and cause bacterial cell lysis (via different mechanism than β-lactams). Spectrum includes staphylococci, streptococci, and enterococci (but not Gram-negative bacteria). Used primarily for treatment of resistant staphylococci and enterococci.	Adverse effects have not been reported in animals. Administer IV; causes severe pain and tissue injury if administered IM or SC. Do not administer rapidly; use slow infusion, if possible (e.g., over 30 minutes). Adverse effects in people include renal injury (more common with older products that contained impurities) and histamine release.	Vancomycin use is not common in animals, but is valuable for treatment of enterococci or staphylococci that are resistant to other antibiotics. Doses are derived from pharmacokinetic studies in dogs. Monitoring of trough plasma concentrations is recommended to ensure proper dose. Maintain trough concentration above 5 µg/mL. Infusion solution can be prepared in 0.9% saline or 5% dextrose, but not alkalinizing solutions.	Vials for injection (0.5 to 10 g).	Dogs: 15 mg/kg q6–8h IV infusion. Cats: 12–15 mg/kg, q8h, IV infusion.

Yohimbine (Yobine)	α_2-adrenergic antagonist. Used primarily to reverse actions of xylazine or detomidine.	High doses can cause tremors and seizures.	Reverses signs of sedation and anesthesia caused by α_2-agonists.	2 mg/mL injection.	0.11 mg/kg IV, or 0.25–0.5 mg/kg SC, IM.

Key to Table Abbreviations:

IM	Intramuscular
IV	Intravenous
OTC	Over the counter (without prescription)
PO	per os (oral)
SC	Subcutaneous
U	Units
mL	milliliter
μg	micrograms

DISCLAIMER FOR DOSE TABLES:
Note: Doses listed are for dogs and cats, unless otherwise listed. Many of the doses listed are extra-label, or are human drugs not approved for animals administered in an extra-label manner. Doses listed are based on best available information at the time of table editing. The author cannot ensure efficacy or absolute safety of drugs used according to recommendations in this table. Adverse effects may be possible from drugs listed in this table of which authors were not aware at the time of table preparation. Veterinarians using this table are encouraged to consult current literature, product labels and inserts, and the manufacturer's disclosure information for additional information on adverse effects, interactions, and efficacy that were not identified at the time these tables were prepared.

APPENDIX III

ENDOCRINE TESTING

ENDOCRINE FUNCTION TESTING PROTOCOLS

ADRENAL GLAND DISORDERS

ACTH STIMULATION TEST

Dogs

Administer 20 IU ACTH gel IM or 0.25 mg synthetic ACTH IV or IM (Cortrosyn, Organon Pharmaceuticals, West Orange, NJ).

ACTH Gel

Serum samples should be obtained before and 2 hours after injection of ACTH for cortisol assay.

Synthetic ACTH

Serum samples should be obtained before and 1 hour after injection of ACTH for cortisol assay.

Cats

Administer 0.125 mg synthetic ACTH IV. Serum samples should be obtained before and 1 hour after injection of ACTH for cortisol assay.

Interpretation

Screening for Cushing's disease

An exaggerated response to ACTH is consistent with Cushing's disease. High normal cut-off values differ slightly between laboratories.

Screening for Hypoadrenocorticism

Pre- and post-cortisol determinations < 1 μg/dl (30 nmol/L) is consistent with hypoadrenocorticism.

Monitoring Mitotane or Ketoconazole Therapy for Cushing's disease

Pre- and post-cortisol determinations should be within the normal basal cortisol range.

LOW-DOSE DEXAMETHASONE SUPPRESSION TEST (LDDST)

Dogs

Administer 0.015 mg/kg dexamethasone (Azium) IV or IM. Obtain serum samples before and 4 and 8 hours after injection of dexamethasone for cortisol assay.

Cats

Administer 0.1 mg/kg dexamethasone (Azium) IV or IM. Obtain serum sample before and 4 and 8 hours after injection of dexamethasone for cortisol assay.

Interpretation

Three Basic Patterns

Lack of Suppression

All cortisol values remain above 1 μg/dL (30 nmol/L). This pattern is consistent with Cushing's disease.

Suppression

Cortisol values fall below 1 μg/dL (30 nmol/L) at 4 and 8 hours. This pattern suggests that the animal does not have Cushing's disease.

Escape from Suppression

Cortisol value falls below 1 μg/dL (30 nmol/L) at 4 hours and rises above 1 μg/dL at 8 hours. This pattern is consistent with pituitary-dependent Cushing's disease.

HIGH-DOSE DEXAMETHASONE SUPPRESSION TEST (HDDST)

Administer 1 mg/kg dexamethasone (Azium) IV or IM. Obtain serum samples before and 4 and 8 hours after injection of dexamethasone for cortisol assay.

Interpretation

Any cortisol determination that falls below 1.5 μg/dL (45 nmol/L) at any point during the 8-hour testing period is considered suppression. Suppression after a high dose of dexamethasone is consistent with pituitary-dependent Cushing's disease. Lack of suppression (all cortisol values remain above 1.5 μg/dL) is diagnostic of a pituitary or adrenal tumor.

THYROID GLAND DISORDERS

TSH STIMULATION TEST

Administer 0.5 U/kg TSH (maximum dose, 5 U) IV. Obtain serum samples before and 6 hours after injection of TSH for T_4 determination.

Interpretation

Post-TSH T_4 levels < 3 μg/dL (35 nmol/L) are consistent with hypothyroidism.

TRH STIMULATION TEST

Administer 0.1 mg/kg TRH IV. Obtain serum samples before and 4 hours after TRH injection for T_4 determination.

Interpretation

An increase in T_4 concentration $< 50\%$ after TRH administration is consistent with hypothyroidism.

T_3 Suppression Test

Obtain a blood sample for determination of T_4 and T_3. The serum is removed and kept refrigerated or frozen. Administer T_3 (Cytomel, Smith, Kline, and French Laboratories) PO at a dosage of 25 μg/cat q8h for 2 days. On the morning of the third day, administer 25 μg of T_3, and 2–4 hours later obtain a second blood sample for T_3 and T_4 determinations. The basal (day 1) and postoral T_3 serum samples should be submitted to the laboratory together to avoid interassay variation.

Interpretation

Serum T_4 concentration after administration of $T_3 >$ than 1.5 μg/dL (20 nmol/L) is consistent with hyperthyroidism.

GASTRINOMA

SECRETIN STIMULATION TEST

Administer 2 units of secretin/kg IV. Take blood samples before administration of secretin and then 2, 5, 10, 15, and 30 minutes later. Assay the samples for gastrin.

Interpretation
Dogs with gastrinomas have a rise in gastrin levels after the injection of secretin. In three reported cases, two dogs had a rise in gastrin levels 2 times baseline 5 minutes after secretin injection, and one dog had a rise in gastrin levels 1.4 times baseline 5 minutes after secretin injection. Normal dogs have a decline in gastrin levels after administration of secretin.

CALCIUM CHALLENGE TEST

Administer 2 mg/kg of calcium gluconate IV over a 1-minute period or administer 5 mg/kg of calcium gluconate as an IV infusion over several hours. Obtain a blood sample before calcium administration and then 15, 30, 60, 90, and 120 minutes after the calcium administration. Assay the samples for gastrin.

Interpretation
Two reported patients with gastrinoma had a doubling of the gastrin level 60 minutes after the calcium infusion.

SEX HORMONE DISORDERS

Gn-RH STIMULATION TEST

Administer 0.5–1.0 μg of Gn-RH/kg IM. Obtain blood samples before Gn-RH administration and 1 hour later. Assay blood samples for testosterone.

Interpretation
Normal dogs have baseline testosterone levels between 0.5–5 ng/mL, and after administration of Gn-RH the testosterone levels rise above 5 ng/mL. Animals with hypoandrogenism have lower values.

HCG STIMULATION TEST

Administer 44 IU of hCG/kg IM. Obtain blood samples before hCG administration and 4 hours later. Assay blood samples for testosterone.

Interpretation
Normal dogs have baseline testosterone levels between 0.5–5 ng/mL, and after administration of hCG, the testosterone levels rise above 5 ng/mL. Animals with hypoandrogenism have lower values.

DIABETES INSIPIDUS

MODIFIED WATER DEPRIVATION TEST

Rule out other causes of polyuria and polydipsia (especially hyperadrenocorticism). Begin water restriction 3 days before abrupt water deprivation.

Day 1 130–165 mL/kg/day
Day 2 100–125 mL/kg/day
Day 3 65–70 mL/kg/day (normal maintenance requirement)

The morning of the fourth day, discontinue food and water. Start the test. Weigh the patient and empty the bladder. Weigh at 1–2 hour intervals. Monitor carefully for dehydration and depression. When 5% of body weight is lost or azotemia develops, empty the bladder and check urine specific gravity. Consider plasma vasopressin determination at this point.

Interpretation
If the urine specific gravity is > 1.025 (dogs) or > 1.030 (cats), stop the test. The patient does not have diabetes insipidus. If the urine specific gravity is not > 1.025 (dogs) or > 1.030 (cats), administer 0.55 U/kg aqueous vasopressin IM (maximum dose, 5 U). Empty the bladder and check urine specific gravity at 30, 60, and 120 minutes postadministration. If urine specific gravity increases < 10%, nephrogenic diabetes insipidus is indicated; if it increases 10–50%, partial central diabetes insipidus is indicated; if it increases 50–80%, complete central diabetes insipidus is indicated.

APPENDIX IV

TESTS OF THE ENDOCRINE SYSTEM*

Hormone	Unit	Dogs	Cats
Adrenocorticotropic hormone, basal (ACTH, plasma)	pmol/L	2–15	1–20
Aldosterone† (plasma)			
Basal	pmol/L	14–957	194–388
Post-ACTH	pmol/L	197–2103	277–721
Cortisol (serum or plasma, urine)			
Basal	nmol/L	25–125	15–150
Post-ACTH	nmol/L	200–550	130–450
Post–low-dose dexamethasone (0.01 or 0.015 mg/kg)	nmol/L	≤ 40	≤ 40
Post–high-dose dexamethasone (0.1 or 1.0 mg/kg)‡	nmol/L	≤ 40	≤ 40
Urinary cortisol-creatinine ratio	$\times 10^{-6}$	8–24†, 10§	—
Insulin, basal (serum)	pmol/L	35–200	35–200
Intact parathormone† (serum)	pmol/L	2–13	0–4
Progesterone (serum or plasma, female)	mmol/L	≤ 3.0 in anestrus, proestrus	≤ 3.0 in anestrus, proestrus
		50–220 in diestrus, pregnancy	50–220 in diestrus, pregnancy
Testosterone (serum or plasma, male)	nmol/L	1–20	1–20
Thyroxine (T_4, serum)			
Basal	nmol/L	12–50	10–50
Post–thyroxine-stimulating hormone (TSH)	nmol/L	> 45	> 45
Triiodothyronine (T_3) suppression‖	nmol/L	—	≤ 20
Triiodothyronine, basal (T_3, serum)	nmol/L	0.7–2.3	0.5–2.0

*Prepared with the assistance of ME Peterson, The Animal Medical Center, New York, NY. Unless indicated otherwise, values in this table are adapted from Kemppainen RJ, Zerbe CA. Common endocrine diagnostic tests: normal values and interpretations. In: Kirk RW, ed. Current veterinary therapy X. Philadelphia: WB Saunders, 1989:961–968. Hormone determinations are variable between laboratories. The laboratory performing the analysis should provide reference values. Before submitting samples for hormone determinations, consult the laboratory for sample specifications, use of anticoagulants, and sample preservation. General sampling conditions are discussed in Reimers TJ. Guidelines for collection, storage, and transport of samples for hormone assay. In: Kirk RW, ed. Current veterinary therapy X. Philadelphia: WB Saunders, 1989:968–973. Factors that affect serum thyroid and adrenocortical hormone concentrations in dogs are discussed in Reimers TJ, Lawler DF, Sutaria PM, Correa MT, Erb HN. Effects of age, sex, and body size on serum concentrations of thyroid and adrenocortical hormones in dogs. Am J Vet Res 1990;51:454.

†Provided by RF Nachreiner, Animal Health Diagnostic Laboratory, Endocrine Diagnostic Section, Michigan State University.

‡This test is used after adrenocortical hyperfunction has been confirmed. It is used to differentiate adrenal tumor (where no suppression is seen) from pituitary-dependent cases (where suppression occurs but is variable).

§From Stolp R, Rijnberk A, Meiher JC, Croughs RJM. Urinary corticoids in the diagnosis of canine hyperadrenocorticism. Res Vet Sci 1983;34:141. Rijnberk A, van Wees A, Mol JA. Assessment of two tests for the diagnosis of canine hyperadrenocorticism. Vet Rec 1988;122:178–180.

‖From Peterson ME, Ferguson DC. Thyroid disease. In: Ettinger SJ, ed. Textbook of veterinary internal medicine. Diseases of the dog and cat. 3rd ed. Philadelphia: WB Saunders, 1989:1632–1675.

From appendices in Bonagura J, ed. Kirk's current veterinary therapy XIII. Philadelphia: WB Saunders, 2000; 1223 (with permission).

APPENDIX V

CONVERSION TABLE FOR HORMONE ASSAY UNITS

	Unit		Conversion factors	
Hormone	Traditional	SI	Traditional to SI	SI to Traditional
Aldosterone	ng/dl	pmol/L	27.7	0.036
Corticotropin (ACTH)	pg/ml	pmol/L	0.22	4.51
Cortisol	µg/dl	mmol/L	27.59	0.36
β-endorphin	pg/ml	pmol/L	0.289	3.43
Epinephrine	pg/ml	pmol/L	5.46	0.183
Estrogen (estradiol)	pg/ml	pmol/L	3.67	0.273
Gastrin	pg/ml	ng/L	1.00	1.00
Glucagon	pg/ml	ng/L	1.00	1.00
Growth hormone (GH)	ng/ml	µg/L	1.00	1.00
Insulin	µU/ml	pmol/L	7.18	0.139
α-Melanocyte-stimulating hormone (α-MSH)	pg/ml	pmol/L	0.601	1.66
Norepinephrine	pg/ml	nmol/L	0.006	169
Pancreatic polypeptide (PP)	mg/dl	mmol/L	0.239	4.18
Progesterone	ng/ml	mmol/L	3.18	0.315
Prolactin	ng/ml	µg/L	1.00	1.00
Renin	ng/ml/hr	ng/L/s	0.278	3.60
Somatostatin	pg/ml	pmol/L	0.611	1.64
Testosterone	ng/ml	nmol/L	3.47	0.288
Thyroxine (T_4)	µg/dl	nmol/L	12.87	0.078
Triiodothyronine (T_3)	ng/dl	nmol/L	0.0154	64.9
Vasoactive intestinal polypeptide (VIP)	pg/ml	pmol/L	0.301	3.33

Contributed by ME Peterson, The Animal Medical Center, New York, NY.
From Appendices. In: Bonagura JD, ed. Current veterinary therapy XIII. Philadelphia: WB Saunders, 2000: 1223 (with permission).

INDEX

Pages in italics denote figures; those followed by a t denote tables

Abscessation, 282–286
  causes, 282–283
  clinical features, 283
  definition/overview, 282
  diagnostics, 284
  differential diagnosis, 283
  etiology/pathophysiology, 282
  pathologic findings, 284–285
  signalment/history, 283
  therapeutics, 285
Acarexx, for ear mites, 211
Acaricides, 177
Accutane. (*see* Isotretinoin)
Acepromazine
  for tick bite paralysis, 183
  withdrawal time prior to intradermal skin testing, 631, 632
Acetaminophen, 654t
Acetylcholinesterase, 220
Acid-fast bacteria. (*see* Mycobacterial infections)
Acne, 71, 164–166, 533, 537
  clinical features, 165
  definition/overview, 164
  diagnostics, 165
  differential diagnosis, 165
  etiology/pathophysiology, 164
  papular and nodular dermatoses, 85, 86
  signalment/history, 164
  therapeutics, 86, 165–166
Acral lick dermatitis, 167–172
  appearance of, *168, 169, 170*
  clinical features, 169
  definition/overview, 167
  diagnostics, 169–170
  differential diagnosis, 169
  etiology/pathophysiology, 167
  signalment/history, 167
  therapeutics, 170–171
Acrodermatitis, 109t
ACTH, 659t, 677, 678
  plasma levels, 607–608
ACTH response test, 41, *55*, 378, 385, 386, 390, 396, 398, 403, 595–601, 674
  complications, 600–601
  definition/overview, 595
  diagnostics, 598–599
  differential diagnosis, 597
  etiology/pathophysiology, 595–596
  laboratory findings, 597–598
  medications and, 599–600
  patient monitoring, 600
  results, 596
  treatment, 599
Acthar. (*see* Corticotropin)
Actinic conditions, papular and nodular, 85, 86
Actinomyces spp. in erosive and ulcerative dermatoses, 62
Actinomycete, 305
Activated charcoal. (*see* Charcoal, activated)
Adenocarcinoma. (*see specific neoplasms*)
Adrenal gland disease. (*see also* Hyperadrenocorticism)
  diagnostics, 674
  in ferrets
    clinical signs, 511, *512*
    definition/overview, 511
    diagnostic tests, 512
    lab findings, 512
    pathophysiology, 511
    prognosis, 512
    treatment, 512
  tumors, 379–381
Adrenal 21-hydroxylase enzyme deficiency, 389, 391, 392
Adrenal hyperplasia-like syndrome, alopecia from, 33t
Adrenal reproductive hormone test, 390
Adrenal sex hormone imbalance, 389
Adrenalectomy, 379, 403
Advantage, 192. (*see also* Imidacloprid)
AIHA. (*see* Autoimmune hemolytic anemia (AIHA))

Albinism, 140
Aldosterone, 677, 678
Allergic disorders
  atopy, 248–252
  contact dermatitis, 107, 257–260, 639
    atopy compared, 250
    clinical features, *258*, 258–259, *259*
    definition/overview, 257
    diagnostics, 259–260
    differential diagnosis, 259
    etiology/pathophysiology, 257
    interdigital dermatitis, 123
    pododermatitis, 111
    signalment/history, 258
  dermatitis
    feline alopecia from, 45, *45*, 58t
    hyposensitization, 633–636
    interdigital dermatitis, 123, *123*, 126t
    intradermal skin testing, preparation, 631–632
    otitis secondary to, 145, *146*, *147*
    overview of, 630
    testing, 630–632
    therapeutics, 59
  pododermatitis, 103, 107, 113
  staphylococcal blepharitis, 627
Allergroom (Allerderm), 587
Allergy
  dust mite, 637
  mold, 638
  testing
    for atopy, 250
    intradermal, 250
    in pruritic dermatoses, 232–233
    serologic, 250
  vaccine, 251, 633–636
    adverse reactions, 633
    how it works, 633
    interactions, 634
    schedule, 635–636
    technique, 633
AllersebT (Allerderm), 588
Allopurinol, for leishmaniasis, 349
Alocetic, for otitis, 150
Alopecia. (*see also* alopecia, canine; alopecia, feline)
  areata, 31, *31*, 32t, 53, *54*, 56t, 561
  cyclic flank, 648
  in dermatomyositis, *526*, 527, *527*, *528*
  in discoid lupus erythematosus, *421*
  in feline skin fragility syndrome, 400–401, *401*, *402*
  in ferrets, 511, *512*
  in growth hormone-responsive dermatoses, 384
  in guinea pigs, 507
  in hyperadrenocorticism, *376*
  in hypothyroidism, *367*, 367–368, *368*
  in leishmaniasis, *347*, *348*
  pruritus and, 232
  in rabbits, 505
  in sebaceous adenitis, 551, 552, *552*
  in sex hormone-responsive dermatoses, 390
Alopecia, canine, 27–42
  clinical features, 28
  definition/overview, 27
  diagnostics, 32t–35t, 41
  differential diagnosis, 28–41
    multifocal, 28–31, *28–31*, 32t
      alopecia aerata, 31, 32t
      demodicosis, 28, *28*, *29*, 32t
      dermatophytosis, 28, 32t
      injection reactions, 28, 32t
      rabies vaccine vasculitis, 28, *30*, 32t
      scleroderma, 31, 32t
      sebaceous adenitis, 31, *31*, 32t
      Staphylococcal folliculitis, 28, *29*, *30*, 32t
    patchy to diffuse, 34t–35t, 38, *39–40*
      anagen/telogen defluxion, 34t, 38
      color mutant alopecia, 34t, 38
      demodicosis, 34t, 38
      dermatophytosis, 34t, 38
      epidermotropic lymphoma, 38, *39*, *40*
      follicular dysplasia, 34t, 38
      hyperadrenocorticism, 34t, 38
      hypothyroidism, 34t, 38, *39*
      keratinization disorders, 35t, 38, *40*
      mycosis fungoides, 35t
      pemphigus foliaceus, 35t, 38
      sebaceous adenitis, 34t, 38
      Staphylococcal folliculitis, 34t, 38
    specific locations, 35t, 38, 41
      black hair follicular dysplasia, 35t, 41
      dermatomyositis, 35t, 41
      melanoderma, 35t, 41
      pinna, 35t, 38
      postclipping, 35t, 38
      seasonal flank alopecia, 35t, 41
      traction alopecia, 35t, 38
    symmetrical, 31, 33t–34t, *36–38*
      castration-responsive dermatosis, 31, 33t
      estrogen-responsive dermatosis, 31, 34t
      growth hormone-responsive dermatosis, 31, 33t, *37*
      hyperadrenocorticism, 31, 33t, *36*
      hyperestrogenism, 31, 33t
      hypogonadism, 31, 33t
      hypothyroidism, 31, 33t
      seasonal flank alopecia, 31
      Sertoli cell tumor, 31, 33t, *38*
      testosterone-responsive dermatosis, 31, 33t
  etiology/pathophysiology, 27
  signalment/history, 27
  therapeutics, 41
  zoonotic potential, 41
Alopecia, feline, 43–60
  clinical features, 44

definition/overview, 43
diagnostics, 55, 56t, 58t
differential diagnosis, 44–55
allergic dermatitis, 45, *45*, 58t
alopecia areata, 53, *54*, 56t
alopecia universalis, 53, 57t
anagen/telogen defluxion, 55, 56t
demodicosis, 55, 56t
dermatophytosis, 55, 56t
diabetes mellitus, 45, *47*, 57t
endocrine alopecia, 44, 46, 58t
epidermotrophic lymphoma, *52*, 53, *53*, 58t
hyperadrenocorticism, 46, *48*, *49*, 57t
hyperthyroidism, 45, *46*, 57t
hypothyroidism, 58t
hypotrichosis, 53, 57t
injection reaction, 56t
obsessive compulsive disorder, *44*, 45, 58t
paraneoplastic alopecia, 46, *50*, 57t
pinnal alopecia, spontaneous, 53, 56t
sebaceous adenitis, 48–49, *50*, *51*, 57t
sex hormone alopecia, 44
squamous cell carcinoma in situ, 49, *51*, *52*, 58t
etiology/pathophysiology, 43
signalment/history, 43
symmetrical, 558–561
clinical features, 558, *559*, *560*
definition/overview, 558
diagnostics, 560–561
differential diagnosis, 560
etiology/pathophysiology, 558
signalment/history, 558
therapeutics, 561
therapeutics, 59
zoonotic potential, 59
Alopecia areata, 561
canine, 31, *31*, 32t
feline, 53, *54*, 56t
Alopecia universalis, 53, 57t
ALP glucocorticoid isoenzyme, 396
Alpha-linolenic acid, 240
Amblyomma americanum, 181, 182
Amblyomma maculatum, 181, 182
Amcinonide, for discoid lupus erythematosus, 422
Amgen, 659t
Aminoglycosides
for anaerobic infections, 296
for bacteremia, *281*
for nocardiosis, 312
ototoxicity from, 156
Aminophylline, for anaphylaxis, 246
Amitraz
for cheyletiellosis, 196
for demodicosis, 41, 59, 207–208, 645
drug interactions, 209
for ear mites, 212
for sarcoptic mange, 201
side effects, 208
toxicosis, 212, 213–216
clinical features, 214
definition/overview, 213
diagnostics, 214
differential diagnosis, 214
signalment/history, 213–214
therapeutics, 215
yohimbine antidote, 208, 215
Amitriptyline, 628
for acral lick dermatitis, 171
for atopy, 252
dosage, 242t
for feline symmetrical alopecia, 561
histamine binding by, 240
for obsessive compulsive disorder, 59
for pruritus, 234
Ammonia tolerance test, 396
Amoxicillin, 654t
for abscessation, 285
for anaerobic infections, 296
for dermatophilosis, 307
for nocardiosis, 312
Amoxicillin/clavulanic acid
for abscessation, 285
for eosinophilic granuloma complex, 266
for pyoderma, 291, 292
Amphotericin B, 654t
for blastomycosis, 343
for coccidiodomycosis, 337–338
for cryptococcosis, 332
precautions, 338
side effects, 338, 654t
Ampicillin, 654t
for dermatophilosis, 307
for nocardiosis, 312
Amyloidosis, 542, 548, 549
ANA. (*see* Antinuclear antibody (ANA))
Anaerobic bacterial infections, 294–296
clinical features, 294–295
definition/overview, 294
diagnostics, 295
differential diagnosis, 295
etiology/pathophysiology, 294
signalment/history, 294
therapeutics, 295–296
Anafranil. (*see* Clomipramine)
Anagen defluxion
canine, 34t, 38
feline, 55, 56t
Anal sac disorders, 157–159
clinical features, 158
definition/overview, 157
diagnostics, 158
differential diagnosis, 158
etiology/pathophysiology, 157
signalment/history, 157–158
therapeutics, 158
Anaphylaxis. (*see* Hypersensitivity reaction)
Ancobon. (*see* Flucytosine)

Andro-Cyp. (*see* Testosterone therapeutics)
Android. (*see* Methyltestosterone)
Andronate. (*see* Testosterone therapeutics)
Angioedema, in cutaneous drug eruptions, 272
Anipryl, 380
Anisocoria, in otitis, 153
Antibiotics. (*see also specific agents*)
  for abscessation, 285
  for acne, 537
  for anaerobic infections, 295–296
  for bacteremia, 280–281
  for eosinophilic granuloma complex, 266
  for interdigital dermatitis, 125, 127
  for lichenoid-psoriasiform dermatosis, 539
  for mycobacterial infections, 302–303
  for nocardiosis, 312
  for otitis, 149–150, 156
  for pyoderma, 291–292
  for schnauzer comedone syndrome, 539
  for sebaceous adenitis, 553
  for vasculitis, 439
Antifungals. (*see also specific agents*)
  for cryptococcosis, 332
  for otitis, 149–150
Antihistamines, 628. (*see also specific agents*)
  adverse effects, 240
  for atopy, 251
  dosages, table of, 241t
  for feline symmetrical alopecia, 561
  for fleas, 187
  food elimination diet trial and, 256
  precautions, 251
  for pruritus, 233, 234, 240
  for sarcoptic mange, 201
  withdrawal time prior to intradermal skin testing, 631, 632
Antimicrobial shampoos, 589–590
  benzoyl peroxide, 589
  chlorhexidine, 589–590
  ethyl lactate, 590
  imidazole, 590
  iodine, 590
Antinuclear antibody (ANA), 617–621
  definition/overview, 617
  diagnostics, 621
  differential diagnosis, 620
  laboratory findings, 620
  pathophysiology, 618
  in pemphigus erythematosus, 411
  signalment, 618
  signs, 618–620
  in systemic lupus erythematosus, 427, 429
  systems affected, 618
  in vasculitis, 439
Antipruritics, topical, 590–591
Antiseborrheic shampoos, 538, 587–589
  benzoyl peroxide, 589
  selenium sulfide, 588–589
  sulfur and salicylic acid, 587–588
  tar, 588
Antisedan, for amitraz toxicosis, 215
Antiseptics, for otitis, 150
Aplasia cutis, 69
Apocrine gland
  adenocarcinoma, 486–488, *487*
  inflammation, 160
Arachidonic acid
  essential fatty acid metabolites effect on, 240
  lipoxygenase inhibitors effect on, 239
  NSAIDS effect on, 239
  pruritus and, 237
Aranofin, in pemphigus, 413
Aristocort. (*see* Triamcinolone)
Arthrocentesis, 621
Aspiration
  of abscess, 284
  fine-needle technique, 4
Aspirin, 655t
  adverse effects, 428, 655t
  for pruritus, 239
  for systemic lupus erythematosus, 428
Astemizole
  adverse effects, 251
  dosage, 241t
Asthenia. (*see* Cutaneous asthenia)
Astringents, for otitis, 150
Atarax. (*see* Hydroxyzine)
Atipamezole
  for amitraz toxicosis, 215
  side effects, 215
Atopy, 248–252
  clinical features, 249
  definition/overview, 248
  diagnostics, 250
  differential diagnosis, 249–250
  etiology/pathophysiology, 248
  pathogenesis of, 238
  pododermatitis, 107
  pruritus from, 232
  signalment/history, 248–249
  therapeutics, 250–252
Atropine
  for anaphylaxis, 246
  for bradycardia, ivermectin-related, 218
  contraindications, 227
  for organophosphate and carbamate toxicity, 223
Auranofin, for bullous pemphigoid, 418
Aurothioglucose
  for bullous pemphigoid, 418
  for eosinophilic granuloma complex, 266
  for pemphigus, 413
Autoantibodies. (*see also* Autoimmune diseases)
  in pemphigoid, 415
  to thyroglobulin and thyroid hormones, 370
Autoimmune diseases. (*see also* Pemphigus)
  bullous pemphigoid, 415–419
  erosive and ulcerative dermatoses, 62, *63*, *64*

exfoliative dermatosis from, 77, 79
otitis from, 145
pemphigus, 407–414
systemic lupus erythematosus, 424–429
Autoimmune hemolytic anemia (AIHA), 622–623
Azathioprine, 655t
adverse effects, 137, 143, 413, 418, 540, 655t
for bullous pemphigoid, 418
contraindications, 444
for discoid lupus erythematosus, 422
for panniculitis, 435
for pemphigus, 412
for pyogranuloma, sterile, 549
for sebaceous adenitis, 540
for systemic lupus erythematosus, 143, 428
toxicity, 428
for uveodermatologic syndrome, 444, 445
for vasculitis, 440
Azithromycin, 655t
Azulfidine. (*see* Sulfasalazine)

Babesia canis, 177
Babesiosis, 177
Bacteremia, 277–281
clinical features, 278
definition/overview, 277
diagnostics, 278–280
etiology/pathophysiology, 277–278
signalment/history, 278
therapeutics, 280–281
Bacterial infections, 643–644
anaerobic, 294–296
erosive and ulcerative dermatoses, 62, 67
folliculitis, 643
alopecia from, 34t, 38
papular and nodular dermatoses, 84
therapeutics, 85
interdigital, *124,* 125, 126t
nail and nailbed, 116, 117t, 120
otitis, 147, 149–150
pododermatitis, *102,* 107, 644
pyoderma, 287–293, 643–644
deep, 643–644
superficial, 643
Bacteroidaceae, 280
Bacteroides, 294, 296
Bactrim, 655t
Barbering, in rabbits, 519–520
clinical signs, 519, *520*
definition/overview, 519
diagnostic tests, 520
etiology/pathophysiology, 519
lab findings, 519
prognosis, 520
treatment, 520
Basal cell tumors, 476–477
clinical features, 476, *477*
definition/overview, 476
diagnostics, 477
differential diagnosis, 477
signalment/history, 476
therapeutics, 477
Baytril. (*see* Enrofloxacin)
Benadryl. (*see* Diphenhydramine)
Benoxaprofen, for pruritus, 239
Benozopyrones, for lymphedema, 572
Benzoyl peroxide
for acne, 86, 165, 166, 537
for acral lick dermatitis, 171
adverse effects, 540
examples of, 589
for exfoliative dermatoses, 81
for interdigital dermatitis, 127
for keratinization disorders, 537–540
for pododemodicosis, 646
properties of, 589
for pyoderma, 291, 292
for sebaceous adenitis, 553
Benzoyl-Plus (EVSCO), 589
Bernese mountain dog, histiocytosis in, *545, 546,* 548, 576, *577*
Beta-endorphin, 678
Betamethasone, 656t
for pemphigus, 413
potency, 239t
Biopsy. (*see also* Cytology)
of abscess, 284
in atopy, 250
in blastomycosis, 343
in bullous pemphigoid, 417
in calcinosis cutis, 599, 605, 611
in coccidiodomycosis, 336
in contact dermatitis, 260
in cryptococcosis, 331, 332
in cutaneous drug eruptions, 272
in dermatomyositis, 528–529
in dermatophytosis, 322
in discoid lupus erythematosus, 422
in eosinophilic granuloma complex, 265
in erosive and ulcerative dermatoses, 72
in feline symmetrical alopecia, 560
fine-needle technique, 4
in flea bite hypersensitivity, 187
in growth hormone-responsive dermatoses, 386
in hepatocutaneous syndrome, 567, 568
in hyperadrenocorticism, 599, 605, 611
in interdigital dermatitis, 125
in leishmaniasis, 348
in mast cell tumors, 468, 469
in mycobacterial infections, 300, 301
in otitis, 148
in panniculitis, 434
in papular and nodular dermatoses, 85
in pemphigus, 412
in pododermatitis, 112, 113
in pox virus infection, 355

    in pruritic dermatoses, 233
    punch, 20–21
    in puppy strangles, 574–575
    in pyoderma, 291
    site selection, 650–651
    skin
        site selection, 20
        technique, 20–21, *21*
        when to biopsy, 19
    in squamous cell carcinoma, 480
    steroid hepatopathy, 395, 397
    in systemic lupus erythematosus, 427
    technique, 651
    in uveodermatologic syndrome, 444
    in vasculitis, 439
    when to biopsy, 650
Black hair follicular dysplasia, 35t, 41
Blastomycosis, 340–345
    clinical features, *341,* 341–342, *342*
    course and prognosis, 344–345
    definition/overview, 340
    diagnostics, 342–343
    differential diagnosis, 342
    etiology/pathophysiology, 340
    prevention/avoidance, 344
    recurrence, 345
    signalment/history, 340–341
    therapeutics, 343–344
    zoonotic potential, 345
Bleomycin, for squamous cell carcinoma, 482
Blepharitis, Staphylococcal, 627
Blood culture
    collection, 279–280
    guidelines, 279
    media, 280
    results, interpretation of, 280
Borrelia burgdorferi, 177, 178
Bowenoid carcinoma (Bowen disease), *51,* 58t. (*see also* Squamous cell carcinoma)
Bowen's disease, 358, *359,* 361
Brainstem auditory-evoked response (BAER), 155
Brush technique, 5, *6, 7*
Bullae osteotomy, 149, 155, 156, 484
Bullous pemphigoid, 415–419
    breed predilection, 88
    chronic form, 415, *416,* 417, 418, 419
    clinical features, 415–417, *416*
    definition/overview, 415
    diagnostics, 417
    differential diagnosis, 417
    etiology/pathophysiology, 415
    of footpad, 109t
    patient monitoring, 418
    pododermatitis, 107
    prognosis, 419
    signalment/history, 415
    therapeutics, 417–418
    vesicles and ulceration, 93, 95
Burn, thermal, 71, *71*
Burrows solution, for interdigital dermatitis, 127
Busipirone, 242t
Buspar. (*see* Busipirone)

Calcinosis, 542, *543, 544,* 549, 550
Calcinosis circumscripta, 110t, 542, *544, 545,* 549, 550
Calcinosis cutis, *377,* 599, 605, 611
Calcium challenge test, 676
Calicivirus. (*see* Feline calicivirus)
Canine distemper virus, in ferrets, 521–522
    clinical signs, 521
    definition, overview, 521
    diagnostic tests, 522
    etiology/pathophysiology, 521
    lab findings, 522
    prognosis, 522
    treatment, 522
Capscarin, for acral lick dermatitis, 171
Carbamate
    contraindications, 188
    toxicity, 220–224
        client education, 223
        clinical features, 221
        definition/overview, 220
        diagnostics, 222
        differential diagnosis, 222
        etiology/pathophysiology, 220–221
        signalment/history, 221
        therapeutics, 222–223
Carbamide peroxide, for otitis, 150
Carboplatin, for melanocytic tumors, 474
Carprofen, for systemic lupus erythematosus, 428
Castration-responsive dermatosis
    alopecia from, 31, 33t
    course and prognosis, 393
    signalment/history, 389
    therapeutics, 392
Ceclor, 656t
Cefaclor, 656t
Cefadroxil, 657t
Cefazolin, *281,* 657t
Cefixime, 657t
Cefotan, 657t
Cefotetan, 657t
Cefoxitin, 296, 657t
Ceftiofur, 658t
Celestone, 656t
Cellulitis, 288, *288*
Cellulitis, canine juvenile, 62, 573–575
    clinical features, 573–574, *574*
    definition/overview, 573
    diagnostics, 574–575
    differential diagnosis, 574
    etiology/pathophysiology, 573
    signalment/history, 573
    therapeutics, 575

Central nervous system, pruritus and, 237
Cephalexin, 658t
for eosinophilic granuloma complex, 266
for otitis, 149
for staphylococcal blepharitis, 627t
Cephalosporins
for acne, 166
for bacteremia, *281*
for pyoderma, 291
Cerumenolytics, for otitis, 150
Ceruminous gland adenocarcinoma, 483–485
clinical features, 483, *484*
course and prognosis, 485
definition/overview, 483
diagnostics, 484
differential diagnosis, 484
patient monitoring, 485
signalment/history, 483
therapeutics, 484
Cetirizine, 241t
Charcoal, activated
for amitraz toxicosis, 215
for pyrethrin/pyrethroid toxicity, 227
Chediak-Higashi syndrome, 583
Cheyletiella parasitovorax, 505–506, *506*
Cheyletiella yasguri, 195
Cheyletiellosis, 194–197
clinical features, 195, *196*
definition/overview, 194
diagnostics, 195–196
differential diagnosis, 195
etiology/pathophysiology, 194, *195*
in rabbits, 505–506, *506*
signalment/history, 194–195
therapeutics, 196
zoonotic potential, 194, 196, 197
CHILD syndrome, 533, 537–538
Chlorambucil
for bullous pemphigoid, 418
for eosinophilic granuloma complex, 266
for epidermotrophic lymphoma, 454
for hypereosinophilic syndrome, 270
for pemphigus, 412
for systemic lupus erythematosus, 137, 143, 428
for vasculitis, 440
Chloramphenicol
adverse effects, 292
for anaerobic infections, 296
pregnancy, use in, 83
for pyoderma, 291
ChlorhexiDerm (DVM), 589
Chlorhexidine
for otitis, 150
otitis from, 153, 156
for pyoderma, 291, 292
shampoos, 589–590
Chlorpheniramine, 628
for acral lick dermatitis, 171
for atopy, 251
dosage, 241t
for feline symmetrical alopecia, 561
for pruritus, 234
Chlorpyrifos, 222
Chlortetracycline, 658t
Chlortrimeton. (*see* Chlorpheniramine)
Cholinesterase activity, 220–222
Chorioptes mites in hedgehogs, 499–500
Chorioretinitis, 331, 332
Chrysotherapy
adverse effects, 413, 418
for bullous pemphigoid, 418
contraindications, 137, 143
for eosinophilic granuloma complex, 266
for pemphigus, 413
Chymotrypsin, pruritus and, 237
Cimetidine, 241t, 658t
for mast cell tumors, 469
for melanocytic tumors, 474
Ciprofloxacin, for tuberculosis, 302
Cisplatin, for squamous cell carcinoma, 481
Claforan, 657t
Claratin. (*see* Loratidine)
Clarithromycin
for mycobacteriosis, atypical, 303
for tuberculosis, 302
Clavamox, 659t
Clavulanic acid, 659t
Clemastine, 628
for atopy, 251
dosage, 241t
Clindamycin
for acne, 166
for anaerobic infections, 296
for otitis, 149
Clofazimine
adverse effects, 303
for leprosy, feline, 302
for mycobacteriosis, atypical, 303
Clomipramine
for acral lick dermatitis, 171
dosage, 242t
Closed-patch testing, 259
Cloxacillin, for pyoderma, 291
CO_2 laser, 266
Coagulation assessment, in steroid hepatopathy, 397
Cobalt 60 radiation therapy, 403
Coccidiodomycosis, 334–339
clinical features, 335–336
complications, 338
course and prognosis, 338–339
definition/overview, 334
diagnostics, 336
differential diagnosis, 336
erosive and ulcerative dermatoses, 62
etiology/pathophysiology, 334
patient monitoring, 338
prevention/avoidance, 338
signalment/history, 335

therapeutics, 336–338
for cats, 337–338
contraindications/precautions, 338
for dogs, 337
zoonotic potential, 339
Cocker spaniel, keratinization disorders in, 533, *534, 535*
Cold agglutinin disease
erosive and ulcerative dermatoses, 62
pododermatitis, 107
Colony-stimulating factor, 659t
Color mutant alopecia, 34t, 38, 76
Comedones, *377,* 533, 539
Complement deficiency, 583
Computed tomography. (*see* CT (computed tomography))
Contact dermatitis, 257–260, 639
atopy compared, 250
clinical features, *258,* 258–259, *259*
contact dermatitis, 260
definition/overview, 257
diagnostics, 259–260
differential diagnosis, 259
etiology/pathophysiology, 257
interdigital dermatitis, 123
pododermatitis, 111
signalment/history, 258
Coombs test, 427, 622–625
definition, 622
diagnostic procedures, 625
differential diagnosis, 623–624
laboratory findings, 624–625
pathophysiology, 622
signalment, 623
signs, 623
systems affected, 622–623
Cortef. (*see* Hydrocortisone)
CortiCalm (Allerderm), 591
Corticosteroids
for acne, 166, 537
for acral lick dermatitis, 171
for actinic conditions, 86
adverse effects, 413, 418
for atopy, 251
for bullous pemphigoid, 418
for contact dermatitis, 260
contraindications, 189, 344
for discoid lupus erythematosus, 422
for eosinophilic granuloma complex, 266
for epidermotropic lymphoma, 59
for exfoliative dermatoses, 82
for fleas, 187
for histiocytosis, 580–581
for hypereosinophilic syndrome, 270
for keratinization disorders, 537–540
for nasal solar dermatitis, 143
for otitis, 149–150
for panniculitis, 434
for pemphigus, 412, 414
for perianal fistula, 162
precautions, 234–235, 251
for pruritus, 233–235, 236, 238–239, 239t
for puppy strangles, 575
for pyoderma, 292
for sebaceous adenitis, 59, 649
for shock, 246
for systemic lupus erythematosus, 428
for uveodermatologic syndrome, 444, 445
withdrawal time prior to intradermal skin testing, 631, 632
Corticotropin, 659t
Corticotropin releasing hormone (CRH) response test, 379
Cortisol, 677, 678
urine cortisol:creatinine ratio, 378, 396, 609–612
Cortrosyn, 659t
Cosyntropin, 659t
Cranial nerve damage, in otitis, 153
Creatinine
urine cortisol:creatinine ratio, 378, 396, 609–612
Cretinism, in congenital hypothyroidism, 369
Crusts, *10,* 20
Cryptococcosis, 329–333
capsular antigen titers, 331, 333
clinical features, *330,* 330–331
definition/overview, 329
diagnostics, 331–332
differential diagnosis, 331
etiology/pathophysiology, 329
signalment/history, 329–330
therapeutics, 332
ulcerative facial dermatitis, *68*
Cryptococcus neoformans, 68, 329
CSF analysis, in otitis, 155
CT (computed tomography)
in hyperadrenocorticism, 379
in otitis, 155
Culture
of abscess, 284
in coccidiodomycosis, 336
in cryptococcosis, 331
in dermatophilosis, 307
in dermatophytosis, *322, 324*
in leishmaniasis, 348
in mycobacterial infections, 301
in nocardiosis, 312
in panniculitis, 434
in pyoderma, 291
in sporotrichosis, 327
Cushing's disease. (*see* Hyperadrenocorticism)
Cutaneous asthenia, 69, 554–557
clinical features, *555,* 555–556, *556*
definition/overview, 554
differential diagnosis, 556
etiology/pathophysiology, 554
signalment/history, 554
therapeutics, 556
Cutaneous basophil hypersensitiviity, 185

Cutaneous cysts, 433
Cutaneous drug eruptions, 271–273
Cutaneous horns, footpad, 110t
Cutaneous lesions
  cytology of, 3–11
  dermahistopathology, 19–21, *22–23*
Cyclic hematopoiesis, 583
Cyclo-oxygenase, 239, 240
Cyclophosphamide, 659t
  adverse effects, 413, 418, 428, 659t
  for bullous pemphigoid, 418
  for eosinophilic granuloma complex, 266
  for epidermotrophic lymphoma, 454
  for hemangiosarcoma, 459
  for histiocytosis, 581
  for mast cell tumors, 469
  for pemphigus, 412
  for systemic lupus erythematosus, 428
Cyclosporine
  adverse effects, 87, 429, 540
  for hypereosinophilic syndrome, 270
  for pemphigus, 412
  for perianal fistula, 162
  for sebaceous adenitis, 85, 540, 553, 649
  for systemic lupus erythematosus, 429
Cyproheptadine, 241t, 628
Cystorellin response test, 391
Cythioate, 188
Cytology, 3–18
  in blastomycosis, 343
  cutaneous and subcutaneous lesions, 3–11
    examination of slides, 6
    indications, 3
    keys to success, 7–9
    magnification recommendations, 8t
    materials, 3
    procedures, sample collection
      fine-needle aspiration, 4
      fine-needle biopsy, 4
      impression smear, 4
      from pustule or papule, 4–5
    slide preparation techniques, 5, *5, 6, 7*
      brush technique, 5, 6, *7*
      squash technique, 5, *5, 7*
    staining slides, 6
  in dermatophilosis, 307
  ear, 12–13
    indications, 12
    keys to success, 13
    materials, 12
    number of infectious agents, evaluation of, 8t, 13
    procedure, 12, *12*
  in erosive and ulcerative dermatoses, 72
  fungal cultures, 16–18
    indications, 16
    materials, 16
    procedure, 16, *17*
  in histiocytoma, 462
  in histiocytosis, 580
  in interdigital dermatitis, 125
  in leishmaniasis, 348
  in *Malassezia* dermatitis, *317*
  in mast cell tumors, 468
  in melanocytic tumors, 472
  in mycobacterial infections, 300, 301
  in nocardiosis, 312
  in otitis, 147, 148, *148*, 155
  in pemphigus, 412
  in pododermatitis, 112
  in pyoderma, 291
  in sex hormone-responsive dermatoses, 391
  in sporotrichosis, 327
  in squamous cell carcinoma, 480
  in steroid hepatopathy, 397
  for yeast, skin scrapings and impression smears, 13–15, *15*, 16t
    indications, 13–15, *15*, 16t
    materials, 13, *13*
    number of yeast, evaluation of, 16t
    procedures, 13–14, *14*
Cytotec. (*see* Misoprostol)
Cytotoxic agents
  adverse effects, 413, 418
  for bullous pemphigoid, 418
  for pemphigus, 412, 414
  for systemic lupus erythematosus, 428
Cytoxan. (*see* Cyclophosphamide)

Dacarbazine, for melanocytic tumors, 474
Dapsone
  adverse effects, 96, 303
  for bullous pemphigoid, 418
  contraindications, 440
  for leprosy, feline, 302
  for linear IgA dermatosis, 96
  patient monitoring, 96
  for pemphigus, 412
  for subcorneal pustular dermatosis, 96
  for vasculitis, 439
Deltasone. (*see* Prednisolone/prednisone)
Demodex canis, *204*, 204–205, 645
Demodex cati, 203
Demodicosis
  clinical features
    alopecia, 28, *28, 29*, 32t
    cats, 55, 56t, 205, 207
    dogs, 28, *28, 29*, 32t, 34t, 38, 205, *205, 206*
  course and prognosis, 209
  definition/overview, 203
  diagnostics, 207
  differential diagnosis, 207
  erosive and ulcerative dermatoses, 62
  etiology/pathophysiology, 203–204
  interdigital dermatitis, 123, *124*, 126t
  nasal, 133
  pododermatitis, *102*, 107

signalment/history
cats, 204–205
dogs, 204
therapeutics, 41, 59, 207–208, 645–646
amitraz, 207–208
generalized therapy, 645–646
ivermectin, 208
localized therapy, 645
milbemycin, 208
pododemodicosis therapy, 646
precautions, 208–209
Depigmenting disorders, 138–143
clinical features, 138
definition/overview, 138
diagnostics, 142
differential diagnosis
albinism, 140
discoid lupus erythematosus, 139, 421, *421*
drug reactions, 140
hypopigmentation, seasonal nasal, 140
nasal solar dermatitis, 139
pemphigus erythematosus, *139*, 139–140, *140*
pemphigus foliaceus, 139
plastic/rubber dish dermatitis, 140, *141*
Schnauzer gilding syndrome, 140
systemic lupus erythematosus, 139
uveodermatologic syndrome, 140, *141*, 441, *442*, *443*
vitiligo, 140, *142*
signalment/history, 138
therapeutics, 143
Depo-Medrol. (*see* Methylprednisolone acetate)
DepoProvera, for pruritus, 239
Depo-testosterone. (*see* Testosterone therapeutics)
Deprenyl, 660t
Derm Cap for sebaceous adenitis, 553
Dermacentor, 177
D. andersoni, 181, 182
D. variabilis, 177, 181, 182
Dermal-Soothe (EVSCO), 591
Dermatohistopathology. (*see* Histopathology)
Dermatomyositis, 525–530
associated conditions, 530
breed predilection, 89
canine juvenile, 69
client education, 529
clinical features, 526–528, *526–528*
complications, 530
course/prognosis, 530
definition/overview, 525
diagnostics, 528–529
differential diagnosis, 528
etiology/pathophysiology, 525
nasal, 133
prevention, 530
signalment/history, 525–526
therapeutics, 529
vesicles and ulceration, *94*, *95*
Dermatopathology. (*see* Histopathology)
Dermatophilosis, 305–308
clinical features, 306
definition/overview, 305
diagnostics, 307
differential diagnosis, 306–307
pathogenesis/etiology, 305
signalment/history, 305–306
zoonotic potential, 308
Dermatophilus congolensis, 305
Dermatophytosis, 319–324, 647
alopecia from
canine, 28, 32t, 34t, 35t, 38, 41
feline, 55, 56t
client education, 324, 647
clinical features, 44, *320*, *321*
definition/overview, 319
diagnostics, 232, 322–323
biopsy, 322
culture, 322, 324
in papular and nodular dermatoses, 85
microscopic examination, 322
pathology, 323
differential diagnosis, 320, 322
in erosive and ulcerative dermatoses, 62
in exfoliative dermatoses, 77, *78*
nasal, 133
pathophysiology, 319
in rabbits, 513–514
risk factors, 320
signalment, 320
therapeutics, 41, 59, 323–324
vaccination, 323
in vesicular and pustular dermatosis, 92
zoonotic potential, 41, 59, 82, 87
Dermazole (Allerderm), 590
DES. (*see* Diethylstilbesterol (DES))
Development inhibitors, insect, 191
Devon Rex hypotrichosis, 53
Dexamethasone, 660t
for anaphylaxis, 246
for eosinophilic granuloma complex, 266
potency, 239t
Dexamethasone suppression test, high-dose, 41, 55, 379, 403, 607–608, 675
Dexamethasone suppression test, low-dose, 41, 55, 378, 381, 403, 602–606, 674–675
definition/overview, 602
diagnostics, 605
differential diagnosis, 603
etiology/pathophysiology, 602–603
follow-up, 605
laboratory findings, 603–604
treatment, 605
Diabetes insipidus, diagnostics for, 676
Diabetes mellitus
cutaneous xanthomatosis and, 104
erosive and ulcerative dermatoses, 69

exfoliative dermatosis, 77
feline alopecia from, 45, *47*, 57t
hyperadrenocorticism-associated, 400, *402*, 403, 404
therapeutics, 59
Diazepam
dosage, 242t
for organophosphate and carbamate toxicity, 223
for pruritus, 234
for pyrethrin/pyrethroid toxicity, 227
Dictoctyl sodium sulfosuccinate, for otitis, 150
Diet trial
challenge and provocation, 255
food elimination, 255
Diethylstilbesterol (DES), 660t
for estrogen-responsive dermatosis, 391
patient monitoring, 392
Diff Quik® stain, 6, 12
Diflucan. (*see* Fluconazole)
Dihydrostreptomycin
adverse effects, 303
for tuberculosis, 302
Dihydrotachysterol, 660t
Dilution alopecia, 76
Diphenhydramine, 628
for anaphylaxis, 246
for atopy, 251
dosage, 241t
for pruritus, 234
shampoo, 591
Dipylidium caninum, 187
Discoid lupus erythematosus, 420–423
clinical features, 421, *421*
complications, 424
course and prognosis, 423
definition/overview, 420
depigmentation, 139
diagnostics, 422
differential diagnosis, 421–422
erosive and ulcerative dermatoses, 62, *64*
etiology/pathophysiology, 420
nasal, 129, *130, 131*
patient monitoring, 423
signalment/history, 420
therapeutics, 422
vesicles and ulceration, 93
Diuretics, for lymphedema, 572
DLE. (*see* Discoid lupus erythematosus)
DMSO
for calcinosis cutis, 549
precautions, 550
Doxepin, 628
for acral lick dermatitis, 171
for atopy, 252
dosage, 241t
precautions for use, 171
for pruritus, 234
Doxorubicin
for epidermotrophic lymphoma, 454
for hemangiosarcoma, 459
for histiocytosis, 581
for melanocytic tumors, 474
Doxycycline
for abscessation, 285
for nocardiosis, 312
Drug eruptions, cutaneous, 271–273
clinical features, 272
definition/overview, 271–273
diagnostics, 272–273
differential diagnosis, 272
etiology/pathology, 271
footpad, 109t
signalment/history, 271
vasculitis from, *438*
Drug-induced disorders. (*see also* Drug eruptions, cutaneous)
depigmentation from, 140
erosive and ulcerative dermatoses, 62, *64, 65*
hypersensitivity
nasal dermatosis, 133
neomycin, 133
Dust mite, 637
Dwarfism, pituitary, 383–386

Ear abalation, 155, 484
Ear cytology, 12–13
indications, 12
magnification recommendation, 8t
materials, 12
number of infectious agents, evaluation of, 8t, 13
procedure, 12, *12*
Ear margin dermatosis, 538
Ear margin dysplasia, 533
Ear mites, 210–212, *212*
clinical features, 210
definition/overview, 210
diagnostics, 211
differential diagnosis, 210–211
signalment/history, 210
therapeutics, 211–212
Ear neoplasia. (*see* Ceruminous gland adenocarcinoma)
Echocardiography, in hypothyroidism, 371
Ectodermal defects, 76
Ectoparasites. (*see also specific parasites*)
in ferrets, 517–518
in guinea pigs, 497–498
in hedgehogs, 499–500
in mice, 503–504
in rabbits, 505–506
Ehlers-Danlos syndrome, 69
Ehrlichia canis, 178
Ehrlichia equi, 178
Ehrlichiosis
canine, 178
granulocytic, 178

Eicosapentaenoic acid, 240
Elavil. (*see* Amitriptyline)
Electromyogram (EMG), 182, 528
Electron microscopy in cutaneous asthenia, 556
Emollients, for exfoliative dermatoses, 82
Endocarditis, 278
Endocrine alopecia
  canine
    estrogen-responsive, 31, 34t
    growth hormone-responsive, 31, 33t, *37*
    hyperadrenocorticism, 31, 33t, 34t, *36*, 38
    hyperestrogenism, 31, 33t
    hypothyroidism, 31, 33t, 34t, 38, *39*
    testosterone-responsive, 31, 33t
  feline, 44, 46, 58t
  therapeutics, 59
Endocrine disorders. (*see also specific disorders*)
  feline skin fragility syndrome, 400–404
  growth hormone-responsive dermatoses, 383–386
  hyperadrenocorticism, 375–382
  hypothyroidism, 365–374
  pododermatitis and, 104, *105*, 107
  sex hormone-responsive dermatoses, 387–393
  steroid hepatopathy, 394–399
Endocrine testing, 674–676, 677
  ACTH stimulation test, 378, 385, 386, 390, 396, 398, 403, 595–601, 674
  calcium challenge test, 676
  Gn-RH stimulation test, 676
  HCG stimulation test, 676
  high-dose dexamethasone suppression test, 41, 55, 379, 403, 607–608, 675
  low-dose dexamethasone suppression test, 41, 55, 378, 381, 403, 602–606, 674–675
  secretin stimulation test, 675–676
  TRH stimulation test, 675
  TSH stimulation test, 675
  water deprivation test, 676
Enilconazole
  for aspergillosis, 137
  for dermatophytosis, 323
  for malassezia dermatitis, 538
Enkephalins, 237
Enrofloxacin, 661t
  for mycobacteriosis, atypical, 303
  for otitis, 149, 150
  for tuberculosis, 302
Enterobacteriaceae, 280
Eosinophilia
  differential diagnoses, 269
  hypereosinophilic syndrome, 268–270
Eosinophilic granuloma, canine, 261–262, 266–267, 542, 549
Eosinophilic granuloma complex, 261–267
  clinical features, 262, *263, 264, 265*
  definition/overview, 261
  diagnostics, 265–266
  differential diagnosis, 262
  etiology/pathophysiology, 261
  of footpad, *103,* 110t
  signalment/history, 262
  therapeutics, 266
Eosinophilic leukemia, 269
Eosinophilic plaque, 103, *103,* 261–262, *263,* 265
Eosinophilic pustulosis
  diagnosis, 92
  therapeutics, 96
Epidermal collarettes, *289*
Epidermal dysplasia, 77, 533, 538
Epidermolysis bullosa acquisita, 107
Epidermotrophic lymphoma, 449–454, *450–452*
  canine alopecia, 38, *39, 40*
  definition/overview, 449
  diagnostics, 453
  differential diagnosis, 453
  etiology/pathophysiology, 449
  exfoliative dermatosis from, 79, *79*
  feline alopecia, *52, 53, 53,* 58t
  prognosis, 454
  signalment/history, 449–450
  therapeutics, 59, 453–454
Epinephrine, 246, 661t, 678
Episoothe (Allerderm), 591
Epitheliogenesis imperfecta, 69
Eqvalan Liquid. (*see* Ivermectin)
Ergamisol. (*see* Levamisole)
Erosive and ulcerative dermatoses, 61–73
  clinical features, 62
  definition, 61
  diagnostics, 71–72
  differential diagnoses, 62, 69
    autoimmune, 62, *63, 64*
    congenital/hereditary, 69
    idiopathic, 71
    immune-mediated, 62, *64, 65, 66, 67*
    infectious, 62, *67, 68*
    metabolic, 69
    miscellaneous, 71, *71*
    neoplastic, 69, *69*
    nutritional, 69
    parasitic, 62, *68*
    physical/conformational, 69
  pathophysiology, 61
  signalment/history, 61
  therapeutics, 72
  zoonotic potential, 72–73
Erythema multiforme, 107
Erythromycin
  for acne, 166
  adverse effects, 292
  for nocardiosis, 312
  for pruritus, 242

for pyoderma, 291
for staphylococcal blepharitis, 627t
Escherichia coli, pyoderma from, 287
Essential fatty acid supplementation. (*see* Fatty acids)
Estrogen, 392, 678. (*see also* Hyperestrogenism)
Estrogen-responsive dermatosis, 31, 34t
course and prognosis, 393
signalment/history, 387
therapeutics, 391–392
Ethambutol
adverse effects, 303
for tuberculosis, 302
Ethyl lactate, 81, 590
Etiderm (Allerderm), 590
Etretinate
for hemangiosarcoma, 459
for sebaceous adenitis, 540
for squamous cell carcinoma, 482
Evening primrose oil, 85, 240, 539, 553
EVSCP-Tar, 588
Excenel, 658t
Exfoliative dermatoses, 74–83
clinical features, 75
definition/overview, 74
diagnostics, 81
differential diagnosis, 75–81
flow chart for, *80*
primary
epidermal dysplasia and ichthyosis, 77
extodermal defects, 76
follicular dysplasia, 76
idiopathic nasodigital hyperkeratosis, 76
idiopathic seborrhea, 75, *75*
sebaceous adenitis, 76, *77*
vitamin A-responsive dermatosis, 76, *76*
zinc-responsive dermatosis, 76
secondary
age, 77
autoimmune skin diseases, 77, 79, *79*
cutaneous hypersensitivity, 77
dermatophytosis, 77, *78*
ectoparasitism, 77, *78*
endocrinopathy, 77
neoplasia, 79, *79*
nutritional disorders, 77
pyoderma, 77
erythroderma, in cutaneous drug eruptions, 271, 272
etiology/pathophysiology, 74
patient monitoring, 82
signalment/history, 74
therapeutics
moisturizers, 82
shampoos, 81–82
systemic therapy, 82
Exotics, 495–522
ferrets
adrenal gland disease, 511–512
canine distemper virus, 521–522
mast cell tumors, 515–516
Sarcoptic mange, 517–518
guinea pigs
ectoparasites, 497–498
ovarian cysts, 507–508
hamsters, Cushing's disease in, 509–510
hedgehogs, chorioptes mites in, 499–500
mice, ectoparasites in, 503–504
rabbits
barbering, 519–520
dermatophytosis, 513–514
fur mites, 505–506
urine scald, 501–502

Facial nerve damage, in otitis, 153
Famotidine, 662t
Fat tissue, panniculitis of, 430–435
Fatty acids
adverse effects, 541
for atopy, 250, 251
essential, 240
precautions, 86
pro-inflammatory, 237
for pruritus, 234, 240
for sebaceous adenitis, 41, 85, 539
Feline calicivirus, 350–353
clinical features, 351, *351*
complications, 353
course and prognosis, 353
definition/overview, 350
diagnostics, 352
differential diagnosis, 351
etiology/pathophysiology, 350
patient monitoring, 352
prevention/avoidance, 352–353
signalment/history, 350–351
therapeutics, 352
vaccination, 352–353
Feline cow pox, 62
Feline hypereosinophilic syndrome. (*see* Hypereosinophilic syndrome)
Feline leprosy. (*see* Leprosy, feline)
Feline paraneoplastic syndrome, 489–493
clinical features, 490, *490, 491*
definition/overview, 489
diagnostics, 492
differential diagnosis, 490, 492
etiology/pathophysiology, 489
prognosis, 492
signalment/history, 489–490
therapeutics, 492
Feline symmetrical alopecia, 558–561. (*see also* Alopecia, feline)
Feminization. (*see* Male feminization)
Ferrets
adrenal gland disease, 511–512

canine distemper virus, 521–522
mast cell tumors, 515–516
clinical signs, 515, *516*
definition/overview, 515
diagnostic tests, 516
etiology/pathophysiology, 515
lab findings, 516
prognosis, 516
treatment, 516
sarcoptic mange, 517–518
clinical signs, 517
definition/overview, 517
diagnostic tests, 518
etiology/pathophysiology, 517
lab findings, 517
prognosis, 518
treatment, 518
Ferritin, serum, 579
Fibrinolysin, pruritus and, 237
Ficin, pruritus and, 237
Fine-needle aspiration
hepatic, 396, 397
technique, 4
Fipronil, for fleas, 187, 192–193
Fistula. (*see* Perianal fistula)
FIV/FeLV-related erosive and ulcerative dermatoses, 62
Flea bite hypersensitivity, 185–187, 189
atopy compared, 249
erosive and ulcerative dermatoses, 62
Flea control products, 190–193
fipronil, 192–193
imidacloprid, 192
insect development inhibitors, 191
lufenuron, 191
insect growth regulators, 190–191
methoprene, 190–191
pyriproxifen, 190
organophosphates, 191–192
pyrethrins/pyrethroids, 191–192
sodium polyborate, 191
Fleas, 185–189
clinical features, 186
definition/overview, 185
diagnostics, 187
differential diagnosis, 186
etiology/pathophysiology, 185
signalment/history, 186
therapeutics, 187–188
Fluconazole, 662t
for coccidiodomycosis, 337–338
for cryptococcosis, 332
Flucytosine, 662t
for cryptococcosis, 332
Flunixin meglumine, for acral lick dermatitis, 171
Fluocinolone
for acral lick dermatitis, 171
for pemphigus, 413
shampoo, 591
Fluoroquinolone
for mycobacteriosis, atypical, 303
for tuberculosis, 302
5-fluorouracil for squamous cell carcinoma, 481
Fluoxetine
for acral lick dermatitis, 171
dosage, 242t
for pruritus, 234
Follicle-stimulating hormone (FSH), for estrogen-responsive dermatosis, 391, 392
Follicular dysplasia, 76
alopecia from, 34t, 38
of black-haired areas, 35t, 41
Folliculitis
in nasal dermatosis, 136
in papular and nodular dermatoses, 84
in pyoderma, 287–292
Food elimination diet, 255
Food reactions, 253–256
clinical features, 254
definition/overview, 253
diagnostics, 255
differential diagnosis, 254–255
etiology/pathophysiology, 253
hypersensitivity
atopy compared, 249
pododermatitis, 107, 113
in pruritic dermatoses, 233
trial courses, 233
prognosis, 256
signalment/history, 254
therapeutics, 255–256
Footpad calcinosis circumscripta, 545
Footpad hyperkeratosis, 107, 108t, 109t, 521, 533, 536, 538, 563, *565*, *566*
Foreign body reaction, 542, 548, 549
glossitis, *11*
interdigital, 123, 125, 126t
Formulary, 654t–673t
Fragility syndrome, feline skin. (*see* Skin fragility syndrome, feline)
Frontline, 177, 192. (*see also* Fipronil)
Frost bite, 71
FS Shampoo, 591
FSH (follicle-stimulating hormone), for estrogen-responsive dermatosis, 391, 392
Fungal infections
blastomycosis, 340–345
coccidiomycosis, 334–339
cryptococcosis, 329–333
culture, in *Malassezia* dermatitis, *317*
dermatophytosis, 319–324
erosive and ulcerative dermatoses, 62, *68*
Malassezia, 314–318
nail and nailbed, 116, 117t, 120, 121
otitis, *147*, 148, *148*, 149–150
Fungizone. (*see* Amphotericin B)

Fur mites, rabbit, 505–506
clinical signs, 505, *506*
definition/overview, 505
diagnostic tests, 506
lab findings, 505
pathophysiology, 505
prognosis, 506
treatment, 506
Furunculosis, 62, *102*, 123, *124*, 127
in nasal dermatosis, 136
in pyoderma, 287–292, *288*
secondary to demodicosis, *206*

Gamma-linolenic acid, 240
Gastrin, 678
Gastrinoma, 675–676
Generic dog food dermatosis
erosive and ulcerative dermatoses, 69
hyperkeratosis of the footpads, 107
Gentamicin, 663t
adverse effects, 292
for bacteremia, *281*
for nocardiosis, 312
for otitis, 150
German short-haired pointers, lupoid dermatosis in, 71
Glossitis, foreign body, *11*
Glucagon, 678
Glucocorticoids. (*see also* Corticosteroids)
anti-inflammatory effects of, 238–239
for bacteremia, *281*
for feline symmetrical alopecia, 561
food elimination diet trial and, 256
hepatopathy from, 394, 398
for keratinization disorders, 538–540
precautions, 398
for pruritus, 238–239
for sarcoptic mange, 201
Glycopyrrolate, for bradycardia, ivermectin-related, 218
GnRH. (*see* Gonadotropin releasing hormone (GnRH))
Gn-RH stimulation test, 676
Gold salts, for systemic lupus erythematosus, 137, 143
Gonadotropin releasing hormone (GnRH)
for hyperestrogenism, 392
response test, 391
Granuloma, idiopathic sterile
nasal, 133
therapeutics, 137
Granulomatous dermatoses. (*see* Sterile nodular/granulomatous dermatoses)
Granulomatous sebaceous adenitis, 551–553, 649
Griseofulvin
absorption enhancement, 323
adverse effects, 120, 137
in pregnancy, 42
vesicular eruption, 89
for dermatophytosis, 41, 59, 323, 324, 514
for nasal dermatosis, 137
for onychomycosis, 120
precautions, 323
Growth hormone therapy, 386, 678
Growth hormone-responsive dermatoses, 383–386
alopecia from, 31, 33t, *37*
definition/overview, 383
diagnostics, 385–386
differential diagnosis, 385
pathogenesis/etiology, 383
signalment/history, 384
therapeutics, 386
Growth regulators, insect, 190–191
Guinea pigs
ectoparasites, 497–498
ovarian cysts, 507–508

Hair, microscopic examination of, 322
Hair follicle neoplasia, 455–456
clinical features, 455, *456*
definition/overview, 455
diagnostics, 456
differential diagnosis, 456
signalment/history, 455
therapeutics, 456
Hair loss. (*see* Alopecia)
Hamsters, Cushing's disease in, 509–510
clinical signs, 509, *510*
definition/overview, 509
diagnostic tests, 510
lab findings, 509
pathophysiology, 509
prognosis, 510
treatment, 510
HCG. (*see* Human chorionic gonadotropin)
HCG stimulation test, 676
HDDST. (*see* Dexamethasone suppression test, high-dose)
Hedgehogs
chorioptes mites in, 499–500
quill loss, *500*
Hemangiosarcoma, 457–460
clinical features, 457, *458*, 459
definition/overview, 457
diagnostics, 459
differential diagnosis, 459
signalment/history, 457
therapeutics, 459
Hemolytic anemia, 622–624
Heparin, 464
Hepatocutaneous syndrome, 104, *105*, 109t, 125, 562–569
clinical features, 563, *563–567*
complications, 569
course and prognosis, 569
definition/overview, 562

diagnostics, 567–568
differential diagnosis, 563
erosive and ulcerative dermatoses, 69
etiology/pathophysiology, 562
pododermatitis, 107
signalment/history, 563
therapeutics, 568–569
Hepatopathy. (*see* Steroid hepatopathy)
Hepatozoon canis, 178
Hepatozoonosis, 178
Hexedene (Allerderm), 589
Hidradenitis suppurativa, 160
High-dose dexamethasone suppression test. (*see* Dexamethasone suppression test, high-dose)
Hismanal. (*see* Astemizole)
Histacalm (Allerderm), 591
Histamine, 237, 464, 469
Histiocytoma, 461–463
clinical features, 461, *462*
definition/overview, 461
diagnostics, 462
differential diagnosis, 462
prognosis, 463
signalment/history, 461
therapeutics, 462
Histiocytosis, 542, 549, 576–581
clinical features, *545*, *546*, 577, *578*, *579*
cutaneous, 62, 66
definition/overview, 576
diagnostics, 579–580
differential diagnosis, 579
etiology/pathophysiology, 576
signalment/history, *545*, 576–577, *577*
therapeutics, 580–581
Histopathology, 19–21, *22–23*
in acral lick dermatitis, 170
in basal cell tumors, 477
in blastomycosis, 343
in canine distemper virus, 522
in ceruminous gland adenocarcinoma, 484
in coccidiodomycosis, 336
in contact dermatitis, 260
in cryptococcosis, 332
in cutaneous asthenia, 556
in dermatomyositis, 528–529
in dermatophytosis, 323
in discoid lupus erythematosus, 422
in eosinophilic granuloma complex, 265–266
in epidermotrophic lymphoma, 453
in feline calcivirus infection, 352
in feline paraneoplastic syndrome, 492
in growth hormone-responsive dermatoses, 386
in hair follicle neoplasia, 456
in hepatocutaneous syndrome, 568
in histiocytoma, 462
in histiocytosis, 580
in hypothyroidism, 371–372
in keratinization disorders, 537
in leishmaniasis, 348–349
in *Malassezia* dermatitis, *317*
in mast cell tumors, 468
in melanocytic tumors, 472, 474
in mycobacterial infections, 301–302
in panniculitis, 430, 434, *434*
in papillomatosis, 360
in pemphigus, 412
in pox virus infection, 355
in sebaceous adenitis, 553
site selection, 650–651
in skin fragility syndrome, 403
in squamous cell carcinoma, 480–481
in steroid hepatopathy, 397
in systemic lupus erythematosus, 428
technique, 651
in uveodermatologic syndrome, 444
in vasculitis, 439
when to biopsy, 650
Hookworm
erosive and ulcerative dermatoses, 62
pododermatitis, 107
Horner's syndrome
in ceruminous gland adenocarcinoma, 485
in otitis, 153, 154, 156
House dust mite, 637
Human chorionic gonadotropin (HCG)
for castration-responsive dermatosis, 392
for hyperestrogenism, 392
Humectants
for exfoliative dermatoses, 82
for ichthyosis, 538
HydraPearls (EVSCO), 587
Hydrocortisone, 663t
for discoid lupus erythematosus, 422
for pemphigus, 413
potency, 239t
Hydrocortisone shampoo, 591
Hydrogen peroxide emetic
for amitraz toxicosis, 215
for organophosphate and carbamate toxicity, 223
for pyrethrin/pyrethroid toxicity, 227
Hydrotherapy, for urine scald in rabbits, 502
Hydroxyurea, for hypereosinophilic syndrome, 270
Hydroxyzine, 628
for acral lick dermatitis, 171
for atopy, 251
dosage, 241t
for pruritus, 234
HyLyt EFA (DVM), 587
Hyperadrenocorticism, 375–382
alopecia from, *401*, *402*
canine, 31, 33t, 34t, *36*, 38
feline, 46, *48*, *49*, 57t
associated conditions, 381

clinical features, *376*, 376–378, *377*, *378*
course and prognosis, 381
definition/overview, 375
diagnostics, 41, 55, 378–379
ACTH response test, 595–600
high-dose dexamethasone suppression test, 607–608
low-dose dexamethasone suppression test, 602–605
urine cortisol:creatinine ratio, 609–612
differential diagnosis, 378
erosive and ulcerative dermatoses, 69
etiology/pathophysiology, 375
exfoliative dermatosis, 77
in feline skin fragility syndrome, 400–404
in hamsters, 509–510
interdigital dermatitis, 123
patient monitoring, 381
pododermatitis, 107
signalment/history, 376
steroid hepatopathy from, 394–398
therapeutics, 379–380
Hyperandrogenism, 388
Hypercholesterolemia, steroid hepatopathy and, 396
Hypereosinophilic syndrome, 62, 268–270
clinical features, 269
definition/overview, 268
diagnostics, 269–270
differential diagnosis, 269
pathogenesis/etiology, 268
signalment/history, 268–269
therapeutics, 270
Hyperestrogenism
alopecia from, 31, 33t
in females
course and prognosis, 393
signalment/history, 387–388, *388*
therapeutics, 392
in males, 388
Hyperkeratosis. (*see also* Keratinization disorders)
in canine distemper virus, 521
footpad, 107, 108t, 109t, 521, 533, 536, 538, 563, *565*, *566*
in growth hormone-responsive dermatoses, 386
in leishmaniasis, 347, *347*
nasal digital, 76, 133, 137, 533, 536, 539
in vitamin A-responsive dermatosis, *535*
Hyperlipidemia
cutaneous xanthomatosis and, 45, *47*, *106*
in hypothyroidism, 369
steroid hepatopathy and, 395, 397, 398
Hypermelanosis of the footpads, 107
Hyperpigmentation
in growth hormone-responsive dermatoses, 384
in hyperadrenocorticism, *376*
in hyperestrogenism, *388*
in hypothyroidism, 368
post-inflammatory, 290
Hypersensitivity reaction, 244–247
clinical features, 245
definition/overview, 244
differential diagnosis, 245–246
etiology/pathophysiology, 244–245
exfoliative dermatoses and, 77
flea bite, 185–187, 189
food, 253–256
otitis from, 145, *146*, *147*
signalment/history, 245
therapeutics, 246
vasculitis from, *437*
Hyperthyroidism
alopecia from, 45, *46*, 57t
exfoliative dermatosis, 77
pododermatitis, 107
therapeutics, 59
Hyphae, microscopic examination of, 16, *17*
Hypoadrenocorticism, diagnostics for, 595–597, 599–600
Hypogammaglobulinemia, 583
Hypogonadism, alopecia from, 31, 33t
Hypomelanosis, 107, 110t
Hypophysectomy, 379
Hypopigmentation, nasal, 133, 140
Hyposensitization, 251, 633–636
adverse reactions, 633
how it works, 633
interactions, 634
schedule, 635–636
technique, 633
Hypotension, therapeutics, 280
Hypothyroidism, 365–374
alopecia from, 31, 33t, 34t, 38, *39*
clinical features, 367–369
cretinism, congenital hypothyroidism, 369
dermatologic, *367*, 367–368, *368*
metabolic, 368
neuromuscular, 368–369
ophthalmic, 369
definition/overview, 365
diagnostics, 369–372
autoantibodies to thyroglobulin and thyroid hormones, 370
echocardiography, 371
pathologic findings, 371–372
radiography, 371
T_4 concentration, endogenous, 370
TRH stimulation test, 371
TSH stimulation test, 370–371
TSH (thyrotropin) concentration, 370
differential diagnosis, 369
etiology/pathophysiology, 365–366
acquired hypothyroidism, 365–366
congenital hypothyroidism, 366

systems affected, 366–367
exfoliative dermatosis, 77
feline, 58
interdigital dermatitis, 123
patient monitoring, 373
prognosis, 373
signalment/history, 366–367
therapeutics, 372–373
Hypotrichosis, feline, 53, 57t
Hytakerol, 660t

Ichthyosis, 77, 533, 538
Idiopathic modular panniculitis, 71
Idiopathic ulcerative dermatosis, 530
IgA deficiency, 583, 585
IgA dermatosis, linear, 89, 93, 96
IgM deficiency, 583
Imidacloprid, for fleas, 187, 192
Imidazoles. (*see also* Ketoconazole; Miconazole)
shampoos, 590
Immune-mediated diseases. (*see also* Pemphigus)
anemia, 622–623
discoid lupus erythematosus, 420–423
erosive and ulcerative dermatoses, 62, *64*, *65*, *66*, *67*
interdigital, 125
nail and nailbed, 116, 117t, 121
pododermatitis, 103, *104*, *105*, 107, 109t
systemic lupus erythematosus, 424–429
uveodermatologic syndrome, 441–445
Immune-mediated hemolytic anemia, 622–623
Immunodeficiency disorders, primary, 582–585
client education, 585
clinical features, 583
course and prognosis, 585
definition/overview, 582
diagnostics, 584
differential diagnosis, 583–584
etiology/pathophysiology, 582–583
patient monitoring, 585
prevention, 585
signalment/history, 583
therapeutics, 584–585
Immunofluorescence
in pemphigus, 412
in systemic lupus erythematosus, 428
Immunohistochemistry
in histiocytosis, 580
in melanocytic tumors, 472
in papillomatosis, 360
in pemphigus, 412
Immunopathologic examination, in discoid lupus erythematosus, 422
Immunotherapy, for atopy, 251
Impetigo, 292
Impression smears
surface, 4
for yeast (*Malassezia* spp.), 13–15, *14*
Imuran. (*see* Azathioprine)
Indolent ulcer, 62, *67*, 261, 262, *264*, *265*, 266
Indulin-like growth factor 1, 385
Infectious dermatoses, 275–361. (*see also specific disease; specific organisms*)
Injection reactions, alopecia from, 28, 32t, 56t
Insect development inhibitors, 191
Insect growth regulators, 190–191
Insulin, 677, 678
Insulin response test, 385
Interceptor. (*see* Milbemycin)
Interdigital dermatitis, 122–127
clinical features, 123
definition/overview, 122
diagnostics, 125, 126t
differential diagnosis, 123–125
multiple feet affected, 123–125
one foot affected, 123
etiology/pathophysiology, 122
signalment/history, 122
therapeutics, 125, 126t, 127
Interferon
for eosinophilic granuloma complex, 266
for epidermotrophic lymphoma, 59, 454
for leishmaniasis, 349
Intertrigo, 69
Intradermal skin testing, 250, 631–632
Iodine Shampoo (EVSCO), 590
Iodism, 327
Irritant contact dermatitis. (*see* Contact dermatitis)
Isoniazid
adverse effects, 303
for tuberculosis, 302
Isotretinoin, 664t
for acne, 86, 166, 537
adverse effects, 87, 166
for epidermotropic lymphoma, 59
for ichthyosis, 538
for schnauzer comedone syndrome, 539
for sebaceous adenitis, 85, 540, 553
Itching. (*see* Pruritus)
Itraconazole, 664t
for blastomycosis, 343, 344
for coccidiodomycosis, 337–338
for cryptococcosis, 332
for dermatophytosis, 41, 59, 324
for nasal dermatosis, 137
for onychomycosis, 120
for sporotrichosis, 327
toxicity, 344
Ivermectin
for cheyletiellosis, 196
in rabbits, 506
for chorioptes mites in hedgehogs, 500
contraindications, 150
for demodicosis, 41, 59, 208, 646

drug interactions, 209
for ear mites, 211
for mouse mange, 504
for otitis, 149–150, 211
precautions, 197, 210, 212
for sarcoptic mange, 201, 233
in ferrets, 518
in guinea pigs, 498
toxicity, 208, 217–219
clinical features, 218
definition/overview, 217
diagnostics, 218
differential diagnosis, 218
etiology/pathophysiology, 217
prognosis, 219
signalment/history, 217
therapeutics, 218
Ivomec. (*see* Ivermectin)
Ixodes, 177, 182–184
I. holocyclus, 180, 182
I. pacificus, 176, 178
I. scapularis, 176, 177, 178

Junctional epidermolysis bullosa, 69

Kallikrein, pruritus and, 237
Kanamycin, 292
Keflex. (*see* Cephalexin)
Keratinization disorders, 75, *75,* 532–541. (*see also* Exfoliative dermatoses)
alopecia from, 35t, 38, *40*
clinical features, 536
definition/overview, 532
diagnostics, 536–537
differential diagnosis, 536
etiology/pathophysiology, 532–533
otitis secondary to, 145, *146*
patient monitoring, 541
signalment/history, 533, 536
breed predilection, 533, *534, 535*
therapeutics, 41, 537–541
for acne, 537
for disorder of cornification in rottweiler, 537–538
ear margin dermatosis, 538
epidermal dysplasia, 538
footpad hyperkeratosis, 538
ichthyosis, 538
lichenoid-psoriasiform dermatosis, 539
nasal digital hyperkeratosis, 539
precautions for use, 540–541
schnauzer comedone syndrome, 539
sebaceous adenitis, 539–540
seborrhea, idiopathic, 538–539
vitamin A-responsive dermatosis, 540
zinc-responsive dermatosis, 540
Keratinocytes, *10*
Keratinophilic mycosis. (*see* Dermatophytosis)
Keratolytic agents, for keratinization disorders, 539, 540
Keratolytic shampoo, for sebaceous adenitis, 41
Ketochlor (DVM), 590
Ketoconazole
absorption enhancement, 323
adverse effects, 120, 137, 338, 380, 541
for blastomycosis, 343
for *Candida paronychia,* 120
for coccidiodomycosis, 337–338
for dermatophytosis, 41, 59, 323
for hyperadrenocorticism, 380, 381, 403
for *Malassezia* dermatitis, 318, 538
for nasal dermatosis, 137
for onychomycosis, 120
for otitis, 149
precautions, 318, 323
for pruritus, 242–243
for sporotrichosis, 327
withdrawal time prior to intradermal skin testing, 631, 632
KOH (potassium hydroxide) preparations, 8t

Laboratory tests, 593–625, 674–676, 677. (*see also specific tests*)
ACTH, plasma levels, 607–608
ACTH stimulation test, 378, 385, 386, 390, 396, 398, 403, 595–601, 674
antinuclear antibody (ANA), 617–621
calcium challenge test, 676
Coombs test, 622–625
Gn-RH stimulation test, 676
HCG stimulation test, 676
high-dose dexamethasone suppression test, 41, 55, 379, 403, 607–608, 675
low-dose dexamethasone suppression test, 41, 55, 378, 381, 403, 602–606, 674–675
lupus erythematosus (LE) cell test, 617–621
secretin stimulation test, 675–676
thyroid, 613–616
TRH stimulation test, 675
TSH stimulation test, 675
urine cortisol:creatinine ratio, 609–612
water deprivation test, 676
Lactophenol cotton blue stain, 16
LDDST. (*see* Dexamethasone suppression test, low-dose)
L-deprenyl, 380, 381, 392, 660t
LE test. (*see* Lupus erythematosus (LE) cell test)
Leishmaniasis, 346–349
clinical features, 347, *347, 348*
definition/overview, 346
diagnostics, 348–349
erosive and ulcerative dermatoses, 62
etiology/pathophysiology, 346
prognosis, 349

signalment/history, 346–347
therapeutics, 349
Leprosy, feline, 297–303
clinical features, 300
diagnostics, 301
differential diagnosis, 300
etiology/pathophysiology, 297
prognosis, 303
signalment/history, 298
therapeutics, 302
Leukocyte adhesion deficiency, 583
Leukoderma, 133, *134,* 140, *142*
Leukotrichia, 133, *134,* 140, *142*
Leukotrienes
glucocorticoid affect on, 239
pruritus and, 237
Levamisole, 664t
Levothyroxine (L-thyroxine)
for growth hormone-responsive dermatoses, 386
for hypothyroidism, 372–373
LH (luteinizing hormone), for estrogen-responsive dermatosis, 391
Lichenification, *534*
Lichenoid-psoriasiform dermatosis, 533, 539
Lick dermatitis. (*see* Acral lick dermatitis)
Lime sulfur
for cheyletiellosis, 196
for demodicosis, 59
for dermatophytosis, 41, 59, 323
for pruritus, 233
for sarcoptic mange, 201, 233
Lincomycin
adverse effects, 292
for pyoderma, 292
Linear IgA dermatosis
breed predilection, 89
diagnosis, 93
therapeutics, 96
Linolenic acid, 240
Liothyronine, 373–373
Lipidemia. (*see* Hyperlipidemia)
Lipoxygenase inhibitors, for pruritus, 239
Loratidine, 241t
Low-dose dexamethasone suppression test. (*see* Dexamethasone suppression test, low-dose)
Lufenuron, 191, 665t
Lupoid dermatosis of German short-haired pointers, 71
Lupoid onchodystrophy, 117t, 121
Lupus. (*see* Discoid lupus erythematosus; Systemic lupus erythematosus)
Lupus erythematosus (LE) cell test, 427, 617–621
definition/overview, 617
diagnostics, 621
differential diagnosis, 620
laboratory findings, 620
pathophysiology, 618
signalment, 618
signs, 618–620
systems affected, 618
Lupus panniculitis, 62
Luteinizing hormone (LH), for estrogen-responsive dermatosis, 391
LymDip. (*see* Lime sulfur)
Lyme disease, 178
Lymphocytic thyroiditis, 365, 371
Lymphodema, 570–572
clinical features, 571
definition/overview, 570
diagnostics, 571
differential diagnosis, 571
etiology/pathophysiology, 570
signalment/history, 570–571
therapeutics, 571
Lymphoma
alopecia from, 38, *39, 40, 52,* 53, *53,* 58t
cutaneous T-cell, 69, *69*
digital, *106*
epidermotropic, 38, *39, 40, 52,* 53, *53,* 58t
nasal, *135*
Lymphosarcoma. (*see* Epidermotrophic lymphoma)
Lysodren. (*see o,p'*-DDD)
LyTar (DVM), 588

Macroconidia, 17, *17*
Malaseb (DVM), 590
Malassezia
cytology, ear, 12–13
dermatitis, 314–318, 642
clinical features, 315, *316, 317*
definition/overview, 314
diagnostics, 317
differential diagnosis, 317
erosive and ulcerative dermatoses, 62
etiology/pathophysiology, 314–315
exfoliative dermatoses, 75
signalment/history, 315
therapeutics, 317–318
magnification recommendation, 8t
otitis, *147,* 148, *148,* 149–150
skin scrapings and impression smears for, 13–15, *15,* 16t
indications, 13–15, *15,* 16t
materials, 13, *13*
number of yeast, evaluation of, 16t
procedures, 13–14, *14*
Malassezia pachydermatis, 314, 634, 642
Male feminization
alopecia from Sertoli cell tumor, 31, 33t, *38*
idiopathic, 388–389
Malogen. (*see* Testosterone therapeutics)
Mange. (*see specific types*)
Mast cell tumors, 69, 464–470
client education, 469
clinical features, 465, *466, 467*

course and prognosis, 470
definition, 464
diagnostics, 468
differential diagnosis, 465
etiology/pathophysiology, 464
in ferrets, 515–516
patient monitoring, 470
signalment/history, 464–465
staging, 468
therapeutics, 468–469
Mechlorethamine, for epidermotrophic lymphoma, 454
Medrol. (*see* Methylprednisolone)
Medroxyprogesterone acetate, for pruritus, 239
Mefoxin. (*see* Cefoxitin)
Megacolon, in hypothyroidism, 371
Megaesophagus, 527
Megestrol acetate
for eosinophilic granuloma complex, 266
for pruritus, 239
Meglumine antimonate, for leishmaniasis, 349
Melanocyte-stimulating hormone (MSH), 678
Melanocytic tumors, 471–475
client education, 474–475
clinical features, 472, *472, 473*
course and prognosis, 475
definition/overview, 471
diagnostics, 472, 474
differential diagnosis, 472
etiology/pathophysiology, 471
patient monitoring, 475
signalment/history, 471
therapeutics, 474
Melanoderma, alopecia from, 35t, 41
6-mercaptopurine, 418, 665t
Methicillin, for pyoderma, 291
Methimazole, for hyperthyroidism, 59
Methocarbamol, for pyrethrin/pyrethroid toxicity, 227
Methoprene, 190–191
Methotrexate, for epidermotrophic lymphoma, 454
Methylprednisolone, 665t
for atopy, 251
for eosinophilic granuloma complex, 266
for pemphigus, 413
potency, 239t
Methylprednisolone acetate, 665t
Methylprednisolone sodium succinate, 413, 665t
Methyltestosterone, 666t
adverse effects, 392, 666t
for estrogen-responsive dermatosis, 391
for growth hormone-responsive dermatoses, 386
precautions, 386
for testosterone-responsive dermatosis, 392
Meticorten. (*see* Prednisolone/prednisone)
Metronidazole
for anaerobic infections, 296
toxicity, 154
Metyrapone, 380, 403
Mice, ectoparasites in, 503–504
clinical signs, 503
definition/overview, 503
diagnostic tests, 504
etiology/pathophysiology, 503
lab findings, 503
treatment, 504
Miconazole
for *Candida paronychia,* 120
for dermatophytosis, 323
for malassezia dermatitis, 538
for otitis, 150
Miconazole Shampoo (EVSCO), 590
Microencapsualtion, of moisturizers, 82
Microsporum canis, 17, 319, 647
Milbemycin, 666t
for demodicosis, 41, 208, 646
drug interactions, 209
for sarcoptic mange, 201
toxicity, 208
Milbolerone, for estrogen-responsive dermatosis, 391
Minocycline, 666t
for nocardiosis, 312
Misoprostol, 628, 667t
for pruritus, 241–242
Mitaban. (*see* Amitraz)
Mites. (*see specific conditions*)
Mitotane. (*see o,p'*-DDD)
Moisturizers
for exfoliative dermatoses, 82
microencapsualtion of, 82
Mold allergy, 638
Mosquito bite hypersensitivity, 62, *68*
Mupirocin
for acne, 86, 165, 166, 537
for acral lick dermatitis, 171
for interdigital dermatitis, 127
for pododemodicosis, 646
Muscle biopsy, 529
Mycobacterial infections, 297–304
clinical features, 299–300
atypical mycobacteriosis, *298, 299,* 300
feline leprosy, 300
tuberculosis, 299
definition/overview, 297
diagnostics, 301–302
atypical mycobacteriosis, 302
feline leprosy, 301
tuberculosis, 301
differential diagnosis, 300–301
atypical mycobacteriosis, 301
feline leprosy, 300
tuberculosis, 300
erosive and ulcerative dermatoses, 62
prognosis, 303
signalment/history, 298–299

atypical mycobacteriosis, 298–299
feline leprosy, 298
tuberculosis, 298
therapeutics, 302–303
atypical mycobacteriosis, 303
contraindications, 303
feline leprosy, 302
tuberculosis, 302
zoonotic potential, 304
Mycoses. (*see* Fungal infections)
Mycosis fungoides, 35t, 69, *69*, 449
Myobia musculi, 503, 504
Myocoptes musculinus, 503, 504
Myopathy, in hypothyroidism, 369
Myositis. (*see* Dermatomyositis)
Myringotomy, 155
Myxedema, 368

Nail and nailbed disorders, 115–121
clinical features, 116
course and prognosis, 121
definition/overview, 115
diagnostics, 119
differential diagnosis, 116, 117t–118t
bacterial infections, 116, 117t
fungal infections, 116, 117t
idiopathic onchodystrophy, 118t
immune-mediated, 116, 117t, *119*
lupoid onchodystrophy, 117t
nail dystrophy, 116
neoplasia, 118t
onychomadesis, 116
onychomycosis, 116
onychorrhexis, 116
paraonychia, 116, *119*
pyonychia, 116, *119*
etiology/pathophysiology, 115
risk factors, 121
signalment/history, 115–116
therapeutics, 119–120
neoplasia, 120
onychomadesis, 120
onychomycosis, 120
onychorrhexis, 120
paronychia, 119–120
Nail dystrophy, 115, 116, 117t, 118t, 120, 121
Naloxone, 237
Naltrexone
for acral lick dermatitis, 171
dosage, 242t
Narcan, 237
Nasal dermatosis, 128–137
clinical features, 129
definition/overview, 128
diagnostics, 136
differential diagnosis, 129
dermatomyositis, 133
dermatophytosis, 133
discoid lupus erythematosus, 129, *130, 131*
drug hypersensitivity, 133
hyperkeratosis, idiopathic, 133
hypopigmentation, 133
nasal solar dermatitis, 129, 137, 139, 143
pemphigus foliaceus, 132, *132*
plastic/rubber dish dermatitis, 133
pyoderma, 133
tumors, 133, *135*
uveodermatologic syndrome, 133, *134*
vitiligo, 133, *134, 135*
zinc-responsive dermatosis, 133
etiology/pathophysiology, 128
signalment/history, 128–129
therapeutics, 136–137
Nasal digital hyperkeratosis, 76, 533, 539
Naxcel, 658t
Nebcin, 671t
Necrolytic dermatitis, superficial (SND), 109t, 125, *563–567*. (*see also* Hepatocutaneous syndrome)
Necrolytic migratory erythema
erosive and ulcerative dermatoses, 69
pododermatitis, 107
Neoplasia. (*see also specific neoplasms*)
basal cell tumors, 476–477
ceruminous gland adenocarcinoma, 483–485
epidermotrophic lymphoma, 449–454
erosive and ulcerative dermatoses, 69
feline paraneoplastic syndrome, 489–493
footpads, 104, 106, *106*, 108t, 111
hair follicle, 455–456
hemangiosarcoma, 457–460
histiocytoma, 461–463
mast cell tumors, 464–470
melanocytic tumors, 471–475
nail and nailbed, 118t, 120, 121
nasal, 133, *135*
squamous cell carcinoma, 478–482
sweat gland/sebaceous gland adenocarcinoma, 486–488
Neosar. (*see* Cyclophosphamide)
Nerve damage, in otitis, 153
Neurological examination, in otitis interna, 153–154
Neuropathy, in hypothyroidism, 368
New methylene blue stain, 6, 16
Niacinamide
for discoid lupus erythematosus, 422
for pemphigus, 413
Nikolsky sign, 410
Nizoral, 403, 590
Nocardia asteroides, 309, 312
Nocardia brasiliensis, 309, 312
Nocardiosis, 309–313
clinical features, 309, *310*, 311, *311*
definition/overview, 309
diagnostics, 312

differential diagnosis, 311
erosive and ulcerative dermatoses, 62
etiology/pathophysiology, 309
signalment/history, 309
therapeutics, 312
Nodular dermatofibrosis, 107, 542, 548, 550
Nodular dermatoses. (*see* Papular and nodular dermatoses; Sterile nodular/granulomatous dermatoses)
Nodules
etiology/pathophysiology, 84
in panniculitis, 431
Non-steroidal anti-inflammatory drugs (NSAIDs)
for bacteremia, *281*
for pruritus, 239
Norepinephrine, 678
Notoedres, 62, *78*
NSAIDs. (*see* Non-steroidal anti-inflammatory drugs (NSAIDs))
NuSal-T (DVM), 588
Nutritional diseases
erosive and ulcerative dermatoses, 69
exfoliative dermatosis, 77
Nylar, 190
Nystagmus, in otitis, 153
Nystatin, for *Candida paronychia,* 120

Oatmeal, colloidal, 233
Oatmeal-based shampoos, 591
Obsessive compulsive disorder
feline alopecia, *44,* 45, 58t
therapeutics, 59
Omega-6/omega-3 fatty acid supplement, 240, 539. (*see also* Fatty acids)
Onchodystrophy
idiopathic, 118t
lupoid, 117t
Onychomadesis, 115, 116, 120, 121
Onychomycosis, 115, 116, 120, 121
Onychorrhexis, 115, 116, 120, 121
o,p'-DDD, 667t
for adrenal 21-hydroxylase enzyme deficiency, 392
adverse effects, 380, 393, 667t
for growth hormone-responsive dermatoses, 386
for hyperadrenocorticism, 379–380, 381, 403, 510
for hyperestrogenism, 392
patient monitoring, 392
Ophthalmic disease
uveodermatologic syndrome, 441–445
Orbifloxacin, for tuberculosis, 302
Organophosphate
for cheyletiellosis, 196
contraindications, 188, 189
for fleas, 188, 191–192
for sarcoptic mange, 201
for ticks, 177
toxicity, 220–224
client education, 223
clinical features, 221
definition/overview, 220
diagnostics, 222
differential diagnosis, 222
etiology/pathophysiology, 220–221
signalment/history, 221
therapeutics, 222–223
Ormetoprim, 667t
Ormetoprim/sulfadimethoxine (Primor), 669t
Otitis externa, 144–150
client instructions, 641
clinical features, 145
definition/overview, 144
differential diagnosis
diagnostics, 148–149
perpetuating factors, 147–148
primary causes, 145
autoimmune diseases, 145
foreign bodies, 145
hypersensitivities, 145, *146, 147*
keratinization disorders, 145, *146*
obstruction, 145
parasites, 145
therapeutics, 149–150
etiology/pathophysiology, 144
in keratinization disorders, 536
signalment/history, 144–145
breed predilections, 144
historical findings, 145
risk factors, 145
Otitis interna, 152–155
clinical features, 153–154
neurological examination findings, 153–154
definition/overview, 152
diagnostics, 154–155
differential diagnosis, 154
etiology/pathophysiology, 152
signalment/history, 152–153
breed predilection, 152
historical findings, 153
risk factors, 153
therapeutics, 155–156
Otitis media
clinical features, 145, 153–154
definition/overview, 144, 152
diagnostics, *147,* 148, *148,* 154–155
differential diagnosis, 145, 154
etiology/pathophysiology, 144, 152
signalment/history, 144–145, 152–153
therapeutics, 149–150, 155–156
Otodectes cynotis, 210, *211.* (*see also* Ear mites)
Ovaban, for pruritus, 239
Ovarian cysts, in guinea pigs, 507–508
clinical signs, 507, *508*
definition/overview, 507

diagnostic tests, 507–508
lab findings, 507
pathophysiology, 507
prognosis, 508
treatment, 508
Ovarian imbalance, 387–388
Oxacillin, 667t
adverse effects, 292
for pyoderma, 291
Oxatomide, for pruritus, 241

Pagetoid reticulosis, 449
Pancreatic exocrine adenocarcinoma, *50*
Pancreatic polypeptide, 678
Panmycin. (*see* Tetracyclines)
Panniculitis, 430–435, 542, *546*, *547*, 548, 549–550
clinical features, 431, *431*, *432*
course and prognosis, 435
definition/overview, 430
diagnostics, 433–434
differential diagnosis, 433
etiology/pathophysiology, 430–431
patient monitoring, 435
signalment/history, 431
therapeutics, 434–435
Papain, pruritus and, 237
Papillomatosis, 357–361
clinical features
cats, 359, *359*
dogs, *358*, 358–359
definition/overview, 357
diagnostics, 360
differential diagnosis, 360
etiology/pathophysiology, 357
prognosis, 360–361
signalment/history, 357–358
cats, 358
dogs, 357–358
therapeutics, 360
Papular and nodular dermatoses, 84–87
definition/overview, 84
diagnostics, 85
differential diagnosis, 84–85
etiology/pathophysiology, 84
patient monitoring, 87
signalment/history, 84
therapeutics, 85–87
acne, canine, 85, 86
actinic conditions, 85, 86
bacterial folliculitis, 84, 85
rhabditic dermatitis, 85, 86
sebaceous adenitis, 84, 85
Papule
etiology/pathophysiology, 84
sample collection from, 4–5
Parakeratotic hyperkeratosis, 133, 136, 307
Paralysis, tick bite, 180–184
Paramite, for sarcoptic mange, 201
Paraneoplastic syndrome, 489–493
alopecia, 46, *50*, 57t
clinical features, 490, *490*, *491*
definition/overview, 489
diagnostics, 492
differential diagnosis, 490, 492
etiology/pathophysiology, 489
pododermatitis in, 110t
prognosis, 492
signalment/history, 489–490
therapeutics, 492
Parasites. (*see also specific parasites*)
in ferrets, 517–518
in guinea pigs, 497–498
in hedgehogs, 499–500
interdigital dermatitis and, 126t
in mice, 503–504
in rabbits, 505–506
Parathormone, 677
Paronychia, *67*, 115, 116, 117t, 118t, *119*, 119–120, 121
Pasteurella multocida, pyoderma from, 287
Pelodera
erosive and ulcerative dermatoses, 62
interdigital dermatitis, 123
pododermatitis, 107
Pemphigoid. (*see* Bullous pemphigoid)
Pemphigus, 407–414
clinical features, 408–410
erythematosus, 408, *409*
foliaceous, 408, *408*, *409*
vegetans, 410
vulgaris, 410, *410*
course and prognosis, 414
definition/overview, 407
diagnostics, 411–412
differential diagnosis
erythematosis, 411
foliaceous, 410–411
vegetans, 411
vulgaris, 411
etiology/pathophysiology, 407
patient monitoring, 413–414
signalment/history, 407–408
therapeutics, 412–413
erythematosus, 413
foliaceous, 412–413
vegetans, 413
vulgaris, 412–413
Pemphigus complex, 90, 92
Pemphigus erythematosus
breed predilection, 88
clinical features, 408, *409*
diagnostics, 411–412
differential diagnosis, 411
nasal, 133
nasal depigmentation, *139*, 139–140, *140*
prognosis, 414
signalment/history, 407–408
therapeutics, 413

Pemphigus foliaceus, 119t
alopecia from, 35t, 38
breed predilection, 88
clinical features, 408, *408, 409*
cytology, *10*
depigmentation from, 139
differential diagnosis, 410–411
erosive and ulcerative dermatoses, 62
etiology/pathophysiology, 407
as exfoliative dermatosis, 77, *79*
nasal, 132, *132*
pathologic findings, 412
pododermatitis, 103, *104,* 107
prognosis, 414
pustular dermatosis, *91*
signalment/history, 407–408
therapeutics, 412–413
Pemphigus vegetans
clinical features, 410
differential diagnosis, 411
pathologic findings, 412
prognosis, 414
signalment/history, 408
therapeutics, 413
Pemphigus vulgaris, *105*
clinical features, 410, *410*
differential diagnosis, 411
erosive and ulcerative dermatoses, 62, *63*
etiology/pathophysiology, 407
pathologic findings, 412
pododermatitis, 107
prognosis, 414
signalment/history, 408
therapeutics, 412–413
vesicular and pustular dermatosis, *94, 95*
Penicillin G, 668t
for anaerobic infections, 296
Penicillin V, 668t
for dermatophilosis, 307
Pentazocine, 242t
Pentoxifylline, 668t
adverse effects/precautions, 260, 440, 529, 668t
for contact dermatitis, 260
contraindications, 529
for dermatomyositis, 529
for keratinization disorders, 538
for pruritus, 243
for vasculitis, 440
Pepsid, 662t
Periactin. (*see* Cyproheptadine)
Perianal fistula, 160–163
clinical features, 161
complications, 162–163
course/prognosis, 163
definition/overview, 160
diagnostics, 161
differential diagnosis, 161
etiology/pathophysiology, 160
signalment/history, 161
therapeutics, 162
Perianal gland hyperplasia, in sex hormone-responsive dermatoses, 390
Permethrin
contraindications, 188
for fleas, 187, 191
Phenergan, 669t
Phenobarbital
for organophosphate and carbamate toxicity, 223
for pyrethrin/pyrethroid toxicity, 227
withdrawal time prior to intradermal skin testing, 631, 632
Phenoxybenzamine, for tick bite paralysis, 183
Phone communication information for dermatology patients, 629
Physostigmine, for ivermectin toxicity diagnosis, 218
Pigmentation. (*see* Hyperpigmentation; Hypomelanosis)
Pilomatricoma, 455–456, *456*
Pinnal alopecia
canine, 35t, 38
spontaneous, 53, 56t
Piperonyl butoxide, 188
Pituitary dwarfism, 383–386
Pituitary-dependent hyperadrenocorticism, 376, 379–381, 397
Pityrosporum canis. (*see Malassezia pachydermatis*)
Plasma cell pododermatitis, 71, 107, 110t, *111*
Plastic food dish hypersensitivity, 133, 140, 141
Pododermatitis, 101–114, 644
clinical features, 102–107
allergic
canine, 103
feline, 103
enndocrine/metabolic
canine, 104, *105*
feline, 104, *106*
environmental, 106
immune-mediated
canine, 103, *104, 105*
feline, 103
infectious
canine, 102
feline, 102–103
miscellaneous, 107
neoplastic
canine, 104
feline, 106, *106*
definition/overview, 101
diagnostics, 112–113
differential diagnosis, 107, 108t–110t, 111
allergic, 107
endocrine/metabolic, 107
environmental, 108t, 111, *112*
immune-mediated, 107, 109t

infectious, 107
neoplastic, 108t, 111
table of, 108t–110t
etiology/pathophysiology, 101
patient monitoring, 113
signalment/history, 101–102
breed predilections, 101
historical findings, 102
Staphylococcal, *67*
therapeutics, 113
Podoplasty, fusion, 127
Polyarteritis nodosa, 438
Polydactylism, 107
Polyflex. (*see* Ampicillin)
Postclipping alopecia, 35t, 38
Potassium iodide, for panniculitis, 435
Pox virus infection, feline, 354–356
definition/overview, 354
differential diagnosis, 355
etiology/pathophysiology, 354
prognosis, 355–356
signalment/history, 354–355
therapeutics, 355
Pralidoxime chloride, for organophosphate and carbamate toxicity, 223
Pramoxine HCl shampoo, 591
Prednisolone sodium succinate, for anaphylaxis, 246
Prednisolone/prednisone, 668t
for acne, 537
adverse effects, 96, 668t
for anaphylaxis, 246
for atopy, 251
for bullous pemphigoid, 418
for canine eosinophilic granuloma, 542, 549
for contact dermatitis, 260
contraindications, 444
for dermatomyositis, 529
for discoid lupus erythematosus, 422
for eosinophilic granuloma complex, 266
for eosinophilic pustulosis, 96
for epidermotrophic lymphoma, 454
for hypereosinophilic syndrome, 270
for keratinization disorders, 537–540
for lichenoid-psoriasiform dermatosis, 539
for linear IgA dermatosis, 96
for mast cell tumors, 469
mitotane use and, 379–380
for otitis, 149
for panniculitis, 434, 549
for pemphigus, 412, 413
potency, 239t
for puppy strangles, 575
for pyogranuloma, sterile, 549
for sex hormone-responsive dermatoses, 392
for systemic lupus erythematosus, 137, 143, 428
for uveodermatologic syndrome, 444, 445
for vasculitis, 439
Pressure point ulcers, 69
Preventic, 177
Primor, 669t
Proactinomyces spp., 309
Progesterone, 669t
for pruritus, 239
testing for, 677, 678
Program, 665t
Prolactin, 678
Promethazine, 669t
Propylene glycol
for footpad hyperkeratosis, 538
for sebaceous adenitis, 85, 539, 553
Prostacyclin, 239
Prostaglandins
glucocorticoid affect on, 239
pruritus and, 237
Prostaphlin. (*see* Oxacillin)
Proteases, pruritus and, 237
Proteus spp., pyoderma from, 287
Protopam, for organophosphate and carbamate toxicity, 223
Protothecosis, 62
Protozoan dermatosis, 346–349
Prozac. (*see* Fluoxetine)
Pruritus, 231–235
clinical features, 232
definition/overview, 231
diagnostics, 232–233
allergy testing, 232–233
biopsy, 233
trial courses, 233
differential diagnosis, 232
etiology/pathophysiology, 231, 237–238
management of, 236–243
signalment/history, 231
therapeutics, 233–234
antihistamines, 240, 241t
erythromycin, 242
fatty acid metabolites, 240
glucocorticoids, 238–239, 239t
ketoconazole, 242–243
lipoxygenase inhibitors, 239
misoprostol, 241–242
NSAIDs, 239
oxatomide, 241
progesterone compounds, 239
psychotropic drugs, 241, 242t
steroids, 234
systemic, 234
topical, 233–234, 243
trental/pentoxifylline, 243
Pseudocholinesterase, 220
Pseudohermaphrodism in miniature schnauzers, 388
Pseudomonas spp.
bacteremia, 278, 280
otitis, 147
pyoderma, 287
Psychogenic alopecia, feline, *44*, 45, 58t

Psychotropic drugs
antihistamine effects of, 240
dosages, table of, 242t
for pruritus, 241
Punch biopsy, 20–21
Puppy strangles, 62. (*see also* Strangles)
Purinethol, 665t
Pustules, *9, 10*. (*see also* Vesicular and pustular dermatoses)
biopsy of, 20
cytology of, *9, 10*
sample collection from, 4–5
Pyoben (Allerderm), 589
Pyoderma, 287–293
clinical features, 288, *288, 289*, 290, *290*
cytology, *9*
deep, 433
definition, 287
diagnostics, 290–291
etiology/pathophysiology, 287
in exfoliative dermatoses, 77
nasal, 133
recurrent, 292
secondary to
atopy, 250
hyperadrenocorticism, *378*
hypothyroidism, 368
signalment/history, 287–288
superficial, 89, *90*
therapeutics, 85, 291–292
Pyogranuloma, 542, *543*, 549
Pyonychia, 115, 116, *119*
Pyrazinamide
adverse effects, 303
for tuberculosis, 302
Pyrethrin
for cheyletiellosis, 196
contraindications, 188
for ear mites, 212
for fleas, 187, 188, 191–192
for ticks, 177
toxicity, 225–227
clinical features, 225–226
definition/overview, 225
diagnostics, 226
differential diagnosis, 226
signalment/history, 225
therapeutics, 226–227
Pyrethroids. (*see* Pyrethrin)
Pyriproxifen, 190
Pythiosis, 62

Rabbits
barbering, 519–520
dermatophytosis, 513–514
fur mites, 505–506
urine scald, 501–502
Rabies vaccine vasculitis, alopecia from, 28, *30*, 32t
Radfordia affinis, 503, 504
Radiation therapy, 403
Radiography
in blastomycosis, 343, 344
bullae, 148, 154
in ceruminous gland adenocarcinoma, 484, 485
in coccidiodomycosis, 336
in feline paraneoplastic syndrome, 492
in hemolytic anemia, 624
in hepatocutaneous syndrome, 567
in histiocytosis, 579–580
in hyperadrenocorticism, 379
in hypothyroidism, 371
in mast cell tumors, 468
in melanocytic tumors, 472
in mycobacterial infections, 301
in squamous cell carcinoma, 480, 482
in steroid hepatopathy, 396
in systemic lupus erythematosus, 427
Radiotherapy
for mast cell tumors, 468
for squamous cell carcinoma, 481
for sweat/sebaceous gland adenocarcinoma, 488
Rat tail, 401, *402*
Relief (DVM), 591
Renin, 678
Retin-A. (*see* Isotretinoin)
Retinoids
for acne, 537
adverse effects, 540
for epidermotrophic lymphoma, 454
for epidermotropic lymphoma, 59
for exfoliative dermatoses, 82
for footpad hyperkeratosis, 538
for ichthyosis, 538
for keratinization disorders, 41
pregnancy, avoidance in, 42, 83, 87
for sebaceous adenitis, 41, 59, 540, 649
for seborrhea, idiopathic, 539
for squamous cell carcinoma, 481
Revolution, for ear mites, 212
Rhabditic dermatitis
papular and nodular dermatoses, 85, 86
therapeutics, 86
Rhipicephalus sanguineus, 176, 177, 178
Rickettsia ricksettsii, 177
Rifampin
adverse effects, 303
for interdigital dermatitis, 127
for leprosy, feline, 302
for tuberculosis, 302
Ringworm. (*see* Dermatophytosis)
Robaxin-V, for pyrethrin/pyrethroid toxicity, 227
Rock Mountain spotted fever, 177
Rodent ulcer, 62, 67
Romanowsky stains, 6
Rotenone, for ear mites, 211

Rottweiler, disorder of cornification in the, 533, 537–538
Rubber dish dermatitis, 140
Rutin, for lymphedema, 572

Sandimmune. (*see* Cyclosporine)
Sarcoptes scabie, 200
Sarcoptic mange, 198–202
  atopy compared, 249
  clinical features, *199,* 199–200
  definition/overview, 198
  diagnostics, *200,* 200–201
  differential diagnosis, 200
  erosive and ulcerative dermatoses, 62
  etiology/pathophysiology, 198
  in ferrets, 517–518
  in guinea pigs, *497,* 497–498
  pruritus from, 233
  signalment/history, 198
  therapeutics, 201
  zoonotic potential, 201–202
Schnauzer comedone syndrome, 533, 539
Schnauzer gilding syndrome, 140
Scleroderma, localized, 31, 32t
Seasonal flank alopecia, 31, 35t, 41
Sebaceous adenitis, 533, 539–540, 551–553, 649
  alopecia from
    canine, 31, 32t, 34t, 38
    feline, 48–49, *50, 51,* 57t
  clinical features, 551–552, *552*
  definition/overview, 551
  diagnostics, 552–553
  differential diagnosis, 552
  etiology/pathophysiology, 551
  exfoliative dermatoses, 76, *77*
  papular and nodular dermatoses, 84, 85
  signalment/history, 551
  therapeutics, 41, 59, 85, 553
Sebaceous gland adenocarcinoma, 486–488
  clinical features, 486, *487*
  definition/overview, 486
  diagnostics, 488
  differential diagnosis, 488
  prognosis, 488
  signalment/history, 486
  therapeutics, 488
SebaMoist (EVSCO), 587
SebHex (EVSCO), 590
Sebolux (Allerderm), 587
Seborrhea
  antiseborrheic shampoos, 587–589
  in hypothyroidism, 368
  idiopathic, 75, *75,* 533, *534,* 538–539
SeboRx (DVM), 588
Secretin stimulation test, 675–676
Seldane. (*see* Terfenadine)
Selegiline hydrochloride, 380
Selenium sulfide, 539, 588–589
Selsun Blue (Ross), 589
Sepsis, 277–281
  clinical features, 278
  definition/overview, 277
  diagnostics, 278–280
  etiology/pathophysiology, 277–278
  signalment/history, 278
  therapeutics, 280–281
Septa, 669t
Serotonin, pruritus and, 237
Sertoli cell tumor
  alopecia from, 31, 33t, *38*
  hyperestrogenism from, 388, *389,* 393
Severe combined immunodeficiency, 583
Sex hormone alopecia
  canine
    estrogen-responsive, 31, 34t
    hyperestrogenism, 31, 33t
    testosterone-responsive, 31, 33t
  feline, 44
Sex hormone disorders, diagnostics for, 676
Sex hormone-responsive dermatoses, 387–393
  clinical features, 390
  course and prognosis, 393
  definition/overview, 387
  diagnostics, 390–391
  differential diagnosis, 390
  patient monitoring, 392
  signalment/history, 387
    adrenal sex hormone imbalance, 389
    castration responsive, 389
    estrogen-responsive, 387
    hyperandrogenism, 388
    hyperestrogenism in females, 384–388, *388*
    hyperestrogenism in males, 388
    male feminizing syndrome, idiopathic, 388–389
    testosterone-responsive, 389
  therapeutics, 391–392
    castration responsive dermatosis, 392
    estrogen-responsive dermatosis, 391–392
    hyperestrogenism, 392
    testosterone-responsive dermatosis, 392
Sézary syndrome, 449
Shampoos, 586–591
  for acne, 537
  antimicrobial, 589–590
    benzoyl peroxide, 589
    chlorhexidine, 589–590
    ethyl lactate, 590
    imidazole, 590
    iodine, 590
  antipruritics, 590–591
  antiseborrheic, 587–589
    benzoyl peroxide, 589
    selenium sulfide, 588–589
    sulfur and salicylic acid, 587–588
    tar, 588
  cleaning, 586–587

client education, 586
for contact dermatitis, 260
for dermatophytosis, 323
for exfoliative dermatoses, 81–82
instructions for clients, 640
for interdigital dermatitis, 127
for *Malassezia* dermatitis, 318
moisturizing, 586–587
Shetland sheepdog, ulcerative dermatosis in, *70*, 71
Siamese cat
hypotrichosis, 53
pinnal alopecia, 53
Silver sulfadiazine, for otitis, 150
Sinequan. (*see* Doxepin)
Skin extensibility index, 556
Skin fragility syndrome, feline, 46, *49*, 400–404
clinical features, 401, *401*, *402*
definition/overview, 400
diagnostics, 403
differential diagnosis, 403
etiology/pathophysiology, 400
signalment/history, 400
therapeutics, 403
Skin scrapings
in erosive and ulcerative dermatoses, 72
in interdigital dermatitis, 125
magnification recommendation, 8t
in otitis, 148
in papular and nodular dermatoses, 85
in pododermatitis, 112
for sarcoptic mange, 200, *200*
for yeast, 13–15
SLE. (*see* Systemic lupus erythematosus)
Slide preparation
brush technique, 5, *6*, *7*
ear cytology, 12, *12*
squash technique, 5, *5*, *7*
Sodium polyborate, 191
Sodium stibogluconate, for leishmaniasis, 349
Solu-Medrol. (*see* Methylprednisolone sodium succinate)
Somatomedin C, 385
Somatostatin, 678
Soriatane
for ichthyosis, 538
for seborrhea, idiopathic, 539
Spherulocytosisaction, 542, 549
Sphinx cat (alopecia universalis), 53, 57t
Splenectomy, for mast cell tumors, 468
Sporanox. (*see* Itraconazole)
Sporothrix schenckii, 325
Sporotrichosis, 325–328
clinical features, 326, *326*
definition/overview, 325
diagnostics, 326–327
differential diagnosis, 326
erosive and ulcerative dermatoses, 62
etiology/pathophysiology, 325
signalment/history, 325–326
therapeutics, 327
zoonotics potential, 327–327
Squamous cell carcinoma, 478–482
client education, 481–482
clinical features, 479, *479*, *480*
course and prognosis, 482
definition/overview, 478
diagnostics, 480–481
differential diagnosis, 479–480
erosive and ulcerative dermatoses, 69
etiology/pathophysiology, 478
feline alopecia, 49, *51*, *52*, 58t
patient monitoring, 482
prevention, 482
signalment/history, 478–479
therapeutics, 86, 480
Squash technique, 5, *5*, *7*
SSKI (supersaturated potassium iodide), for sporotrichosis, 327
Staining cytology slides, 6
Staphylococcal infections
antibiotics for, 291–292
bacteremia, 280
blepharitis, 627
erosive and ulcerative dermatoses, 62, *67*
folliculitis
alopecia from, 28, *29*, *30*, 32t, 34t
therapeutics, 41
hypersensitivity, *437*
interdigital, *124*, 125
otitis, 147
pododermatitis, *67*
pyoderma from, 287, 291, 634
Staphylococcus aureus, 280
Staphylococcus intermedius, 89, 147, 280, 287, 291–292, 634, 643
Steinerma carpocapsae, 188
Sterile nodular panniculitis, 430, 431, 433, 434, 435
Sterile nodular/granulomatous dermatoses, 542–550
associated conditions, 550
complications, 550
definition/overview, 542
diagnostics, 548–549
differential diagnosis, 548
etiology/pathophysiology, 542, *543–548*
patient monitoring, 550
signalment/history, 548
therapeutics, 549–550
Steroid hepatopathy, 394–399
associated conditions, 398
clinical features, 395
definition/overview, 394
diagnostics, 396
biochemistry, 396
CBC, 396
imaging, 396–397
pathologic findings, 397

procedures, 397
differential diagnosis, 395–396
etiology/pathophysiology, 394–395
patient monitoring, 398
prevention/avoidance, 398
prognosis, 398
signalment/history, 395
therapeutics, 397
Steroids. (*see* Corticosteroids)
Stomatitis, *11*
Strangles, 62, 573–575
clinical features, 573–574, *574*
definition/overview, 573
diagnostics, 574–575
differential diagnosis, 574
etiology/pathophysiology, 573
signalment/history, 573
therapeutics, 575
Streptokinase, pruritus and, 237
Streptomyces spp., 62
Subcorneal pustular dermatosis
breed predilection, 89
diagnosis, 92, *92*
therapeutics, 96
Subcutaneous lesions, cytology of, 3–11
Sulfadiazine
for abscessation, 285
for eosinophilic granuloma complex, 266
for nocardiosis, 312
Sulfamethoxazole/trimethoprim, 266, 285, 292, 296, 655t, 669t
Sulfasalazine
adverse effects, 96
contraindications, 440
drug interactions, 440
patient monitoring, 96
for subcorneal pustular dermatosis, 96
for vasculitis, 439
Sulfonamides
for abscessation, 285
for eosinophilic granuloma complex, 266
for nocardiosis, 312
for otitis, 149
pregnancy, use in, 83
SulfOxyDex (DVM), 589
Sulfur/salicylic acid
for exfoliative dermatoses, 81
for keratinization disorders, 538
shampoos
examples of, 587–588
properties of, 587
Sunlight, affect on
bullous pemphigoid, 415, 417
discoid lupus erythematosus, 420, 423
pruritus, 238
uveodermatologic syndrome, 441
Sunscreens, in squamous cell carcinoma, 482
Superficial necrolytic dermatitis (SND), 109t, 125, *563–567*. (*see also* Hepatocutaneous syndrome)
Supravital stains, 6
Suprax, 657t
Sweat gland adenocarcinoma, 486–488
clinical features, 486, *487*
definition/overview, 486
diagnostics, 488
differential diagnosis, 488
prognosis, 488
signalment/history, 486
therapeutics, 488
Syndactylism, 107
Systemic lupus erythematosus, 424–429
antinuclear antibody (ANA) test, 617–621
clinical features, 425, *425*, *426*, 427
definition/overview, 424
depigmentation, 139
differential diagnosis, 427–428
erosive and ulcerative dermatoses, 62
etiology/pathophysiology, 424–425
systems affected, 424–425
exfoliative dermatosis, 79
lupus erythematosus (LE) cell test, 617–621
nasal, 129, *131*, *132*
pathologic findings, 428
patient monitoring, 429
pododermatitis, 107
prognosis, 429
signalment/history, 425
therapeutics, 137, 143, 428–429
vesicles and ulceration, 93, *93*

T_4 concentration, endogenous, 370
Tagamet. (*see* Cimetidine)
Tail gland hyperplasia, in sex hormone-responsive dermatoses, 390
Taktic-EC. (*see* Amitraz)
Talwin. (*see* Pentazocine)
Tamoxifen
adverse effects, 393
for hyperestrogenism, 392
Tapazole, for hyperthyroidism, 59
Tar shampoos
adverse effects, 540
examples of, 588
for exfoliative dermatoses, 82
properties of, 588
for seborrhea, 539
Tattoos, in squamous cell carcinoma, 482
Tavist. (*see* Clemastine)
Telogen defluxion
canine, 34t, 38
feline, 55, 56t
Temaril. (*see* Trimeprazine)
Terfenadine, 241t, 669t
Testex. (*see* Testosterone therapeutics)
Testicular tumors
hyperandrogenism from, 388, 393
hyperestrogenism from, 388, *389*, 393
Testosterone, testing for, 677, 678

Testosterone therapeutics, 670t. (*see also* Methyltestosterone)
  for castration-responsive dermatosis, 392
  patient monitoring, 392
  for testosterone-responsive dermatosis, 392
Testosterone-responsive dermatosis
  alopecia from, 31, 33t
  signalment/history, 389
  therapeutics, 392
Tetracyclines, 670t
  adverse effects, 313, 670t
  for discoid lupus erythematosus, 422
  for nocardiosis, 312
  for pemphigus, 413
Thallium toxicosis, 71
Thermal burn, 71, *71*
Thiamine deficiency, 154
Thromboxane, glucocorticoid affect on, 239
Thymic deficiency, 583
Thyrogobulin, autoantibodies to, 370
Thyroid hormones, 613–616, 671t. (*see also* Hyperthyroidism; Hypothyroidism)
  associated conditions affecting, 616
  definition/overview, 613
  diagnostics, 615, 675
  etiology/pathophysiology, 613–614
  laboratory findings, 614–615
  risk factors, 614
  systems affected, 614
Thyroiditis, lymphocytic, 365, 371
Thyrotoxicosis, 373
Thyrotropin. (*see* TSH (thyroid-stimulating hormone))
Thyroxine, 677, 678
Thytropar. (*see* TSH (thyroid-stimulating hormone))
Ticarcillin, 671t
Ticarcillin/clavulanate, 671t
Tick bite paralysis, 178, 180–184
  client education, 183–184
  clinical features, 181–182
  definition/overview, 180
  diagnostics, 182
  differential diagnosis, 182
  etiology/pathophysiology, 180
  geographic distribution, 181
  incidence/prevalence, 181
  signalment/history, 181
  therapeutics, 182–183
Ticks, 175–179
  clinical features, 176
  conditions associated with, 177–178 (*see also specific conditions*)
    babesiosus, 177
    ehrlichiosis, 178
    hepatozoonosis, 178
    Lyme disease, 178
    Rocky Mountain spotted fever, 177
    tick paralysis, 178
  control, 177
  definition/overview, 175
  diagnostics, 176
  etiology/pathophysiology, 175–176
  signalment/history, 176
  therapeutics, 176–177
  zoonotic potential, 1787
Timentin, 671t
T-Lux (Allerderm), 588
Tobramycin, 671t
Top Spot, 192. (*see also* Fipronil)
Touch imprints, 4
Toxic epidermal necrolysis, 62, *64*, 107
Toxicity. (*see specific compounds or products*)
Traction alopecia, 35t, 38
Tramisol. (*see* Levamisole)
Trental, 668t
  for pruritus, 243
Tretinoin
  for acne, 86, 166, 537
  for nasal digital hyperkeratosis, 539
Trexan. (*see* Naltrexone)
TRH stimulation test, 371, 675
TRH (thyroid-releasing hormone), 366
Triamcinolone, 672t
  for eosinophilic granuloma complex, 266
  for pemphigus, 413
  potency, 239t
Tribrissen, 669t
Trichoepithelioma, 455–456
Trichophyton gypseum, 319
Trichophyton mentagrophytes, 319, 513, 647
Triiodothyronine, 677, 678
Trimeprazine, 241t, 628
Trimethoprim-sulfa, 669t
  for abscessation, 285
  adverse effects, 292, 669t
  for anaerobic infections, 296
  for eosinophilic granuloma complex, 266
  for pyoderma, 292
Trimtabs. (*see* Triamcinolone)
Trixacarus caviae, 497–498
Trypsin, pruritus and, 237
TSH stimulation test, 370–371, 675
TSH (thyroid-stimulating hormone), 366, 671t
  concentration, 370
  TSH stimulation test, 370–371, 675
Tuberculosis, 297–304
  clinical features, 299
  diagnostics, 301
  differential diagnosis, 300
  etiology/pathophysiology, 297
  signalment/history, 298
  therapeutics, 302
  zoonotic potential, 304
Tzanck preparation, 4, 72, 85

Ulcers. (*see also* Erosive and ulcerative dermatoses)
  biopsy of, 20

in systemic lupus erythematosus, *425, 426*
Ultrasonography
of abscess, 284
in adrenal gland disease, 512
in feline paraneoplastic syndrome, 492
in hemolytic anemia, 625
in hepatocutaneous syndrome, 567
in hyperadrenocorticism, 379
in mast cell tumors, 468
in steroid hepatopathy, 397
Ultraviolet light
bullous pemphigoid exacerbation by, 415, 417
in discoid lupus erythematosus, 420, 423
pruritus and, 238
Unasyn, 654t
Universal Medicated shampoo (Vet Solutions), 590
Uremia, in erosive and ulcerative dermatoses, 69
Urinary incontinence, in sex hormone-responsive dermatoses, 390
Urine cortisol:creatinine ratio, 609–612
complications, 611–612
definition/overview, 609
diagnostics, 611
differential diagnosis, 610
etiology/pathophysiology, 609–610
laboratory findings, 610–611
patient monitoring, 611
treatment, 611
Urine scald, rabbit
clinical signs, 501, *502*
definition/overview, 501
diagnostic tests, 502
lab findings, 501
pathophysiology, 501
prognosis, 502
treatment, 502
Urticaria, in cutaneous drug eruptions, 272
Uveodermatologic syndrome, 133, *134*, 140, *141*, 441–445
clinical features, 441, *442, 443*, 444
definition/overview, 441
diagnostics, 444
differential diagnosis, 444
etiology/pathophysiology, 441
patient monitoring, 444–445
signalment/history, 441
therapeutics, 444

Vaccination
for dermatophytosis, 323
feline calcivirus, 352–353
Lyme disease, 178
papillomavirus, 360
Vaccine, allergy, 251, 633–636
adverse reactions, 633
how it works, 633
interactions, 634
schedule, 635–636
technique, 633
Valium. (*see* Diazepam)
Vancomycin, 672t
Vasculitis, 436–440
causes and risk factors, *438*, 438–439
clinical features, *437*, 437–438, *438*
in cutaneous drug eruptions, 272, 273
definition/overview, 436
diagnostics, 439
differential diagnosis, 439
erosive and ulcerative dermatoses, 62
of footpad, 109t
patient monitoring, 440
pododermatitis, 107
prognosis, 439
signalment/history, 436–437
in systemic lupus erythematosus, 428
therapeutics, 439–440
Vasoactive intestinal polypeptide (VIP), 678
Vesicular and pustular dermatoses, 88–97
clinical features, 89
definition/overview, 88
diagnostics, 95
biopsy, 20
differential diagnosis
pustular
dermatophytosis, 92
eosinophilic pustulosis, sterile, 92
linear IgA dermatosis, 93
pemphigus complex, 90, *91*, 92
pyoderma, superficial, 89, *90*
subcorneal pustular dermatosis, 92, *92*
vesicles/ulceration
bullous pemphigoid, 93, 95
dermatomyositis, *94*, 95
discoid lupus erythematosus, 93
pemphigus vulgaris, *94*, 95
systemic lupus erythematosus, 93
etiology/pathophysiology, 88
signalment/history, 88–89
therapeutics, 95–96
Vestibular disease
idiopathic, 154
in otitis, 145, 153, 156
Vetalog. (*see* Triamcinolone)
Vinblastine, for mast cell tumors, 469
Vincristine
for epidermotrophic lymphoma, 454
for hemangiosarcoma, 459
for histiocytosis, 581
for hypereosinophilic syndrome, 270
for mast cell tumors, 469
Viral infections
canine papillomatosis, 357–361
feline calcivirus, 350–353
feline pox virus, 354–356
Vitamin A, 660t

for exfoliative dermatoses, 82
pregnancy, use in, 83
Vitamin A-responsive dermatosis, 76, *76*, 533, *535*, 540
Vitamin D
for exfoliative dermatoses, 82
for keratinization disorders, 41
Vitamin E
for dermatomyositis, 529
for discoid lupus erythematosus, 422
for hemangiosarcoma, 459
for panniculitis, 434, 550
for squamous cell carcinoma, 482
Vitiligo, 133, *134*, *135*, 140
Vogt Kayanagi Harada-like syndrome, *134*, 441–445

Walking dandruff. (*see* Fur mites, rabbit)
Warts. (*see* Papillomatosis)
Water deprivation test, 676
West Highland white terrier, ichthyosis in, 77
Wood's lamp examination, 232, 322
Wright's stain, 6

Xanthoma, cutaneous, 542, *548*, 549, 550
Xanthomatosis, cutaneous, 45, *47*, 104, *106*
footpad, 110t
pododermatitis, 107
Xeroderma, 586
Xerosis, 540
X-linked severe combined immunodeficiency, 583

Yeast. (*see also Malassezia*)
ear cytology, 12–13
magnification recommendation, 8t
otitis, *147*, 148, *148*, 149–150
secondary to atopy, 250
skin scrapings and impression smears for, 13–15, *15*, 16t
indications, 13–15, *15*, 16t
materials, 13, *13*
number of yeast, evaluation of, 16t
procedures, 13–14, *14*
Yohimbine, 673t
for amitraz toxicosis, 208, 215
side effects, 215, 673t
Yorkshire terriers, alopecia of, 35t, 41

Zinc-responsive dermatosis, 76, 533, 540
erosive and ulcerative dermatoses, 69
hyperkeratosis and, 109t
nasal, 133
pododermatitis, 107, 109t
Zithromax, 655t
Zoonoses
blastomycosis, 345
cheyletiellosis, 194, 196, 197
coccidiodomycosis, 339
dermatophilosis, 308
dermatophytosis, 41, 59, 82, 87
erosive and ulcerative dermatoses, 72–73
sarcoptic mange, 201–202
sporotrichosis, 326, 327
tuberculosis, 304
Zyrtec. (*see* Cetirizine)